The Parasomnias and Other Sleep-Related Movement Disorders

The Parasomnias and Other Sleep-Related Movement Disorders

Edited by

Michael J. Thorpy
Director, Sleep-Wake Disorders Center, Montefiore Medical Center and Professor of Neurology,
Albert Einstein College of Medicine, Bronx, New York, USA

Giuseppe Plazzi
Assistant Professor of Neurology, Università di Bologna and Chief of the Sleep Laboratory,
Dipartimento di Scienze Neurologiche, Università di Bologna, Bologna, Italy

CAMBRIDGE UNIVERSITY PRESS

CAMBRIDGE UNIVERSITY PRESS
Cambridge, New York, Melbourne, Madrid, Cape Town, Singapore,
São Paulo, Delhi, Dubai, Tokyo

Cambridge University Press
The Edinburgh Building, Cambridge CB2 8RU, UK

Published in the United States of America by
Cambridge University Press, New York

www.cambridge.org
Information on this title:
www.cambridge.org/9780521111577

© Cambridge University Press 2010

This publication is in copyright. Subject to statutory exception
and to the provisions of relevant collective licensing
agreements, no reproduction of any part may take place
without the written permission of Cambridge University Press.

First published 2010

Printed in the United Kingdom at
the University Press, Cambridge

*A catalog record for this publication is available from the
British Library*

Library of Congress Cataloging in Publication data
The parasomnias and other sleep-related movement disorders /
editors, Michael Thorpy, Giuseppe Plazzi.
   p. ;   cm.
Includes bibliographical references and index.
ISBN 978-0-521-11157-7 (hardback)
1. Sleep disorders.   2. Sleepwalking.   I. Thorpy, Michael J.
II. Plazzi, Giuseppe.   III. Title.
[DNLM: 1. Parasomnias.   2. Movement Disorders.
WM 188 P223 2010]
RC547.P37   2010
616.8′498 – dc22   2009048604

ISBN 978-0-521-11157-7 Hardback

Cambridge University Press has no responsibility for the
persistence or accuracy of URLs for external or third-party internet
websites referred to in this publication, and does not guarantee that
any content on such websites is, or will remain, accurate or
appropriate.

To the extent permitted by applicable law, Cambridge University
Press is not liable for direct damages or loss of any kind resulting
from the use of this product or from errors or faults contained in it,
and in every case Cambridge University Press's liability shall be
limited to the amount actually paid by the customer for the
product.

Every effort has been made in preparing this publication to provide
accurate and up-to-date information which is in accord with
accepted standards and practice at the time of publication.
Although case histories are drawn from actual cases, every effort
has been made to disguise the identities of the individuals involved.
Nevertheless, the authors, editors and publishers can make no
warranties that the information contained herein is totally free
from error, not least because clinical standards are constantly
changing through research and regulation. The authors, editors and
publishers therefore disclaim all liability for direct or consequential
damages resulting from the use of material contained in this
publication. Readers are strongly advised to pay careful attention to
information provided by the manufacturer of any drugs or
equipment that they plan to use.

Contents

Contributors   page vii
Preface   x
Credits and Acknowledgments   xii
Foreword by Elio Lugaresi   xiii

Section 1: Introduction

1. **Parasomnias: a short history**   3
   Shannon S. Sullivan and Christian Guilleminault
2. **Epidemiology of parasomnias**   7
   Maurice M. Ohayon
3. **Neuroimaging of parasomnias**   13
   Eric A. Nofzinger
4. **Clinical evaluation of parasomnias**   19
   Imran M. Ahmed and Michael J. Thorpy
5. **Video-polysomnography of parasomnias**   34
   Stefano Vandi
6. **Parasomnias due to medications or substances**   42
   Rosalind D. Cartwright
7. **Parasomnias due to medical and neurological disorders**   54
   Marco Zucconi and Alessandro Oldani
8. **Trauma, post-traumatic stress disorder, and parasomnias**   64
   Thomas A. Mellman and Anissa M. Maroof
9. **Sexsomnias**   70
   Nikola N. Trajanovic and Colin M. Shapiro
10. **Medico-legal consequences of parasomnias**   81
    Irshaad O. Ebrahim and Colin M. Shapiro

Section 2: Disorders of arousal

11. **Confusional arousals**   99
    Gregory Stores
12. **Sleepwalking**   109
    Antonio Zadra and Jacques Montplaisir
13. **Sleep terrors**   119
    Meredith Broderick and Christian Guilleminault

Section 3: Parasomnias usually associated with REM sleep

14. **REM sleep behavior disorder**   131
    Raffaele Manni and Michele Terzaghi
15. **Recurrent isolated sleep paralysis**   142
    James Allan Cheyne
16. **Nightmare disorder**   153
    Michael Schredl

Section 4: Other parasomnias

17. **Sleep-related dissociative disorder**   163
    Christina J. Calamaro and Thornton B. A. Mason
18. **Sleep enuresis**   175
    Oliviero Bruni, Luana Novelli, Elena Finotti and Raffaele Ferri
19. **Catathrenia (sleep-related groaning)**   184
    Roberto Vetrugno, Giuseppe Plazzi and Pasquale Montagna

Contents

20. **Sleep-related hallucinations and exploding head syndrome** 194
    Satish C. Rao and Michael H. Silber

21. **Sleep-related eating disorder** 202
    John W. Winkelman

Section 5: Sleep-related movement disorders and other variants

22. **Restless legs syndrome (RLS) and periodic leg movements (PLM)** 213
    Richard P. Allen

23. **Sleep starts** 229
    Sudhansu Chokroverty and Divya Gupta

24. **Fragmentary myoclonus** 237
    Pasquale Montagna and Roberto Vetrugno

25. **Sleep-related leg cramps** 244
    Renee Monderer and Michael J. Thorpy

26. **Sleep-related bruxism** 252
    Nelly Huynh

27. **Propriospinal myoclonus** 261
    Giuseppe Plazzi and Roberto Vetrugno

28. **Sleep-related rhythmic movement disorder** 270
    Timothy F. Hoban

29. **Sleep panic arousals** 278
    Ravi Singareddy and Thomas W. Uhde

30. **Sleep-related epilepsy** 289
    Carl W. Bazil

Section 6: Therapy of parasomnias

31. **Pharmacotherapy and parasomnias** 301
    Rafael Pelayo and Deepti Sinha

32. **Behavioral and psychiatric treatment of parasomnias** 312
    Shelby F. Harris and Michael J. Thorpy

33. **Hypnotherapy and parasomnias** 323
    Gina Graci

Index 330

Color plate section is between pages 210–11.

Contributors

Imran M. Ahmed
Sleep-Wake Disorders Center, Montefiore Medical Center, Bronx, New York, USA.

Richard P. Allen
Neurology and Sleep Medicine, Johns Hopkins University, Asthma and Allergy Bldg, Hopkins Bayview Circle, Baltimore, Maryland, USA.

Carl W. Bazil
The Neurological Institute, Columbia University, New York, NY, USA.

Meredith Broderick
Stanford University Sleep Disorders Clinic, Stanford, California, USA.

Oliviero Bruni
Center for Pediatric Sleep Disorders, Department of Developmental Neurology and Psychiatry, University of Rome La Sapienza, Rome, Italy.

Christina J. Calamaro
Assistant Professor, University of Maryland School of Nursing, Department of Family and Community Health, Baltimore, Maryland, USA.

Rosalind D. Cartwright
Neuroscience Program, Graduate College, Rush University Medical Center, Chicago, Illinois, USA.

James Allan Cheyne
University of Waterloo, Ontario, Canada.

Sudhansu Chokroverty
JFK Medical Center, New Jersey Neuroscience Institute, Seton Hall University, Edison, New Jersey, USA.

Irshaad O. Ebrahim
The London Sleep Centre, London, UK.

Raffaele Ferri
Sleep Research Centre, Department of Neurology, Oasi Institute (IRCCS), Troina, Italy.

Elena Finotti
Sleep Disorders Center, Department of Neurological Sciences, University of Bologna, Italy.

Gina Graci
Northwestern University, Feinberg School of Medicine, Robert H. Lurie Comprehensive Cancer Center, Chicago, Illinois, USA.

Christian Guilleminault
Stanford University Sleep Disorders Clinic, Stanford, California, USA.

Divya Gupta
JFK Medical Center, New Jersey Neuroscience Institute, Seton Hall University, Edison, New Jersey, USA.

Shelby F. Harris
Sleep-Wake Disorders Center, Montefiore Medical Center, Bronx, New York, USA.

Timothy F. Hoban
The Michael S. Aldrich Sleep Disorders Center, Department of Pediatrics, Women's Hospital, Ann Arbor, Missouri, USA.

Nelly Huynh
Sleep Diagnostic Center, Stanford University, Stanford, California, USA.

Raffaele Manni
Unit of Sleep Medicine and Epilepsy, IRCCS C. Mondino, Institute of Neurology Foundation, Pavia, Italy.

Contributors

Anissa M. Maroof
Department of Psychiatry, Howard University, Washington, DC, USA.

Thornton B. A. Mason
Division of Neurology, Wood Center, The Children's Hospital of Philadelphia, Philadelphia, Pennsylvania, USA.

Thomas A. Mellman
Department of Psychiatry, Howard University, Washington, DC, USA.

Renee Monderer
Sleep-Wake Disorders Center, Montefiore Medical Center, Bronx, New York, USA.

Pasquale Montagna
Department of Neurological Sciences, University of Bologna Medical School, Bologna, Italy.

Jacques Montplaisir
Centre d'étude du sommeil, Hôpital du Sacré-Coeur, Université de Montréal, Montréal, Québec, Canada.

Eric A. Nofzinger
Sleep Neuroimaging Research Program, University of Pittsburgh School of Medicine, Pittsburgh, Pennsylvania, USA.

Luana Novelli
Center for Pediatric Sleep Disorders, Department of Developmental Neurology and Psychiatry, Sapienza University, Rome, Italy.

Maurice M. Ohayon
Stanford Sleep Epidemiology Research Center, Stanford University School of Medicine, Palo Alto, California, USA.

Alessandro Oldani
Sleep Disorders Center, Department of Clinical Neurosciences, H. San Raffaele Turro, Milan, Italy.

Rafael Pelayo
Department of Pediatrics, Psychiatry, and Behavioral Science, Stanford University School of Medicine, Stanford, California, USA.

Giuseppe Plazzi
Department of Neurological Sciences, University of Bologna, Bologna, Italy.

Satish C. Rao
Sleep Disorders Center, Mayo Clinic College of Medicine, Rochester, Minnesota, USA.

Michael Schredl
Central Institute of Mental Health, Mannheim, Germany.

Colin M. Shapiro
Sleep and Alertness Clinic, University Health Network, Toronto, Ontario, Canada.

Michael H. Silber
Sleep Disorders Center, Mayo Clinic College of Medicine, Rochester, Minnesota, USA.

Ravi Singareddy
Department of Psychiatry (H073), Penn State College of Medicine, Hershey, Pennsylvania, USA.

Deepti Sinha
Department of Pediatrics, Psychiatry, and Behavioral Science, Stanford University School of Medicine, Stanford, California, USA.

Gregory Stores
University of Oxford, c/o North Gate House, Dorchester on Thames, Oxon, UK.

Shannon S. Sullivan
Stanford University Sleep Disorders Clinic, Stanford, California, USA.

Michele Terzaghi
Unit of Sleep Medicine and Epilepsy, IRCCS C. Mondino, Institute of Neurology Foundation, Pavia, Italy.

Michael J. Thorpy
Sleep-Wake Disorders Center, Montefiore Medical Center, and Albert Einstein College of Medicine, Bronx, New York, USA.

Nikola N. Trajanovic
Sleep and Alertness Clinic, University Health Network, Toronto, Ontario, Canada.

Thomas W. Uhde
Department of Psychiatry (H073), Penn State College of Medicine, Hershey, Pennsylvania, USA.

Stefano Vandi
Department of Neurological Sciences, University of Bologna, Bologna, Italy.

Roberto Vetrugno
Department of Neurological Sciences, University of Bologna, Bologna, Italy.

John W. Winkelman
Division of Sleep Medicine, Brigham and Women's Hospital, Harvard Medical School, Boston, Massachusetts, USA.

Antonio Zadra
Centre d'étude du sommeil, Hôpital du Sacré-Coeur, Université de Montréal, Montréal, Québec, Canada.

Marco Zucconi
Sleep Disorders Center, Department of Neurology, Scientific Institute and University Ospedale San Raffaele, Vita-Salute University, Milan, Italy.

Preface

Intense medical and scientific interest in an increasing number of topics in sleep medicine has led to the production of this volume on *Parasomnias and Other Sleep-Related Movement Disorders*. Although parasomnias are ubiquitous in childhood and occur across all ages, this is the first publication to focus on this topic in detail. There is growing recognition that sleep disorders represent a major public health concern, and understanding the basic, translational, clinical and psychosocial aspects of sleep disorders is essential to the process of becoming a skilled clinical practitioner.

The earliest reported descriptions of some of the parasomnias such as sleepwalking and nightmares have been known since antiquity; however, new parasomnias have been described, such as REM sleep behavior disorder and catathrenia [1]. There have been numerous developments in the field of abnormal movement disorders during sleep that have led to a better understanding of the clinical features, the diagnostic criteria and subsequently, treatments.

These developments have continually deepened our understanding of parasomnias as pathophysiological conditions and have also drawn attention to the impact on the lives of those who have these conditions. Parasomnias can be severe, chronic, debilitating and disabling neurological disorders, often having early age of onset [2]. They frequently involve abnormal involuntary behaviors during sleep, leading to injuries, emotional distress and even medico-legal liability [3]. Despite their prominent symptoms and impact on patients' health-related quality of life, parasomnias remain under-recognized and under-appreciated disorders, perhaps because of their predominantly nighttime occurrence. Patients with parasomnias often suffer from a constellation of other co-morbid medical and/or psychiatric conditions [4].

In children and adolescents, the psychological and social complications of parasomnias can be widespread and potentially severe. Parasomnias can affect patients' academic and vocational performance, as well as social and recreational activities. Accordingly, this volume addresses issues in the etiology, pathophysiology, diagnosis, differential diagnoses and management of parasomnias including psychosocial ramifications and effects on quality of life.

In the last decade, significant advances in elucidating the pathophysiology of some of the parasomnias have been made. However, effective treatments are often lacking, and there is the need for specific and effective treatments for many of the disorders. A large number of medications have been effective in some patients, even though few are FDA-approved in the USA for most of the parasomnias. Behavioral interventions, hypnosis and psychiatric treatments can be effective for some. Strategies for the management of the risk for injury of both the patient or bed partner, such as securing the environment, are discussed in this volume.

The nature and mechanisms of parasomnias remain largely unknown; however, the latest research evidence is covered here. The parasomnias are often misdiagnosed because similar symptoms exist and overlap with some of the movement disorders [5]. Those disorders that should be considered in the differential diagnoses are discussed in detail with an emphasis on the differentiating features.

The volume is broadly divided into six main sections: **Section I**: *Introductory chapters*; **Section II**: *Disorders of arousal*; **Section III**: *Parasomnias usually associated with REM sleep*; **Section IV**: *Other parasomnias*; **Section V**: *Sleep-related movement disorders and other variants*, and **Section VI**: *Therapy of parasomnias*.

In its first section, the basic, translational, and clinical background of parasomnias is reviewed. In this regard, the first three introductory chapters cover the historical, epidemiological, and neuroimaging of parasomnias.

In the second section of the book, the clinical aspects of the disorders of arousal that commonly occur in children, including confusional arousals, sleepwalking and sleep terrors, are discussed.

The third section deals with the parasomnias usually associated with REM sleep. Issues relating to the REM sleep behavior disorder, recurrent isolated sleep paralysis and nightmare disorder are presented.

The fourth section deals with a group of parasomnias under the group heading of "other parasomnias". This section addresses less commonly recognized and less understood parasomnias such as sleep-related dissociative disorders, sleep-related groaning and sleep-related eating disorder.

The fifth section deals with sleep-related movement disorders and other variants that are often included in the differential diagnosis of the parasomnias.

The sixth section discusses the pharmacologic, behavioral and psychiatric management of the parasomnias.

The reader will find that in addition, this volume contains detailed discussions of important secondary issues including the importance of medico-legal aspects, safety, education, counselling and recognition of psychiatric and cognitive comorbidities.

It has been the editors' objective to provide a comprehensive and authoritative guide for clinicians that is presented in a manner which is both readable and easily understood. It is our hope that we have succeeded in accomplishing this goal.

This volume is intended primarily for sleep disorders specialists and sleep researchers. However, it is suitable for psychiatrists, neurologists, and any professionals and researchers interested in the interdisciplinary field of sleep medicine. It will be of considerable interest to general practitioners, and physicians who evaluate and treat sleep disorders. It will also be equally interesting to psychiatry and neurology residents and fellows, clinical psychologists, advanced graduate medical students, neuropsychologists, house officers, and other mental health and social workers who want to get an overall understanding of abnormal behaviors during sleep. Additionally, because of the growing medico-legal aspects of the parasomnias, this book has interest to the legal profession.

In as much as research findings in many areas are rapidly broadening our understanding of parasomnias, it is anticipated that future editions of this volume of *Parasomnias and Other Sleep-Related Movement Disorders* will take these developments into account.

Michael J. Thorpy
Giuseppe Plazzi

References

1. Schenck CH, Mahowald MW. Rapid eye movement sleep parasomnias. *Neurol Clin* 2005; **23**: 1107–26.
2. Stores G. Aspects of parasomnias in childhood and adolescence. *Arch Dis Child* 2009; **94**: 63–9.
3. Ebrahim IO, Fenwick P. Sleep-related automatism and the law. *Med Sci Law* 2008; **48**: 124–36.
4. Lam SP, Fong SY, Ho CK, Yu MW, Wing YK. Parasomnia among psychiatric outpatients: A clinical, epidemiologic, cross-sectional study. *J Clin Psychiatry* 2008; **69**: 1374–82.
5. Nobili L. Nocturnal frontal lobe epilepsy and non-rapid eye movement sleep parasomnias: Differences and similarities. *Sleep Med Rev* 2007; **11**: 251–4.

Credits and Acknowledgments

Parasomnias and Other Sleep-Related Movement Disorders provides scientific and clinical information on abnormal movement disorders during sleep for all health care workers interested in disorders of sleep. It is our pleasure to acknowledge the contributions of those who were instrumental in the production of this book.

Our sincere appreciation goes to Elio Lugaresi, Professor Emeritus, University of Bologna, Italy, who agreed to write the foreword. We wish to express our appreciation for his contribution.

We would like to express our deep appreciation to all the contributors for their scholarly contributions that facilitated the development of this book. The expertise of contributors to *Parasomnias and Other Sleep-Related Movement Disorders* reflects the broad diversity and knowledge concerning parasomnia research, which has continued to grow over the last several decades. These authors represent the cutting edge of basic and applied parasomnia research as well as providing the most recent information regarding how such knowledge can be used in clinical settings. Their informed opinions and insights have significantly contributed to our scientific understanding of parasomnias and have provided important interpretations regarding future research directions.

The highly talented publishing team at Cambridge University Press made this project an especially pleasurable one. Their guidance, technical expertise, and commitment to excellence were invaluable.

Finally, and most importantly, we want to thank our spouses, families and colleagues for their support, and understanding during the development of this book.

Michael J. Thorpy
Giuseppe Plazzi

Foreword

Henry Roger, a French neurologist based in Marseilles, published a monograph of the lessons he gave in the academic years 1900–31 (H. Roger, *Troubles du Sommeil*. Paris: Masson et Cie editeurs, 1932). The two main chapters of his book concerned the insomnias and hypersomnias, while a short chapter was devoted to what Roger termed the parasomnias, "les petits troubles de la fonction hypnique" (unusual, but common sleep events of little clinical relevance). Among the parasomnias, Roger included nocturnal episodes known for centuries, such as sleep terror, sleepwalking, nightmares and enuresis, as well as disturbing dreams giving rise to agitated loud comments (*reves parlès*) and episodes of violent motor agitation recurring nightly.

I think the dreams accompanied by somniloquy correspond to what we nowadays call REM behavior disorder (RBD), whereas the violent nocturnal motor attacks resemble the epileptic nocturnal frontal lobe seizures described by my group in the early 1980s by the name of nocturnal paroxysmal dystonia.

The same chapter also describes the muscle jerks arising on falling asleep. Roger noted that these movements may occur sporadically and be of little clinical relevance, but may also recur at very short intervals preventing sleep onset. Plainly, Roger's detailed description of myoclonias arising on falling asleep refers to what we currently call hypnic jerks, nocturnal myoclonus and propriospinal myoclonus.

This preamble serves to make my point that a neurologist working early in the last century and basing his observations on accurate history-taking alone had described the majority of unusual events related to sleep. It was decades before the multiform semiological, etiopathogenetic and clinical aspects of these events were identified and investigated by countless sophisticated sleep laboratories.

The objective and systematic study of the parasomnias only got underway after Dement and Kleitman first described the polygraphic features of human sleep in 1957. In the 1960s, this was followed by the discovery of nocturnal myoclonus and the demonstration that arousal disorders are a benign condition. However, landmark breakthroughs were to come in the 1970s–1980s when polysomnographic recordings performed under audiovisual control became a routine means of sleep investigation. Use of this technique led to the discovery of RBD, nocturnal frontal lobe seizures, and many other sleep disorders previously ignored or misinterpreted.

The 33 chapters of this extraordinary book document the striking development of sleep medicine in recent decades. We now know, for example, that the term "parasomnias" does not cover all the unusual events arising during sleep. Some sleep-related movement disorders and nocturnal variants of epilepsy, in fact, cannot be included among the "petits troubles de la fonction hypnique."

For these reasons, I am sure this book will be useful to neurologists, psychiatrists, psychologists, child neurologists and all those hoping to broaden their knowledge of these fascinating topics.

The book's editors, Michael Thorpy and Giuseppe Plazzi, are to be complimented for having entrusted each chapter to a leading expert in the field. They also have the merit for the difficult task of editing to bridge the stylistic gaps typical of multi-author works.

Wishing the volume the success it deserves, I also congratulate the publisher for taking on this task at such a difficult time.

Elio Lugaresi

Section 1: Introduction

Introduction

Parasomnias: a short history

Shannon S. Sullivan and Christian Guilleminault

If the notions of dream and nightmare are centuries old, going back to ancient Egyptian and Jewish civilizations, the distinction between nightmares and parasomnias is recent. It is interesting to note that already in 1932 Kouretas and Scouras [1] reported the complete absence of muscle tone during nightmares in one of their patients, but Kleitman in his seminal monograph places "nightmares, night terrors, somniloquy, bruxism and jactitation, enuresis, numbness and hypnalgia, and personality dissociation" under the terminology "parasomnia" [2]. The term "parasomnia", derived from the greek "para" meaning "around" and the latin "somnus" meaning "sleep", had been coined in 1932 by the French researcher Henri Roger who published a monograph entitled "Les Troubles du Sommeil-Hypersomnies, Insomnies, and Parasomnies" [3]. In this monograph, Roger gave an excellent description of an episode of sleep terror in a child, and also described a somnambulistic episode. Kleitman's review of previous literature shows that the difference between nightmares and sleep terrors was not well perceived before Roger; rather, many syndromes now understood to be within the rubric "parasomnia" had been investigated independently.

As parasomnias became distinguishable from nightmares, a possible link between such episodic nocturnal phenomena and seizure disorders was proposed. Henri Gastaut in Marseille, France, wanted to understand whether a relationship existed between the common parasomnias and seizures. To resolve this question, the Marseille team monitored individuals with abnormal nocturnal behavior and normal matched controls during nocturnal sleep. In 1965, Gastaut and Broughton reported some of their findings and hypothesized that most "episodic phenomena," as they called events, were non-epileptic in nature and occurred out of NREM sleep, predominantly during slow wave sleep [4]. These authors confirmed the clinical description of sleep terrors reported by Kanner in 1935 [5]. However, they indicated that many of these phenomena occurred during NREM sleep stages 3 and 4, including enuresis. They even performed cystometric recordings during sleep in children and reported that the enuretic episodes occurred when the cystic pressure waves reached 120 cm H_2O. Jacobson et al. [6] and Kales and Jacobson [7] focused more on sleepwalking episodes and had similar findings to Gastaut and colleagues, indicating the occurrence of events during NREM sleep, particularly stages 3 and 4. They emphasized subjects' "indifference to environment" during episodes, and the "complete amnesia" of the events the following morning. The authors made the interesting observation that a sleepwalking event could be induced by having a known somnambulistic child stand up in slow wave sleep.

These studies were presented and discussed at the 15th European Meeting on Electro-encephalography held in 1967 in Bologna, Italy, a meeting organized by Lugaresi and Gastaut and attended by European and North American researchers. Thereafter, in 1968 Broughton questioned the pathophysiological mechanisms underlying sleepwalking, sleep terrors, and head-banging [8]. He dissociated them formally from nocturnal epilepsy, emphasizing the well-demonstrated presence of sleep disturbance and occurrence in NREM sleep – and more particularly stage 4 sleep; he termed such events "disorders of arousal". He also differentiated nocturnal enuresis from the other phenomena.

During the same period several authors emphasized the familial nature of the disorders. Kales and Jacobson [7] indicated that sleepwalking was found in families; in 1980, Kales et al. suggested a two-threshold multifactorial mode of inheritance [9]. Bakwin (1970) found that monozygotic twins were concordant for sleepwalking considerably more than dizygotic twins ($p = 0.06$) [10]. In 1972, Hallstrom suggested an autosomal dominant pattern of heredity for sleep terrors [11]. None of these studies fully explained observed patterns of inheritance, despite the fact that familial patterns were seen in parasomnias. In 1971, Klackenberg, in his classic longitudinal study which followed about 200 children from birth in 1955 until age 16 in Stockholm [12], made an interesting observation: children who would become somnambulistic later in life had much more restless sleep at the age of 4–5 years. Another important finding of this longitudinal study was that somnambulism and sleep terrors could be very rare or chronic. In the "chronic" or "habitual" sleepwalkers, enuresis occurred from 5 until 16 years of age and represented 2.5% of the sample. This number is of interest, as another epidemiologic study found similar results. Ohayon et al., based on a representative sample of the adult population, found that sleepwalking affects 2.5% of the population [13]. Hublin et al., on the other hand, indicated that 25% of children with a history of sleepwalking will sleepwalk as adults [14].

The following 20 years focused on pharmacological treatment of parasomnias with emphasis on the use of benzodiazepines, with variable results. A short report by an English orthodontist was completely ignored. Timms, who performed rapid maxillary expansion on children with a narrow hard palate, but who did not routinely perform sleep studies, described clinical amelioration of symptoms that today would suggest the presence of sleep-disordered breathing [15]. He also described the elimination of chronic sleepwalking events following rapid maxillary expansion.

In 1999, Ohayon et al. in their epidemiological studies on sleepwalking and sleep terrors found that obstructive sleep apnea syndrome was the most common sleep disorder associated with parasomnias between the ages of 15 and 24 years [13]. In 2002, Espa et al. reported a similar association in a small number of subjects focusing on sleepwalking, as did Guilleminault et al., investigating sexual violence and confusional arousal [16,17]. Around the same time, Ohayon et al. reported an important relationship between bruxism and the presence of sleep-disordered breathing (SDB) [18]. Goodwin et al., in the pediatric Tuscon sleep cohort, also identified a frequent association between SDB and sleepwalking in 2004 [19].

Investigations of sleep EEG in parasomnias became more focused. In 1995, Zucconi et al., using a cyclic alternating pattern (CAP) scoring system, indicated that various parasomnias were associated with an abnormally elevated CAP rate [20]. This finding was confirmed by Guilleminault et al. both in children and in young adult sleepwalkers [21,22].

Another type of investigation of the sleep EEG was performed by Gaudreau et al. [23] and Guilleminault et al. [24] using quantified EEG. Both of these groups showed that subjects with chronic parasomnias had a significant decrease in delta power during the first NREM–REM sleep cycle, and lower than expected delta power in the second cycle. Guilleminault et al. compared quantified EEG and CAP analyses and showed that the results were concordant when these two analyses were applied to the same subjects [21]. The conclusions drawn by these authors were that sleep EEG analyses indicated an "instability of NREM sleep." The investigations of Guilleminault et al. of children and adults [25] with chronic parasomnias showed that: (1) the individuals with chronic parasomnia presented such an instability of NREM sleep every night, with or without the presence of the parasomnia; (2) the subjects presented with another sleep disorder (most commonly SDB) which was responsible for the instability of NREM sleep; (3) the presence of an additional factor (e.g. stress, alcohol, fever, sleep deprivation) was needed to provoke the parasomnia episode; and (4) treatment of the underlying sleep disorder (including rapid maxillary distraction as noted by Timms) alleviated the instability of NREM sleep and eliminated or improved the parasomnia.

Recent work on bruxism suggests that teeth-grinding may be an attempt to protect against the occurrence of sleep apnea, which raises the question of whether this symptom should be placed in the same category as the others, despite the fact that it is also associated with NREM sleep instability. Understanding of parasomnias has evolved over time and will continue to evolve. As suggested by Guilleminault et al., to the extent that parasomnias are triggered by unstable NREM sleep caused by SDB, the heritability of parasomnias may be related to the underlying familial facial traits involved in the development of SDB [26].

Epileptic disorders were shown to be rarely involved in abnormal behavior during NREM sleep, but when sleep-related seizure disorders are present, specific seizure entities are implicated. In sleep-related seizure disorder, polysomnographic studies have demonstrated that a frontal lobe locus is most common, and less frequently the mesiotemporal region is involved. Pedley and Guilleminault [27] tried to chronicle distinguishing characteristics between NREM parasomnias and sleep-related seizures, but such differences are based on statistical analyses and may not be true for every event. The stereotypy of the abnormal behavior of a seizure disorder is the most constant finding. Seizures are also more likely to occur out of stage 2 NREM and during the second half of the night. Studies from the 1970s and 1980s have demonstrated that nocturnal seizures represent a bit less than 1% of the abnormal behavior during sleep.

Finally, nocturnal polysomnography has allowed the dissociation of NREM from REM sleep abnormal behavior. The initial description of what is now known as "REM sleep behavior disorder" (RBD) came from Japanese researchers. It was related to the disappearance of the normal atonia of REM sleep reported during delirium secondary to alcohol intoxication [28]; it was again described by Japanese researchers in psychiatric patients [29]. In 1986, Quera-Salva and Guilleminault presented cases of olivo-pontocerebellar degeneration and REM without atonia associated with the acting out of dreams [30].

In the same year, Schenk et al. reported the presence of other neurological syndromes, particularly parkinsonianism, and called it a "new category of parasomnia" [31]. In 1987 these authors presented idiopathic cases and named the syndrome "REM sleep behavior disorder" [32]. Aspects of these cases resembled the 1965 report by Jouvet and Delorme of cats with bilateral, symmetrical dorsolateral pontine brainstem lesions of the peri-locus coeruleus who displayed loss of REM sleep atonia along with the development of abnormal oneiric behavior, thought to be related to dream enactment [33].

Further investigation indicated that many patients with Parkinson's Disease and multisystem atrophy manifested this disorder, and that it could also be observed with brainstem lesions involving the descending pathways leading to the active inhibition of REM sleep. Drugs such as tricyclic antidepressants, which are known to inhibit these pathways, were also shown to lead to iatrogenic RBD.

The continuous work of Schenk and Mahowald [34] and investigations of the Mayo Clinic group [35] combining polysomnographic studies and pathologic investigations at death revealed that many patients initially considered "idiopathic" developed Parkinson's Disease or Lewy body dementia sometimes 10–15 years after the RBD diagnosis. Systematic autopsy showed that subjects with RBD but without any other neurologic disorder already had the presence of Lewy bodies in the medulla. Progressively, the notion emerged that RBD is commonly related to Lewy bodies [36] and that a progressive rostral invasion of neurons occurs over time, leading to the development of associated neurological syndromes. RBD is often considered to be a synucleinopathy with risk of developing another neurological syndrome in the years to come.

Questions still have to be answered. Are all RBD related to a synucleinopathy? Probably not; but the percentage of RBD that is associated with synucleinopathy is unknown, despite preliminary data which indicate that this association is common. Are other neurodegenerative diseases involved in RBD? Alzheimer's Disease has been reported in association with RBD, but this seems rare to exceptional; other neurodegenerative diseases are involved more frequently. Whether idiopathic RBD truly exists is still an unanswered question.

References

1. Kouretas D, Scouras P. Sur un trouble particulier du sommeil: le cauchemar. *Encephale* 1932, 7: 622–7.
2. Kleitman N. *Sleep and Wakefulness*. Chicago: University of Chicago Press, 1939; 280–9.
3. Roger H. *Les Troubles du Sommeil*. Paris: Masson et Cie, 1932; 275–83.
4. Gastaut H, Broughton J. A clinical and polysomnographic study of episodic phenomena during sleep. *Biol Psychiatry* 1965; 7: 197–221.
5. Kanner L. *Child Psychiatry*. Springfield, IL: Thomas, 1935; 281.
6. Jacobson A, Kales A, Lehmann D, Zweizig JR. Somnambulism: all-night electroencephalographic studies. *Science* 1965; **148**: 975–7.
7. Kales A, Jacobson A. Clinical and electrophysiological studies of somnambulism. In Gastaut H, Lugaresi E, Berti-Ceroni G, Coccagna G (Eds), *Proceedings of the 15th European meeting on encephalography: The abnormalities of sleep in man*. Bologna: Aulo Gaggi, 1967; 295–302.
8. Broughton RJ. Sleep disorders: disorders of arousal? Enuresis, somnambulism, and nightmares occur in confusional states of arousal, not in "dreaming sleep". *Science* 1968; **159**: 1070–8.
9. Kales A, Soldatos CR, Bixler EO, *et al.* Hereditary factors in sleepwalking and night terrors. *Br J Psychiat* 1980; **137**: 111–8.
10. Bawkin H. Sleep-walking in twins. *Lancet* 1970; **2**(7670): 446–7.

11. Hallstrom T. Night terror in adults through three generations. *Acta Psychiatr Scand* 1972; **48**: 350–2.
12. Klackenberg G. A prospective longitudinal study of children. *Acta Pediatr Scand* 1971; **224** (suppl): 179–85.
13. Ohayon M, Guilleminault C, Priest R. How frequent are night terrors, sleep walking and confusional arousals in the general population. Their relationship to other sleep and mental disorders. *J Clin Psychiatry* 1999; **60**: 268–76.
14. Hublin C, Kaprio J, Partinen M, Heikkila K, Koskenvuo M. Prevalence and genetics of sleepwalking: a population-based twin study. *Neurology* 1997; **48**: 177–81.
15. Timms DJ. Some medical aspects of rapid maxillary expansion. *Br J Orthodontics* 1974; **1**: 127–32.
16. Espa F, Dauvilliers Y, Ondze B, Billiard M, Besset A. Arousal reactions in sleepwalking and night terrors in adults: the role of respiratory events. *Sleep* 2002; **25**: 871–5.
17. Guilleminault C, Moscovitch A, Yuen K. Atypical sexual behavior during sleep. *Psychosom Med* 2002; **64**: 328–36.
18. Ohayon MM, Li KK, Guilleminault C. Risk factors for sleep bruxism in the general population. *Chest* 2001; **119**: 53–61.
19. Goodwin JL, Kaeming KL, Fregosi RF, *et al.* Parasomnias and sleep disordered breathing in Caucasian and Hispanic children – the Tucson children's assessment of sleep apnea study. *BMC Medicine* 2004; 2–14.
20. Zucconi M, Oldani A, Ferini-Strambi L, Smirne S. Arousal fluctuation in non rapid-eye-movement parasomnia: the role of the cyclic alternating pattern as a measure of sleep instability. *J Clin Neurophysiol* 1995; **12**: 147–54.
21. Guilleminault C, Kirisoglu C, Rosa A da, Lopes MC, Chan A. Sleepwalking, a disorder of NREM sleep instability. *Sleep Med* 2006; **7**: 163–70.
22. Guilleminault C, Lee JH, Chan A, Lopes MC, Huang YS, Rosa A da. NREM sleep instability in recurrent sleepwalking in prepubertal children. *Sleep Med* 2005; **6**: 515–21.
23. Gaudreau H, Joncas S, Zadra A, Montplaisir J. Dynamics of slow-wave activity during the NREM sleep of sleepwalkers and control subjects. *Sleep* 2000; **23**: 755–60.
24. Guilleminault C, Poyares D, Abat F, Palombini L. Sleep and wakefulness in somnambulism, a spectral analysis study. *J Psychosomat Res* 2001; **51**: 411–6.
25. Guilleminault C, Kirisoglu C, Bao G, Arias V, Chan A, Li K. Adult chronic sleepwalking and its treatment based on polysomnography. *Brain* 2005; **128**: 1062–9.
26. Guilleminault C, Palombini L, Pelayo R, Chervin RD. Sleepwalking and sleep terrors in prepubertal children: what triggers them? *Pediatrics* 2003; **111**: e17–25.
27. Pedley TA, Guilleminault C. Episodic nocturnal wanderings responsive to anticonvulsant drug therapy. *Ann Neurol* 1977; **2**: 30–5.
28. Tachibana M, Tanaka K, Hishikawa Y, Kaneko Z. A sleep study of acute psychotic states due to alcohol and meprobamate addiction. *Adv Sleep Res* 1975; **2**: 177–205.
29. Hishikawa Y, Sugita Y, Iijima S, *et al*. Mechanisms producing "stage-1 REM" and similar dissociation of REM sleep and their relation to delirium. *Adv Neurol Sci (Tokyo)* 1981: **25**: 1129–47.
30. Quera-Salva MA, Guilleminault C. Olivo-ponto-cerebellar degeneration, abnormal sleep and REM sleep without atonia. *Neurology* 1986; **36**: 577.
31. Schenck CH, Bundlie SR, Ettinger MG, Mahowald MW. Chronic behavioral disorders of human REM sleep: a new category of parasomnia. *Sleep* 1986; **9**: 293–308.
32. Schenck CH, Bundlie SR, Patterson AL, Mahowald MW. Rapid eye movement sleep behavior disorder. A treatable parasomnia affecting older adults. *JAMA* 1987; **257**: 1786–9.
33. Jouvet M, Delorme F. Locus coeruleus et sommeil paradoxal. *CR Soc Biol* 1965; **159**: 895–9.
34. Schenck CH, Bundlie SR, Mahowald MW. Delayed emergence of a parkinsonian disorder in 38% of 29 older men initially diagnosed with idiopathic rapid eye movement sleep behavior disorder. *Neurology* 1996; **46**: 388–93.
35. Boeve BF, Silber MH, Saper CB, *et al*. Pathophysiology of REM sleep behaviour disorder and relevance to neurodegenerative disease. *Brain* 2007; **130**: 2770–88.
36. Uchiyama M, Isse K, Tanaka K, *et al*. Incidental Lewy body disease in a patient with REM sleep behavior disorder. *Neurology* 1995; **45**: 709–12.

Section 1 Chapter 2

Introduction

Epidemiology of parasomnias

Maurice M. Ohayon

Introduction

Parasomnias are sleep disorders characterized by abnormal behavioral or physiological events occurring at different sleep stages. These disorders have seldom been investigated in the adult general population although, as we will see, they are very frequent. Many of these parasomnias are accompanied with behaviors that can be potentially dangerous to the sleeper or to others, leading sometimes to dramatic consequences, such as self-mutilation, murder or suicide.

Parasomnias presented in this chapter are those included in the latest International Classification of Sleep Disorders (ICSD-2) [1]. They are divided into three main categories: disorders of arousal, parasomnias associated with REM sleep, and other parasomnias. There are 15 possible diagnoses of parasomnias. For many of them, information about their prevalence and incidence is limited or inexistent.

Disorders of arousal

Arousal parasomnias occur mainly during NREM sleep. This group consists of confusional arousals, sleepwalking and sleep terrors. These parasomnias occur primarily in childhood and normally cease by adolescence. A same individual may experience more than one type of arousal parasomnias. However, epidemiological figures for these co-occurrences are yet to be determined.

Confusional arousals

Confusional arousals, or sleep drunkenness, correspond to a mental confusion occurring upon wakening, be it at night or in the morning. Physiologically speaking, cerebral reactivation to external stimuli is altered in the transitional period from NREM sleep to wakefulness. The sleeper appears awake but behavior may be very inappropriate, marked by memory deficits, disorientation in time and space and slow mentation and speech. An episode can be triggered by a forced awakening. Complex behaviors may occur, resulting in potentially dangerous situations for the sleeper and others.

Confusional arousals have received little attention in epidemiological studies. In children, Laberge et al. [2] have estimated that about 17% of children between 3 and 13 years are experiencing occasional or frequent episodes of confusional arousals. In our study, we have estimated their frequency in the general population to be 4.2%; decreasing from 6.1% in the 15–24 age group to 3.3% in the 25–34 and stabilizing around 2% after 35 years old [3]. No other figure exists for comparative purposes. Although confusional arousals are suspected to have a genetic component, genetic epidemiological prevalence is yet to be determined.

The phenomenon, however, has generated much more interest from a forensic standpoint. The first review of the literature devoted to assaults committed in a state of confusional arousal was completed in 1905 by Gudden [4]. It included 18 cases among which 10 resulted in homicides. In 1943, a similar review by Schmidt [5] covered 35 cases (15 homicides and 20 bodily injuries). Thirty later years, A. Bonkalo [6] reviewed cases of murder committed during confusional arousals that occurred from 1791 to 1974. He identified approximately 20 cases, mostly perpetrated by men. More recently, B. Raschka [7] has brought the case of a man of 54 years that, for no apparent reason, had assaulted two police officers shortly after they had awakened him in his car. Polysomnographic findings indicated that the man suffered from obstructive sleep apnea syndrome. It was concluded that the combination

The Parasomnias and Other Sleep-Related Movement Disorders, ed. M. J. Thorpy and G. Plazzi. Published by Cambridge University Press. © Cambridge University Press 2010.

of this disorder with alcohol intake and sudden arousal had prompted the violent behavior.

Several studies and case reports [7–10] have underscored the association between sleep apnea and violent behavior. One of these found that cerebral hypoxia provoked by recurrent breathing pauses during sleep could, over the long term, cause excessive daytime sleepiness, road accidents, impulsive behaviors at awakening, and even cerebral damage [10]. Being suddenly awakened when in a relative state of cerebral anoxia can produce a confusional state that can translate into violent behavior [7].

Precipitant factors of confusional arousals include sleep deprivation, consumption of alcohol, hypnotics or tranquilizers prior to bedtime, or a sudden awakening from sleep [3,11,12].

Sleepwalking

Sleepwalking is a parasomnia that occurs in NREM sleep stages 3 and 4, usually in the first third of the principal sleep episode. This disorder is characterized by automatic behavior during which the sleepwalker is usually unaware of his surroundings and almost entirely unresponsive to external stimuli. Sleepwalkers may leave their bed, walk around their bedrooms and perform semi-purposeful acts. They may also carry out complex motor automatisms, such as driving a car. There is always complete amnesia for the episode at awakening.

Sleepwalking is more common in childhood, with a prevalence ranging from 5 to 30% for occasional or frequent episodes of somnambulism [13,14]. The disorder, however, can also appear for the first time in adulthood [10,15]. The prevalence of sleepwalking oscillates between 2 and 5% in the adult general population according to some authors [14,16–18]. As for confusional arousals, prevalence significantly decreases with age from 4.9% in the 15–24-year age group to 0.5% in the ≥65-year age group [18]. A strong familial occurrence has often been reported in sleepwalking; for example, in a prospective study, Abe *et al.* reported a sleepwalking occurrence of 14% in children aged between 8 and 10 years who had one of their parents with a sleepwalking history and 2% of sleepwalking in children with non-sleepwalking parents [19].

It is not uncommon for sleepwalkers to inflict injury to themselves or others during an episode. Rauch and Stern described two cases of self-inflicted injury [20]. One involved a 34-year-old man who fell 20 feet into some bushes, lacerating his head and fracturing his tenth thoracic vertebra. The other involved a 20-year-old man who smashed through a glass door, resulting in a severe laceration of his right wrist. Several cases of murder while sleepwalking have also been documented. Studying 100 patients who claimed amnesia for their crime at the time of hospitalization, Hopwood and Shell identified one case of somnambulistic homicide: a fireman who battered his wife to death with a shovel during a sleepwalking episode [21]. More recently, Broughton *et al.* described the extraordinary case of a man who, during a sleepwalking episode, drove his car several kilometers to the home of his wife's parents before killing them [22].

Sleep terrors

Sleep terrors, too, are parasomnias that occur in NREM sleep stages 3 and 4. Typically, these episodes begin with an abrupt awakening from sleep accompanied by a panicky scream. The individual is generally inconsolable during an episode. At awakening, there is complete or partial amnesia of the frightening dream.

Like sleepwalking, sleep terrors occur more commonly in childhood, but less frequently than sleepwalking. Between 1 and 6.5% of children are afflicted by sleep terrors [23,24], and as many prepubertal children have recurrent episodes [25]. Occurrence of a few episodes of sleep terrors in childhood is estimated to occur in 20–30% [26]. In the adult general population, the prevalence of sleep terrors has been estimated to be about 1% for weekly episodes [27] and around 2% for less frequent episodes [18,27].

One of the earliest reports of murder during a sleep terror episode is the case of Esther Griggs, who in 1858 threw her baby out of a window. She was apparently dreaming her house was on fire at the time and was actually attempting to save her baby. We can find in the literature several cases of sleepwalking/sleep terror episodes that resulted in murder or serious injury [28–30]. The individual typically has no or only fragmentary memory of the dream being acted out. From the accounts of those who remember their dreams in part, certain recurring themes emerge. These include defending oneself against attacks from others or beasts, trying to escape a danger, or trying to protect a loved one against potential danger.

Sleepwalking and sleep terrors can be triggered by stress, sleep deprivation, alcohol ingestion, and almost all sedative medications (hypnotics, tranquilizers, antihistamines, stimulants).

Parasomnias associated with REM sleep

This group of parasomnias is composed of three disorders occurring essentially during REM sleep. These disorders are nightmare disorder, recurrent isolated sleep paralysis and REM sleep behavior disorder (RBD).

Nightmare disorder

Nightmares are frightening dreams occurring generally during REM sleep and often resulting in awakening the dreamer. This disorder is frequent in children. It affects boys and girls equally. Nightmares occur always or often in 2–11% of children and now and then in 15–31% [31]. About a third of adults with recurrent nightmares have onset of the symptom during childhood [16]. Nightmares have been reported to occur at least once a week in 5% of the adult population [32] and always or often in 1–5% [26]. Women are 2–4 times more frequently affected than men. There are persistent genetic effects on the disposition to nightmares in about 45% of childhood and 37% of adult nightmares [33].

Recurrent isolated sleep paralysis

Sleep paralysis is one of the main symptoms associated with narcolepsy, but it can also occur individually (i.e. isolated sleep paralysis). Téllez-Lòpez et al. [34] found that 11.3% of their general population sample had sleep paralysis episodes at least sometimes. Where more narrowly defined populations are concerned, Goode [35] and Everett [36] observed rates of 4.7% and 15.4%, respectively, for self-reported sleep paralysis in medical students, and Bell et al. [37] noted a prevalence of 41% in Black Americans. In a study of adults living on the northeast coast of Newfoundland, Ness [38] reported a rate of 62% for "old hag" attacks, as sleep paralysis is popularly known in that part of Canada. An epidemiological study performed with 8085 subjects between 15 and 99 years of age found that 6.2% had at least one episode of sleep paralysis in their lifetime; 0.8% experienced severe sleep paralysis (at least one episode per week); and 1.4% moderate sleep paralysis (at least one episode per month) [39].

REM sleep behavior disorders

REM sleep behavior disorders (RBD) were first described in the late 1970s by Japanese researchers and labeled as such by Schenck et al. [43]. This sleep disorder is characterized by a loss of generalized skeletal muscle REM-related atonia and the presence of physical dream enactment. The individual has no consciousness of acting out a dream, but is generally able to recount the dream upon awakening. This syndrome often results in behavior dangerous to oneself or others [40–42]. Their initial sample [40] included four men and one woman, all aged 60 years or over. Four of them had neurological disorders. Most of these cases had excessive slow-wave sleep for their age. This is not, however, a *sine qua non* condition. Indeed, Tachibana et al. [43] reported seven cases of RBD without neurological or psychiatric disorder that had a normal quantity of slow-wave sleep. In all studies, this disorder is observed almost exclusively in men.

According to Schenck and Mahowald [44], prodromal symptoms of RBD appeared 10–40 years before the full manifestation of the disorder in 25% of the studied cases. This prodrome is characterized by sleep talking, yelling, or limb-jerking during sleep.

The mechanism underlying this disorder is not yet fully understood. Polysomnographic recordings of individuals with RBD showed a reduction of the tonic phenomena of REM sleep and the activation of the phasic phenomena. Destruction of the brainstem regions responsible for the REM sleep atonia has been hypothesized as responsible of such phenomena.

The prevalence of RBD in the general population is little-documented. Ohayon et al. [45] estimated it at 0.5% in the general population using minimal criteria proposed by the International Classification of Sleep Disorder (ICSD). However, as many as 2% of the general population reported experiencing violent behaviors during sleep, with a male predominance [45].

Other parasomnias

This group of parasomnias comprises sleep-related dissociative disorders, sleep enuresis, catathrenia, exploding head syndrome, sleep-related hallucinations, sleep-related eating disorder, unspecified parasomnia, parasomnia due to a drug or substance and parasomnia due to a medical condition.

Epidemiological data on this group of parasomnias are scarce. Prevalence in the general population is unknown for most of the parasomnias. Catathrenia, or sleep-related groaning, is a newly described parasomnia occurring in both REM and NREM sleep [46].

Sleep enuresis

Sleep enuresis, also called nocturnal bedwetting, is characterized by recurrent involuntary voiding during the night. It is considered primary when the individual never experienced a dry period for at least six consecutive months.

Sleep enuresis is relatively common in childhood ($\geq$5 years old) and progressively decreases with age. At 4–5 years of age, the prevalence of sleep enuresis is estimated to be between 20 and 30%. At 7 years, it decreases to about 10%, and further decreases to around 3% in 12-year-olds. The prevalence during adolescence and adulthood is around 2% [31,47,48]. Sleep enuresis in prepubertal children is twice as frequent among boys than girls. In adulthood, the prevalence is comparable in both sexes. However, in the elderly, this problem affects women more frequently than men.

Sleep enuresis has a strong hereditary component. When both parents have a history of sleep enuresis in childhood, 77% of the children suffer from enuresis. When only one of the parents has a positive history, nearly half the children have sleep enuresis [1].

Sleep-related hallucinations

Sleep-related hallucinations refer to hallucinations occurring at sleep onset (hypnagogic hallucinations) or upon awakening (hypnopompic hallucinations). Hypnagogic hallucinations are common in the general population with a prevalence of 25–37% [49,50]. The prevalence of hypnopompic hallucinations is around 7–13% [49,50]. Both hypnagogic and hypnopompic hallucinations significantly decrease with age, being twice less frequent in elderly subjects ($\geq$65 years). These hallucinations are also more frequent among women than men. About 30% of those experiencing sleep-related hallucinations are frightened by them [50].

Conclusions

Our knowledge about the prevalence and incidence of parasomnias is still limited compared to dyssomnias. Most of the available data are based on the main symptoms of parasomnias, not the diagnoses.

Information about the associated factors and triggers of an episode is also limited. As shown, parasomnias are frequent in the general population; more than 30% of individuals experiences at least one type of parasomnia. The consequences on daytime functioning and the emotional distress experienced following a parasomnia episode are undocumented at the epidemiological level. Therefore, it is difficult to ascertain what proportion of these individuals are in need of treatment.

At the genetic level, there is growing evidence that many parasomnias have a genetic component. Therefore, epidemiological genetic links need to be studied. Ethnicity also could play a role in some parasomnias. However, with the exception of sleep paralysis, the role of race has not been investigated.

References

1. American Academy of Sleep Medicine. *The International Classification of Sleep Disorders: Second Edition, Diagnostic and Coding Manual.* Westchester, IL: American Academy of Sleep Medicine, 2005.
2. Laberge L, Tremblay RE, Vitaro F, Montplaisir J. Development of parasomnias from childhood to early adolescence. *Pediatrics* 2000; **159**: 1070–8.
3. Ohayon MM, Priest RG, Zulley J, Smirne S. The place of confusional arousals in sleep and mental disorders: general population findings (13057 subjects). *J Nerv Ment Dis* 2000; **188**: 340–8.
4. Gudden D. Die physiologische und pathologische schlorftrunkenheit. *Arch Psychiat* 1905; **40**: 989–1015.
5. Schmidt G. Die Verbrechen in der schlaftrunkenheit. *J Neurol Psychiatry* 1943; **176**: 208–53.
6. Bonkalo A. Impulsive acts and confusional states during incomplete arousal from sleep: criminological and forensic implications. *Psychiatr Q* 1974; **48**: 400–09.
7. Raschka LB. Sleep and violence. *Can J Psychiatry* 1984; **29**: 132–4.
8. Nofzinger EA, Wettstein. Homicidal behavior and sleep apnea: a case report and medicolegal discussion. *Sleep* 1995; **18**: 776–82.
9. Schenck CH, Mahowald MW. A polysomnographically documented case of adult somnambulism with long-distance automobile driving and frequent nocturnal violence: parasomnia with continuing danger as a noninsane automatism? *Sleep* 1995; **18**: 765–72.

10. Schenck CH, Milner DM, Hurwitz TD, Bundlie SR, Mahowald MW. A polysomnographic and clinical report on sleep-related injury in 100 adult patients. *Am J Psychiatry* 1989; **146**: 1166–73.

11. Lemoine P, Lamothe P, Ohayon M. Violence, sleep and benzodiazepines. *Am J Foren Psychiatry* 1997; **18**: 17–26.

12. Roth B, Nevsimalova S, Rechtschaffen A. Hypermania with 'sleep drunkenness'. *Arch Gen Psychiatry* 1972; **26**: 456–62.

13. Jacobson A, Kales JD, Kales A. Clinical and electrophysiological correlates of sleep disorders in children. In Kales A (Ed), *Sleep: Physiology and Pathology*. Philadelphia: JB Lippincott, 1969; 109–18.

14. Hublin C, Kaprio J, Partinen M, Heikkila K, Koskenvuo M. Prevalence and genetics of sleepwalking: a population-based twin study. *Neurology* 1997; **48**: 177–81.

15. Guilleminault C, Leger D, Philip P, Ohayon MM. Nocturnal wandering and violence: review of a sleep clinic population. *J Foren Sci* 1998; **43**: 150–5.

16. Bixler EO, Kales A, Soldatos CR, Kales JD, Healey S. Prevalence of sleep disorders in the Los Angeles metropolitan area. *Am J Psychiatry* 1979; **136**: 1257–62.

17. Cirignotta F, Zucconi M, Mondini S, Lenzi PL, Lugaresi E. Enuresis, sleepwalking and nightmares: an epidemiological survey in the republic of San Marino. In Guilleminault C, Lugaresi E (Eds), *Sleep/Wake Disorders: Natural History, Epidemiology, and Long-Term Evolution*. New York, NY: Raven Press, 1983; 237–41.

18. Ohayon MM, Guilleminault C, Priest RG. Night terrors, sleepwalking, and confusional arousals in the general population: their frequency and relationship to other sleep and mental disorders. *J Clin Psychiatry* 1999; **60**: 268–76.

19. Abe K, Amatomi M, Oda N. Sleepwalking and recurrent sleeptalking in children of childhood sleepwalkers. *Am J Psychiatry* 1984; **141**: 800–01.

20. Rauch PK, Stern TA. Life-threatening injuries resulting from sleepwalking and night terrors. *Psychosomatics* 1986; **27**: 62–4.

21. Hopwood J, Snell HK. Amnesia in relation to crime. *J Mental Sci* 1933; **79**: 27–41.

22. Broughton R, Billings R, Cartwright R, *et al*. Homicidal somnambulism: a case report. *Sleep* 1994; **17**: 253–64.

23. Simonds JF, Parraga H. Prevalence of sleep disorders and sleep behaviors in children and adolescents. *J Am Acad Child Adolesc Psychiatry* 1982; **21**: 383–8.

24. Broughton RJ. Parasomnias. In Chokroverty S (Ed), *Sleep Disorders Medicine*. Stoneham, MA: Butterworth-Heinemann, 1994; 381–99.

25. Thorpy MJ, Glovinsky PB. Parasomnias. *Psychiatr Clin North Am* 1987; **10**: 623–39.

26. Partinen M. Epidemiology of sleep disorders. In Kryger MH, Roth T, Dement WC (Eds), *Principles and Practice in Sleep Medicine*. Philadelphia: WB Saunders, 1994; 437–52.

27. Hublin C, Kaprio J, Partinen M, Koskenvuo M. Nightmares: familial aggregation and association with psychiatric disorders in a nationwide twin cohort. *Am J Med Genet* 1999; **88**: 329–36.

28. Hartmann E. Two case reports: night terrors with sleepwalking – a potential lethal disorder. *J Nerv Ment Dis* 1983; **171**: 503–05.

29. Crisp AH, Matthews BM, Oakey M, Crutchfield M. Sleepwalking, night terrors, and consciousness. *Br Med J* 1990; **300**: 360–2.

30. Kavey NB, Whyte J, Resor SR Jr, Gidro Frank S. Somnambulism in adults. *Neurology* 1990; **40**: 749–52.

31. Partinen M, Hublin C. Epidemiology of sleep disorders. In Kryger MH, Roth T, Dement WC (Eds), *Principles and Practice in Sleep Medicine*. Philadelphia: WB Saunders, 2000; 558–79.

32. Ohayon MM, Morselli PL, Guilleminault C. Prevalence of nightmares and its relationship to psychopathology and daytime functioning in insomnia subjects. *Sleep* 1997; **20**: 340–8.

33. Hublin C, Kaprio J, Partinen M, Koskenvuo M. Limits of self-report in assessing sleep terrors in a population survey. *Sleep* 1999; **22**: 89–93.

34. Téllez-Lòpez A, Sánchez EG, Torres FG, Ramirez PN, Olivares VS. Hábitos y trastornos del dormir en residentes del área metropolitana de Monterrey. *Salud Mental* 1995; **18**: 14–22.

35. Goode GB. Sleep paralysis. *Arch Neurol* 1962; **2**: 228–34.

36. Everett HC. Sleep paralysis in medical students. *J Nerv Ment Dis* 1963; **3**: 283–7.

37. Bell CC, Shakoor B, Thompson B, *et al*. Prevalence of isolated sleep paralysis in black subjects. *J Natl Med Assoc* 1984; **76**: 501–08.

38. Ness RC. The Old Hag phenomenon as sleep paralysis: a biocultural interpretation. *Cult Med Psychiatry* 1978; **2**: 15–39.

39. Ohayon MM, Zulley J, Guilleminault C, Smirne S. Prevalence and pathological associations of sleep paralysis in the general population. *Neurology* 1999; **52**: 1194–200.

40. Schenck CH, Bundlie SR, Ettinger MG, Mahowald MW. Chronic behavioral disorders of human REM sleep: a new category of parasomnia. *Sleep* 1986; **9**: 293–308.

41. Schenck CH, Bundlie SR, Patterson AL, Mahowald MW. Rapid eye movement sleep behavior disorder. A treatable parasomnia affecting older adults. *JAMA* 1987; **257**: 1786–9.

42. Schenck CH, Hurwitz TD, Mahowald MW. REM sleep behavior disorder: an update on a series of 96 patients and a review of the world literature. *J Sleep Res* 1993; **2**: 224–31.

43. Shimizu T, Jnami Y, Sugita Y, *et al*. REM sleep without muscle atonia (stage 1-REM) and its relation to delirious behavior during sleep in patients with degenerative diseases involving the brain stem. *Jpn J Psychiatr Neurol* 1990; **44**: 681–92.

44. Schenck CH, Mahowald MW. Injurious sleep behavior disorders (parasomnias) affecting patients on intensive care units. *Intens Care Med* 1991; **17**: 219–24.

45. Ohayon MM, Caulet M, Priest RG. Violent behaviour during sleep. *J Clin Psychiatry* 1997; **58**: 369–78.

46. Vetrugno R, Provini F, Plazzi G, Vignatelli L, Lugaresi E, Montagna P. Catathrenia (nocturnal groaning): a new type of parasomnia. *Neurology* 2001; **56**: 681–3.

47. Stein MA, Mendelsohn J, Obermeyer WH, Amromin J, Benca R. Sleep and behavior problems in school-aged children. *Pediatrics* 2001; **107**: E60; 1–9.

48. Yeung CK, Sihoe JD, Sit FK, Bower W, Sreedhar B, Lau J. Characteristics of primary nocturnal enuresis in adults: an epidemiological study. *BJU Int* 2004; **93**: 341–5.

49. Ohayon MM, Priest RG, Caulet M, Guilleminault C. Hypnagogic and hypnopompic hallucinations: pathological phenomena? *Br J Psychiatry* 1996; **169**: 459–67.

50. Ohayon MM, Priest RG, Zulley J, Smirne S, Paiva T. Prevalence of narcolepsy symptomatology and diagnosis in the European general population. *Neurology* 2002; **58**: 1826–33.

Section 1 Introduction
Chapter 3
Neuroimaging of parasomnias

Eric A. Nofzinger

Introduction

In the past few decades, structural and functional neuroimaging methods have emerged as a way to assess brain function in health and in pathology. These methods allow for the quantification of a variety of aspects of brain structure and function including regional brain volumes, metabolism, blood flow, white matter tract integrity, brain iron concentrations and receptor binding. Given that sleep is regulated by the brain and may ultimately serve brain function, these tools may provide important information regarding abnormal brain function in sleep disorder patients such as those with parasomnias. If so, such assessments may serve an important function in the evaluation and management of parasomnia patients and in the development of new pharmacologic agents to treat parasomnias. This chapter will briefly review the use of structural and functional neuroimaging in the assessment and management of parasomnias.

Neuroimaging studies of healthy human sleep

Neuroimaging studies have revealed reliable broad changes in cerebral activity across the sleep wake cycle. Globally, brain activity decreases from waking to NREM sleep, then increases to waking levels again during REM sleep [1–17]. Preclinical studies support a deafferentation of the cortex at the level of the thalamus and the occurrence of intrinsic thalamocortical electrical oscillations in NREM sleep. Studies across several laboratories and using various imaging methods have demonstrated that from waking to NREM sleep there are relative regional reductions in activity in the heteromodal association cortex in the frontal, parietal and temporal lobes as well as in the thalamus. This suggests that the thalamocortical circuits that play an important role in NREM sleep function are those involving regions that support waking, conscious, goal-directed behavior. Preclinical work shows that REM sleep is associated with an electrophysiologically active cortex, with selective activation of cholinergic networks that originate in the brainstem and basal forebrain and that densely innervate the limbic and paralimbic cortex. Consistent with this, in relation to waking and NREM sleep, REM sleep is associated with increased relative activity in the pontine reticular formation, as well as limbic (e.g. amygdala and hypothalamus) and paralimbic cortex (e.g. ventral striatum, anterior cingulate and medial prefrontal cortex). This suggests that REM sleep may play an important role in emotional behavior, given the important involvement of these structures in the regulation of affect and in motivated behavior.

Restless legs syndrome (RLS)/periodic limb movement disorders of sleep (PLMD)

The majority of the work in the area of neuroimaging and parasomnias and sleep-related movment disorders has been in the area of RLS and PLMD. The scope of the work performed to date has been both driven by, and constrained by, clinical manifestations of the disorder and by the measurements currently available using neuroimaging tools.

The most extensive work has been performed in the area of central dopaminergic dysfunction in these disorders. A series of studies measured central dopamine D2-receptor occupancy with [123I]-labeled (S)-2-hydroxy-3-iodo-6-methoxy-([1-ethyl-2-pyrrolidinyl]methyl) benzamide (IBZM) and SPECT in patients with PLMD [18–20]. They found lower striatal [123I]IBZM binding in patients with PLMD and higher binding following dopaminergic therapy. Michaud et al. report the results of pre- and post-synaptic dopaminergic status using [123I]beta-CIT and [123I]IBZM SPECT, respectively, in ten patients with both RLS and PLMD [21]. They found no differences in DA transporter binding, but lower striatal D2-receptor binding in patients ($p = .006$). They suggest that this indicates a decreased number of D2-receptors or a decreased affinity of D2-receptors for IBZM. This supports a central striatal D2 receptor abnormality in the pathophysiology of RSL/PLMD. Tribl et al. [22] assessed patients with idiopathic RLS (iRLS) and periodic limb movements in sleep (PLMS) who had exhibited a good response to dopaminergic and non-dopaminergic treatment, and ten healthy sex- and age-matched controls using 123I-IBZM and SPECT. The patients showed no significant differences in striatal to frontal IBZM binding to D2 receptors compared to controls. These findings show the normal function of striatal D2 receptors in successfully treated patients with iRLS and PLMS. Eisensehr [23] studied 14 drug-naive and 11 levodopa-treated patients with idiopathic restless legs syndrome (RLS), and 10 controls age-matched to each RLS group with polysomnography (PSG), [(123)I]-(N)-(3-iodopropen-2-yl)-2beta-carbomethoxy-3beta-(4-chlorophenyl) tropane ((123)I-IPT) SPECT, and [(123)I]-(S)-2-hydroxy-3-iodo-6-methoxy-[(1-ethyl-2-pyrrolidinyl)methyl] benzamide ((123)I-IBZM) SPECT. Drug-naive and levodopa-treated patients with RLS and controls showed similar striatal dopamine transporter and dopamine D(2)-receptor binding, the latter declining with age. The authors conclude that striatal dopamine transporter and receptor density is normal in drug-naive and levodopa-treated patients with RLS.

Cervenka et al. assessed 16 RLS patients naive to dopaminergic drugs and 16 matched control subjects with PET [13]. [11C]Raclopride and [11C]FLB 457 were used to estimate D2-receptor availability in the striatum and extrastriatal regions, respectively. Examinations were performed both in the morning (starting between 10:00 and 12:00 h) and evening (starting at 18:00 h). In the striatum, patients had significantly higher [11C]raclopride binding potential (BP) values than controls. In extrastriatal regions, [11C]FLB 457 BP was higher in patients than controls, and in the regional analysis the difference was statistically significant in subregions of the thalamus and the anterior cingulate cortex. The study supports involvement of the dopamine system in both striatal and extrastriatal brain regions in the pathophysiology of RLS. Increased D2-receptor availability in RLS may correspond to higher receptor densities or lower levels of endogenous dopamine, either of which would support the hypothesis of hypoactive dopaminergic neurotransmission in RLS.

Restless legs syndrome has been associated with iron depletion and serum ferritin levels have been shown to be decreased by 13% per allele of a common variant in an intron of BTBD9 on chromosome 6p21.2 found to be associated with RLS. Neuroimaging methods allow for the regional quantification of brain iron content, prompting sleep neuroimaging researchers to assess brain iron content in patients with RLS. Allen et al. studied brain iron insufficiency in RLS [24]. Using a special MRI measurement ($R2'$), the authors assessed regional brain iron concentrations in 10 subjects (5 with RLS, 5 controls). $R2'$ was significantly decreased in the substantia nigra, and somewhat less significantly in the putamen, both in proportion to RLS severity. The results show the potential utility of this MRI measurement, and also indicate that brain iron insufficiency may occur in patients with RLS in some brain regions. A replication and extension study by the same group in 22 early-onset and 19 late-onset RLS subjects showed a reduced mean iron index from the substantia nigra in early-onset, but not late-onset RLS patients [14]. These data support a role of low brain iron in the SN in at least those RLS patients with early-onset. A small study by Godau et al. also demonstrated brain iron deficiency in RLS patients using MRI T2 relaxometry and sonographically assessed echogenicity in multiple brain regions, suggesting the possible involvement of other brain regions in addition to the substantia nigra [14]. In a larger study of late-onset RLS patients, Astrakas et al. also found low substantia nigra iron content in the substantia nigra using MRI T2 relaxometry. Low brain iron content, therefore, especially in the basal ganglia, appears to be a replicable neuroimaging finding in patients with RLS [1].

Neuroimaging methods allow for the determination of brain volumetric changes in patient samples to see if structural cerebral abnormalities may play a role in the disorder. Etgen et al. assessed 51 RLS patients and 51 age- and sex-matched controls using high-resolution T1-weighted magnetic resonance imaging, and analyzed differences between patient and control groups using voxel-based morphometry [16]. They demonstrated an increase in size of the pulvinar of the thalamus in the patient group, raising the possibility that the thalamus may play a role in the abnormal sensory experience or may reflect a chronic increase in afferent input of behaviorally relevant information in RLS patients. A second group from another lab performed a similar study, but using mostly medication-naive RLS patients to eliminate a possible confound of medication use on pulvinar size [8]. They were unable to replicate the prior finding of an increase in pulvinar size in RLS patients. Another study found volumetric reductions in primary sensorimotor cortex, extending into primary motor cortex, that correlated with RLS symptom severity and disease duration [7], raising the possibility that an alteration in sensorimotor cortices may play a role in the pathophysiology of RLS. In a related study, this group used diffusion tensor imaging (DTI) to assess cerebral white matter tract disruption in 45 RLS patients and 30 healthy controls [3]. They found reduced fractional anisotropy (FA), a measure of white matter tract integrity, in multiple tracts associated with primary and associate motor and somatosensory cortices, again raising the possibility that RLS may be associated with a neocortical abnormality. Across all studies assessing regional cerebral volumes, however, individual findings have not been replicated, raising questions as to whether the disorder is associated with volumetric changes in the cerebral cortex.

Low-dose opioid treatment has been used in the management of some RLS patients. One study examined opioid receptor availability in 15 patients with primary RLS and 12 age-matched healthy controls using PET and [11C]diprenorphine, a non-selective opioid receptor ligand [15]. While no mean group differences were noted between patients and controls, correlational analyses showed negative correlations between pain scores and ligand binding in the orbitofrontal cortex and anterior cingulated gyrus. These findings suggest that the more severe the RLS symptoms, the greater the release of endogenous opioids in the medial pain system.

The subjective experience of RLS is one of discomfort that can be quantified and related to brain function. Bucher *et al.* assessed the pathophysiology of periodic limb movements and sensory leg discomfort in RLS using high-resolution functional magnetic resonance imaging [25]. During sensory leg discomfort there was mainly bilateral activation of the cerebellum and contralateral activation of the thalamus. During the combined periodic limb movement and sensory leg discomfort conditions, patients also showed activity in the cerebellum and thalamus. In contrast to the sensory leg discomfort condition alone, the combined condition was associated with additional activation in the red nuclei and brainstem close to the reticular formation. Voluntary imitation of periodic limb movements by patients and control subjects was not associated with brainstem activity, but with additional activation in the globus pallidus and motor cortex. These findings indicate that cerebellar and thalamic activation may occur because of sensory leg discomfort and that the red nucleus and brainstem are involved in the generation of periodic limb movements in patients with RLS. A novel study by Spiegelhalder *et al.* correlated an indirect measure of discomfort with regional brain function using fMRI [6]. They found an inverse correlation between discomfort and brain activity in somatosensory pathways, raising the possibility that a central sensory processing pathology may be associated with RLS. Further studies in this area are needed to clarify and extend these preliminary findings.

Sleepwalking

Only one nuclear medicine study has studied regional brain function associated with sleepwalking. Bassetti *et al.* performed 99mTc ECD SPECT studies during stages 3 and 4 sleep one night before and one night during a sleepwalking episode [26] (Figure 3.1). They reported increased blood flow in the cerebellar vermis and the posterior cingulate cortex during sleepwalking. In relation to healthy wakefulness, the sleepwalking episode was associated with a decline in frontoparietal association cortices as would be typical of NREM sleep, albeit in the absence of declines in thalamic blood flow. They interpret the results to reflect both unconsciousness, as reflected by a loss of frontoparietal function, and a persistence of motor generators, as reflected by preserved thalamocingulate circuits, in sleepwalking behavior.

REM sleep behavior disorder

Shirakawa *et al.* reported the results of a [123-I] IMP SPECT study of 20 patients with REM sleep behavior disorder (RBD) in comparison with 7 healthy controls [27]. They reported decreased blood flow in the upper frontal lobe and pons. They suggest that these findings may be associated with the pathogenesis of RBD, especially the decreased blood flow in the pons as this is

Section 1: Introduction

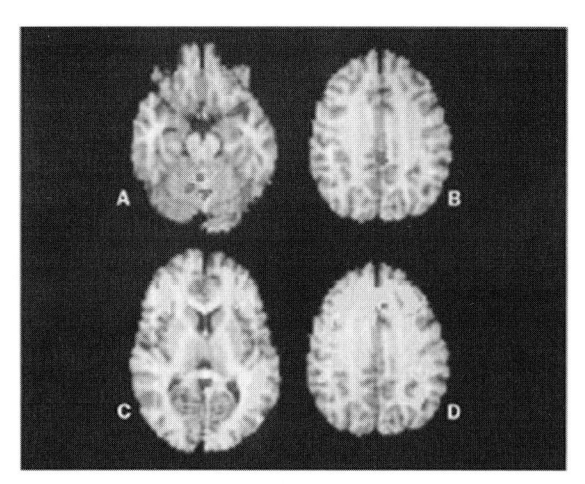

Figure 3.1 The color version of this figure can be found in the color plate section. SPECT findings during sleepwalking after integration into the appropriate anatomical magnetic resonance image.

The highest increases of regional cerebral blood flow (>25%) during sleepwalking compared with stage 3 to 4 NREM sleep are found in the anterior cerebellum – i.e. vermis (A) and in the posterior cingulate cortex (Brodmann area 23 [Tallarch coordinate $x = -4$, $y = -40$, $z = 31$] (B)). However, in relation to data from normal volunteers during wakefulness ($n = 24$), large areas of frontal and parietal association cortices remain deactivated during sleepwalking, as shown in the corresponding parametric maps (2-threshold = –3). Note the inclusion of the dorsolateral prefrontal cortex (C), mesial frontal cortex (D), and left angular gyrus (C) within these areas.

theoretically thought to play a role in RBD. Eisensehr et al. studied pre- and post-synaptic dopaminergic status using [123I]-IPT and [123I]-IBZM SPECT, respectively, in 5 patients with RBD, 7 age- and sex-matched controls, and 14 Parkinson's patients [28]. They found decreased DA transporter binding in RBD in relation to controls, although not as severe as in Parkinson's patients, and no change in striatal D2-receptor binding in RBD. They suggest that this supports a central striatal dopamine transporter abnormality in the pathophysiology of RBD. Albin et al. assessed [11C]-dihydrotetrabenazine (DTBZ) PET in 6 patients with RBD and in 19 age- and sex-matched controls [29]. They found decreased DTBZ binding in RBD in relation to controls. This study supports a loss of dopaminergic midbrain neurons in chronic RBD; however, it remains unclear whether this is primary or a secondary effect of the pontine abnormality in RBD. Gilman et al. assessed the severity of RBD and the density of striatal monoaminergic terminals using PET with (+)-[11C]dihydrotetrabenazine ([11C]DTBZ) and SPECT with (–)-5-[123I]iodobenzovesamicol ([123I]IBVM) to measure the density of [123I]IBVM in patients with multiple-system atrophy (MSA) and in controls [30]. The MSA subjects showed decreased mean [11C]DTBZ binding in the striatum and decreased [123I]IBVM binding in the thalamus. Moreover, in the MSA group, striatal [11C]DTBZ binding was inversely correlated with the severity of REM atonia loss. They concluded that decreased nigrostriatal dopaminergic projections may contribute to RBD in MSA.

Mazza et al. performed cerebral blood flow evaluation using (99m)Tc-ethylene cysteinate dimer (ECD) SPECT on eight patients with polysomnographically confirmed RBD and nine age-matched controls [11]. They found increased perfusion in the pons and putamen bilaterally and in the right hippocampus. In addition, they observed decreased perfusion in the frontal (Brodmann area [BA] 4, 6, 10, 43, 44, 47 bilaterally and left BA 9, 46) and temporoparietal (BA 13, 22, 43 bilaterally and left BA 7, 19, 20, 21, 39, 40, 41, 42) cortices. They concluded that these abnormalities are consistent with the anatomic metabolic profile of Parkinson's disease.

Eisensehr et al. hypothesized that subclinical RBD shows a less severe reduction of striatal dopamine transporters than clinically manifest RBD [31]. To test this, they studied striatal postsynaptic dopamine D2-receptors with (S)-2hydroxy-3iodo-6-methoxy-([1-ethyl-2-pyrrolidinyl]methyl) benzamide labeled with iodine 123 (IBZM) and the striatal presynaptic dopamine transporters with (N)-(3-iodopropene-2-yl)-2beta-carbomethoxy-3beta-(4-chlorophenyl) tropane labeled with iodine 123 (IPT) using single-photon emission computed tomography (SPECT) in the following groups: 8 patients with idiopathic subclinical RBD, 8 patients with idiopathic clinically manifest RBD, 11 controls, and 8 patients with PD stage Hoehn & Yahr I. They found that the IPT uptake was highest in controls. There was a significant decrease in IPT uptake from controls to patients with subclinical RBD, from patients with subclinical RBD to clinically manifest RBD, and from patients with clinically manifest RBD to patients with PD. This study suggests that there is a continuum of reduced striatal dopamine transporters involved in the pathophysiologic mechanisms causing increased muscle activity during REM sleep in patients with subclinical RBD.

Iranzo et al. investigated whether 1H-MRS can detect hypothesized brainstem abnormalities in patients with idiopathic RBD. No significant differences in N-acetylaspartate/creatine, choline/creatine and myoinosito/creatine ratios were found between patients and controls. These results do not suggest that marked mesopontine neuronal loss or 1H-MRS detectable metabolic disturbances occur in idiopathic RBD [32].

Caselli *et al.* assessed whether healthy adults reporting dream-enactment behavior (DEB+) have a reduced cerebral metabolic rate for glucose (CMRgl) in regions preferentially affected in patients with dementia with Lewy bodies (DLB) [33]. DEB was associated with significantly lower CMRgl in several brain regions known to be preferentially affected in both DLB and Alzheimer's disease (parietal, temporal, and posterior cingulate cortices) and in several other regions, including the anterior cingulate cortex. The DEB-associated CMRgl reductions were significantly greater in the APOE e4 non-carriers than in the carriers. They concluded that cognitively normal persons with DEB have reduced CMRgl in brain regions known to be metabolically affected by DLB, supporting further study of DEB as a possible risk factor for the development of DLB.

Summary

At this time, the majority of efforts in parasomnia and sleep-related movement disorder imaging research have been in the area of RLS/PLMD. Among the more consistent findings are those involving the role of dopamine and iron in the pathophysiology of the disorder, supporting the role of these systems in the clinical management of the disorder. Extensive research in this area is needed in order to further clarify pathophysiology, predictors of response to treatments, treatment mechanisms and clarifying the role of sensory processing within sleep in the clinical manifestations of these disorders.

References

1. Astrakas LG, Konitsiotis S, Margariti P, *et al.* T2 relaxometry and fMRI of the brain in late-onset restless legs syndrome. *Neurology* 2008; **71**: 911–6.
2. Desseilles M, Dang-Vu T, Schabus M, *et al.* Neuroimaging insights into the pathophysiology of sleep disorders. *Sleep* 2008; **31**: 777–94.
3. Unrath A, Muller HP, Ludolph AC, *et al.* Cerebral white matter alterations in idiopathic restless legs syndrome, as measured by diffusion tensor imaging. *Mov Disord* 2008; **23**: 1250–5.
4. Godau J, Klose U, DiSanto A, *et al.* Multiregional brain iron deficiency in restless legs syndrome. *Mov Disord* 2008; **23**: 1184–7.
5. Unger MM, Moller JC, Stiasny-Kolster K, *et al.* Assessment of idiopathic rapid-eye-movement sleep behavior disorder by transcranial sonography, olfactory function test, and FP-CIT-SPECT. *Mov Disord* 2008; **23**: 506–99.
6. Spiegelhalder K, Feige B, Paul D, *et al.* Cerebral correlates of muscle tone fluctuations in restless legs syndrome: a pilot study with combined functional magnetic resonance imaging and anterior tibial muscle electromyography. *Sleep Med* 2008; **9**: 177–83.
7. Unrath A, Juengling FD, Schork K, *et al.* Cortical grey matter alterations in idiopathic restless legs syndrome: an optimized voxel-based morphometry study. *Mov Disord* 2007; **22**: 1751–6.
8. Hornyak M, Ahrendts JC, Spiegelhalder K, *et al.* Voxel-based morphometry in unmedicated patients with restless legs syndrome. *Sleep Med* 2007; **9**: 22–6.
9. Nielsen T, Levin R. Nightmares: a new neurocognitive model. *Sleep Med Rev* 2007; **11**: 295–310.
10. Dang-Vu TT, Desseilles M, Petit D, *et al.* Neuroimaging in sleep medicine. *Sleep Med* 2007; **8**: 349–72.
11. Mazza M, Soucy JP, Gravel P, *et al.* Assessing whole brain perfusion changes in patients with REM sleep behavior disorder. *Neurology* 2006; **67**: 1618–22.
12. Reimold M, Globas C, Gleichmann M, *et al.* Spinocerebellar ataxia type 1, 2, and 3 and restless legs syndrome: striatal dopamine D2 receptor status investigated by [11C]raclopride positron emission tomography. *Mov Disord* 2006; **21**: 1667–73.
13. Cervenka S, Palhagen SE, Comley RA, *et al.* Support for dopaminergic hypoactivity in restless legs syndrome: a PET study on D2-receptor binding. *Brain* 2006; **129**: 2017–28.
14. Earley CJ, Barker PB, Horska A, *et al.* MRI-determined regional brain iron concentrations in early- and late-onset restless legs syndrome. *Sleep Med* 2006; **7**: 395–6.
15. von Spiczak S, Whone AL, Hammers A, *et al.* The role of opioids in restless legs syndrome: an [11C]diprenorphine PET study. *Brain* 2005; **128**: 906–17.
16. Etgen T, Draganski B, Ilg C, *et al.* Bilateral thalamic gray matter changes in patients with restless legs syndrome. *Sleep Med* 2005; **7**: 395–6.
17. Mrowka M, Jobges M, Berding G, *et al.* Computerized movement analysis and beta-CIT-SPECT in patients with restless legs syndrome. *J Neural Transm* 2005; **112**: 693–701.
18. Staedt J, Stoppe G, Kogler A, *et al.* Dopamine D2 receptor alteration in patients with periodic

19. Staedt J, Stoppe G, Kogler A, *et al.* Nocturnal myoclonus syndrome (periodic movements in sleep) related to central dopamine D2-receptor alteration. *Eur Arch Psychiatry Clin Neurosci* 1995; **245**: 8–10.

20. Staedt J, Stoppe G, Kogler A, *et al.* Single photon emission tomography (SPET) imaging of dopamine D2 receptors in the course of dopamine replacement therapy in patients with nocturnal myoclonus syndrome (NMS). *J Neural Transm Gen Sect* 1995; **99**: 187–93.

21. Michaud M, Soucy JP, Chabli A, *et al.* SPECT imaging of striatal pre- and postsynaptic dopaminergic status in restless legs syndrome with periodic leg movements in sleep. *J Neurol* 2002; **249**: 164–70.

22. Tribl GG, Asenbaum S, Happe S, *et al.* Normal striatal D2 receptor binding in idiopathic restless legs syndrome with periodic leg movements in sleep. *Nucl Med Commun* 2004; **25**: 55–60.

23. Eisensehr I, Wetter TC, Linke R, *et al.* Normal IPT and IBZM SPECT in drug-naive and levodopa-treated idiopathic restless legs syndrome. *Neurology* 2001; **57**: 1307–09.

24. Allen RP, Barker PB, Wehrl F, *et al.* MRI measurement of brain iron in patients with restless legs syndrome. *Neurology* 2001; **56**: 263–5.

25. Bucher SF, Seelos KC, Oertel WH, *et al.* Cerebral generators involved in the pathogenesis of the restless legs syndrome. *Ann Neurol* 1997; **41**: 639–45.

26. Bassetti C, Vella S, Donati F, *et al.* SPECT during sleepwalking. *Lancet* 2000; **356**: 484–5.

27. Shirakawa S, Takeuchi N, Uchimura N, *et al.* Study of image findings in rapid eye movement sleep behavioural disorder. *Psychiatry Clin Neurosci* 2002; **56**: 291–2.

28. Eisensehr I, Linke R, Noachtar S, Schwarz J, Gildehaus FJ, Tatsch K. Reduced striatal dopamine transporters in idiopathic rapid eye movement sleep behaviour disorder. Comparison with Parkinson's disease and controls. *Brain* 2000; **123**: 1155–60.

29. Albin RL, Koeppe RA, Chervin RD, *et al.* Decreased striatal dopaminergic innervation in REM sleep behavior disorder. *Neurology* 2000; **55**: 1410–2.

30. Gilman S, Koeppe RA, Chervin RD, *et al.* REM sleep behavior disorder is related to striatal monoaminergic deficit in MSA. *Neurology* 2003; **61**: 29–34.

31. Eisensehr I, Linke R, Tatsch K, *et al.* Alteration of the striatal dopaminergic system in human narcolepsy. *Neurology* 2003; **60**: 1817–9.

32. Iranzo A, Santamaria J, Pujol J, Moreno A, Deus J, Tolosa E. Brainstem proton magnetic resonance spectroscopy in idiopathic REM sleep behavior disorder. *Sleep* 2002; **25**: 867–70.

33. Caselli RJ, Chen K, Bandy D, *et al.* A preliminary fluorodeoxyglucose positron emission tomography study in healthy adults reporting dream-enactment behavior. *Sleep* 2006; **29**: 927–33.

Section 1 Chapter 4

Introduction

Clinical evaluation of parasomnias

Imran M. Ahmed and Michael J. Thorpy

Introduction

There are 15 different parasomnias discussed in the International Classification of Sleep Disorders, 2nd edition (ICSD-2). They are undesirable physical or experiential events that accompany sleep. These disorders consist of abnormal sleep-related movements, behaviors, emotions, perceptions, dreaming, and autonomic nervous system functioning. They are disorders of arousal, and sleep stage transition. Many of the parasomnias are manifestations of central nervous system activation and autonomic nervous system changes with skeletal muscle activity. There are also other sleep-related movement disorders that are not parasomnias but need to be considered in the differential diagnosis. These sleep-related movement disorders are listed as a separate category from parasomnias in the ICSD-2, and include, among others, restless legs syndrome (RLS), periodic limb movement disorder (PLMD), sleep-related leg cramps, sleep-related bruxism, and sleep-related rhythmic movement disorder. In addition, parasomnias can often occur in conjunction with other sleep disorders, such as obstructive sleep apnea syndrome or narcolepsy, and it is not uncommon for several parasomnias to occur in the same patient [1] (Table 4.1).

Parasomnias can contribute to impaired academic or occupational performance, disturbances of mood and social adjustment. Marriages and relationships may be adversely affected by the disordered sleep of a spouse or bed partner [2]. Often, parasomnias may be markers of other disorders; for instance, somnambulism can be provoked by obstructive sleep apnea. Accordingly, complaints of abnormal movements or behaviors need to be taken seriously and an evaluation of these problems requires a systematic approach. An evaluation should include a careful sleep history taken from the patient and often, more importantly, the patient's bed partner or caregiver [3]. Additionally, information about the patient's comorbid illnesses, past medical history, social history and psychosocial conditions, family history, physical examination and appropriate sleep studies are valuable when forming a differential diagnosis.

History

Chief complaint

Assessment begins with the presenting sleep complaint. These sleep disturbances may include abnormal sleep-related movements, behaviors, emotions, perceptions, dreaming, hallucinations and autonomic nervous system disturbances. They may occur in otherwise normal individuals and often do not require further extensive evaluation; however, when they result in injuries, sleep disruption, excessive daytime sleepiness, and adverse medical or psychosocial consequences to the patient and/or bed partner, a comprehensive evaluation is warranted [4,5]. Occasionally, patients with parasomnias who live or sleep alone may suspect some abnormality with their sleep. They may awaken with unexplained injuries or awaken to find their room/home inexplicably disheveled, or awaken in a different place from where they went to bed. More often they are unaware of their behaviors during sleep, and for that reason are frequently brought to a physician's attention by family members, caregivers, or bed partners.

Characterizing the sleep disturbance

With the complaint in mind, a thorough history should be taken, which includes information characterizing

---

The Parasomnias and Other Sleep-Related Movement Disorders, ed. M. J. Thorpy and G. Plazzi. Published by Cambridge University Press. © Cambridge University Press 2010.

Table 4.1 Classification of parasomnias and parasomnia-like events.

Parasomnias		
ICD-9-CM	DSM IV-TR	Classification
Disorders of arousal		
327.41		Confusional arousals
307.46	307.46	Sleepwalking
307.46	307.46	Sleep terrors
Parasomnias usually associated with REM sleep		
327.42	307.47	REM sleep behavior disorder
327.43		Recurrent isolated sleep paralysis
307.47	307.47	Nightmare disorder
Other parasomnias		
300.15	300.15	Sleep-related dissociative disorders
788.36	307.6	Sleep enuresis
327.49		Catathrenia (sleep-related groaning)
327.49		Exploding head syndrome
368.16		Sleep-related hallucinations
327.49	307.50	Sleep-related eating disorder
327.40	307.47	Parasomnia, unspecified
292.85	292.85	Parasomnia due to a drug or substance
291.82	291.82	Parasomnia due to alcohol
327.44	327.44	Parasomnias due to medical condition
Sleep-related movement disorders		
ICD-9-CM	DSM IV-TR	Classification
333.99		Restless legs syndrome
327.51		Periodic limb movement disorder
327.52		Sleep-related leg cramps
327.53		Sleep-related bruxism
327.59		Sleep-related rhythmic movement disorder
327.59		Other sleep-related movement disorder, unspecified
327.59 or 292.85	292.85	Sleep-related rhythmic movement disorder ... due to drug or substance
327.59		... due to medical condition
Isolated symptoms, apparently normal variants and unresolved issues		
ICD-9-CM	DSM IV-TR	Classification
307.49		Sleep talking
307.47		Sleep starts, hypnic jerks
781.01		Benign sleep myoclonus of infancy
781.01		Hypnagogic foot tremor and alternating leg muscle activation
781.01	307.47	Propriospinal myoclonus at sleep onset
781.01	307.47	Excessive fragmentary myoclonus
Sleep disorders associated with conditions classified elsewhere		
ICD-9-CM	DSM IV-TR	Classification
345		Sleep-related epilepsy
Other psychiatric and behavioral disorders frequently encountered in the differential diagnosis of sleep disorders (DSM IV-TR codes are utilized here)		
DSM IV-TR		
	300.xx	Panic disorder w/ or w/o agoraphobia (or nocturnal panic disorder)
	309.81.1	Post-traumatic stress disorder

the specific sleep problem, differentiating between various possible sleep disorders, and assessing the patient's functional status and psychological disposition. Ideally, this should be done via interviews with the patient as well as the caregiver, bed partner, or other observer. If the patient can bring in a video of the event, it can greatly improve the understanding of the important features.

A description of the abnormal sleep phenomena is a useful starting point in defining the sleep problem. If the feature involves abnormal movements during sleep, further information may help identify sleep-related movement disorders like rhythmic movement disorder of sleep or periodic limb movement disorder. If the complaint involves disturbed dreaming, the possibility of REM sleep parasomnias, such as RBD or nightmare disorders, can be entertained. Assessing the events that could have initiated the abnormal behavior (e.g. a fever may precipitate sleep terrors or confusional arousals) as well as identifying the disturbance's frequency, duration, clinical course, severity, and provocative/exacerbating factors all further characterize the sleep complaint. It is useful to know if there is any dream recall after awakening from the event. It is also important to differentiate normal sleep phenomena from sleep disorders.

Time of the event

Knowledge of the timing of parasomnias and parasomnia-like events is useful in forming a differential diagnosis. Some occur during sleep–wake transitions, either prior to sleep onset (e.g. hypnic jerks) or upon awakening from sleep (e.g. rhythmic movement disorder), while others occur during wakefulness (e.g. sleep-related dissociative disorder). Certain parasomnias may occur preferentially during NREM sleep or REM sleep, and some may occur at any time during the sleep cycle. The typical NREM parasomnias (confusional arousals, sleepwalking, sleep terrors) usually occur during slow-wave sleep (or during transition to and from slow-wave sleep) and thus occur during the first half of the night, as there is a greater amount and density of slow-wave sleep at this time. It is likely that disturbances that occur within an hour or so of falling asleep are NREM parasomnias [4,6,7]. Similarly, abnormal behaviors occurring during the latter half of the night or during early morning hours are likely to be REM parasomnias, since REM sleep is most prominent during this time. In addition, parasomnias usually only occur 1–2 times per night; therefore, episodes that reportedly occur several times during the night should suggest an alternative diagnosis (e.g. seizures or dissociative sleep disorder). Generally, dream recall is vague at best when the patient is awoken from an NREM parasomnia, and is relatively vivid and detailed when the patient is awoken from a REM parasomnia. A person is typically confused and disoriented when awoken from an NREM parasomnia (occurring in slow-wave sleep) and is alert and oriented when awoken from a REM parasomnia [4,6,7]. Unfortunately, like many things in medicine, these guidelines are not strict rules and many exceptions do occur.

Normal behaviors

Certain sleep phenomena that occur infrequently can be considered normal; however, if the same phenomena were to happen often or compromise an individual's physical, psychological or emotional health, then it is considered a disorder. For instance, most people have had or will have a nightmare at some point in their life, but it is only considered a disorder if it is (among other things) occurring frequently. Other sleep disturbances are considered normal if they only occur in certain situations; for example, individuals can normally experience episodes of sleep-related hallucinations or sleep paralysis in the setting of sleep deprivation. Occasionally, when a person prematurely awakens from an extended sleep period, there is an internal drive to continue to sleep. The individual is drowsy, disoriented and may have difficulty concentrating or experience automatic behaviors. This normal "sleep inertia" or "sleep drunkenness" resembles confusional arousals, and the term is often used interchangeably with this NREM parasomnia. Other sleep phenomena, such as somniloquy (sleep talking) and hypnic jerks (sudden and brief contraction of limb muscles at sleep onset) are very common in the general population and are normal if they occur as isolated events [1]. On the other hand, somniloquy may represent part of a prodrome to REM sleep behavior disorder [1,4] or co-occur with obstructive sleep apnea; hence, detailed questioning is necessary. Hypnic jerks may be confused with a myoclonic epilepsy if one fails to inquire about a history of myoclonus during wake.

Precipitating factors

Many events can provoke or exacerbate a parasomnia. As a general rule, anything that causes sleep fragmentation or increases slow-wave sleep could also result in a parasomnia in a predisposed individual. Consequently, many medical, neurologic, psychiatric and even other sleep disorders that disrupt sleep have an increased propensity to cause parasomnias (Tables 4.2 and 4.3). For instance, anxiety and mood disorders have been associated with confusional arousals [7–9]; migraines and strokes have been linked to somnambulism [1,10]; hyperthyroidism and febrile illnesses are also associated with sleepwalking [11–13]; and obstructive sleep apnea and periodic limb movement

Section 1: Introduction

Table 4.2 Some common medical/sleep disorders associated with parasomnias.

Circadian rhythm disorders (e.g. shift work) [61,62]	Confusional arousals, sleep paralysis, bruxism
Disorders of hypersomnia (e.g. narcolepsy) [63]	Confusional arousals, REM sleep behavior disorder (rbd), sleep-related eating disorder, sleep-related hallucinations
Insomnia	Confusional arousals, sleep-related hallucinations, nightmares
Obstructive sleep apnea [14–17]	Disorders of arousal, sleep enuresis, sleep-related eating disorder
Periodic limb movement disorder [14–17]	Sleep-related eating disorder
Restless legs syndrome [64]	Sleep-related eating disorder
Hyperthyroidism [11–13]	Sleepwalking
Migraines [1,10]	Sleepwalking
Head injury [1]	Sleepwalking
Encephalitis [65]	Sleepwalking, sleep-related eating disorder
Stroke [1,10]	Sleepwalking, RBD
Febrile illness [11–13]	Sleepwalking
Parkinson's disease/parkinsonism [66,68]	RBD, sleep-related hallucinations, sleepwalking
Dementia w/ Lewy body dz [67, 68]	RBD, sleep-related hallucinations
Tourette's syndrome [68]	RBD
Autism [68]	RBD
Diabetes mellitus [69]	Sleep enuresis
Urinary tract infections [59,60]	Sleep enuresis
Chronic constipation [70]	Sleep enuresis
Seizures	Sleep enuresis
Visual loss [18,53,54]	Sleep-related hallucinations
Brainstem or diencephalic pathology [54,68] (e.g. tumor, or peduncular hallucinosis)	Sleep-related hallucinations, RBD

Table 4.3 Psychiatric disorders associated with parasomnias.

Anxiety [1,7–9,19,20,22,24,26]	Confusional arousals, sleep terrors, sleep-related hallucinations
Bipolar disorder [1,7–9,19,20,22,24,26]	Confusional arousals, sleep terrors, sleep-related hallucinations
Depression [1,7–9,19,20,22,24,26]	Confusional arousals, sleep terrors, sleep-related hallucinations
Post-traumatic stress disorder/acute stress disorder [24–27]	Nightmares

disorder have been associated with REM sleep behavior disorder [14–17].

Sleep fragmentation is only one of the possible mechanisms through which these disorders are thought to instigate parasomnias; other mechanisms are also suspected. Occasionally, parasomnias arise during recovery from increased sleep pressure or sleep deprivation, i.e. during rebound slow wave sleep or rebound REM sleep (e.g. sleepwalking can occur in a severe sleep apnea patient during recovery sleep after CPAP (continuous positive airway pressure) therapy is initiated). Although studies are limited, the occurrence of parasomnias in children is believed by some to be part of a developmental process, whereas in adults there appears to be a higher association with psychological disorders and in the older adult, a physiologic etiology is more probable [1,4,6,7]. Parasomnias may also result from physical and/or emotional stress, sleeping in unfamiliar surroundings, forced awakenings, perimenstrual symptoms, medications (e.g. lithium, neuroleptics, anticholinergics, sedatives/hypnotics), recreational drugs (stimulants),

Table 4.4 Other possible triggers for parasomnias [1,4,6,7].

Insufficient sleep	Confusional arousals, sleepwalking, sleep paralysis, sleep-related hallucinations
Recovery from insufficient sleep	Confusional arousals
Forced awakenings	Confusional arousals
Travel	Sleepwalking
Sleep in unfamiliar surroundings	Sleepwalking
Physical/emotional stress	Sleepwalking, ?sleep paralysis, sleep enuresis
PMS?	Sleepwalking
Environmental stimuli	Sleepwalking

and alcohol (Tables 4.4 and 4.5). (For more information on medications and parasomnias see Chapter 6.)

Other defining elements

Further characterization of the sleep complaint includes assessing the patient's functional status and mood during the day. Many parasomnias in children, for instance, usually require no more than reassurance for treatment; however, if the patient is depressed, has poor school attendance or has suboptimal school performance that is attributed to the sleep disturbance, then pharmaceutical intervention may be more appropriate.

In addition, there are many disorders that may mimic parasomnias; hence, a physician needs to inquire about other disorders considered in the differential diagnosis of parasomnias. For example, a history of visual loss/impairment may suggest Charles Bonnet syndrome in a patient with a complaint of hallucinations [18], or a history of head injury may be present in a patient suspected of having parasomnia-like seizures. Other disorders in the differential for parasomnias will be discussed later in the text.

Psychiatric assessment

As mentioned above, there appears to be an association between psychiatric disorders and some of the parasomnias. Accordingly, it is prudent to inquire about comorbid or prior history of psychiatric disorders, such as bipolar disorder, anxiety disorders, mood disorders, and psychotic disorders. In adults, studies fail to demonstrate a definite relationship between psychiatric disorders and sleepwalking/sleep terrors; however, many of these patients have or had at one time either a bipolar, a non-psychotic depressive or an anxiety disorder [1,8,9,19,20]. Confusional arousals, in contrast, are more prone to occur in patients with these psychiatric disorders. Similar to confusional arousals, sleep paralysis is also associated with psychopathology. It has been associated with bipolar disorder and the use of anxiolytic medications [1,8,9,19–23]. Sleep-related hallucinations and sleep-related dissociative disorder are also linked to anxiety and mood disorders [9,24–26].

Identification of the presence of any psychological trauma or history of such trauma, e.g. physical, sexual, or emotional abuse, difficult divorce, loss of a loved one, etc., is important when trying to understand the possible sources of a parasomnia. There is a predisposition to sleep-related dissociative disorder in victims of physical or sexual abuse or post-traumatic stress disorder (PTSD) [25–27]. Secondary sleep enuresis is also noted in these patients [1]. Nightmares are a common finding in PTSD patients, so much so that it is included as part of its diagnostic criteria [28]. Some studies even suggest that mental stress can precipitate sleep paralysis episodes; however, this is contradicted in other studies.

Certain personality profiles are more common in some parasomnias; hence, performing the Minnesota Multiphasic Personality Inventory in select patients may be helpful. For instance, nightmares have an increased prevalence in individuals with a more borderline personality profile [26].

Unfortunately, despite these strong associations, there is evidence (although studies are limited) that treatment of the comorbid psychiatric disorder does not necessarily improve some of the parasomnias [1,8,9,19,20]. Nevertheless, the comorbid disorders may complicate management of the parasomnia.

Family history

Some parasomnias appear to have familial tendencies. Genetic factors play an important role in predisposition to all of the arousal disorders (confusional arousals, somnambulism, and sleep terrors) [4,30–32]. For most of the other parasomnias, further studies are required to identify or confirm genetic influences. With regard to the REM parasomnias, it is suggested that REM sleep behavior disorder may be hereditary. Some studies found genetic factors that

Section 1: Introduction

Table 4.5 Some drugs that trigger or exacerbate parasomnias.

Drug/substance/medication	Associated parasomnia(s)
Psychotropic medications [44]	Disorders of arousal, sleep-related eating disorder
Phenothiazines	
Anticholinergics	
Lithium [58]	also Sleep enuresis
Drugs of abuse [1,74]	Confusional arousals, sleep-related hallucinations, sleep-related eating disorder
Alcohol [44]	Disorders of arousal, sleep-related eating disorder
Past alcohol use	Sleep-related hallucinations
Alcohol cessation	Sleep-related eating disorder
Antidepressants [1,44,48]	REM sleep behavior disorder, nightmares, sleepwalking
Venlafaxine	
Selective serotonin reuptake inhibitors	
Tricyclic antidepressants	
Mirtazapine	
Other antidepressants (except bupropion)	
Buproprion	Only associated with sleepwalking
Anxiolytics [1,8,9,19–23,44]	
Isolated sleep paralysis	
Hypnotics [71,72]	Sleep-related eating disorder, sleepwalking
Zolpidem	
Triazolam	
Other medications and substances [59,60,73]	
Caffeine	Sleep enuresis
Diuretics	Sleep enuresis
Smoking cessation	Sleep-related eating disorder
Other medication groups listed [1,74,75]	Nightmares
Dopamine receptor agonists	
Antihypertensives	
Drugs affecting GABA	
Drugs affecting acetylcholine	
Drugs affecting histamine	
Withdrawal from REM-suppressant drugs	

predispose individuals to nightmares. Genetic factors also dispose patients to the co-occurrence of other parasomnias with nightmares [1,33]. A maternal form of transmission has been identified in two families with recurrent isolated sleep paralysis [33]. There is also a strong suspicion for the familial basis for primary enuresis as there is an increased prevalence among parents, siblings, or other relatives of child patients [34].

Legal implications

Sleep-related injury or violence has forensic and legal implications. A thorough and careful sleep and psychiatric history are essential when there is the potential of legal action. Violent sleep-related behaviors or injuries have been well documented as part of confusional arousals, sleepwalking/sleep terrors, and REM sleep behavior disorder. Examples of such behaviors range from property damage related to sleep terrors/somnambulism, somnambulistic motor vehicle accidents to homicides, attempted homicides or suicides associated with sleepwalking, to sexual battery during episodes of sexsomnias, to punching/bruising a bed partner during an episode of REM sleep behavior disorder [35–40]. These behaviors occur as a result of an overlap of features of NREM sleep and/or REM sleep with wake [41,42]. They are believed to originate from brainstem and other more "primitive" structures without the benefits of control, elaboration and modification proffered by "higher" (cortex) neural structures [4,40].

It is often very difficult to differentiate violent parasomnias from mindful criminal acts; some key distinguishing features should be kept in mind. The timing of the episode should be in association with the patient's sleep. Events occurring during a period of sustained wakefulness are not parasomnias. Violent parasomnias usually have a prodrome of PSG abnormalities, milder behaviors or injurious episodes during sleep [4,40,42,43]. They are typically of brief duration, sudden and unexpected without apparent motivation or evidence of premeditation. A trigger or precipitating factor can often be identified, e.g. sleep deprivation, sleep-disordered breathing, alcohol, or an external noise [44]. The targets of the violent act are usually victims of circumstance; i.e. they were targeted because they happened to be in the wrong place during the parasomnia episode or were the ones who triggered the episode, they were not sought out as targets [45]. Furthermore, the behaviors do not coincide with the patient's waking personality. Some degree of amnesia or misperception is typical and there is often evidence of the patient's lack of awareness during the event. With regard to the NREM parasomnias, there is usually amnesia of the episode; however, some partial, fragmented recall of events is possible. With REM sleep behavior disorder, the recall may be of the patient's dream. For example, a patient described punching and kicking her bed partner while she was dreaming of fighting off an attacker. When the bed partner retaliated by holding down the patient's arms or throwing cold water on her, the patient recalled the events as additional attackers restraining her or having acid thrown on her face by one of the attackers, respectively. After awakening from a violent parasomnia, the patient is often confused and/or frightened of the situation they have found themselves in; they do not attempt to run away or hide their actions [35–40]. Even during the episodes, the witnessed actions appear to be inappropriate automatic behaviors [35–40]. Formal sleep studies complete with continuous, audiovisual monitoring, extensive surface EEG electrodes and all four-limb EMG electrodes are necessary.

There are also potential legal implications for some non-violent parasomnias. Recurrent sleep-related hallucinations may mislead a patient to believe a crime has occurred [46]. One case report describes an episode where a 23-year-old woman accuses a driver of sexual assault during a car ride home. Subsequent investigations and studies revealed that the patient had a vivid hypnagogic hallucination. Another case report describes vivid hallucinations that led to marital discord and workplace conflict in a 45-year-old patient with undiagnosed narcolepsy with cataplexy.

Although a standardized approach and assessment of patients for a parasomnia with legal consequences is not available, all the components for parasomnia evaluation discussed above are essential.

Sleep questionnaires

There are no available standardized sleep questionnaires for parasomnias; however, other associated symptoms can be assessed by this modality. Sleep questionnaires can be helpful to the physician to more quickly collect extensive information regarding sleep–wake habits. The Epworth Sleepiness Scale is a valuable instrument for determining the presence of daytime sleepiness over time [47]. The patient scores the likelihood of falling asleep in eight situations on a rating scale of 0 to 3 leading to a maximum score of 24. Patients with a score of 10 or higher should be considered to have significant daytime sleepiness, and those over 15 have severe daytime sleepiness. Other sleep questionnaires such as the Pittsburgh Sleep Quality Index, the Stanford Sleepiness Scale, the Karolinska Sleepiness Scale, or the fatigue severity scale may be useful in some patients depending upon the associated complaint.

Of most importance is the sleep log or diary that documents, over a period of approximately 2 weeks, the time of sleep onset, wake time, awakenings, naps, and the occurrence of any abnormal events. Utilizing this form, the physician can readily identify possible triggers for a parasomnia, such as disruption of the sleep–wake schedule.

Physical examination

The goal of the physical examination is to uncover medical, neurologic, psychiatric or sleep disorders

Table 4.6 Important components of the physical examination in a patient with parasomnias.

Vital signs:	Blood pressure (hypertension), pulse, respiratory rate, pulse oximetry on room air, height, weight
Examination of head, eyes, ears nose, throat (HEENT)	Crowded oropharynx: tonsils, soft palate, uvula, tongue
	Retrognathic or micrognathic, small maxilla, small oral space
	Chronic nasal congestion, enlarged turbinates, deviated nasal septum
Neck	Neck circumference, enlarged thyroid
Cardiovascular	Signs of heart failure (pedal edema, enlarged heart, jugular venous pulsations, etc.)
	Arrhythmias
	Carotid artery pulsations, bruits
	Distal pulses
Pulmonary	Anterior–posterior diameter of chest wall
	Ventilation/accessory muscle use
	Cyanosis
	Adventitious respiratory sounds
Neurologic	Mini mental state exam
	Assess for CNS disease (e.g. Parkinson's disease, stroke, seizures, brainstem pathology)
Psychiatric	Appearance, attitude, behavior and psychomotor activity
	Speech (rate, amount, tone, impairments), mood/affect
	Perception (hallucinations, illusions, depersonalization and/or derealization)
	Thought process (loose associations, tangential thinking, circumstantiality, blocking, perseveration, echolalia, flight of ideas)
	Thought content (delusions, obsessions, suicidal/homicidal thoughts)

associated with parasomnias, or to identify other disorders that may be confused for a parasomnia. Accordingly, the examination should ideally be comprehensive for most patients with parasomnias and then focus on neurological, cardiovascular, and psychiatric evaluations (Table 4.6). The examination should always include determination of the patient's blood pressure and vital signs. The patient's body habitus is important to assess, especially when trying to evaluate for obstructive sleep apnea; therefore, the patient's height, weight (i.e. Body Mass Index) and neck circumference should be obtained as well as a determination of the distribution of body fat (e.g. abdominal, neck, etc.). In some patients, an evaluation of thyroid size may prove pertinent, as a prominent thyroid may contribute to airway obstruction during sleep. In the patient with obstructive sleep apnea (OSA) syndrome, an evaluation of the upper airway is also important, particularly to determine if there is a narrow airway and/or if there is the presence of enlarged tonsillar tissue or a large tongue. The size and shape of the soft palate and uvula should be determined.

An examination of the cardiovascular system should assess for irregular heart rhythms and heart rates, especially in patients with cardiac parasomnias, such as sleep-related cardiac arrhythmias. The jugular venous and carotid pulsations should be observed and the carotid auscultated for bruits. Evidence of heart failure on exam suggests an etiology for the sleep disruption or may indicate the severity of a sleep disorder (e.g. right heart failure in OSA patients).

Respiratory breaths should be observed for rate, rhythm, depth, and effort of breathing and any adventitious sounds need to be auscultated. Prolonged expiration suggests narrowed lower airways from pulmonary disorders, such as asthma or chronic obstructive pulmonary disease (COPD). Asthmatic patients often complain of sleep-related exacerbation of their breathing (nocturnal asthma). In addition, these disorders can cause nocturnal arousals/awakenings, thus potentially triggering other parasomnias. Other features, including increased anteroposterior diameter of the chest wall and the use of accessory respiratory muscles, on exam are consistent with COPD. The chest should be ausculated for any adventitious sounds, such as wheezing, and the patient examined for cyanosis.

A thorough neurological examination will evaluate for any cognitive impairment or focal neurologic abnormalities. A mini mental state exam or a more thorough neuropsychologic testing may help identify (and monitor) patients with a dementing disorder. Focal abnormalities may suggest an etiology for the parasomnia or an associated neurologic disorder, such as seizures, strokes or other structural lesions of cortical, subcortical, or brainstem regions. Strategically located lesions in these regions predispose patients to sleep disruption or the development of REM sleep behavior disorder [1,4]. The examination should also assess for signs of parkinsonism/Parkinson's disease (bradykinesia, tremor, cogwheel rigidity, postural instability).

Differential diagnosis (Table 4.7)

As discussed earlier, the abnormal movements, behaviors, or experiences during sleep can be mistaken with normal sleep events and should be differentiated. For instance, *hypnic jerks* (sleep starts) are occasionally associated with a hallucination or vocalization and can be confused with certain parasomnias, such as nightmares or REM sleep behavior disorder (RBD). Hypnic jerks usually occur during sleep–wake transitions whereas RBD occurs during the latter half of the night from REM sleep. Hypnic jerks are brief, usually single, body or body segment muscle contractions, whereas in RBD the involved muscle activities can be complex, appearing semi-purposeful and of longer duration. Nightmares also usually occur during REM sleep; however, when following traumatic situations, they can occur at sleep onset [1,4,28]. Unlike hypnic jerks, they typically result in awakenings and have associated anxiety.

Certain parasomnias are brought on by medical disorders, other sleep disorders, medications, recreational drugs, alcohol or sleep deprivation. These are usually classified as *Parasomnias due to a drug or substance* or *Parasomnia due to a medical condition* (see Chapters 6 and 7, respectively). For instance, OSA can fragment sleep, resulting in arousals from deep sleep causing confusional arousals or sleepwalking.

Table 4.7 Common differential diagnosis of abnormal behaviors/movements during sleep.

1. NREM parasomnias
   A. Confusional arousals
   B. Sleep terrors
   C. Sleepwalking
2. REM parasomnias
   A. REM sleep behavioral disorder
   B. Nightmares
3. Sleep starts/hypnic jerks
4. Periodic limb movement during sleep disorder
5. Sleep-related bruxism
6. Sleep-related eating disorder
7. Sleep-related epilepsy/nocturnal seizures
8. Parasomnia due to drug or substance
9. Parasomnia due to a medical condition
10. Parasomnia overlap syndrome
11. Status dissociatus
12. Post-traumatic stress disorder
13. Nocturnal panic disorder
14. Conversion disorder
15. Munchausen by proxy
16. Malingering
17. Sleep-related dissociative disorder

Beta-blockers used for treatment of hypertension can induce nightmares in some individuals [48,49]. Sleep enuresis can result from conditions ranging from a urinary tract infection and diabetes mellitus to seizures and sickle cell disease (sleep enuresis in these cases is diagnosed as *secondary sleep enuresis*, not *Parasomnia due to...*) [1]. Patients with PTSD and acute stress disorder often have nightmares.

Disorders of arousal

Included in the differential of parasomnias are other parasomnias. There is often considerable overlap of features between the disorders of arousal (i.e. confusional arousals, sleep terrors and sleepwalking) as well as between these NREM parasomnias and the REM parasomnia, RBD. This overlap is often more pronounced in adults than in children [4,6]. An example of such overlap of NREM features is seen in this case where the parents of a child with confusional arousals described their child as awaking from sleep with episodes of confusion occasionally associated with crying or screaming. Another child's sleep terror events were typified by intense screaming that was occasionally associated with getting up out of bed and running across the room. Accordingly, most experts consider the three NREM parasomnias part of a spectrum of disorders, with confusional arousals on one end, sleepwalking in the middle and sleep terrors at the other end. Clinical differentiation between the three can be difficult at times, especially in adults.

REM parasomnias

REM parasomnias, such as nightmares and REM sleep behavior disorder (RBD), could also be confused with other parasomnias. Nightmares can resemble sleep terrors and RBD can clinically look like sleepwalking. As discussed earlier, REM parasomnias differ from NREM parasomnias in that they usually occur out of REM sleep towards the latter half of the night, with clear recollection of dream content and minimal or no post-event disorientation. Nightmares, unlike sleep terrors, are often associated with anxiety and subsequently having difficulty returning to sleep. REM sleep behavior disorder manifests as dream enactment behavior occurring during REM sleep. Sleepwalking usually occurs during slow-wave sleep; however, it can also represent dream enactment in some patients (especially adults). Although the guidelines outlined here are helpful, differentiation between these two disorders can become difficult. A polysomnogram capturing the episodes may be required [5,50]. Some patients may meet the diagnostic criteria for both NREM parasomnias and RBD; these patients are diagnosed with *Parasomnia overlap disorder*. In patients with a subtype of RBD, *status dissociatus*, the distinguishing polysomnographic features of the different stages of sleep and wake become blurred. This usually occurs in patients with other neurologic comorbid pathology, such as dementia, HIV infection with involvement of brain, narcolepsy, etc. (clinically presenting as RBD and/or an NREM parasomnia), and should be considered among the differential in patients with parasomnias [51]. These and other REM and NREM parasomnias will be further differentiated in later chapters.

Seizure disorders

There are some disorders that present with clinical symptoms that resemble certain parasomnias. The most notorious of these disorders are *nocturnal seizures*. Seizures can mimic almost all of the parasomnias and should be ruled out by history and/or by formal electrographic studies. Complex partial seizures, particularly involving the mesial frontal lobe or temporal lobe of the cortex, can bear a resemblance to confusional arousals, sleep terrors, sleepwalking, or RBD. There are also rare cases of seizures manifesting as nightmares [52]. More commonly, visual hallucinations have been described in patients with posterior parietal or occipital lobe seizures, resembling sleep-related hallucinations. Atonic seizures have been confused with sleep paralysis episodes during waking hours, and certainly nocturnal urinary incontinence and vocalizations are common in seizures and can easily be mistaken for sleep enuresis or catathrenia, respectively.

There are some components in the clinical history that can help differentiate seizures from some of the parasomnias. Nocturnal seizures often manifest as abnormal stereotypic repetitive behaviors. They can occur multiple times throughout the night and occasionally during the waking period. They are often responsive to anti-epileptic medications. In contrast, the NREM parasomnias only occur once or twice a night and usually only during the first half of the night. They do not occur during wakefulness and are not generally responsive to anti-epileptic therapy. Often, the only definitive way to distinguish seizures from parasomnias is to capture the target event during a polysomnogram with extended electroencephalogram (EEG) channels or during long-term video-EEG monitoring and identifying an electrographic ictal correlate to the episode. Unfortunately, this does not always happen; some seizures do not have surface EEG electrographic correlates and occasionally the target episodes do not occur during the monitoring period. In such situations adjunctive information such as the presence or absence of spikes during EEG recordings (including a standard EEG with sleep, hyperventilation, and photic stimulation) are valuable.

Other medical and psychiatric disorders

There are multiple other disorders resembling parasomnias. Charles Bonnet hallucinations and midbrain/diencephalic pathology (peduncular hallucinosis) mimic sleep-related hallucinations [18,53,54]; the excessive eating behaviors in Kleine–Levin syndrome and Klüver–Bucy syndrome can look like sleep-related eating disorder; compression neuropathies and the familial periodic paralyses have features similar to sleep paralysis; and certain *headache syndromes* (e.g. migraines) can resemble exploding head syndrome.

There are also a number of psychiatric disorders that have symptoms that are confused with certain parasomnias and thus should be considered in the differential. The excessive eating behaviors seen in bulimia nervosa and anxiety disorders can mislead one to a diagnosis of sleep-related eating disorder. Nocturnal panic attacks can be misdiagnosed as sleep terrors or nightmares. Conversion disorders can mimic recurrent isolated sleep paralysis. Malingering and Munchausen by proxy are other disorders to consider in the differential of parasomnias. Sleep-related dissociative disorder is categorized in the ICSD-2 under parasomnias as it has nocturnal behaviors that are similar to the behaviors seen in both NREM and REM parasomnia; however, it meets the Diagnostic and Statistical Manual of Mental Disorders, 4th edition text revision (DSM-IV-TR) diagnostic criteria for a dissociative disorder.

Laboratory investigations

Need for extensive evaluation

Parasomnias (especially the disorders of arousal) are primarily diagnosed via clinical history; occasionally patients provide home videotapes of the events that are helpful in making a diagnosis. Most parasomnias do not require further investigations. When they (1) are, however, potentially violent or injurious to the patient or others; (2) have forensic implications; (3) cause significant social or familial disruption; (4) have daytime consequences to the patient, e.g. excessive daytime sleepiness or behavioral difficulties; (5) are associated with medical, psychiatric, or neurologic symptoms or findings; (6) are vaguely described such that a diagnosis can not be definitively made; and/or (7) seizures are suspected, then further laboratory work up is warranted [4,5,7,50].

Polysomnogram

Routine polysomnograms (i.e. with standard sleep apnea montage) and unattended sleep studies have serious limitations in the evaluation of parasomnias and are considered inappropriate in this setting. The polysomnograms should be preferably performed at sleep centers with technologists and physicians experienced in monitoring for parasomnias/seizures, reviewing the raw data of these patients, and interpreting the results [5]. In addition to the physiological parameters monitored in a routine polysomnogram, continuous audiovisual monitoring while using multiple channel electroencephalography (EEG) and multiple montages and the capability for EEG analysis at the standard EEG speed of 30 mm s^{-1} is required to evaluate for possible seizures or epileptiform discharges in suspected parasomnia patients. In addition, multiple EMG electrode placements over several muscle groups (e.g. chin electrodes, bilateral leg electrodes and bilateral arm electrodes) should be placed in suspected RBD patients to increase the yield of detecting the abnormal tone or phasic movements during REM sleep. These polysomnograms are often diagnostic when the target events are captured; however, if the target event did not occur during the study period, indirect support for a diagnosis may still be obtained from the recording.

Electroencephalogram

If sleep-related seizures are suspected, a routine EEG with sleep, hyperventilation and photic stimulation is required. If negative (i.e. no interictal epileptiform activity), then an EEG with sleep deprivation is necessary. Often the EEG can turn out normal even in patients known to have seizures. This is especially common with patients with mesial frontal lobe seizures [3]. Accordingly, after about three EEGs that are unrevealing, a prolonged daytime EEG or long-term video-EEG monitoring for 24 h or longer may be needed if seizures are clinically suspected. In some cases, invasive intracranial recording may be necessary.

Neuroimaging

Neuroimaging [55] is important when there is suspicion that a neurologic illness is associated with the parasomnia. For example, an MRI of the brain especially with visualization of the brainstem is valuable when looking for strategically located structural lesions that may cause, for instance, REM sleep behavior disorder. In addition, an MRI of the brain with thin cuts through the temporal lobe is required for patients with seizures.

Other studies

Evoked potential studies may be useful when evaluating the functional integrity of the brainstem in select parasomnia patients [56]. Pulmonary function tests can help identify and determine the severity of pulmonary disorders that may be responsible for some parasomnias; while a 12-lead EKG or 24 h Holter monitoring can help identify ischemic heart disease or cardiac arrhythmias.

Urine screening may be necessary, particularly in young people, when drug abuse is the suspected etiology or trigger for the parasomnia. Selected blood tests may be useful as well. Thyroid function tests may be indicated if the patient has features suggesting hypo- or hyperthyroidism. A serum ferritin level may be helpful in supporting a diagnosis of restless legs syndrome or periodic limb movement disorder. An arterial blood gas can provide insight to a patient's acid-base status as well as pulmonary function.

Education and treatment

After all the necessary steps in the evaluation of parasomnias are complete, the patient and patient's family need to be educated about the diagnosis as well as its pathophysiology, precipitating and relieving factors. In children, they should be informed that parasomnias, such as the disorders of arousal, are a neurodevelopmental phenomenon and are not indicative of a psychological disturbance. The patient and patient's family should be reassured that these disorders usually remit by adolescence [1,4,7] and do not result in psychological trauma. Similarly, for nightmares, it should be explained that most children will have a nightmare (especially between the ages of 3 and 6 years) and it is a normal part of cognitive development [57]. In most cases the nightmares are isolated events and, if frequent, usually remit as the child grows up. Most adults with parasomnias appreciate a discussion about the pathophysiology of the disorder. Patients and their families need to be able to identify stressors, traumatic events, or other triggers (e.g. sleep deprivation or febrile illness) that may be contributing to the parasomnias. The parents of a child with a parasomnia need to be taught how to react to or act both during the event and during waking hours. For instance, minimizing intervention during an episode of sleep terrors helps prevent exacerbation of the agitation and prolongation of the event. A discussion of the night's events should be avoided in patients with a disorder of arousal as this can cause them unnecessary anxiety [57,58]; however, in patients with recurrent nightmares a discussion would be a necessary first step in therapy, e.g. imagery reversal therapy (see Chapter 11). Patients and/or their families need to be educated as to when pharmaceutical therapy would be indicated. They must be instructed on the appropriate expectations of treatment, i.e. behavioral or medical therapy may considerably improve the parasomnias; however, occasional episodes may persist. Parasomnias in adults are usually more difficult to treat.

Proper sleep hygiene is the cornerstone of treatment for many of the parasomnias. Patients should also be instructed to allow adequate time for sleep and to maintain a regular sleep–wake schedule. The sleep environment should be kept safe; keeping sharp objects away from the bed, securing windows, doors, and staircases, removing clutter from the floors, and placing a mattress on the floor near the bed are useful for many patients, as is sleeping close to the ground, etc. Alarms or bells on doors would notify families when an event is occurring. For patients with sleep enuresis, incontinence bed alarms are beneficial. As indicated earlier, awakening or interfering with a patient during a disorder of arousal should be avoided, as this may worsen the episode. Guiding a sleepwalker without awakening him/her, for example, back to bed is more appropriate. Most importantly, the underlying disorder or trigger of the parasomnia needs to be treated appropriately. For patients with nightmares, an avoidance of frightening or overstimulating images, especially prior to bedtime, and a reduction of stressors will diminish the reoccurrence of this parasomnia [57]. Some patients may also require medication to manage their parasomnia. A more detailed discussion of pharmaceutical therapy and other more specific behavioral therapies for the different parasomnias is beyond the scope of this chapter and will be addressed in later chapters.

Summary

This chapter outlines the approach to a patient with a parasomnia. It begins with a thorough history-taking, keeping in mind the Parasomnia Classification in the ICSD-2 and the differential diagnosis of abnormal behaviors and events during sleep. The history is aimed at obtaining a detailed account of the subjective and objective sequences of events as well as the timing and circumstances in which the events occurred. The clinical evaluation and physical examination should uncover medical, neurologic, psychiatric or sleep disorders associated with parasomnias, or identify other disorders that may be confused for a parasomnia. Further assessment with comprehensive sleep studies may be required in some patients. Seizures should always be considered in the differential of parasomnias and formal EEG studies should be performed where appropriate. Patients should be educated on the diagnosis. Proper sleep hygiene should be discussed as well as avoidance of triggers such as inadequate sleep time. Pharmaceutical therapy may be required in some patients.

References

1. American Academy of Sleep Medicine. International Classification of Sleep Disorders – 2. Chicago, IL: American Academy of Sleep Medicine, 2005.
2. Yeh SB, Schenck CH. A case of marital discord and secondary depression with attempted suicide resulting from REM sleep behavior disorder in a 35-year-old woman. *Sleep Med* 2004; **5**: 151–4.
3. Kellinghaus C, Lüders HO. Frontal lobe epilepsy. *Epileptic Disord* 2004; **6**: 223–39.
4. Mahowald M. Parasomnias. *Med Clin N Am* 2004; **88**: 669–78.
5. Kushida C, Littner MR, Morgenthaler T, *et al*. Practice parameters for the indications for polysomnography and related procedures: an update for 2005. *Sleep* 2005; **28**: 499–521.
6. Reading P. Parasomnias: the spectrum of things that go bump in the night. *Pract Neurol* 2007; **7**: 6–15.
7. Stores G. Parasomnias of childhood and adolescence. *Sleep Med Clin* 2007; **2**: 405–17.
8. Ohayon M, Priest R, Zulley J, Smirne S. The place of confusional arousals in sleep and mental disorders: Findings in a general population sample of 13,057 subjects. *J Nerv Ment Dis* 2000; **188**: 340–8.
9. Abad VC, Guilleminault C. Sleep and psychiatry. *Dialogues Clin Neurosci* 2005; **7**: 291–303.
10. Barabas G, Ferrari M, Matthews WS. Childhood migraine and somnambulism. *Neurology* 1983; **33**: 948–9.
11. Ajlouni KM, Ahmad AT, El-Zaheri MM, *et al*. Sleepwalking associated with hyperthyroidism. *Endocr Pract* 2005; **11**: 5–10.
12. Dorus E. Sleepwalking and febrile illness. *Am J Psychiatry* 1979; **136**: 1620.
13. Kales JD, Kales A, Soldatos CR, Chamberlin K, Martin ED. Sleepwalking and night terrors related to febrile illness. *Am J Psychiatry* 1979; **136**: 1214–5.
14. Iranzo A, Santamaría J. Severe obstructive sleep apnea/hypopnea mimicking REM sleep behavior disorder. *Sleep* 2005; **28**: 203–06.
15. Wetter TC, Pollmächer T. Restless legs and periodic leg movements in sleep syndromes. *J Neurol* 1997; **244**(Suppl 1): S37–45.
16. Manconi M, Ferri R, Zucconi M, Fantini ML, Plazzi G, Ferini-Strambi L. Time structure analysis of leg movements during sleep in REM sleep behavior disorder. *Sleep* 2007; **30**: 1779–85.
17. Haba-Rubio J, Janssens JP, Rochat T, Sforza E. Rapid eye movement-related disordered breathing: Clinical and polysomnographic features. *Chest* 2005; **128**: 3350–7.
18. Gilmour G, Schreiber C, Ewing C. An examination of the relationship between low vision and Charles Bonnet syndrome. *Can J Ophthalmol* 2009; **44**: 49–52.
19. Szelenberger W, Niemcewicz S, Dabrowska AJ. Sleepwalking and night terrors: Psychopathological and psychophysiological correlates. *Int Rev Psychiatry* 2005; **17**: 263–70.
20. Gau SF, Soong WT. Psychiatric comorbidity of adolescents with sleep terrors or sleepwalking: A case-control study. *Aust NZ J Psychiatry* 1999; **33**: 734–9.
21. Khazaal Y, Krenz S, Zullino DF. Bupropion-induced somnambulism. *Addict Biol* 2003; **8**: 359–62.
22. Landry P, Warnes H, Nielsen T, Montplaisir J. Somnambulistic-like behaviour in patients attending a lithium clinic. *Int Clin Psychopharmacol* 1999; **14**: 173–5.
23. Mehl RC, O'Brien LM, Jones JH, Dreisbach JK, Mervis CB, Gozal D. Correlates of sleep and pediatric bipolar disorder. *Sleep* 2006; **29**: 193–7.
24. Ulloa RE, Birmaher B, Axelson D, *et al*. Psychosis in a pediatric mood and anxiety disorders clinic: Phenomenology and correlates. *J Am Acad Child Adolesc Psychiatry* 2000; **39**: 337–45.
25. Tyler KA, Cauce AM, Whitbeck L. Family risk factors and prevalence of dissociative symptoms among homeless and runaway youth. *Child Abuse Negl* 2004; **28**: 355–66.
26. Johnson JG, Cohen P, Kasen S, Brook JS. Dissociative disorders among adults in the community, impaired functioning, and axis I and II comorbidity. *J Psychiatr Res* 2006; **40**: 131–40. Epub 2005 Dec 6.
27. Roe-Sepowitz D, Bedard LE, Pate K. The impact of child abuse on dissociative symptoms: A study of

incarcerated women. *J Trauma Dissoc* 2007; **8**: 7–26.

28. American Psychiatric Association. Diagnostic and Statistical Manual of Mental Disorders, Fourth Edition, Text Revision. Arlington, VA: American Psychiatric Association, 2000.

29. Semiz UB, Basoglu C, Ebrinc S, Cetin M. Nightmare disorder, dream anxiety, and subjective sleep quality in patients with borderline personality disorder. *Psychiatry Clin Neurosci* 2008; **62**: 48–55.

30. Hublin C, Kaprio J, Partinen M, Heikkila K, Koskenvuo M. Parasomnias: Co-occurrence and genetics. *Psychiatr Genet* 2001; **11**: 65–70.

31. Hublin C, Kaprio J, Partinen M, Heikkila K, Koskenvuo M. Prevalence and genetics of sleepwalking; A population based twin study. *Neurology* 1997; **48**: 177–81.

32. Kales A, Soldatos C, Bixler E, et al. Hereditary factors in sleepwalking and night terrors. *Br J Psychiatry* 1980; **137**: 111–8.

33. Hublin C, Kaprio J, Partinen M, Koskenvuo M. Nightmares: Familial aggregation and association with psychiatric disorders in a nationwide twin cohort. *Am J Med Genet* 1999; **88**: 329–36.

34. Loeys B, Hoebeke P, Raes A, Messiaen L, De Paepe A, Vande Walle J. Does monosymptomatic enuresis exist? A molecular genetic exploration of 32 families with enuresis/incontinences. *BJU Int* 2002; **90**: 76–83.

35. Lauerma H. Fear of suicide during sleepwalking. *Psychiatry* 1996; **59**: 206–11.

36. Broughton R, Billings R, Cartwright R, et al. Homicidal somnambulism: a case report. *Sleep* 1994; **17**: 253–64.

37. Cartwright R. Sleepwalking violence: A sleep disorder, a legal dilemma, and a psychological challenge. *Am J Psychiatry* 2004; **161**: 1149–58.

38. Bornemann M, Mahowald MW, Schenck C. Parasomnias: Clinical features and forensic implications. *Chest* 2006; **130**: 605–10.

39. Mahowald M, Schenck C, Rosen G, Hurwitz T. The role of a sleep disorder center in evaluating sleep violence. *Arch Neurol* 1992; **49**: 604–07.

40. Mahowald MW, Bundhe SR, Hurwitz TD, Schenck CH. Sleep violence – forensic science implications: Polygraphic and video documentation. *J Forensic Sci* 1990, **35**: 413.

41. Mahowald MW, Schenck CH. Dissociated states of wakefulness and sleep. *Neurology* 1992; **42**: 44.

42. Pressman MR. Hypersynchronous delta sleep EEG activity and sudden arousals from slow-wave sleep in adults without a history of parasomnias: Clinical and forensic implications. *Sleep* 2004; **27**: 706–10.

43. Kayumov L, Pandi-Perumal SR, Fedoroff P, Shapiro CM. Diagnostic values of polysomnography in forensic medicine. *J Forensic Sci* 2000; **45**: 191–4.

44. Pressman MR. Factors that predispose, prime and precipitate NREM parasomnias in adults: Clinical and forensic implications. *Sleep Med Rev* 2007; **11**: 5–30; discussion 31–3.

45. Pressman MR. Disorders of arousal from sleep and violent behavior: The role of physical contact and proximity. *Sleep* 2007; **30**: 1039–47.

46. Szucs A, Jansky J, Hollo A, Migleczi G, Halasz P. Case report: Misleading hallucinations in unrecognized narcolepsy. *Acta Psychiatr Scand* 2003; **108**: 314–7.

47. Johns MW. A new method for measuring daytime sleepiness: The Epworth sleepiness scale. *Sleep* 1991; **14**: 540–5.

48. Brismar K, Mogensen L, Wetterberg L. Depressed melatonin secretion in patients with nightmares due to beta-adrenoceptor blocking drugs. *Acta Med Scand* 1987; **221**: 155–8.

49. Maebara C, Ohtani H, Sugahara H, Mine K, Kubo C, Sawada Y. Nightmares and panic disorder associated with carvedilol overdose. *Ann Pharmacother* 2002; **36**: 1736–40.

50. Aldrich M, Jahnke B. Diagnostic value of video-EEG polysomnography. *Neurology* 1991; **41**: 1060–6.

51. Mahowald MW, Schenck CH. Status dissociatus – a perspective on states of being. *Sleep* 1991; **14**: 69–79.

52. Huppertz HJ, Franck P, Korinthenberg R, Schulze-Bonhage A. Recurrent attacks of fear and visual hallucinations in a child. *Child Neurol* 2002; **17**: 230–3.

53. Silber MH, Hansen MR, Girish M. Complex nocturnal visual hallucinations. *Sleep Med* 2005; **6**: 363–6.

54. Benke T. Peduncular hallucinosis: A syndrome of impaired reality monitoring. *J Neurol* 2006; **253**: 1561–71. Epub 2006 Sep 27.

55. Desseilles M, Dang-Vu T, Schabus M, Sterpenich V, Maquet P, Schwartz S. Neuroimaging insights into the pathophysiology of sleep disorders. *Sleep* 2008; **31**: 777–94.

56. Raggi A, Manconi M, Consonni M, et al. Event-related potentials in idiopathic rapid eye movements sleep behaviour disorder. *Clin Neurophysiol* 2007; **118**: 669–75. Epub 2007 Jan 5.

57. Mindell JA, Owens JA. Sleepwalking and sleep terrors. In *A Clinical Guide to Pediatric Sleep: Diagnosis and Management of Sleep Problems*. Philadelphia, PA: Lippencott Williams and Wilkins, 2003; 88–96.

58. Landry P, Warnes H, Nielsen T, Montplaisir J. Somnambulistic-like behaviour in patients attending a

lithium clinic. *Int Clin Psychopharmacol* 1999; **14**: 173–5.

59. Jalkut MW, Lerman SE, Churchill BM. Enuresis. *Pediatr Clin North Am* 2001; **48**: 1461–88.

60. Rasmussen PV, Kirk J, Borup K, Nørgaard JP, Djurhuus JC. Enuresis nocturna can be provoked in normal healthy children by increasing the nocturnal urine output. *Scand J Urol Nephrol* 1996; **30**: 57–61.

61. Ahlberg K, Jahkola A, Savolainen A, *et al.* Associations of reported bruxism with insomnia and insufficient sleep symptoms among media personnel with or without irregular shift work. *Head Face Med* 2008; **4**: 4.

62. Ohayon MM, Priest RG, Zulley J, Smirne S. The place of confusional arousals in sleep and mental disorders: Findings in a general population sample of 13,057 subjects. *J Nerv Ment Dis* 2000; **188**: 340–8.

63. Nightingale S, Orgill JC, Ebrahim IO, de Lacy SF, Agrawal S, Williams AJ. The association between narcolepsy and REM behavior disorder (RBD). *Sleep Med* 2005; **6**: 253–8.

64. Provini F, Antelmi E, Vignatelli L, *et al.* Association of restless legs syndrome with nocturnal eating: A case-control study. *Mov Disord* 2009; **24**: 871–7.

65. Hughes JR. A review of sleepwalking (somnambulism): The enigma of neurophysiology and polysomnography with differential diagnosis of complex partial seizures. *Epilepsy Behav* 2007; **11**: 483–91. Epub 2007 Oct 10.

66. Poryazova R, Waldvogel D, Bassetti CL. Sleepwalking in patients with Parkinson disease. *Arch Neurol* 2007; **64**: 1524–7.

67. Gold G. Dementia with Lewy Bodies: Clinical diagnosis and therapeutic approach. *Front Neurol Neurosci* 2009; **24**: 107–13. Epub 2009 Jan 26.

68. Thomas A, Bonanni L, Onofrj M. Symptomatic REM sleep behaviour disorder. *Neurol Sci* 2007; **28**(Suppl 1): S21–36.

69. Ferrara P, Rigante D, D'Aleo C, *et al.* Preliminary data on monosymptomatic nocturnal enuresis in children and adolescents with type 1 diabetes. *Scand J Urol Nephrol* 2006; **40**: 238–40.

70. Kasirga E, Akil I, Yilmaz O, Polat M, Gözmen S, Egemen A. Evaluation of voiding dysfunctions in children with chronic functional constipation. *Turk J Pediatr* 2006; **48**: 340–3.

71. Yang W, Dollear M, Muthukrishnan SR. One rare side effect of zolpidem – sleepwalking: A case report. *Arch Phys Med Rehabil* 2005; **86**: 1265–6.

72. Dolder CR, Nelson MH. Hypnosedative-induced complex behaviours: Incidence, mechanisms and management. *CNS Drugs* 2008; **22**: 1021–36.

73. Schenck CH, Hurwitz TD, O'Connor KA, Mahowald MW. Additional categories of sleep-related eating disorders and the current status of treatment. *Sleep* 1993; **16**: 457–66.

74. Obermeyer WH, Benca RM. Effects of drugs on sleep. *Neurol Clin* 1996; **14**: 827–40.

75. Hensel J, Pillmann F. Late-life somnambulism after therapy with metoprolol. *Clin Neuropharmacol* 2008; **31**: 248–50.

76. Khazaal Y, Krenz S, Zullino DF. Bupropion-induced somnambulism. *Addict Biol* 2003; **8**: 359–62.

Section 1 Chapter 5

Introduction

Video-polysomnography of parasomnias

Stefano Vandi

Introduction

The fundamental elements of video-polysomnography are suggested by its name: video (watching patients and their body movements) polysomnography (recording the state of wakefulness or the different stages of sleep). The dual function of this type of recording in patients with parasomnias serves for diagnosis or research. Diagnostic recording needs concomitant video and polysomnographic parameters to highlight the elements useful to establish the diagnosis and exclude other pathologies. Research video-polysomnography recording includes additional parameters that can add to our knowledge of sleep and wake.

The number and quality of transducers and electrodes should be adjusted to the patient so as to allow body movements and sufficient comfort, thereby increasing the probability of recording all aspects of a pathological event. Great attention should be paid to how electrodes, transducers and their cables are applied so that they will resist strong motor events [1] and ensure the continuity of the recording during the episode (Figures 5.6 and 5.7). In addition, the video recording should display the whole patient without losing information during the events because the patient is out of the screen.

Recording room

Little attention is paid to the recording room, but it is one of the most important aspects of polysomnography. Patients should be in a sufficiently comfortable environment to allow them to fall asleep easily and sleep for a long time. The room must be completely darkened with the exception of a small light, if required, to orientate the patient. It must also be soundproofed to prevent disturbance from outside noise. The room temperature must be regulated and maintained at a level to allow the patient to sleep without blankets (Figure 5.5) which would invalidate the video recording.

Particular attention must be paid to any sharp corners on fittings or furniture that could harm the patient during a violent motor event if the patient stands up and walks. Unless it is monitored by a technician, the main door to the recording room must be secured so as to not allow access to a potentially dangerous environment. The door should not be able to be opened by the patient during an event. The recording area that is supervised by a technician must be outside the sleeping room, but close enough to allow the technician to intervene to prevent injury to a patient during an event, or to allow communication with the patient to assess their awareness.

Video recording

The aim of the video recording is to allow the patient's motor events to be visualized for diagnosis and to be reviewed at a later date. The video should be synchronized with the polysomnographic parameters [2].

Video-polysomnography was originally developed with an analogical system. The use of a mixer allowed simultaneous recordings from two different cameras: one framed the patient and the other framed the traces of ink pens on the recording paper. The limitation of this technique was the irreversibility of the final product: the patient's frame and polysomnographic tracing (numbers of channels and EEG derivations) could not be modified.

Nowadays, digital polysomnographic recording systems can allow the video to be modified off-line to enlarge the patient's details, select the most important polysomnographic parameters and allow modification

Figure 5.1 Camera mounted on the wall in front of the patient: correct framing of the patient both lying and sitting.

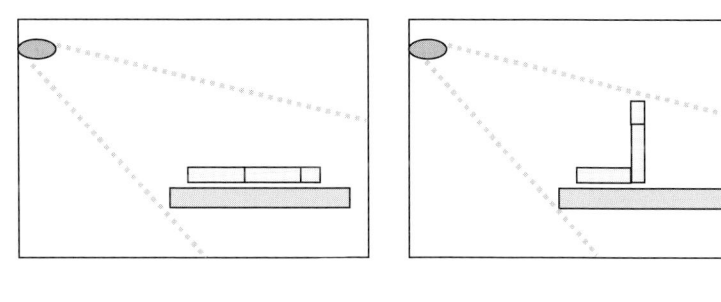

Figure 5.2 Camera mounted on the ceiling: correct framing of the patient while lying but not sitting.

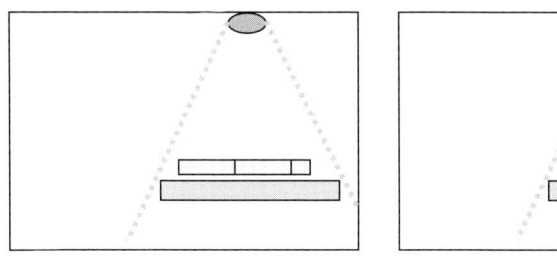

of the amplitude with appropriate filter settings and also to modify the EEG derivations [3].

The digital video recording should be fully integrated into the recording system to allow the complete management of all the components: cameras, environmental microphone and video settings.

The camera should have the following features:

- high resolution (a high number of pixels allows images to be enlarged off-line without loss of quality);
- sensitive to infrared lights (the recording is performed in the dark with an infrared light);
- autofocus (the patient can get out of bed and move around the room thereby changing the distance from the lens);
- automatic and rapid adjustment of the iris (with a slowly adjusting iris, a sudden onset of room light could cause loss of images for several seconds);
- remote adjustment of the zoom;
- the camera should be wall mounted in front of the patient, 2 or 3 m from the floor (Figure 5.1) at an angle of 45°. If the camera is placed too low, the patient's face will not be visible while lying in bed, whereas mounted on the ceiling the patient's face is not visible while sitting in bed (Figure 5.2);
- remote control of the camera movement;
- silent (the autofocus and iris adjustments and the camera movements should be very silent because even a slight noise could awaken the patient).

Multiple room cameras – for example, one side camera and one above the patient – will give more information from different recording angles. Some video-polygraphic recorders can manage more than one camera at the same time.

Infrared lights are essential for video recording in the dark. They should be placed on side walls (at an angle of 45° to the camera) or above or below the camera, so as not to form shadows (Figure 5.3).

The environmental microphone adds sound to the video recording. The microphone should be positioned near the patient's head to limit outside noises. A tracheal microphone can pick up tracheal vibrations, converting them into a written tracing.

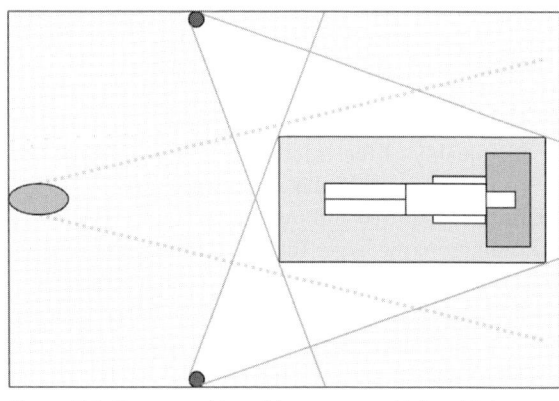

Figure 5.3 Correct position of the camera and infrared lights.

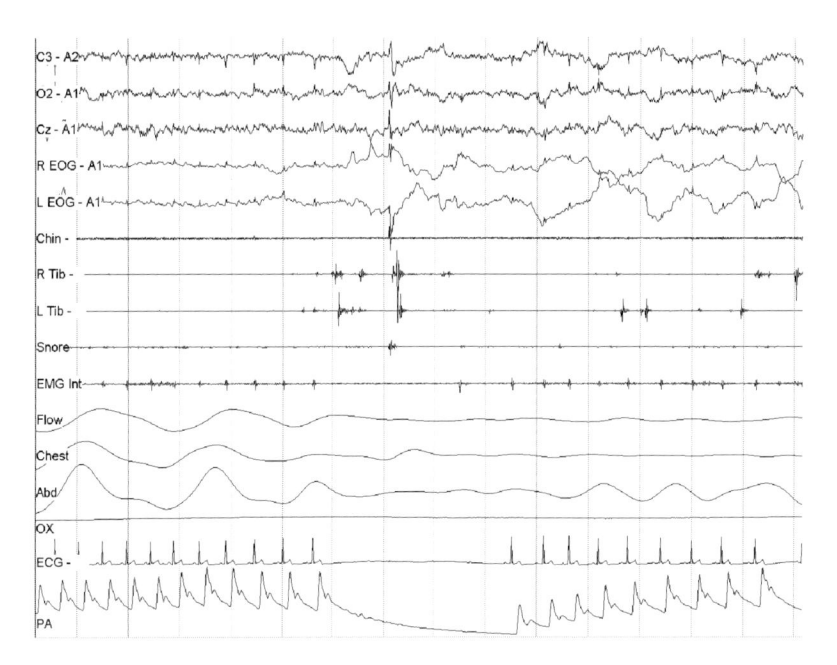

Figure 5.4 Thirty-second polysomnographic recording: a REM sleep stage showing respiratory and cardiac changes.

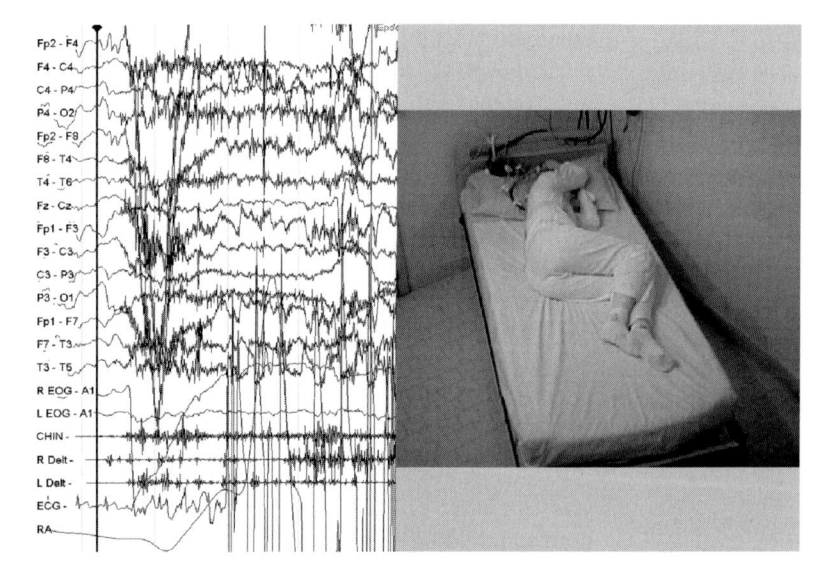

Figure 5.5 The frame refers to the vertical black line on the tracings. The patient is sleeping (SWS) without blankets to highlight body movements.

The quality of the video recording is managed by the recording system and is directly proportional to the quantity of acquired and memorized data. The higher the resolution, the larger the file. One night of recording (7–8 h), with a medium–high video resolution, would be around 8 Gigabytes of data. Large files are difficult to review, manage and store, so a compromise must be reached between file size and quality of the video recording by adjusting the resolution.

Polysomnographic recording

In addition to video recording, video-polysomnography includes the acquisition of parameters essential for the recognition of the different sleep stages. Video-polysomnography also yields information on the cardiocirculatory system, respiratory system and body movements.

The equipment used for this recording is the polysomnograph. Unlike an EEG, the polysomnograph

Figure 5.6 The patient suddenly awakens and sits up: movements are not retained by the cables.

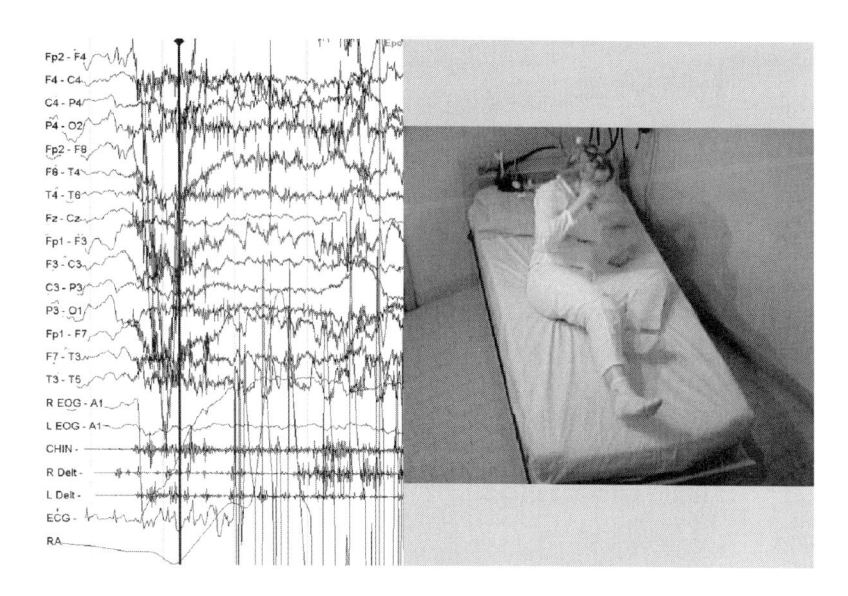

can simultaneously record referential and differential AC and DC channels. An important feature of the polysomnograph is to have a very small head box so that the patient is not disturbed by the box during motor activity. The cable between the head box and the polysomnograph should be light and long enough for the patient to move freely about the room.

An alternative solution could be a telemetry recording: a wireless system where parameters are recorded via radio signal. The patient can leave the room and the recording can be supervised on the screen unless the patient is out of the transmission signal area. The video would need to be integrated with additional cameras. A limitation of telemetry is the size and weight of the battery and signal transmission system.

Recording quality is greatly influenced by the techniques used to apply electrodes and transducers and by the structural features of the system. Devices with high CMRR (common-mode rejection ratio) are preferable because they are able to delete common mode input signals (230 V – 50/60 Hz). Another feature is the amplifier input impedance that should be high enough to record good signals if electrode impedance is too high. The subsequent step to signal acquisition is the digitalizing process, defined by digital resolution and sampling rate.

Digital resolution

The digital resolution defines the vertical reading points, hence the resolution: the higher the number of points, the greater the graphic resolution of the tracing which is defined by the number of bits in the polysomnograph. The latest polysomnographs have more than 16 bits, which allows an optimal resolution and avoids the risk of saturation (excessive amplitude) of the tracing.

Previous 12-bit recording systems required a maximal scale to be set specific for each parameter to obtain an adequate resolution: the higher the number of bits, the better the quality of the system. New polysomnographs do not need to set the amplitude during acquisition. Only the display setting is required which includes the sensitivity, the low-frequency filter (LFF) and the high-frequency filter (HFF). The latter three parameters can be edited both on-line and off-line.

Sampling rate

The sampling rate defines the horizontal reading points, providing a complete acquisition of the coordinates to digitize the signal. The number of bits cannot be changed, but the sampling rate can be set by the technician. The sampling rate should be at least twice the typical frequency of the recorded parameter. In EEG recording, where the basic frequency is 64 Hz, a sampling rate of 128 Hz could be adequate. Otherwise, in EMG recording, it would not be sufficient because of its higher frequency.

A 20-channel polysomnographic recording with a 128 Hz sampling rate lasting 7–8 h (one night) produces about a 100-Mb file. The size of this file is irrelevant compared to the 7–8 Gb file produced by video

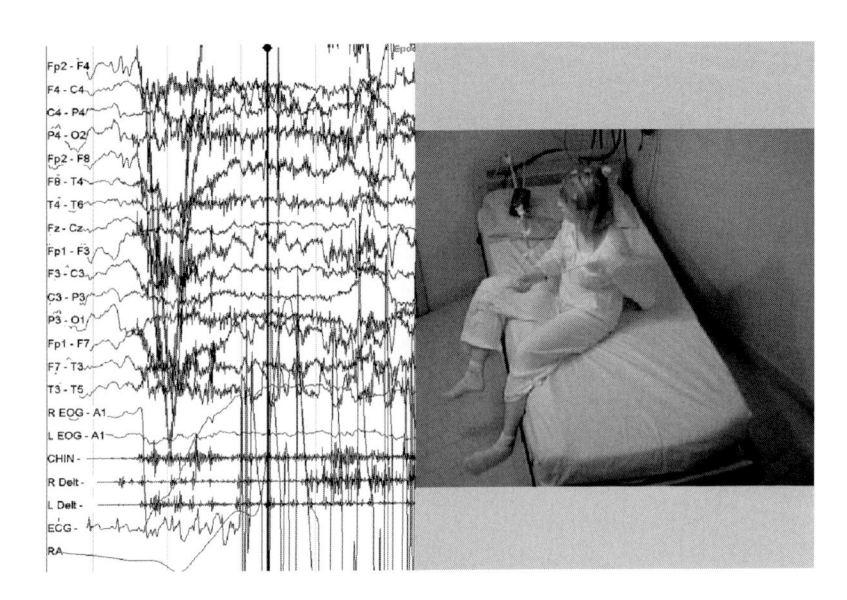

Figure 5.7 The patient sits on the bed: she is confused and pulls off the ECG cable.

recording. Therefore the sampling rate currently used is 256–512 Hz, which adds most information to the recorded parameters. Even though this sampling rate may seem excessive for routine recordings, it offers useful data for future analysis and the files are not difficult to manage or store. Some polysomnographs have sampling rates that go beyond 1024–2048 Hz.

Recorded parameters

Sleep

The basic purpose of video-polysomnography is to recognize and score sleep stages. This is made possible by recording from at least three EEG channels: one frontal, one central and one occipital [4]. The recommended derivations are between EEG electrodes and the contralateral mastoid [5]. This produces a tracing that highlights the main features of sleep stages.

The recording needs to be integrated with two electrooculogram (EOG) channels whose derivations are given by a right electrode (placed above the outer canthus of the eye) and a left electrode (placed below the outer canthus of the eye). Both electrodes are referred to the same mastoid. These derivations detect the rapid eye movements during the REM stage and the slow eye movements before falling asleep (SEM).

The information necessary for sleep scoring is completed with the electromyogram (EMG) of the submental muscle. The EMG is recorded by two electrodes, one placed on the muscle and the other placed on the chin. The recording of two tracings from the same parameter reduces false information [6]. EOG and chin EMG are fundamental parameters for sleep scoring especially in pathological conditions of sleep (Figure 5.4).

EOG: AC Channel (input), LFF 0.1 Hz – HFF 35 Hz (display setting).

Electroencephalogram

A video-polysomnographic recording could be performed to differentiate a parasomnia from epilepsy, in which case many EEG channels are required [6]. Generally a full set of electrodes according the 10–20 system is used, with the opportunity to reproduce different montages. Pre-cabled caps are not recommended for night recordings because of their instability during movements and their poor tolerance for the patient over a long period of time. The best recordings are performed using disc electrodes glued onto the patient's with collodium or adhesive paste.

EEG: AC Channel (input), LFF 0.3 Hz – HFF 70 Hz (display setting).

Motor activity

For the diagnosis and the study of parasomnias, it could be necessary to identify and describe the motor activity [7]. This is possible by recording the EMG of each skeletal muscle to evaluate the start, intensity and end of the muscle contraction. The EMG can be recorded with disc electrodes taped to the skin.

Electrode cables also need to pass under pyjamas or alternatively be fixed in place with an elastic band.

The second most recorded muscle, after the submental muscle, is the anterior tibial muscle, which detects foot movements and is essential during the recording of periodic limb movements (PLM). It is also advisable to monitor agonist and antagonist muscles on both sides of the body.

The sampling rate used in the EMG recording should be very high, at least 1024 Hz: this setting will determine the temporal sequence of movements with an accuracy of a thousandth of a second. Listed below are the muscles usually monitored in the study of parasomnias:

Face	Orbicularis oculi
	Orbicularis oris
	Frontalis
	Masseter
Neck	Sternocleidomastoid
	Mylohyoid
	Splenius capitis
	Cricoarythenoid muscles
Upper limbs	Deltoid
	Biceps brachii
	Triceps brachii
	Flexor carpi radialis
	Long radial extensor of wrist
Trunk	Rectus abdominis
	External oblique
Lower limbs	Anterior tibialis
	Gastrocnemius
	Biceps femoris
	Flexor digitorum brevis
	Extensor digitorum brevis

EMG: AC Channel (input), LFF 20 Hz – HFF 100 Hz (display setting).

Respiratory activity

Monitoring respiratory activity will help to disclose abnormal changes which could occur before or during critical events and provides information on snoring, respiratory rate and obstructive or central apneas or hypopneas. For this purpose, the sensors mostly used are an oronasal thermal sensor or a nasal air pressure sensor to detect the oronasal airflow. Both thoracic and abdominal expansions are recorded with respiratory effort transducers. A complementary sensor for the detection of respiratory effort is diaphragmatic and intercostal EMG.

Respiratory noise is detected by a tracheal microphone which highlights the snoring and picks up any sleep talking.

A further device used to define the severity of respiratory events is a pulse oximeter. It is advisable not to use an adhesive probe but an ear clip or a finger clip probe. The probe should be easy to remove during major motor events that would take the patient far from the instrument.

When severe hypoventilation is expected, it is advisable to use a transcutaneous capnograph to monitor PO_2 and PCO_2. The signal is detected by a probe placed over a muscle: the heat produced by the probe allows the gas to evaporate. The reliability of the parameter could be compromised by excessive movement.

When high negative inspiratory and positive expiratory pressures are expected, they can be quantified by detection of endoesophageal pressure. The measurement is obtained by a latex probe placed in the esophagus passing through the nose. The other end of the probe is connected to a pressure transducer which provides a voltage value proportional to the respiratory effort. This type of probe is not tolerated by all patients and in some cases it is necessary to remove it to allow sleep.

Respiration: AC Channel (input), LFF 0.01 Hz – HFF 10 Hz (display setting).

Respiratory noise: AC Channel (input), LFF 20 Hz – HFF 100 Hz (display setting).

Oximeter: DC Channel (input), HFF 30 Hz (display setting).

Capnograph: DC Channel (input), HFF 30 Hz (display setting).

Endoesophageal pressure: DC Channel (input), HFF 30 Hz (display setting).

Other autonomic parameters
ECG

A basic parameter in every polysomnographic recording is the electrocardiogram (ECG) that gives information on heart rate, tachycardia or bradycardia and other specific cardiac abnormalities (Figure 5.4). Using just one channel, it is advisable to use a Lead II that produces a QRS complex higher in amplitude than

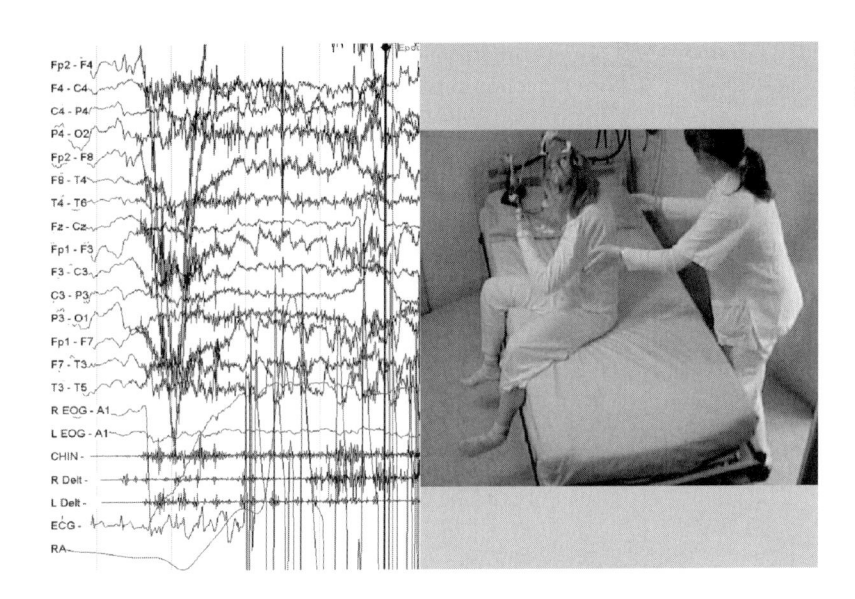

Figure 5.8 The patient tries to tear off the EEG electrodes: The technician intervenes to limit the action.

other derivations. This facilitates the scoring and automatic analysis.

ECG: AC Channel (input), LFF 0.5 Hz – HFF 70 Hz (display setting).

Blood pressure

The ECG could be integrated with blood pressure (BP) monitoring. The signal is detected by placing two cuffs over the patient's fingers: the alternative functioning of the cuffs allows continuous blood pressure recording. This detection system severely limits patients' movements so it should only be used when there is little motor activity.

BP: DC Channel (input), HFF 70 Hz (display setting).

Finger plethysmograph

By detecting blood flow in the finger, the finger plethysmograph (FP) provides an indication of vasodilation and vasoconstriction that can be related to heart rate and blood pressure.

FP: AC Channel (input), LFF 0.5 Hz – HFF 70 Hz (display setting).

Sympathetic skin response

The sympathetic skin response (SSR) is detected by disc electrodes placed on the palm of the hand or the sole of the foot. The skin is very thick in these areas, so it may be difficult to obtain low skin impedance. A reliable signal is possible even with resistances that may go beyond 50 ohm, but they must be equal between them. The SSR potential can be spontaneous or evoked.

SSR: AC Channel (input) LFF 0.1 Hz – HFF 10 Hz (display setting).

Enuresis

To monitor enuresis, an enurometer may be required. This instrument reports any loss of urine on a graphic tracing, but no information is given on the quantities of urine or release time. The probe is positioned close to the genitals so that it will get wet during enuresis. The probe must be replaced after each enuresis episode.

Enuresis: DC Channel (input), HFF 10 Hz (display setting).

Technical assistance

The polysomnographic technician performs several tasks during an overnight recording:

- supervision of the recording to ensure the perfect functioning of electrodes and transducers;
- integration of the recording with additional electrodes if new events occur during the night;
- intervention during an event to prevent injury to the patient;
- intervention during the recording to verify space and time orientation in the patient; and
- intervention during the recording to question the patient about the event (Figure 5.8).

References

1. Coccagna G. *Il sonno e I suoi disturbi*. Second edition. Padova: Piccin, 2000.
2. Tinuper P, Grassi C, Bisulli F, et al. Split-screen synchronized display. A useful video-EEG technique for studying paroxysmal phenomena. *Epileptic Disord* 2004; **6**: 27–30.
3. Hunter J, Jasper HH. A method of analysis of seizure pattern and electroencephalogram: A cinematographic technique. *Electroencephalogr Clin Neurophysiol* 1949; **1**: 113–4.
4. AASM. *The AASM Manual for the Scoring of Sleep and Associated Events: Rules, Terminology and Technical Specifications*. Westchester, IL: American Academy of Sleep Medicine, 2007.
5. Rechtschaffen A, Kales A. *A Manual of Standardized Terminology, Techniques and Scoring System for Sleep Stages of Human Subjects*. US Department of Health, Education, and Welfare Public Health Service-NIH/NID, 1968.
6. Montagna P, Provini F, Vetrugno R. Propriospinal myoclonus at sleep onset. *Neurophysiol Clin* 2006; **36**: 351–5. Epub 2007 Jan 26. Review.
7. Frauscher B, Gschliesser V, Brandauer E, et al. Video analysis of motor events in REM sleep behaviour disorder. *Mov Disord* 2007; **22**: 1461–70.
8. Provini F, Plazzi G, Tinuper P, et al. Nocturnal frontal lobe epilepsy. A clinical and polygraphic overview of 100 consecutive case. *Brain* 1999; **122**: 1017–31.

Section 1
Chapter 6

Introduction

Parasomnias due to medications or substances

Rosalind D. Cartwright

Introduction and history

Before reviewing what we now know concerning the medications and substances associated with the parasomnias, we need to look at the criteria set out in the ICSD-R [1] and ICSD-2 [2] that define a diagnosis of a parasomnia due to a drug or substance. These two publications agree on three principles.

- The first principle is that there must be a close relationship between exposure to a drug, medication or biological substance and the onset of parasomnia signs and symptoms.
- Second, that the emergent parasomnia can be a *de novo* parasomnia, the aggravation of a chronic intermittent parasomnia, or the reactivation of a previous parasomnia.
- Third, the parasomnias most predictably associated with medications or biological substances are the disorders of arousal (DOA), sleep-related eating disorder (SRED), REM behavior disorder (RBD) and the parasomnia overlap disorder.

However, the two diagnostic manuals differ markedly in the list of medications implicated. The ICSD-R focused on those associated with the NREM parasomnias, particularly sleepwalking (SW), while the ICSD-2 lists those "reported to trigger" an "acute or chronic" REM parasomnia, particularly REM behavior disorder (RBD). Neither defines what "substances" are or may be at issue. Although there is a good deal of literature on the relation of the imidazopyridine agents to SW and SRED starting as early as 1994, zolpidem (Ambien) and eszopiclone (Lunesta) are not mentioned. This review will cover the medications as listed to be associated with both the NREM and REM parasomnias in addition to the evidence from the newer drugs and two of the substances that have been the subject of some debate: caffeine and alcohol. Although there is some evidence that stopping smoking also has a triggering effect, the cases are very few.

The principles noted above leave several issues to be clarified as we review the literature of an association between some medication or substance and a parasomnia symptom. The first is the meaning of "close" in relation to the onset of symptoms. Arbitrarily we will adopt a criterion window of up to 3 days after the initiation of a new medication or an escalation in dosage, granting that, in most cases, this timing will be shorter. The reason this is important is a second problem: many patients involved in these studies are taking multiple medications which were not stopped, and ethically should not be stopped, before a new medication was started. Ideally, in the best of all worlds, all patients would have other medications discontinued so that the efficacy of some new agent can be assessed without the possibility of drug interaction effects. Keeping the timing short between the beginning of a new medication or substance or its escalation or discontinuation and the onset of parasomnia symptoms, reduces the probability that the relation between the agent and symptoms is a chance association. However, that still leaves open the interaction question. The interaction may in fact be what is efficacious for the treatment of the originally diagnosed disorder, but is also responsible for the initiation of the new, undesirable parasomnia problem. This is the case in at least one of the case studies we will review.

The next issue stems from the second criterion listed above: the emergence of a *de novo* parasomnia.

This opens the question of the meaning of "*de novo*". Are there true parasomnias without a genetic-based predisposing factor? The long-held understanding that "genetics play an important role in the parasomnias" has been based on family studies [3], twin studies [4], and HLA typing genetic studies [5]. The latter studies were conducted before the more precise methods, the single nucleotide polymorphisms (SNIPs) techniques, were available to identify the genetic component involved in those not identified by the *DQB1* genes. The concordance of sleepwalking in identical twins is not 100% [4], leaving room for other variables to account for why one twin is spared, or perhaps delayed in expressing their sleepwalking symptoms. There may be a different genetic abnormality involved in the late-emerging parasomnias that is responsive to specific chemical agents. Perhaps it is time to apply the SNIPs method for more specific gene studies in those "*de novo*" cases to clarify this issue. Until then, the meaning of "*de novo*" will have to rest on the imprecise criterion of the absence of a known childhood or family history.

The third principle suggests that those disorders that share the same sleep abnormality will be responsive to medications and substances that affect that specific sleep stage or sleep marker. For the DOA sleepwalkers and sleep terror patients, those who show the signature delta sleep arousals in the first third of the night's sleep, or by low slow-wave activity (SWA) [6–8], would be expected to be responsive to those medications and substances that affect a change in the percent of delta sleep, i.e. slow-wave sleep (SWS), and/or an increase in the number of arousals from that sleep stage. The second group, the SRED and also the sleep-related sexual events (sexsomnia), in which the parasomnia behaviors have been noted to occur during SWS but also at other times of the night, suggests we look broadly for the sleep changes associated with the emergence or exacerbation of SRED events following the initiation or withdrawal of some medication or substance. The REM parasomnia RBD is identified with the loss of the defining muscle atonia of REM sleep allowing arousals with motor behavior to occur. Here, movements of other kinds intrude into all of sleep, the periodic limb movements of sleep (PLMD), for example. This indicates that we should look for bursts of muscle activity or movements prior to or during REM sleep arousals, and increases in other motor behaviors throughout the night following a new RBD diagnosis, in conjunction with the introduction or escalation of a medication or increase or discontinuation of a substance.

Given all of these issues, there will not be many of the early studies that meet a standard of having been designed to give a clear answer to the question of whether the parasomnia is closely related to the introduction or change in a medication, nor will the sleep data have been collected or analyzed to address the additional issues we have raised. Much of the early literature consists of single case reports or a series of cases, without any data concerning the intervening changes in sleep architecture. These are, however, useful for us to review to identify those medications which appear to be related to the onset or exacerbation of parasomnia symptoms and so are candidates for further more precise studies. Some of this follow-up work has been performed in better-designed studies and has had sleep data collected and reported. We will begin this review with some of these early observational studies starting with the NREM parasomnias.

NREM parasomnias associated with medications

Sleepwalking is not the only NREM parasomnia that has been observed to be associated with a medication or substance. It is, however, the most common of this group, the one most familiar to psychiatrists, who noted this as a side effect following the initiation or escalation of some medications used for treating their patients, particularly those with bipolar depression in manic episodes, schizoaffective patients and those anxiety patients presenting with insomnia. Single case reports and some case series were published following the introduction of anti-psychotic, anti-depressant, anti-anxiety and sleep-inducing agents. Some of these also included observations about the effects of reducing or stopping various medications and substances.

As sleepwalking is also the "first step" in an SRED event, as typically the patient will walk to the kitchen in a non-conscious state before eating, and as it is associated with some of the same medications as have been implicated in DOA, it will be included as a subtype of sleepwalking.

The *International Classification of Sleep Disorders: Revised Diagnostic and Coding Manual* [1] states under "predisposing factors" that in SW "thioridazine hydrochloride, chloral hydrate, lithium carbonate, prolixin, perphenazine and desipramine hydrochloride can exacerbate or induce sleepwalking." Thus, sleepwalking has been associated with a wide spectrum of medications which are prescribed for a broad range of patients. The incidence of sleepwalking following the initiation of these medications is unknown. The prevalence, as estimated in the general population by Ohayon *et al.* is 2% [9], and in psychiatric out-patients 8.5% by Lam *et al.* [10], who point out that there are lessons to be learned for prescribing physicians from what is probably a profound under estimate of this "side effect" of sedating anti-depressants and non-benzodiazapine hypnotics.

Psychiatric patients have been a sample of convenience for examining the frequency of sleepwalking in response to initiating and/or withdrawing from a single or combinations of psychotropic drugs with or without a sleep-promoting pharmacological agent. These are most often small sample, uncontrolled observational studies. In addition, there have been some large sample studies of psychiatric patients using questionnaire methods comparing those reporting parasomnia symptoms to those who do not. Here the parasomnia is a secondary diagnosis. These rarely involved sleep studies. Those that do are more often not psychiatric patients but those with a primary complaint of a parasomnia symptom who have been referred to a sleep disorder service for diagnosis. These patients are likely to be studied in the laboratory as part of their diagnostic work-up. Their sleep may then be compared to age-matched controls without a parasomnia history in between-group designs. Other designs are within subjects' nights on and off a medication, or a comparison of nights with two different medications, or a medication compared to a placebo. The third type of sample uses laboratory animals for investigating the effects on EEG of drugs and substances implicated in the parasomnia.

NREM parasomnias with medications in psychiatric patients

There is a long history of case reports implicating almost all psychotropic medications and hypnotics as being associated with sleepwalking in psychiatric patients. Generalizations, based on case reports, are difficult to make given the frequency of multiple medications in any one case, and the differences between these combinations in case series. What we will cover here are the published reports in which a sleepwalking event occurred closely following the initiation of a medication and its resolution on withdrawal from that drug.

Lithium carbonate and mood stabilizers

Case reports of sleepwalking following the initiation of lithium carbonate have probably the longest history. Lithium is still used for the control of symptoms in bipolar depression, particularly for those with difficult-to-control manic episodes. It is also used for control of Kleine–Levin syndrome, which appears to be a bipolar variant in some cases. The primary symptom of this disorder is episodic long periods of hypersomnia up to 20 of the 24 h a day, which then may be followed by short periods of insomnia. The hypersomnia phase may be accompanied with hyperphagia and hypersexuality in young males. Lithium is also used to treat cases of episodic hypersomnia in young females who generally lack the hyperphagia and hypersexuality symptoms of the males. These cases that do not meet the criteria of being menstrually related are known as the sleeping beauties. Both genders have been treated with valproic acid and/or lithium for their "mood stabilizing" effect. Lithium has also been used in the treatment of schizoaffective disorder patients.

One early report of sleepwalking by Huapaya is often quoted [11]. Only one of the seven cases in this report involved lithium. The author notes that all seven were out-patients, who had in common that they were on a combination of medication including hypnotics, neuroleptics, anti-depressants, minor tranquilizers, stimulants, and anti-histamines, and that some used alcohol in addition to their drugs. We will review the one case in which lithium was given to illustrate the difficulty of concluding anything about the contribution of this medication to the initiation of sleepwalking and/or its cessation.

Case #6 a 40-year-old man with no previous history of sleepwalking, diagnosed as endogenous depression for which he had been prescribed lithium, maprotiline and perphenazine during the day. His night-time medications were: 2 mg perphenazine and 30 mg oxazepam. On these he reported sleepwalking, including finding himself walking in the street at night. His daytime medications were then changed to lithium, protriptyline and diazepam. At night he was given 25 mg amitriptyline and 300 mg of methyprylon. On this regimen he continued to be depressed and was still sleepwalking. His daytime medications were then changed, increasing the protriptyline to 50 mg. The diazepam and methyprylon were discontinued. His night-time medications were perphenazine 2 mg and flurazepam 30 mg. His sleepwalking was then reported to have stopped. He was followed up for 10 months with no recurrence of the sleepwalking.

I have quoted this case in some detail not only to illustrate the multiple medication involved in this and many of the psychiatric cases, but the difficulty of concluding anything about the role of lithium, as it was never specified whether it was withdrawn when the other daytime drugs were discontinued. If it was, there would be some indication that it played a role in this patient's sleepwalking, but that remains undetermined in this case.

Another early publication by Charney *et al.* reviewed nine cases of "somnambulistic-like episodes secondary to combined lithium-neuroleptic treatment" [12]. Five were diagnosed as bipolar manic and six as schizoaffective disorder. Again, since all these patients were on lithium plus four different other medications, it is difficult to sort out which drug at which dosage is related to the sleepwalking. The episodes began between 2 days and 2 weeks after the lithium plus another medication was started. For seven of the nine patients, the lag was 2–3 days. The cessation of sleepwalking was noted in one case when lithium was increased and one when it was decreased. This study, too, does not give clear evidence of the role of lithium in the reported sleepwalking.

Another single case study of a schizoaffective patient by Glassman, Darko and Gillin also involves sleepwalking which occurred only when taking a combination of lithium, chlorpromazine, triazolam and benztropine [13]. In this case, a sleep study was done while the patient was on these medications. An episode occurred out of Stage 2 sleep. In this case, the authors conclude that CNS-active medications have a role in triggering pathological sleep phenomena in predisposed individuals. The basis for that inference was that a brother of the patient also had a sleepwalking episode following "exposure to a substance affecting the CNS."

A questionnaire study of 389 patients attending a lithium clinic by Landry *et al.* found that 27 patients (6.9%) reported sleepwalking and related the onset of this to their treatment with lithium alone or in combination with other psychotropic drugs [14]. Forty-five patients (11.6%) reported they had childhood sleepwalking, and 12 of these (27%) had their childhood sleepwalking reactivated by this medication. This study suggests that lithium may induce sleepwalking and that those with a childhood history appear to be at increased risk of reactivating sleepwalking while taking this and other psychotropic drugs. Only one publication included sleep data from the laboratory suggesting that lithium may be related to an arousal from SWS typical of this parasomnia. This study by Kupfer *et al.* examined lithium in affective disorder patients [15]. They reported specific sleep effects. One of these, a delay of the onset of REM sleep, may implicate an increase in SWS prior to the first REM, a characteristic of SW events.

In sum, there has not been a published sleep laboratory study of lithium, used as a single medication, in patients on and off the drug. At present, the evidence is only suggestive that those who have a childhood history of parasomnias or a family history are at increased risk of developing sleepwalking within 3 days of the initiation of lithium above the rate reported in the general psychiatric patient population [10].

Other neuroleptics

Again, this literature has the problem that several different medications are usually given in combination to treat psychiatric patients. We will summarize those where there is evidence of the onset of sleepwalking within 3 days of the initiation of a specific medication and that the episodes ceased when the medication was withdrawn. There are three such cases reported by Charney *et al.* [12].

* In one case sleepwalking was initiated with thioridazine, which stopped when the drug was withdrawn and began again when it was re-started.

Luchins *et al.* reported a large series of sleep studies conducted on one schizoaffective patient [16].

* The patient had stabbed her daughter to death during a sleepwalking episode. She was studied both on and off thioridazine. Of the 29 sleep study nights, 10 were on thioridazine. The patient had events on five of these nights. On 19 nights without this medication, no episode was recorded. The nights on the drug, her REM time was increased significantly and Stage 4 was increased but did not reach the $p < .05$ level of significance.

It is unfortunate that the scoring of combined SWS (Stages 3 + 4) was not calculated, as this is the conventional scoring of delta sleep today, and may have reached significance in this case. Also, there was no report of the number of arousals during Stage 4 sleep. Both have been indicated as characteristic of the sleep of sleepwalkers [17].

There were two cases involving perphenazine that could be identified as responsible for the initiation of

Section 1: Introduction

sleepwalking which ceased when the drug was discontinued. Landry *et al.* noted one case when sleepwalking began on chlorprothixene and did not recur when this was reduced in dosage [14]. A second case was treated on methaqualone along with several others. This patient had repeated sleepwalking episodes on the combination but stopped when methaqualone was discontinued. Huapaya also reported two cases which implicated methaqualone with sleepwalking which took place when the patients were on a combination of medications but stopped when this medication was withdrawn [11].

There were only four medications that could be identified as being associated with the initiation of sleepwalking and its cessation when the drug was discontinued: thioridazine, perphenazine, chlorprothixene and methaqualone. Only the one report by Luchins *et al.* included sleep studies on and off these medications to inform us of the nature of the sleep and the changes in the sleep stages on these medications [16]. No information was included on whether these sleep stage increases were normalized when the drugs were discontinued.

There are two cases reported by Kolivakis *et al.* in which olanzapine was administered as a single drug [18]. Sleepwalking occurred when the dosage was 20 mg. A second study by Paquet *et al.* reports that when olanzapine was added to the patient's ongoing lithium to control a manic episode, sleepwalking began a "few days after this addition" [19]. These cases are notable in that olanzapine has been shown to increase SWS by Sharpley *et al.* [20].

It would be helpful to know the effects on the percent of SWS and on the number of arousals in SWS for all medications found to trigger sleepwalking as a test of the prevailing model of the NREM parasomnias being related to increases in the amount and depth of SWS and to arousals from this sleep stage [17].

Anti-depressants

An early paper by Flemenbaum used questionnaires to study the effect of a tricyclic anti-depressant versus an anti-psychotic medication in association with pavor nocturnus [21]. There is some confusion in this report as to whether these are nightmares, perhaps a REM parasomnia, or sleep terrors, an NREM parasomnia disorder. The publication included no data about the time of night that the episodes occurred. The aim was to study the difference between administering the medication as a single night-time dose or as divided doses during the day. The author reports that of $N = 76$ psychiatric in-patients, of $N = 19$ who had a single night-time dose of either or both of the two classes of drugs, $N = 14$ (73%) had frightening dreams whereas only $N = 7$ (10.5%) had frightening dreams when given divided doses. There was also no report of what medications were being compared. The author does mention that most had flurazepam HCl which he states interferes little with the sleep EEG, and "most on the tricyclic antidepressants had that as a single medication while others had this in combination with perphenazine–amtriptyline or chlorpromazine, thioridazine etc." In support of this being a parasomnia of SWS, the author states that 8 of 11 given an anti-depressant as a single night-time medication reported confusion and physiological arousal on awakening from the frightening dream, and one woman had a sleepwalking episode for the first time in her life.

There are four recent single case studies of an anti-depressant associated with the onset of sleepwalking. Two included information showing a marked decrease or cessation of episodes when the medication was reduced or stopped. In both, the drug involved was paroxetine. Alao *et al.* [22] and Kawashima *et al.* [23] both showed no sleepwalking at 10 mg, but at 20 mg sleepwalking occurred and increased in frequency beginning in the first few hours of sleep. In the study by Alao *et al.* [22], when paroxetine was replaced by sertraline and it was increased from 50 mg to 100 mg, sleepwalking reappeared. Amitriptyline has also been associated with sleepwalking at higher dosages. Ferrandiz-Santos *et al.* reported a case in which there was no sleepwalking until the drug was escalated to 150 mg [24].

Summarizing the anti-depressant medications and their effects on sleep, few studies give the effects on SWS. From the few that do, it appears that the tricyclics and SSRIs have opposite effects on SWS. The SSRIs generally decrease and the tricyclics increase this sleep stage, and therefore the latter might be expected to initiate or increase the frequency of sleepwalking according to the Broughton model [17].

NREM parasomnias with medications in sleep disorder patients

Benzodiazepines and sleepwalking

This class of medications has yielded more information concerning their effects on sleep from studies conducted on and off these agents. This is not surprising since some of these are newer drugs than those we reviewed above, although they were sometimes used in combination to control night-time sleep disturbances associated with the psychiatric disorders. The primary use for the benzodiazepines is the treatment of insomnia. Those presenting with sleep onset difficulty, problems with sleep maintenance, or early morning awakening difficulty of more than 2 weeks duration, without an accompanying psychiatric diagnosis, are the typical patients for these studies. These patients are more often seen as out-patients in a sleep disorder service, where sleep studies are likely to be conducted as part of the diagnostic work up. In 1999, the number of prescriptions written for this class of medications was reported to be over 100 million.

Borbely *et al.* looked into the effects on EEG sleep stages of three benzodiazepines for eight healthy young subjects in comparison to their night on a placebo [25]. The drugs involved were: flunitrazepam 2 mg, flurazepam 30 mg and triazolam 0.5 mg. All drugs reduced Stage 1 and REM sleep percents and decreased the number of stage shifts. They all increased the percent of Stage 2 sleep. A spectral analysis scoring showed that all three drugs reduced the low frequency activity in the range of 0.25–10.0 Hz in Stages 2, 3 + 4 and REM. These changes persisted into the next night off the drug. The authors point out that this power spectral analysis scoring provides specific changes in the sleep missed by the more conventional scoring based on the percentage of sleep spent in each stage per hour of sleep. The reduction of low-frequency activity in the first third of the drug night was maintained for the remainder of the night. Although these sleepers were all healthy without a parasomnia history, these findings add to the possibility that these drugs may help to inform us about their role in those with a sleepwalking history, as the benzodiazepines are noted by Mendelson [26] to be "profound suppressors of slow wave sleep." This, then, is opposite to the model of increases in SWS being a priming factor for NREM parasomnias as outlined by Broughton [17]. The prediction would be that if those who have had a prolonged suppression of SWS while on a benzodiazepine were to be abruptly withdrawn, they would experience a rebound of SWS, making the initiation of a NREM parasomnia activity more likely. We will discuss the apparent contradiction of the traditional model of NREM parasomnia in the Conclusion section below.

Benzodiazepines and sleep eating disorder (SRED)

There are several studies relating triazolam with SRED. Poitras reported a case series of three who complained of sleep eating on this medication, all with amnesia for the event [27]. Menkes reported a single case in which the sleepwalking began with the first prescription [28]. In another single case offered by Laurema [29], triazolam was alternated with midazolam in a man with severe insomnia and PLMD. He had nine episodes of wandering in the house and sleep eating followed by amnesia and some bizarre behaviors including finding shoe polish in his refrigerator. Schenck *et al.* reported a study of the sleep data of nine SRED patients with documented SW in the laboratory [30]. These were seen to arise abruptly from Stages 2 and 3 + 4, or in another three cases had an excessive number of abrupt spontaneous arousals. These authors report that the percent of Stages 3 + 4 were "robust" for both nights of recorded sleep with a Night 1 mean of 23.4 (5.5) and Night 2 mean of 26.2 (8.4). Only one of those in the SW group was on triazolam during the two sleep study nights; all others were off their medications.

Schenck reported a case of a woman who had escalated her triazolam dose from .25 to .75 mg without informing her physician. This was followed immediately by nightly sleepwalking with cooking, binge eating bizarre foods and wandering into her neighbor's yard with amnesia for all these events. Her daytime behavior was unaffected as she continued to work as a postmistress. All abnormal behaviors ceased when triazolam was discontinued.

SRED is not the only parasomnia reported to follow starting triazolam. A 29-year-old woman with severe insomnia got up in the "middle of the night and dressed herself" according to Regenstein *et al.* [31]. Lemoine *et al.* had a single case of a 19-year-old female who arose during the night and stabbed a woman in her care 35 times [32]. She was also taking temazepam and clorazepate, which were prescribed.

In summary, the benzodiazepine that has been most clearly associated with SRED is triazolam, although it is associated with the initiation of several other NREM parasomnias as well, as are other benzodiazepines. However, it should be noted that another medication in this class, clonazepam, has been the treatment most consistently effective in the control of these behaviors. As this medication has an effect of increasing sleep continuity and reducing the percent of SWS, it will be interesting to look into the sleep architecture of those who do not respond well to this treatment, and even more interesting will be to examine the sleep characteristics of those who remit without further drug treatment once this medication associated with the onset of their NREM parasomnia has been discontinued. Such research needs to be done routinely, as both drug and substance effects on sleep can be long-lasting. Such data will inform us about the nature of the baseline sleep architecture once a washout is complete.

Nonbenzodiazapines with sleepwalking, sleep eating and sleepsex

Zolpidem tartrate has been responsible for an explosion of publications dating from 1994 to the present devoted to the association of this sleep aid to the initiation of SW, SRED, and sexsomnia, both in those with a reactivation of a previous childhood parasomnia event and others for whom the parasomnia is a *de novo* event. The earliest case was reported by Mendelson [33], which was a well-designed research study conducted in a sleep laboratory.

*The subject was a 20-year-old volunteer for a research study. He had no medical or psychiatric history and no history of alcohol or drug use. He did have a history of some sleepwalking as a child but none since then. His baseline sleep study was normal with 420 minutes of sleep and sleep efficiency of 97%, SWS of 16%. The first experimental night he was given flurazepam 30 mg and was awakened with increasingly loud auditory tones until an awakening took place. No SW events took place in response to these stimuli. One week later he was given zolpidem 10 mg at 60 minutes before bedtime. Ten minutes after sleep onset he was awakened by the auditory tones. This produced a normal awakening. When the tones were begun during Stage 4 sleep, he was observed to get out of bed and walk on top of the bed. The technician entered the room and reported that the subject was confused with no memory of having walked about. He returned to sleep within 3 minutes. The third night he was given a placebo and had a normal sleep study. He had only a vague morning memory of the sleepwalking event.

There are several single clinical case studies of zolpidem now in the literature. One case reported by Harazin and Berigan [34] had never experienced sleepwalking but did have episodes while taking zolpidem which stopped when this medication was discontinued. Yang *et al.* also reported that a male in-patient in his mid 50s with no history of SW, a previous history of alcoholism and traumatic brain injury, experienced insomnia following hip surgery [35]. He was given zolpidem on two non-consecutive nights. He walked on both nights, but not on the intervening nights when no zolpidem was administered, and did not resume SW once off this medication. Sattar *et al.* published another *de novo* case in which there was no prior childhood or family history of sleepwalking [36].

*A 47-year-old male patient who had been diagnosed with bipolar disorder and treated with citalopram 40 mg daily and zolpidem 5 mg at bedtime.

When he developed a manic episode, valproic acid was added. Two days after, a sleepwalking event occurred approximately one hour after sleep onset, when he found himself at an open window with no memory of getting out of bed. When valproic acid was discontinued, the sleepwalking stopped. On rechallenge with valproic acid, the SW resumed. Zolpidem was then withdrawn and sleepwalking did not recur. The authors conclude that since the patient was taking two medications known to increase SWS and although the patient refused a sleep study, they suggest this combination of valproic acid and zolpidem may be responsible for producing the sleepwalking.

Other parasomnia behaviors have also been reported on zolpidem which stopped when the medication was discontinued. In most cases this involved SRED behavior. Morganthaler and Silber reported a series of five cases all complaining of insomnia [37]. The mean age was 55. Following being given zolpidem, four of the five began SRED, and this increased in severity in the fifth case. All episodes stopped when this medication was withdrawn. This too was the story in a case reported by Sansome *et al.* [38]. This 51-year-old female had no prior history of sleepwalking but had multiple medical problems including restless legs syndrome (RLS), diabetes, depression and migraine for which she was treated with metformin, sumatriptan, and citalopram and had been stable on these for over a year. Zolpidem was added for her complaint of insomnia. SRED events began with amnesia the next morning documented by her accusing her husband of leaving empty food packages on the countertops. Tsai *et al.* state that three females were being treated for insomnia with zolpidem [39]. These patients reported engaging in repetitive compulsive cleaning, shopping and eating. All episodes stopped when this medication was discontinued.

Tsai *et al.* recently completed a large, retrospective study of 255 psychiatric patients who were taking psychotropic medication and zolpidem averaging 10 mg for more than 6 months [40]. Interviews were conducted on both the patients and family members. Thirteen (5.1%) reported various parasomnia behaviors following starting zolpidem, all with no recall of these behaviors. These included one who walked to her boyfriend's house, others used the telephone, sleep eating took place, and watching television. All were amnestic for these events.

Landolt et al. conducted a positron emission tomography (PET) study of eight young men who had a baseline night then 40 h of sleep deprivation with zolpidem 20 mg or placebo [41]. They report sleep deprivation with placebo increased the power of SWS (1.25–7.00 Hz) in comparison to the baseline night. The sleep deprivation with zolpidem decreased power in the 3.75–10 Hz and 14.25–16.0 Hz range. They found that in comparison to the baseline night, zolpidem attenuated power in the whole range of 1.75–11 Hz and that sleep deprivation and zolpidem had different effects on EEG power spectra. Here is the first real replication of the Push/Pull model of NREM parasomnia as proposed by Espa et al. [7]. This requires a revision of the traditional simpler increase of SWS model.

Erman et al. have recently reported a multisite study comparing eszopiclone and zolpidem for the control of insomnia [42]. The eszopiclone was delivered at four different dosages and the zolpidem at a 10 mg dose; a matching placebo was also involved at each drug dose level. Patients were screened to exclude any with chronic or unstable medical conditions, a psychiatric diagnosis or sleep disorder other than primary insomnia by a two-night sleep study. Patients were randomized by order of the eszopiclone dosage of 1, 2, 2.5, and 3 mg. Patients were aged 21–64 years with a mean age of 40.6 years. Sleep studies were conducted with a washout period of 3–7 days between nights. Results showed eszopiclone at 2.5 and 3 mg were significantly different from the placebo in reducing the amount of wake time after sleep onset (WASO) and increased sleep efficiency (SE). These findings were not different from zolpidem 10 mg. Our interest is in the side effects of this medication. These were only significantly higher than placebo for a category of all CNS adverse effects. There was no follow-up of events or side effects after this acute study, nor was there any report of changes off these medications.

Since there have been so many published reports of NREM parasomnia events on zolpidem, both the regular and controlled release (CR) formulation, it is curious that there have been only occasional reports of sleep driving, sleep eating, sleepsex and nightmares on a similar medication. It is well known that the filing of a class action suite in the US led to a relabeling of zolpidem to include a warning of parasomnia events, and a similar action was taken in Australia. It may be that eszopiclone is not a trigger for these events, or they have not been assessed. This question was addressed recently in a critique of studies supported by pharmaceutical companies by Kripke [43].

Substances associated with NREM parasomnias

Alcohol

The association of alcohol ingestion and non-conscious behavior arising out of SWS sleep has become a topic of considerable controversy around the question of legal responsibility. Should an alcohol-induced behavioral arousal from SWS be treated as an NREM parasomnia, in which SW events with or without aggression or sexual behavior are conducted without awareness, motivation or planning, followed by retrograde amnesia and remorse? These characteristics conform to the criteria of an NREM parasomnia as defined by Bonkalo on which the ISDC-R indications for this diagnosis are based [44]. Or, as some argue, since the consumption of alcohol is a voluntary act, with perhaps known consequences, should not NREM parasomnias that follow be treated as one for which the defendant bears full responsibility? Aside from the legal argument is the scientific argument: does the SWS arousal into a non-conscious complex motor behavior *require* an increase in SWS and a higher arousal threshold as a necessary condition, or is this model of NREM parasomnia now in need of revision? The grounds for this debate have been evidence of the effects of alcohol on sleep, particularly on SWS, in the first two hours of the night. This evidence has been found to be extremely variable in different subject groups: non-drinkers, social drinkers and alcohol abusers, and whether the abusers are now abstinent or not, and for how long.

There has been some speculation about the effects on REM sleep during acute withdrawal from alcohol addiction and its resemblance to the REM without atonia (RWA), a hallmark of RBD. The REM sleep under these circumstances has been noted to have a higher eye movement density and more body movements, with more arousals [45]. These signs in the sleep study along with the presence of hallucinations have been argued to parallel the dream enactment symptom from REM arousals in the RBD patients. This will await further research including long-term follow-up of dry alcoholics. At this time the data appear to support that this resemblance to RBD does not persist in those who have been dry over one year.

On top of the need to clarify the acute and chronic effect on sleep of alcohol in different groups and the effects of its abrupt withdrawal are the ethical considerations concerning the protection of human subjects of administering alcohol in research protocols, which has delayed further studies. The evidence of long-term alcohol having the effect of reducing SWS in amount and depth was found to be a strong predictor of SW with violence in the one large study of persons with clinical histories of SW and/or sleep terrors (ST) [46]. However, these results were based on a single night of study with only 24 h of restriction on alcohol. This study does indicate the need for better-controlled designs including controls for age effects on SWS and the use of the more refined spectral analysis scoring of SWS. The percent of alpha rating introduced in the Moldofsky *et al.* study as a measure of self-awareness during sleep is a useful addition to differentiate malingering in criminal cases [46].

Caffeine

The effects of caffeine abuse on NREM parasomnias has also been debated in recent publications, with a similar argument being proposed by Pressman that since caffeine reduces SWS it cannot be considered as having a triggering effect for a SW event [47]. This argument is counteracted by another study showing that the effects of sleep deprivation with caffeine reduces SWA compared to sleep deprivation alone [48], and evidence in the human study of SW and/or ST, where a history of caffeine abuse (more than 6 cups per day) and SWS sleep < 2% differentiated SW with violence toward others from those who were non-violent SW [46].

It appears that chronic alcohol, caffeine and zolpidem reduce SWS and increase arousals from this sleep stage, although there are differences at different dosages of caffeine [49]. These substances also reverse the effect of sleep deprivation which increases SWS and take longer to recover the lost SWS following lifting the restriction on sleep. Since all three have been implicated in SW events [46,50], it seems prudent that we consider them as possibly associated with NREM parasomnia events and in need of well-designed further research.

REM behavior disorder and associated medications

Although a large number of medications and some substances are listed as triggers of both acute and chronic RBD in the ICSD-2 [2], there is actually very little published support at this time that anti-depressants, MAOI, anti-anxiety medications, and beta-blockers, are responsible for the onset of this disorder in the absence of significant neuropathology. There is better support for the emergence of an RBD following an abrupt withdrawal of imipramine, alcohol and amphetamine abuse. The ICSD-2 manual also states "Caffeine and chocolate abuse have also been implicated in causing or unmasking, RBD" [2]. The studies showing evidence for caffeine abuse and for the association of venlafaxine were both published as abstracts from meetings which are not included in the publicly searchable databases for scientific literature [51].

Nash *et al.* report that mirtazapine induces RBD in parkinsonism [52]. This medication has listed as side effects nightmares and RLS on the drug information site. Schenck *et al.* have noted that patients treated for depression and obsessive–compulsive disorder with fluoxetine develop RBD [53].

Fluoxetine

In a report by Schenck *et al.* [53], a review of 2650 sleep studies of patients treated with fluoxetine or tricyclic anti-depressants and patients without those medications including 70 diagnosed with RBD and 30 with no sleep diagnosis, the authors found 41 (1.5%) were treated with fluoxetine. There was a significant association between fluoxetine and prominent eye movements in NREM sleep in 48.8% of the 20 out of 41 patients who were on this medication. This was a much higher rate than for those on tricyclics 5.8%, 3 out of 52. This intrusion of eye movements on fluoxetine was higher than those diagnosed with RBD 4.3%, 3 out of 70, and for normal sleepers 3.3%, 1 out of 30. The authors conclude that this medication, as a powerful serotonin re-uptake inhibitor, results in the release of saccadic eye movements in NREM sleep. One patient with obsessive–compulsive disorder had a history of developing RBD soon after beginning fluoxetine therapy. This disorder persisted in spite of the discontinuation of the medication. A study by Armitage, Trivedi and Rush examined 41 depressed patients before and after being treated with 30 mg of fluoxetine for 4–5 weeks [54]. They report 34% of the patients (14 patients) had increased eye movements and muscle tone in all sleep stages. They, too, suggest this is an effect of the increased serotonin availability. Dorsey, Lukas and Cunningham compared the sleep of nine depressed patients on 10–80 mg of fluoxetine to six unmedicated depressed patients [55]. The fluoxetine group had lower SE, more NREM arousals and eye movements than the control group. Also, four of the nine of those treated with fluoxetine had significant PLMD, which was not found in any of the controls. It appears that this medication is associated with disruptive motor control in sleep and that this is associated with more arousals. However, there is no clear evidence of the dream enactment so characteristic of the RBD diagnosis. This calls into question the similarity to the RBD disorder.

Conclusions

At this point in time, the state of our knowledge concerning the association of various medications and substances to parasomnia behaviors points to the need for an increased research effort to clarify many issues. We are faced with an escalation in the number of reports of these undesirable and even dangerous sleep-related, non-conscious behaviors, implicated in starting, escalating or stopping some medication or substance, at the same time as there is an increase in the number of medications and substances that are being used to promote sleep. Clearly there is a need to rethink some of the assumptions that have prevailed in the literature since early work was done. This is particularly true of the work on the effects of alcohol on sleep. Many of these original studies have been cited over and over without having been replicated with more power, better-controlled designs, and more precise scoring of effects. The development of new drugs has made the need for testing their effects in studies with longer follow-up times apparent, as there is evidence of slow recovery of sleep following acute withdrawal effects. These need to be performed independent of funding by pharmacological companies, as many fund only less-expensive studies of acute effects.

With the increasing number of parasomnias being now listed as overlap disorders [56], with evidence of abnormal behaviors following arousals from both NREM and REM sleep, there is a breakdown of the distinction between these two classes of parasomnias. Clearly, there is a need to look into causes other than the traditional sleep stage proportions and the effects of stress-related or medication-induced sleep deprivation.

As noted earlier, the refinement of methods for genetic studies is an avenue that needs to be pursued to clarify the so-called *de novo* parasomnias. The assumption that there is an underlying genetic vulnerability responsible for allowing motor activity to interrupt sleep into abnormal behaviors has not been disproven – it does need to be tested further. Also the model that the SWS arousals of parasomnias require sleep deprivation or some other agent to increase the push for more of this sleep is questionable, as the increase is not sufficient to provoke an arousal unless there is also an opposing outside pull of an arousing stimulus (auditory tones) or an internal arousing agent (caffeine, zolpidem, or, in some cases, alcohol). The presence of these opposing drives appears to be the necessary condition for the abnormality of the arousal, possibly in those with some genetic vulnerability [57]. This requires power density scoring to demonstrate the abnormality when no behavioral arousal has taken place. There remains much work to be done.

References

1. American Academy of Sleep Medicine. *International Classification of Sleep Disorders, Revised: Diagnostic and Coding Manual*. Rochester, Mn: American Academy of Sleep Medicine, 2001.
2. American Academy of Sleep Medicine. *International Classification of Sleep Disorders, 2nd edition: Diagnostic and Coding Manual*. Westchester, IL: American Academy of Sleep Medicine, 2006.
3. Kales A, Soldatos CR, Bixler EO, *et al*. Hereditary factors in sleepwalking and night terrors. *Br J Psychiatry* 1980; **137**: 111–8.
4. Hublin C, Kaprio J, Heikkila K, *et al*. Prevalence and genetics of sleepwalking: A population-based twin study. *Neurology* 1997; **48**: 177–81.
5. Lecendreux M, Bassetti C, Dauvilliers Y, *et al*. HLA and genetic susceptibility to sleepwalking. *Mol Psychiatry* 2003; **8**: 114–7.
6. Gaudreau H, Joncas S, Zadra A, *et al*. Dynamics of slow wave sleep during the NREM sleep of sleepwalkers and control subjects. *Sleep* 2000; **23**: 755–60.
7. Espa F, Ondze B, Deglise P, *et al*. Sleep architecture, slow wave activity and sleep spindles in adult patients with sleepwalking and sleep terrors. *Clin Neurophys* 2000; **111**: 929–39.

8. Guilleminault C, Poyares D, Abat F, *et al.* Sleep wakefulness in somnambulism: A spectral analysis study. *J Psychosom Res* 2001; **51**: 411–6.

9. Ohayon M, Guilleminault C, Priest RG. Night terrors, sleepwalking and confusional arousals in the general population: Their frequency and relationship to other sleep and mental disorders. *J Clin Psychiatry* 1999; **60**: 268–76.

10. Lam SP, Fong SYY, Ho CKW, *et al.* Parasomnia among psychiatric outpatients: A clinical, epidemiologic, cross-sectional study. *J Clin Psychiat* 2008; **69**: 1374–82.

11. Huapaya LVM. Seven cases of somnambulism induced by drugs. *Am J Psychiatry* 1979; **136**: 985–6.

12. Charney DS, Kales A, Soldatos CR, *et al.* Somnambulistic-like episodes secondary to combined lithium–neuroleptic treatment. *Br J Psychiatry* 1979; **135**: 418–24.

13. Glassman JN, Darko D, Gillin JC. Medication-induced somnambulism in a patient with schizoaffective disorder. *J Clin Psychiatry* 1986; **47**: 523–4.

14. Landry P, Warnes H, Nielsen T, *et al.* Somnambulistic-like behavior in patients attending a lithium clinic. *Int Clin Psychopharm* 1999; **14**: 173–5.

15. Kupfer DJ, Reynolds CF III, Weiss BL, *et al.* Lithium carbonate and sleep in affective disorders: Further considerations. *Arch Gen Psychiatry* 1974; **30**: 79–84.

16. Luchins DJ, Sherwood PM, Gillin CJ, *et al.* Filicide during psychotropic-induced somnambulism: A case report. *Am J Psychiatry* 1978; **135**: 1404–05.

17. Broughton RJ. NREM arousal parasomnias. In Kryger MH, Roth T, Dement WC (Eds), *Principles and Practice of Sleep Medicine*, 3rd edition. Philadelphia, PA: W.B. Saunders Co., 2000; 693–706.

18. Kolivakis TT, Margolese HC, Beauclair L, *et al.* Olanzapine-induced somnambulism. *Am J Psychiatry* 2001; **158**: 1158.

19. Paquet V, Strul J, Servais L. Sleep-related eating disorder induced by olanzapine. *J Clin Psychiatry* 2002; **63**: 597.

20. Sharpley AL, Vassallo CM, Cowann JP. Olanzapine increases slow-wave sleep: Evidence for blockade of central 5HT2c receptors in vivo. *Biol Psychiatry* 2000; **47**: 468–70.

21. Flemenbaum A. Pavor nocturnes: A complication of single daily tricyclic or neuroleptic dosage. *Am J Psychiatry* 1976; **133**: 570–2.

22. Alao AO, Yolles JC, Armenta WC, *et al.* Somnambulism precipitated by selective-reuptake inhibitors. *Pharm Techno* 1999; **15**: 204–07.

23. Kawashima T, Yomada S. Paroxetine-induced somnambulism. *J Clin Psychiatry* 2003; **64**: 483.

24. Fernando-Santos JA, Mataix-Sanjuan AL. Amytriptyline and somnambulism. *Ann Pharmacother* 2000; **34**: 1208.

25. Borbely AA, Mattmann P, Strauch I, *et al.* Effect of benzodiazepine hypnotics on all-night sleep EEG spectra. *Hum Neurobiol* 1985; **4**: 189–94.

26. Mendelson WB. Hypnotic medications: Mechanisms of action and pharmacological effects. In Kryger MH, Roth T, Dement W (Eds), *Principles and Practice of Sleep Medicine*, 4th edition. Philadelphia, PA: WB Saunders Co., 2005; 444–51.

27. Poitras R. A propos d'épisodes d'amnesies anterogrades associes a l'utilisation du triazolam. *Union Med Can* 1980; **109**: 427–9.

28. Menkes DB. Triazolam-induced nocturnal bingeing with amnesia. *Austral NZ J Psychiatry* 1992; **26**: 320–1.

29. Laurema H. Nocturnal wandering caused by restless legs and short-acting benzodiazepines. *Act Psychiatry Scand* 1991; **83**: 492–3.

30. Schenck CH, Hurwitz TD, Bundlie SR, *et al.* Sleep-related eating disorders: Polysomnographic correlates of a heterogeneous syndrome distinct from daytime eating disorders. *Sleep* 1991; **14**: 419–31.

31. Regenstein QA, Reich P. Agitation observed during treatment with newer hypnotic drugs. *J Clin Psychiatry* 1985; **46**: 280–3.

32. Lemoine P, Lamothe P, Ohayon MM. Violence, sleep and benzodiazepines. *Am J Foren Psychiatry* 1997; **18**: 17–26.

33. Mendelson WB. Sleepwalking associated with zolpidem. *J Clin Psychopharmacol* 1994; **34**: 150.

34. Harazin J, Berigan TR. Zolpidem tartrate and somnambulism. *Mil Med* 1999; **164**: 669–70.

35. Yang W, Dollear M, Muthukrishnan SR. One rare side effect of zolpidem – sleepwalking: A case report. *Arch Phys Med Rehabil* 2005; **86**: 1265–6.

36. Sattar SP. Somnambulism due to probable interaction of valporic acid and zolpidem. *Ann Pharmacother* 2003; **37**: 1429–33.

37. Morganthaler TI, Silber MH. Amnestic sleep-related eating disorder is associated with zolpidem. *Sleep Med* 2002; **3**: 323–7.

38. Sansone RA, Sansone LA. Zolpidem, somnambulism, and nocturnal eating – Letter to the editor. *Gen Hospital Psychiatry* 2008; **30**: 90–1.

39. Tsai MJ, Tsai YH, Huang YB. Compulsive activity and antegrade amnesia after zolpidem use. *Clin Toxicol* 2007; **45**: 179–81.

40. Tsai YH, Yang B, Chen CC, et al. Zolpidem-induced amnesia and somnambulism: Rare occurrences? *Eur Neuropsychopharm* 2009; **19**: 74–6.

41. Landolt H-P, Finelli LA, Roth C, et al. Zolpidem and sleep deprivation: Different effect on EEG power spectra. *J Sleep Res* 2000; **9**: 175–83.

42. Erman MK, Zamit G, Rubens R, et al. A polysomnographic placebo-controlled evaluation of the efficacy and safety of eszopiclone relative to placebo and zolpidem in the treatment of primary insomnia. *J Clin Sleep Med* 2008; **4**: 229–34.

43. Kripke DF. Who should sponsor sleep disorders pharmaceutical trials? *J Clin Sleep Med* 2007; **3**: 671–3.

44. Bonkalo A. Impulsive acts and confusional states during incomplete arousal from sleep: Criminological and forensic implications. *Psychiatry Quar* 1974; **48**: 400–09.

45. Tachibana M, Tanka K, Hishikawa Y, et al. A sleep study of acute psychotic states due to alcohol and meprobamate addiction. *Adv Sleep Res* 1975; **2**: 177–205.

46. Moldofsky H, Gilbert R, Lue FA, et al. Sleep-related violence. *Sleep* 1995; **18**: 731–9.

47. Pressman M, Mahowald MW, Schenck CH, et al. Alcohol-induced sleepwalking or confusional arousal as a defense to criminal behavior: A review of scientific evidence, methods and forensic considerations. *J Sleep Res* 2007; **16**: 198–212.

48. Shwierin B, Borbely AA, Tobler I. Effects of N6-cyclopentyladenosine and caffeine on sleep regulation in the rat. *Eur J Pharmacol* 1996; **300**: 163–71.

49. Wurts SW, Edgar DM. Caffeine during sleep deprivation: sleep tendency and dynamics of recovery sleep in rats. *Pharmacol Biochem Behav* 2000; **65**: 155–62.

50. Howard C, D'Orban PT. Violence in sleep: Medico-legal issues and two case reports. *Psychol Med* 1987; **17**: 915–25.

51. Stolz SE, Aldrich MS. REM behavior disorder associated with caffeine abuse. *Sleep Res Online* 1991; **20**: 341.

52. Nash JR, Wilson SJ, Potokar JP, et al. Mitrazapine induces REM sleep behavior disorder (RBD) in parkinsonism. *Neurology* 2003; **61**: 1161.

53. Schenck CH, Mahowald MW, Kim SW, et al. Prominent eye movements during NREM sleep and REM sleep behavior disorder associated with fluoxetine treatment of depression and obsessive–compulsive disorder. *Sleep* 1992; **15**: 226–35.

54. Armitage R, Triveti M, Rush AJ. Fluoxetine and oculomotor activity during sleep in depressed patients. *Neuropsychopharmacology* 1995; **12**: 159–65.

55. Dorsey, CM, Lukas SE, Cunningham SI. Fluoxetine-induced sleep disturbance in depressed patients. *Neuropsychopharmacology* 1996; **14**: 437–42.

56. Schenck CH, Boyd J, Mahowald MW. A parasomnia overlap disorder involving sleepwalking sleep terrors, and REM sleep behavior disorder in 33 polysomnographically confirmed cases. *Sleep* 1997; **20**: 972–81.

57. Cartwright R. Letter to the Editor re: Pressman M. Factors that predispose, prime and precipitate NREM parasomnias in adults. *Sleep Med Revs* 2008; **12**: 77–80.

Section 1 Chapter 7

Introduction

Parasomnias due to medical and neurological disorders

Marco Zucconi and Alessandro Oldani

According to the International Classification of Sleep Disorders (ICSD 2005), there are 12 core categories of parasomnias, mainly classified according to the sleep state of origin [1]. The last three categories consist of parasomnias: unspecified, due to drug or substance, and due to medical conditions. The essential feature of this last diagnosis is that a parasomnia emerges as a manifestation of an underlying neurological or medical condition. Some authors categorize the parasomnias as "primary" (disorders of the sleep state per se) and "secondary" (organ-system disorders that appear during sleep) [2]. The secondary sleep parasomnias can be further classified by the organ system involved:

- Central Nervous System
    headaches, tinnitus, seizures

- Cardiopulmonary
    cardiac arrhythmias, nocturnal angina pectoris, nocturnal asthma, respiratory dyskinesias, miscellaneous

- Gastrointestinal
    gastroesophageal reflux, diffuse esophageal spasm, abnormal swallowing

- Miscellaneous
    nocturnal muscle cramps, nocturnal pruritus, night sweats, nocturnal tongue biting, benign nocturnal alternating hemiplegia of childhood

Nevertheless, these secondary phenomena represent different events and symptoms arising from specific organ systems and occurring preferentially during the sleep period rather than sleep-related manifestations of an underlying medical or neurological disorder.

The REM sleep behavior disorder (RBD) is the parasomnia most commonly associated with an underlying neurological condition (the so-called "symptomatic RBD") and will be analyzed in detail in Chapter 14. Another parasomnia often associated with different medical conditions such as delirium tremens, Morvan's fibrillary chorea, fatal familial insomnia and sporadic Creutzfeldt–Jakob disease, is called "agrypnia excitata" [3,4].

Hypnagogic and hypnopompic visual hallucinations can occur with neurological disorders such as narcolepsy, dementia with Lewy bodies, midbrain and diencephalic pathology, and Parkinson's disease.

The disorders of arousal are the most frequent of the NREM sleep parasomnias. They may be triggered by prior sleep deprivation, alcohol, emotional stress and febrile illness [5,6]. Several medication-induced cases have been reported with sedative-hypnotics, stimulants, neuroleptics, and anti-histamines, often in combinations [6–9]. In some women, disorders of arousal can be both exacerbated or alleviated by pregnancy, suggesting hormonal effects [10–12]. These factors appear to be triggering events in susceptible individuals rather than causes of parasomnia. Similarly, a number of medical, neurological and sleep disorders may trigger the parasomnia episodes.

Symptomatic REM sleep behavior disorder

REM sleep behavior disorder (RBD), the most interesting REM parasomnia, can be associated with neurological disorders and medical diseases.

Neoplasms of the brainstem [13], acute or chronic multiple sclerosis (MS) [14,15], acute focal pontine inflammatory lesions [16], Guillain–Barré syndrome (GBS) [17], amyotrophic lateral sclerosis (ALS) [18], and autosomal dominantly inherited spinocerebellar ataxia type 2 and 3 (SCA2, SCA3) [19,20], generally involve brainstem structures of importance in the pathogenesis of RBD. However, RBD has been described in other neurological diseases not associated with brainstem impairment, such as Morvan's chorea [21], fatal familial insomnia [22], and limbic encephalitis [23], suggesting that other areas might be implicated in the pathophysiology of RBD, as well as in neurodevelopmental disorders such as autism [24], Tourrette's syndrome [25], and group A xeroderma pigmentosus [26].

RBD usually occurs in the setting of neurodegenerative diseases such as Lewy body dementia (LBD), Parkinson's disease (PD), and multiple system atrophy (MSA), and it may precede the development of parkinsonism by many years [27]. Since the first descriptions of the RBD association with neurodegenerative diseases, it appeared that the association of this parasomnia had a predilection for synucleinopathies (PD, LBD, MSA) instead of tauopathies such as Alzheimer's disease (AD), progressive supranuclear palsy (PSP), corticobasal degeneration (CBD), Pick's disease or frontotemporal dementia (FTD) [27–30]. However, recently some studies described RBD or REM sleep without atonia (RSWA) in different patients with tauopathies [27,30,31], leading to doubt about the special association of RBD and synucleinopathies.

RBD in Parkinson's disease

The presence of clinical RBD in PD varies from 15 to 34% and this percentage increases, if we add the polysomnographic features of RSWA, as suggested by some authors [27,32], up to around 50% of patients. It can appear first, simultaneously or after the onset of PD [33]. As a prognostic factor, RBD in PD seems associated with a major risk of cognitive impairment and slowing of the waking EEG [34], and, as a clinical correlate, PD patients with RBD are less likely to be tremor-predominant as well as have a lower UPDRS rating score due to less tremor [35]. Moreover, in a recent study, the Canadian group of Jacques Montplaisir found an increased frequency of falls and a lower response to medication in PD patients affected by RBD, while motor complications or other motor manifestations are similar to PD patients without RBD [35]. These results were found in a small group of PD patients in which the RBD status was confirmed by video-polysomnography. Larger cohorts of PD patients have been evaluated and the findings were dissimilar without differences between motor subtypes, but higher Hoehn and Yahr scores and only marginally longer disease duration in PD with RBD [36]. However, in these types of studies the diagnosis of RBD is only "probable" because PSG data were not available and the assessment was by clinical history. The same method has been used in a retrospective chart review study, finding a longer disease duration, higher doses of dopaminergic drugs and higher frequency of dyskinesia and fluctuations in PD with RBD compared to non-RBD patients, although with the same UPDRS score [37]. Taken together, these data, at least those in PSG-confirmed RBD and PD patients, seem to indicate that the parkinsonism has less tremor with a reduced response to dopaminergic drugs and more falls, characteristics suggesting a different form of disease other than pure PD, such as MSA or other more rare parkinsonisms [35]. Moreover, the observation of RBD in juvenile-onset parkinsonism with Parkin gene mutation (Park2) where α-synuclein deposits are generally absent [38], indicates that it is not only synuclein deposition that can cause RBD in neurodegenerative disorders.

RBD in Lewy body dementia

The association between RBD and LBD has been demonstrated although through case reports and a few case series, as no systematic studies have been performed. The suggested prevalence was about 70% of the examined patients [39–41], and this strong association is the basis to consider RBD as a criterion suggestive for the diagnosis of LBD [42]. It has to be remembered that the only autopsy case of RBD (idiopathic) has shown Lewy bodies in the central nervous system (CNS) with predominance in the brainstem [43]. A pathophysiological hypothesis has been proposed for the progression of the symptoms and signs in some synucleinopathies (PD, LBD): the synucleinopathy involvement follows a caudorostral direction across the CNS, and is responsible for the appearance of the RBD in the early stage of the disease when degeneration is more important at the brainstem level with rostral progression and development of the full-blown illness later [29].

Section 1: Introduction

RBD in multiple system atrophy

Several reports have confirmed the strong association between RBD and MSA [44–46]. In some of these reports the clinical features of RBD have been confirmed by video-polysomnography, indicating a high prevalence of the parasomnia: in up to 70% of the cases if the polysomnographic features of RSWA are included, and with a strong female prevalence compared to the preponderance of male RBD patients seen in the other diseases. Generally, the parasomnia precedes by years the onset of the disease and in some cases may be the first symptom, appearing even 10 years before full-blown MSA [44]. The high prevalence of RBD in MSA is not completely understood, but it could be because of the involvement of the brainstem (the pons in particular), which is very common in MSA and implicates pathological modification of the structures controlling REM sleep muscle atonia [47].

RBD has been associated with MSA and disautonomic involvement, and not with pure autonomic failure (PAF), a different form of synucleinopathy but with some clinically similar features [48]. However, a recent study demonstrated the REM parasomnia in a few PAF patients, raising the issue that PAF may be an initial form of degeneration in patients who subsequently develop PD or LBD [49], or alternatively many patients with MSA, DLB and PD may have autonomic involvement with RBD in the clinical or subclinical course of the degenerative disease [50].

RBD in Alzheimer's disease

RBD has been described and associated with several neurodegenerative diseases, but the presence in AD is considered rare, and with no pathological confirmation. In the past, some cases described as RBD associated with probable AD or, in one case, with autopsy-confirmed AD have been subsequently ascribed to LBD or the LB variant of AD, on the basis of careful anatomic–pathological examination [51]. A more recent clinical study of a series of 15 patients with probable AD, with video-PSG confirmation, revealed one case of RBD and three cases of RSWA [30]. Although no histopathologic data were available to confirm the diagnosis of AD, and the Lewy body variant of AD cannot be ruled out, these findings seem to suggest that RBD is rare but RSWA may be present in clinically probable AD, which is considered a typical tauopathy. Moreover, recently one case of a possible new parasomnia has been described: stage 1–2 NREM movement behavior disorder associated with a progressive dementia, characterized by abnormal and violent sleep-associated behaviors, emerging from REM and NREM sleep and lasting throughout the sleep duration. The main difference from RBD was the EEG-PSG pattern, which contains elements of stage 2 NREM and abnormal continuous rapid eye movements, and muscle twitches longer than myclonus. The REM sleep was similar to RSWA. The authors hypothesized that it was an early stage of an evolving status dissociatus, associated with a neurodegenerative disease, possibly AD of moderate severity, associated with a frontal lobe syndrome [31].

RBD in progressive supranuclear palsy

RBD has been described in this type of tauopathy for many years [18,33,52], with a prevalence similar to that in PD. A recent detailed clinical–polysomnographic study of 15 patients with PSP found the presence of RSWA in 27% of the cases, with two of them showing complex behaviors during video-PSG indicating RBD [53].

RBD in other tauopathies

In corticobasal degeneration, characterized by akinesia, cortical myoclonus and the "alien limb" sign, RSWA and one case of full-RBD have been reported as case reports, but there are no studies on series or consecutive patients [54,55]. There are no published reports of RBD or RSWA in primary progressive aphasia (PPA), Pick's disease or frontotemporal dementia (FTD). We recently observed a series of 15 patients with clinical dementia (7 with FTD, 8 with other types of dementia, 5 with LBD, 2 with vascular type and 1 with probable AD), in whom the video-PSG examination showed no RBD episodes or RSWA in the FTD patients, whereas two patients (with clinical LBD) showed RBD during the recording, and one patient (with probable AD) had RSWA [56]. Our results are consistent with the strong association of RBD with synucleinopathies rather than tauopathies. However, although rare, RBD, or at least RSWA, may be part of degenerative disorders of the tau type.

In other syndromic parkinsonisms, such as pallidonigral degeneration or OPCA, there is no report of clear association with RBD or RSWA [57].

There is a large body of evidence that RBD is associated with synucleinopathy degeneration; however, the rare presence of this parasomnia in other neurodegenerative disorders suggests that the localization of the degeneration (in the brainstem and pons), rather than the specific type of neuronal degeneration, is important in producing RBD and RSWA [27,28].

RBD in other neurological disorders

RBD has been reported in other neurological disorders, but mainly by case reports. In addition, SCA3, ALS and MS where the parasomnia has been described in patients with clear evidence of lesions in the pons, the occurrence of RBD has been reported in *epilepsy* in association with a late-onset cryptogenic sleep-related generalized form of seizures. Besides the similarity of the two motor type of episodes (parasomnia and seizure), the relationship may be in the sleep fragmentation and instability of RBD that leads to an increase in likelihood of seizures [58].

In *Guillan–Barré syndrome* (GBS), besides the autonomic dysfunction, RBD, hallucinations and vivid dreams have been described [29]. Recently, mental status abnormalities were correlated with sleep structure changes in a large, prospective controlled study [17], with the finding of a high percentage of REM sleep abnormalities such as sleep onset REM period, abnormal eye movement during NREM sleep, and a high percentage of RSWA, and some evidence of status dissociatus.

Post-traumatic stress disorder (PTSD) shows some alterations of REM sleep structure (twitches, PLMS) resembling those typical of RBD, and one report found a high incidence of comorbidity between the two disorders [59], with the hypothesis of disturbed REM sleep phasic mechanisms in PTSD. However, in PTSD, besides insomnia, nightmares and other REM parasomnias, and night terrors, an NREM parasomnia is the more frequent sleep disorder reported [60].

In *limbic encephalitis*, the documentation by PSG of RBD enhances the possibility that, besides other areas implicated in the pathogenesis, different mechanisms (autoimmune-mediated mechanisms) may be implicated, since the remission of the inflammatory syndrome has been associated with a partial resolution of RBD [23]. Recently a case of RBD in a patient with an isolated focal inflammatory lesion in the dorsomedial pontine tegmentum has been described [16]. Moreover, in this unusual case, a narcoleptic syndrome was associated with the RBD.

Pharmacologically induced RBD

Different medications have been associated with RBD or RSWA, particularly psychotrophic and antihypertensive drugs. Amongst the CNS agents, the first reports involved tricyclic antidepressants such as clomipramine [61], imipramine [62], and others, whilst some case reports indicated an improvement of RBD symptoms following the administration of such drugs (imipramine, desipramine, carbamazepine) [13,63]. In some earlier reports, the REM sleep alteration was identified and named as stage 1-REM with PSG characteristics similar to RSWA and often accompanied by vivid dreams [64]. Also, monoamino oxidase inhibitors (MAOI) such as selegiline and phenelzine have shown potential to induce RBD in PD patients [65] and healthy young subjects [66]. More recently, RBD symptoms or RSWA have been reported in patients treated with serotoninergic drugs (venlafaxine, fluoxetine, mirtazapine, paroxetine, sertraline and citalopram) [67,68]. A systematic PSG study showed that the percentage of patients treated with selective serotoninergic reuptake inhibitors (SSRI) developed more submental EMG activity during REM sleep than controls. These patients are at greater risk with increasing age. PD patients treated for depression with SSRIs or patients with depression or obsessive–compulsive disorders have been reported to develop RBD or RSWA. In particular, fluoxetine and mirtazapine appear to be the drugs at most risk to trigger RBD episodes [67,69]. On the other hand, a few reports have shown that administration of paroxetine improved RBD [70]. Bisoprolol, a selective β1 adrenoreceptor blocking agent, utilized for treatment of hypertension, has been described to provoke REM sleep EMG activity [71], as well as tramadol, an analgesic opioid derivative, SSRI and α-2-adrenoreceptor antagonist [29]. However, clonidine has been shown to improve nocturnal symptoms in a single patient with idiopathic RBD [29].

Hallucinations and RBD have been reported in patients with PD and AD, respectively, treated with dopamine agonists and cholinergic drugs [72,73]. Withdrawal from drugs such as barbiturates [74], meprobamate, alcohol [75], and nitrazepam have been reported to be associated with reduced REM muscle atonia and oneiric behaviors, as has intoxication with biperidin, or excessive use of caffeine or chocolate [76–79].

Hypnagogic and hypnopompic hallucinations

Hallucinations, both diurnal and nocturnal, have been described in PD associated with cognitive decline and RBD. A temporal association has been reported to exist between hallucinations and abnormal daytime sleep onset REM periods, short and fragmented REM sleep or RBD [80–82]. Dysfunction of the cholinergic system, with ponto-geniculo-occipital circuits, has been hypothesized as the basis for nocturnal and diurnal hallucinations, and the link with RBD seems to indicate that this parasomnia may be a risk factor for hallucinatory behaviors and also cognitive decline in PD [83]. Hypnagogic hallucinations and vivid dreams have been described in a high proportion of patients with GBS during the intensive care unit (ICU) period, appearing to correlate with lower levels of CSF hypocretin-1 and autonomic dysfunction, compared to ICU patients without GBS [17]. Patients with hallucinations had abnormal REM sleep structure and characteristics including REM sleep without atonia and REM sleep behavior disorder. Moreover, atypical NREM sleep features were present, such as abnormal eye movements indicating possible status dissociatus-like parasomnia.

Nocturnal eating syndrome (NES) and sleep-related eating disorder (SRED) in obesity and mental illness

NES, characterized by a circadian delay in the timing of feeding relative to the normal circadian time of sleep onset, may contribute to the development of obesity, as many subjects had normal weight prior to the development of NES and subsequently gained weight [84]. However, to date it is not clear whether night eating contributes to weight gain, and also the extent to which overweight status or obesity promotes NES.

Concerning the association between NES and mental disorders: obese subjects with NES had higher depression scores and lower self-esteem on the appropriate scales, and a circadian decline of mood in the afternoon (after 4 p.m.), in an opposite way to endogenous depression patients [85]. NES is common in psychiatric outpatients [86]. However, mental disorders seem independent from the binge eating disorder.

SRED, characterized by recurrent episodes of eating after an arousal from night-time sleep with adverse consequences, is associated with being overweight as well as obesity, and as with NES some authors have claimed that the excess weight could be related to the nocturnal eating [84]. SRED is also linked to comorbid mental disorders such as anxiety, a history of repeated abuse, and PTSD. Also depression of mood is common in SRED [87]. There are no data about the direction of the correlation between the two.

Sleep disordered breathing and parasomnias

In the last two decades, some studies have demonstrated that arousals secondary to apneas, hypopneas and irregular breathing can be the trigger for sleepwalking and related disorders in both children and adults [88–90]. Apnea-induced arousals from NREM sleep with complex behavior may be indistinguishable from primary disorders of arousal. Guilleminault and colleagues reported that of 49 children with the dual findings of sleepwalking and sleep-disordered breathing, 45 were completely cured of sleepwalking with successful treatment of the sleep-disordered breathing [89]. Similar results have been noted with treatment of adult sleepwalkers with sleep apnea syndrome following treatment with CPAP or ENT surgery [88]. Alternatively, CPAP therapy of obstructive sleep apneas may result in slow-wave sleep rebound and emergent sleepwalking and other arousal disorders. In 1991, Millman and colleagues reported the case history of a 33-year-old obese white man who, during his first night with nasal CPAP, abruptly sat up and began to walk across the room. He was observed to be in stage 4 sleep during this episode. A similar episode of sleepwalking occurred the same night during stage 3 sleep. He was prescribed nasal CPAP at 15 cmH$_2$O pressure to use at home, and no further episodes of sleepwalking were reported [91].

Migraine and parasomnias

Between 1983 and 1986, there were reports of an increased incidence of somnambulism in children with migraine [92]. In recent years, Casez and colleagues evaluated 100 consecutive patients with cephalalgia [93]. Their study showed that sleepwalking is significantly linked with migraine, but not with other types of headache: 32.8% of patients with migraine had a history of somnambulism during childhood, whereas only 5.1% of patients without migraine had a similar history (the same incidence of the general population). In the migraine group, neither the different subtypes of migraine nor the mean age at onset had a significant association with somnambulism. The authors did not suggest that migraine and somnambulism are part of the same pathology, but that migraine and somnambulism may follow a common pathway, either chemical or topographic. Finally, in 2006, Evans reported the rare case of a 26-year-old female with recurrent episodes of sleep paralysis followed by a migraine headache [94].

Infective diseases and parasomnias

Since 1979, despite the well-known association between sleepwalking and febrile illness [94,95], the only study of the relation between infective disease and parasomnia was in 2006 [96]. Eidlitz-Markus and Zeharia assessed the neurologic complications of pertussis infection by reviewing the clinical records of all children (aged 7–18 years) with serology-positive pertussis infection admitted at the Schneider Children's Medical Center of Israel from 1995 to 2005. The review yielded 60 patients with a diagnosis of pertussis, of whom 6 (10%) had undergone an electroencephalogram due to the presence of neurological symptoms (i.e. suspicion of epilepsy); the clinical neurological findings were the same in all cases: the parents reported that at 1–2 h after falling asleep at night the child would wake up and make several attempts to breathe. These efforts were accompanied by high-pitched sounds and sounds of suffocation. Usually, the child got out of bed, agitatedly walked around the room, then returned to bed and continued to sleep. The episodes lasted 1–2 min and occurred a few times per night. None of the children remembered any of these events the next morning. The authors suggested that this description was clinically compatible with partial arousal parasomnia. In all cases, the sleep symptoms resolved within 10 weeks, along with resolution of the pertussis infection symptoms. There was no recurrence of the parasomnia episodes during six months of follow-up. The authors discussed the possibility that the pertussis toxin directly induced the partial arousal that manifested as a parasomnia. Alternatively, other authors have suggested that the respiratory effort, such as occurs in pertussis, could be responsible for many of the arousal parasomnia episodes, mimicking sleep-disordered breathing [97].

Other diseases and parasomnias

In 2005, Ajlouni and colleagues [98] described eight cases of patients with new-onset sleepwalking episodes that coincided with the start of thyrotoxicosis. The cause-and-effect relationship between the two conditions, was supported by: (a) the disappearance of the sleepwalking with successful achievement of euthyroidism; (b) the absence of family history of parasomnias; (c) the adult onset; and (d) the relapse of sleepwalking in two patients when their thyrotoxicosis became poorly controlled as a result of noncompliance with medications.

In 2008, Mouzas and colleagues reported a significantly higher occurrence of self-reported sleepwalking, nocturnal enuresis, night illusions, sleep terrors and nightmares than that of a control group in 116 patients suffering from vitiligo [99]. They underlined the relationship between parasomnias during early life and later development of vitiligo, suggesting the hypothesis that a neural mechanism involving the serotoninergic systems may potentially be involved in the etiopathology of vitiligo.

Parkinson's disease and parasomnias

An association of sleepwalking with Parkinson's disease has been reported in the literature in the last decade, including a series of 100 consecutive patients with Parkinson's disease [100,101]. Night walking was also reported in 10 of 93 patients with REM sleep behavior disorder of different origins, including Parkinson's disease. Five of these 10 patients had an underlying unspecified neurodegenerative disorder [33]. Recently, Poryazova and colleagues reported the occurrence of adult-onset (*de novo*) sleepwalking in a series of six patients with idiopathic Parkinson's disease [102]. All patients had at least one concomitant sleep–wake disorder, including REM sleep behavior disorder (four patients) and insomnia (four patients). The authors' conclusion was that the neurodegenerative changes associated with Parkinson's disease at the brainstem level can affect the ascending control of state transition and the descending control of locomotion and muscle tone, together giving rise to various sleep-associated behavioral disturbances including sleepwalking, REM sleep behavior disorder and overlap parasomnia.

References

1. American Academy of Sleep Medicine. *International Classification of Sleep Disorders: Diagnostic and Coding Manual*, 2nd edition. Westchester, IL: American Academy of Sleep Medicine, 2005.
2. Mahowald MW. Other parasomnias. In Kryger MH, Roth T, Dement WC (Eds), *Principles and Practice of Sleep Medicine*. Philadelphia, PA: Elsevier Saunders, 2005; 917–25.
3. Montagna P, Lugaresi E. Agrypnia excitata: A generalized overactivity syndrome and a useful concept in the neurophysiology of sleep. *Clin Neurophysiol* 2002; **113**: 552–60.
4. La Morgia C, Parchi P, Capellari S, *et al*. "Agrypnia excitata" in a case of sporadic Creutzfeldt–Jakob disease VV2. *J Neurol Neurosurg Psychiatry* 2009; **80**: 244–6.
5. Vela Bueno G, Dobladez Blanco B, Vaquero Cajal E. Episodic sleep disorder triggered by fever – A case presentation. *Waking Sleeping* 1980; **4**: 243–51.
6. Nino-Murcia G, Dement WC. Psychophysiological and pharmacological aspects of somnambulism and night terrors in children. In Meltzer HY (Ed), *Psychopharmacology: The Third Generation of Progress*. New York, NY: Raven Press, 1987; 873–9.
7. Warnes H, Osivka S, Montplaisir J. Somnambulistic-like behaviour induced by lithium-neuroleptic treatment. *Sleep Res* 1993; **22**: 287.
8. Mendelson WB. Sleepwalking associated with zolpidem. *J Clin Psychopharmacol* 1994; **14**: 150.
9. Harazin J, Berigan TR. Zolpidem tartrate and somnambulism. *Mil Med* 1999; **164**: 669–70.
10. Schenk CH, Mahowald MW. Two cases of premenstrual sleep terrors and injurious sleep-walking. *J Psychosom Obstet Gynecol* 1995; **16**: 79–84.
11. Snyder S. Unusual case of sleep terror in a pregnant patient. *Am J Psychiatry* 1986; **143**: 391.
12. Berlin RM. Sleepwalking disorder during pregnancy: A case report. *Sleep* 1988; **11**: 298–300.
13. Mahowald MW, Shenck CH. REM sleep parasomnias. In Kryger MH, Roth T, Dement WC (Eds), *Principles and Practice of Sleep Medicine*, 4th edition. Philadelphia, PA: Elseviers Saunders, 2005; 897–916.
14. Plazzi G, Montagna P. Remitting REM sleep behaviour disorder as the initial sign of multiple sclerosis. *Sleep Med* 2002; **3**: 437–9.
15. Tippmann-Peikert M, Boeve BF, Keegan BM. REM sleep behaviour disorder initiated by acute brainstem multiple sclerosis. *Neurology* 2006; **66**: 1278–9.
16. Mathis J, Hess CW, Bassetti C. Isolated mediotegmental lesion causing narcolepsy and rapid eye movement sleep behaviour disorder: A case evidencing a common pathway in narcolepsy and rapid eye movement sleep behaviour disorder. *J Neurol Neurosurg Psychiatry* 2007; **78**: 427–9.
17. Cochen V, Arnulf I, Demeret S, *et al*. Vivid dreams, hallucinations, psychosis and REM sleep in Guillain–Barré syndrome. *Brain* 2005; **128**: 2535–45.
18. Sforza E, Krieger J, Petiau C. REM sleep behaviour disorder: Clinical and physiopathological findings. *Sleep Med Rev* 1997; **1**: 57–69.
19. Friedman JH, Fernandez HH, Sudarsky LR. REM behavior disorder and excessive daytime somnolence in Machado–Joseph disease (SCA-3). *Mov Disord* 2003; **18**: 1520–2.
20. Boesch SM, Frauscher B, Brandauer E, *et al*. Disturbance of rapid eye movement sleep in spinocerebellar ataxia type 2. *Mov Disord* 2006; **21**: 1751–4.
21. Liguori R, Vincent A, Clover L, *et al*. Morvan's syndrome: Peripheral and central nervous system and cardiac involvement with antibodies to voltage-gated potassium channel. *Brain* 2001; **124**: 2417–26.
22. Lugaresi E, Provini F, Montagna P. The neuroanatomy of sleep. Considerations on the role of the thalamus in sleep and proposal for a caudorostral organization. *Eur J Anat* 2004; **8**: 85–93.
23. Iranzo A, Graus F, Clover L, *et al*. Rapid eye movement sleep behavior disorder and potassium channel antibody-associated limbic encephalitis. *Ann Neurol* 2006; **59**: 178–82.
24. Thirumulai SS, Shubin RA, Robinson R. Rapid eye movement sleep behaviour disorder in children with autism. *J Child Neurol* 2002; **17**: 173–8.
25. Trajanovic NN, Voloh I, Shapiro C, *et al*. REM sleep behaviour disorder in a child with Tourette's Syndrome. *Can J Neurol Sci* 2004; **31**: 572–5.
26. Kohyama J, Shimohira M, Kondo S, *et al*. Motor disturbance during REM sleep in a group A xeroderma pigmentosum. *Acta Neurol Scand* 1995; **92**: 91–5.
27. Gagnon JF, Postuma R, Mazza S, *et al*. Rapid-eye-movement sleep behaviour disorder and neurodegenerative diseases. *Lancet Neurol* 2006; **5**: 424–32.
28. Iranzo A, Molinuevo JL, Santamaria J, *et al*. Rapid-eye-movement sleep behaviour disorder as an early marker for a neurodegenerative disorder: A descriptive study. *Lancet Neurol* 2006; **5**: 572–7.

29. Thomas A, Bonanni L, Onofrj M. Symptomatic REM sleep behaviour disorder. *Neurol Sci* 2007; **28**: S21–36.

30. Gagnon JF, Petit d, Fantini ML, *et al.* REM sleep behavior disorder and REM sleep without atonia in probable Alzheimer Disease. *Sleep* 2006; **29**: 1321–5.

31. Arnulf I, Mabrouk T, Mohamed K, *et al.* Stages 1–2 non-rapid eye movement sleep behavior disorder associated with dementia: A new parasomnia? *Mov Disord* 2005; **20**: 1223–8.

32. Gagnon JF, Bedard MA, Fantini ML, *et al.* REM sleep behavior disorder and REM sleep without atonia in Parkinson's disease. *Neurology* 2002; **59**: 585–9.

33. Olson EJ, Boeve BF, Silber MH. Rapid eye movement sleep behaviour disorder: Demographic, clinical and laboratory findings in 93 cases. *Brain* 2000; **123**: 331–9.

34. Vendette M, Gagnon JF, Decary A, *et al.* REM sleep behaviour disorder predicts cognitive impairment in Parkinson disease without dementia. *Neurology* 2007; **69**: 1843–9.

35. Postuma RB, Gagnon JF, Vendette M, *et al.* REM sleep behaviour disorder in Parkinson's disease is associated with specific motor features. *J Neurol Neurosurg Psychiatry* 2008; **79**: 1117–21.

36. Scaglione C, Vignatelli L, Plazzi G, *et al.* REM sleep behaviour disorder in Parkinson's disease: A questionnaire-based study. *Neurol Sci* 2005; **25**: 316–21.

37. Gjerstad MD, Boeve B, Wentzel-Larsen T, *et al.* Occurrence and clinical correlates of REM sleep behaviour disorder in patients with Parkinson's disease over time. *J Neurol Neurosurg Psychiatry* 2008; **79**: 387–91.

38. Kumru H, Santamaria J, Tolosa E, *et al.* Relation between subtype of Parkinson's disease and REM sleep behavior disorder. *Sleep Med* 2007; **8**: 779–83.

39. Boeve BF, Silber MH, Ferman TJ, *et al.* REM sleep behavior disorder and degenerative dementia: An association likely reflecting Lewy body disease. *Neurology* 1998; **51**: 363–70.

40. Boeve BF, Silber MH, Ferman TJ, *et al.* Association of REM sleep behavior disorder and neurodegenerative disease may reflect an underlying synucleinopathy. *Mov Disord* 2001; **16**: 622–30.

41. Boeve BF, Silber MH, Parisi JE, *et al.* Synucleinopathy pathology and REM sleep behavior disorder plus dementia or parkinsonism. *Neurology* 2003; **61**: 40–5.

42. McKeith IG, Perry EC, Perry RH, *et al.* Report of the second dementia with Lewy body international workshop: Diagnosis and treatment. Consortium on dementia with Lewy bodies. *Neurology* 1999; **53**: 902–05.

43. Uchiyama M, Isse K, Tanaka K, *et al.* Incidental Lewy body disease in a patient with REM behaviour disorder. *Neurology* 1995; **45**: 709–12.

44. Plazzi G, Corsini R, Provini F, *et al.* REM sleep behavior disorders in multiple system atrophy. *Neurology* 1997; **48**: 1094–7.

45. Tachibana N, Kimura K, Kitajima K, *et al.* REM sleep motor dysfunction in multiple system atrophy: With special emphasis on sleep talk and its early clinical manifestation. *J Neurol Neurosurg Psychiatry* 1997; **63**: 678–81.

46. Iranzo A, Santamaria J, Rye D, *et al.* Characteristics of idiopathic REM sleep behavior disorder and that associated with MSA and PD. *Neurology* 2005; **65**: 247–52.

47. Vetrugno R, Provini F, Cortelli P, *et al.* Sleep disorders in multiple system atrophy: A correlative video-polysomnographic study. *Sleep Med* 2004; **5**: 21–30.

48. Plazzi G, Cortelli P, Montagna P, *et al.* REM sleep behaviour disorder differentiates pure autonomic failure from multiple system atrophy with autonomic failure. *J Neurol Neurosurg Psychiatry* 1998; **64**: 683–5.

49. Weyer A, Minnerop M, Abele M, *et al.* REM sleep behavioral disorder in pure autonomic failure (PAF). *Neurology* 2006; **66**: 608–09.

50. Kauffman H, Nahm K, Purohit D, *et al.* Autonomic failure as the initial presentation of Parkinson disease and dementia with Lewy bodies. *Neurology* 2004; **63**: 1093–5.

51. Shenck CH, Mahowald MW, Anderson ML, *et al.* Lewy body variant of Alzheimer disease (AD) identified by post-mortem ubiquitin staining in a previously reported case of AD associated with REM sleep behaviour disorder. *Biol Psychiatry* 1997; **42**: 527–8.

52. Montplaisir J, Petit D, Decary A, *et al.* Sleep and quantitative EEG in patients with progressive supranuclear palsy. *Neurology* 1997; **49**: 999–1003.

53. Arnulf I, Merino-Andreu M, Bloch F, *et al.* REM sleep behaviour disorder and REM sleep without atonia in patients with progressive supranuclear palsy. *Sleep* 2005; **28**: 349–54.

54. Kimura K, Tachibana N, Aso T, *et al.* Subclinical REM sleep behavior disorder in a patient with corticobasal degeneration. *Sleep* 1997; **20**: 891–4.

55. Wetter TC, Brunner H, Collado-Seidel W, *et al.* Sleep and periodic limb movements in corticobasal degeneration. *Sleep Med* 2002; **3**: 33–6.

56. Zucconi M, Marcone A, Iannaccone S, *et al.* REM sleep behaviour in dementia: Preliminary results in

clinically diagnosed frontotemporal dementia. *Sleep* 2004; **27**(suppl): A317.

57. Boeve BF, Lin SC, Strongosky A, et al. Absence of rapid eye movement sleep behavior disorder in 11 members of the pallidopontonigral degeneration kindred. *Arch Neurol* 2006; **63**: 268–72.

58. Manni R, Terzaghi M. REM behaviour disorder associated with epileptic seizures. *Neurology* 2005; **64**: 883.

59. Husain AM, Miller PP, Carwile ST. REM sleep behavior disorder: Potential relationship to post traumatic stress disorder. *J Clin Neurophysiol* 2001; **18**: 148–57.

60. Costa CS, Macedo CR, Lopes EA, et al. Study of posttraumatic stress disorder (PTSD): Causes, neuro-psychic consequences and concomitant symptoms in patients with sleep disorders. *Sleep* 2006; **29**(suppl): A0874.

61. Bental E, Lavie P, Sharf B. Severe hypermotility during sleep treatment of cataplexy with clomipramine. *Isr J Med Sci* 1979; **15**: 607–09.

62. Matsumoto M, Mutoh F, Nahoe H, et al. The effects of imipramine on REM sleep behaviour disorder in three cases. *Sleep Res* 1991; **20**: 35.

63. Bamford CR. Carbamazepine in REM sleep behaviour disorder. *Sleep* 1993; **16**: 33–4.

64. Niiyama Y, Shimizu T, Abe M, et al. Cortical reactivity in REM sleep with tonic mentalis EMG activity induced by clomipramine: An evaluation by slow vertex response. *Electroencephalogr Clin Neurophysiol* 1993; **86**: 247–51.

65. Louden MB, Morehead MA, Schmidt HS. Activation by selegiline (Eldepryle) of REM sleep behavior disorder in parkinsonism. *W V Med J* 1995; **91**: 101.

66. Akindele MO, Evns JI, Oswald I. Mono-amine oxidase inhibitors, sleep and mood. *Electroencephalogr Clin Neurophysiol* 1979; **29**: 47–56.

67. Shenck CH, Mahowald MW, Kim SW, et al. Prominent eye movements during NREM sleep and REM sleep behavioural disorder associated with fluoxetine treatment of depression and obsessive–compulsive disorder. *Sleep* 1992; **15**: 226–35.

68. Winkelman JW, James L. Serotoninergic antidepressants are associated with REM sleep without atonia. *Sleep* 2004; **27**: 317–21.

69. Onofrj M, Luciano AL, Thomas A, et al. Mirtazapine induces REM sleep behavior disorder (RBD) in parkinsonism. *Neurology* 2003; **60**: 113–5.

70. Yamaoto K, Uchimura N, Habukawa M, et al. Evaluation of the effects of paroxetine in the treatment of REM sleep behavior disorder. *Sleep Biol Rhythms* 2006; **4**: 190.

71. Iranzo A, Santamaria J. Bisoprolol-induced rapid eye movement sleep behavior disorder. *Am J Med* 1999; **107**: 390–2.

72. Onofrj M, Thomas A, D'Andreamatteo G, et al. Incidence of RBD and hallucination in patients affected by Parkinson's disease: 8-year follow-up. *Neurol Sci* 2002; **23**(suppl 2): S91–4.

73. Carlander B, Touchon J, Ondze B, et al. REM sleep behaviour disorder induced by cholinergic treatment in Alzheimer's disease. *J Sleep Res* 1996; **5**(suppl 1): 28.

74. Silber MH. REM sleep behavior disorder associated with barbiturate withdrawal. *J Sleep Res* 1996; **25**: 371.

75. Tachibana M, Tanaka K, Hishikawa Y, et al. A sleep study of acute psychotic states due to alcohol and meprobamate addiction. *Adv Sleep Res* 1975; **2**: 177–205.

76. Sugano T, Suenaga K, Endo S, et al. Withdrawal delirium in a patient with nitrazepam addiction. *Jpn J EEG EMG* 1980; **8**: 34–5.

77. Atsumi Y, Kojima T, Matsu'ura M, et al. Polygraphic study of altered consciousness effect of biperiden on EEG and EOG. *Annu Rep Res Psychotrop Drugs* 1977; **9**: 171–81.

78. Stolz SE, Aldrich MS. REM sleep behaviour disorder associated with caffeine abuse. *Sleep Res* 1991; **20**: 341.

79. Vorona RD, Ware JC. Exacerbation of REM sleep behaviour disorder by chocolate ingestion: A case report. *Sleep Med* 2002; **3**: 365–7.

80. Arnulf I, Bonnet AM, Damier P, et al. Hallucinations, REM sleep and Parkinson's disease: A medical hypothesis. *Neurology* 2000; **55**: 281–8.

81. Comella CL, Tanner CM, Ristanovic RK. Polysomnographic sleep measures in Parkinson's disease patients with treatment-induced hallucinations. *Ann Neurol* 1993; **34**: 710–4.

82. Manni R, Pacchetti C, Terzaghi M, et al. Hallucinations and sleep–wake cycle in PD: A 24-hour continuous polysomnographic study. *Neurology* 2002; **59**: 1979–81.

83. Sinforiani E, Zangaglia R, Manni R, et al. REM sleep behavior disorder, hallucinations and cognitive impairment in Parkinson's disease. *Mov Disord* 2006; **21**: 462–6.

84. Howell MJ, Shenck CH, Crow SJ. A review of nighttime eating disorders. *Sleep Med Rev* 2009; **13**: 23–34.

85. Gluck ME, Geliebter A, Satov T. Night eating syndrome is associated with depression, low self-esteem, reduced daytime hunger, and less weight loss in obese outpatients. *Obes Res* 2001; **9**: 264–7.

86. Striegel-Moore RH, Dohm FA, Hook JM, et al. Night eating syndrome in young adult women: Prevalence and correlates. *Int J Eat Disord* 2005; **37**: 200–06.

87. Vetrugno R, Manconi M, Ferini-Strambi L, et al. Nocturnal eating: Sleep related eating disorder or night eating syndrome? A video-polysomnographic study. *Sleep* 2006; **29**: 949–54.

88. Guilleminault C, Kirisoglu C, Bao G, et al. Adult chronic sleepwalking and its treatment based on polysomnography. *Brain* 2005; **128**: 1062–9.

89. Guilleminault C, Palombini L, Pelayo R, et al. Sleepwalking and sleep terrors in prepubertal children: What triggers them? *Pediatrics* 2003; **111**: 17–25.

90. Goodwin JL, Kaemingk KL, Fregosi RF, et al. Parasomnias and sleep disordered breathing in Caucasian and Hispanic children – the Tucson children's assessment of sleep apnea study. *BMC Med* 2004; **28**: 14.

91. Millman RP, Kipp GJ, Carskadon MA. Sleepwalking precipitated by treatment of sleep apnea with nasal CPAP. *Chest* 1991; **99**: 750–1.

92. Barabas G, Ferrari M, Schemp Matthews W. Childhood migraine and somnambulism. *Neurology* 1983; **3**: 948–9.

93. Casez O, Dananchet D, Besson G. Migraine and somnambulism. *Neurology* 2005; **65**: 1334–5.

94. Evans RW. Exploding head syndrome followed by sleep paralysis: A rare migraine aura. *Headache* 2006; **46**: 682–3.

95. Kales JD, Kales A, Soldatos CR, et al. Sleepwalking and night terrors related to febrile illness. *Am J Psychiatr* 1979; **136**: 1214–5.

96. Eidlitz-Markus T, Zeharia A. Adolescent pertussis-induced partial arousal parasomnia. *Pediatric Neurology* 2006; **35**: 264–7.

97. Espa F, Dauvilliers Y, Ondze B, et al. Arousal reactions in sleepwalking and night terrors in adults: The role of respiratory events. *Sleep* 2002; **25**: 32–6.

98. Ajlouni KM, Ahmad AT, El-Zaheri MM, et al. Sleepwalking associated with hyperthyroidism. *Endocr Pract* 2005; **11**: 5–10.

99. Mouzas O, Angelopoulos N, Papaliagka M, et al. Increased frequency of self-reported parasomnias in patients suffering from vitiligo. *Eur J Dermatol* 2008; **18**: 165–8.

100. Costantino AEA, Waters C. Somnambulism in Parkinson's disease: Another sleep disorder to deal with. *Neurology* 2002; **58**(suppl 3): A432.

101. De Cock VC, Vidaileht M, Leu S, et al. Restoration of normal motor control in Parkinson's disease during REM sleep. *Brain* 2007; **130**: 450–6.

102. Poryazova R, Waldogel D, Bassetti CL. Sleepwalking in patients with Parkinson Disease. *Arch Neurol* 2007; **64**: 1524–7.

Introduction

Chapter 8: Trauma, post-traumatic stress disorder, and parasomnias

Thomas A. Mellman and Anissa M. Maroof

Introduction

Post-traumatic stress disorder (PTSD) is unique among psychiatric conditions in requiring an antecedent stressful event while also being defined as a specific syndrome. The type of life stressors that have been linked to PTSD are defined as severely threatening, often involving threats to life and/or physical integrity. The Diagnostic and Statistical Manual (DSM-IV) further requires that the traumatic event be experienced with fear, helplessness or horror [1]. Symptoms of PTSD include re-experiencing the trauma in the form of intrusive recollections, nightmares, and sometimes flashbacks; emotional numbing and avoidance of trauma reminders; and symptoms of increased arousal that include difficulty initiating and maintaining sleep. To meet diagnostic criteria, these symptoms must last for more than one month and lead to significant distress or impairment. According to the National Comorbidity Study, 10% of women and 5% of men in the United States have had PTSD during their lifetime. PTSD developed in 8% of the men and 20% of the women exposed to qualifying trauma. Kessler *et al.* also determined that the highest risk traumas for developing PTSD were sexual assault and military combat. PTSD was found to have a chronic course in approximately one-third of those affected, along with high rates of psychiatric comorbidity, with major depression, substance use disorders, and other anxiety disorders being the most frequently represented conditions [2].

Difficulties with sleep are a prominent feature of the disorder. The DSM-IV criteria specifically include nightmares with trauma-related content and difficulty with sleep initiation and maintenance. While there is some uncertainty and controversy about the nature of sleep disturbances in PTSD, studies that will be subsequently reviewed indicate that there can be more to sleep disturbance in PTSD than nightmares and insomnia, including awakening with fear in the absence of dream recall, excessive motor activity and dream enactment.

Parasomnias are defined in the fourth edition of *Principles and Practice of Sleep Medicine* as undesirable physical or behavioral phenomena that occur during sleep [3]. They are categorized based on whether they are associated with REM or NREM sleep. Behaviors observed in parasomnias include ambulating, talking, screaming and shaking. Parasomnias associated with REM sleep are sometimes attributed to the physical acting out of dreams. Thus, there is overlap between phenomena observed in PTSD and parasomnias. In addition, there have been anecdotal observations and some limited documentation of parasomnias in association with trauma exposure and PTSD. Since we view parasomnia-like experiences as part of a continuum of PTSD-related sleep phenomena, we have included sections reviewing findings regarding insomnia, nightmares, and polysomnographic evaluations of REM and NREM sleep. We then discuss observations of motor activity during sleep in PTSD and the limited information available on complex sleep-related behaviors.

Trauma, PTSD, and insomnia

Insomnia is common in the aftermath of trauma and can persist and contribute to dysfunction among those who develop PTSD. Green found insomnia to be the most frequent symptom endorsed by survivors within 1–4 months of several natural disasters [4]. In the National Vietnam Veterans Readjustment study, 44% of the veterans with PTSD endorsed difficulty with sleep initiation either "sometimes" or "very frequently", compared with 6% of veterans without PTSD, and 5% of civilians and 91% of veterans with PTSD reported this degree of difficulty with sleep maintenance compared with 63% of the veterans without PTSD, and 53% of the civilians [5]. A community survey conducted by Ohayon and Shapiro determined that 41–47% of the participants with PTSD had difficulty initiating or maintaining sleep compared to 13–18% of those without PTSD [6].

In contrast to the consistency of these subjective reports, findings regarding the presence of objective indices of impaired sleep initiation and maintenance in PTSD have been mixed. A recent meta-analysis of 20 polysomnographic studies found that patients with PTSD exhibited more stage 1 sleep, less SWS, and greater REM density compared to those without PTSD [7]. The possibility that an ameliorative effect of a sleep laboratory has influenced sleep laboratory findings in PTSD (e.g. feeling safe due to being observed; arousal having been conditioned to home environments) is suggested by two recent studies that utilized home monitoring and found associations of PTSD with increased sleep latency and reduced sleep efficiency [8,9].

Sleep-disordered breathing can be an underlying cause for disrupted sleep patterns. Krakow and colleagues reported very high rates of sleep breathing disorders (apnea and upper airway resistance syndrome) in a group of female research participants seeking treatment for PTSD related to sexual assault [10]. They subsequently noted improvement of PTSD symptoms with treatment of sleep breathing disorders. A study that recruited PTSD cases from a community sample, however, did not find elevated rates of sleep apnea or other primary sleep disorders [11].

Trauma, PTSD, and nightmares

Sleep disturbances and nightmares are a normal and characteristic response to trauma [12]; however, they tend to be transient features that resolve with time. In some individuals, sleep disturbances and nightmares endure typically as a feature of PTSD. Dreams have been theorized to have an adaptive role in emotional processing and mood regulation [13]. Recurring nightmares appear to represent an impairment of this process.

Nightmares are among the most prominent complaints of patients with PTSD. DeFazio et al. found that 68% of combat veterans with PTSD reported ongoing nightmares [14]. This contrasts rates for nightmares of 8% reported for subjects without PTSD [15]. Neylan et al. studied veterans with and without PTSD, and found that 52% of those with PTSD reported experiencing nightmares either "sometimes" or "very frequently", compared to 5% of veterans without PTSD [5]. Dreams that represent traumatic experiences have been characterized as highly specific to and a "hallmark" of PTSD [16]. Several studies have documented persisting nightmares representing combat experiences [5,17–19]. However, dream content during the chronic phase of PTSD can represent threat in other contexts and reflect a variety of themes and situations [20,21]. In a study that evaluated spontaneously recalled dreams during the early aftermath of trauma, Mellman et al. found that surgical patients who reported distressing dreams that they rated as similar to their memory of the trauma had more severe PTSD symptoms concurrently and at follow-up [22].

PTSD and REM sleep

The prominence of disturbing nightmares that represent traumatic experiences in PTSD and the relationship between REM sleep and dream mentation has focused investigators on the role of this sleep stage in the disorder. In their seminal paper, Ross et al. inferred that PTSD-related nightmares are related to REM sleep due to their often being disturbing, vivid, affect-laden, and associated with sleep paralysis and "hypnopompic hallucinations" [16]. Many of the findings from PSG studies of PTSD relate to REM sleep. The meta-analysis performed by Kobayashi et al. noted increased eye movement density with PTSD [7]. This finding has also been noted in major depressive disorder (MDD); however, in a study by Ross et al., in individuals with MDD increased REM density was observed earlier in the night during the first REM period, while those with PTSD had increased REM density through the entire night [23]. Other findings relate to peripheral motor activity. Ross et al. found a higher incidence of phasic EMG bursts in their PTSD patients relative to controls, and related this finding to phenomena observed in REM behavior disorder (RBD) [23]. An earlier report of PSG findings in trauma survivors noted excessive, at times "violent" movements during REM sleep [24].

There are also findings suggesting disruption to REM sleep continuity with PTSD. While nightmares and anxious awakenings can be preceded by NREM sleep in PTSD, findings from Mellman et al. [17] and Woodward et al. [25] indicate that the majority are preceded by REM sleep. Breslau *et al.* reported more frequent transitions from REM sleep to stage one or awake, in a community sample with either lifetime only (i.e. remitted) or current PTSD, compared with trauma-exposed and trauma-unexposed controls [11]. A recent clinical study from Japan noted "REM interruption" in association with PTSD [26]. In a study that uniquely obtained PSG recordings within a month of trauma exposure, Mellman *et al.* found that the patients who were developing PTSD had shorter continuous periods of REM sleep prior to stage shifts or arousals [27]. Thus, there is also converging evidence for disruptions of REM sleep continuity (symptomatic awakenings, increased awakening/arousals, and motor activity) and increased REM activation with PTSD.

PTSD and body/limb movement during sleep

In a survey from Inman *et al.* that compared 35 Vietnam veterans with PTSD and 37 individuals with insomnia, the PTSD group was more likely to report waking up with the covers torn apart, restless legs in bed, and excessive body movement during sleep [28]. Lavie and Hertz reported that individuals with "combat neurosis", now called PTSD, following the Yom Kippur War showed higher rates of body movement during stage 2 sleep compared to controls [29]. Other studies with objective sleep measures have also reported increased body movements during sleep in patients with PTSD relative to controls including limb movements [17,30] and the aforementioned phasic EMG activity during REM sleep [23]. One limitation to these finding is that these studies include older age males who have a higher propensity to develop body/limb movements during sleep, usually as a result of their medical illness. Thus, it is difficult to differentiate whether these movements observed during sleep in PTSD patients are secondary to their PTSD or a primary sleep disorder such as periodic limb movements.

PTSD and parasomnias

These preceding sections indicate the overlap between parasomnias and sleep-related phenomena described in PTSD (vivid dreams, disrupted REM sleep, and excessive motor activity). Documentation of parasomnias per se with PTSD in the clinical research literature is limited. In a series of 33 cases presenting with parasomnias, Schenk *et al.* describe a case where the onset of "violent parasomnias" coincided with the onset of PTSD and major depression in a veteran of military combat. Humphreys *et al.* described 28 children in whom domestic violence was associated with sleep disruption [31]. One of the children manifested "sleepwalking" which began at the same time as PTSD symptoms.

In their survey of 35 patients with combat-related PTSD and 37 patients with insomnia, Inman *et al.* reported that endorsements of "sleep talking", "yelling or shouting during sleep", and "waking up with covers torn apart" were greater in the PTSD group [28]. The survey responses were scaled from "1" (not at all) to "7" (always). Mean endorsements for these items ranged between 4.2 and 5.6, indicating a relatively frequent pattern of occurrence. Mellman *et al.* surveyed 58 combat veterans of whom 37 were found to meet criteria for PTSD [17]. More of the veterans with PTSD endorsed thrashing/violent movements during sleep, night terrors, and sleep paralysis. These episodes were endorsed as occurring weekly or more by 59%, 38%, and 24% of the veterans with PTSD, respectively.

As indicated in a previous section much of the focus in the PTSD literature has been on REM sleep phenomena. Parasomnia disorders that relate specifically to the REM stage include RBD. RBD features limb or body movements associated with dream mentation, and harmful sleep behaviors, acting out of dreams, and/or disruption of sleep continuity by abnormal behavior. Overlap of REM and NREM related parasomnias is indicated by the Schenk *et al.* case series, where 16 of the 33 cases had both RBD and sleep walking or sleep terrors [32]. In their paper reporting increased phasic motor bursts during REM sleep, Ross *et al.* proposed a link between this phenomenon and RBD [24]. Overlap between clinical populations diagnosed with RBD and PTSD is preliminarily suggested in a report by Husain *et al.*, where a comorbid diagnosis of PTSD was noted in 56% of 27 outpatients who met criteria for RBD [33]. In the case described by Schenck *et al.* with PTSD, the patient had violent movements during sleep, and EMG activity similar to that described in RBD was observed [32].

Sleep paralysis is also a phenomenon of REM sleep where the suppression of motor tone that is normally confined to REM sleep persists into awakening. As noted above, a preliminary survey of combat veterans found increased frequencies of sleep paralysis among those with PTSD. Hinton *et al.* reported high rates of sleep paralysis in a population of Cambodian refugees that was highly trauma exposed [34]. Rates were significantly elevated among the PTSD patients, where 65% (30/46) had monthly episodes of sleep paralysis compared with 15% (8/54) of those who did not have PTSD. Sleep paralysis was also associated with PTSD severity in their study. In contrast, Mellman *et al.* did not find an association between sleep paralysis and PTSD in an adult African American population attending primary care clinics, but did find an association with trauma exposure [35].

Summary and implications

Clinicians who work with patients with PTSD are frequently made aware of complaints of restless sleep, a propensity toward thrashing and violent movements during sleep, and physical enactments related to dream activity. None the less, clinical research data characterizing these phenomena and their overlap with parasomnia disorders is quite limited. As noted in the preceding section, descriptions of parasomnia cases have noted co-occurrence with PTSD, and preliminary surveys of individuals with PTSD have reported endorsement of parasomnia-like experiences at rather high frequencies. Clearly, further research is indicated to determine the frequency, associated features, risk factors, and treatment response of complex sleep-related behaviors with PTSD.

Clinicians who evaluate patients with sleep disorders would be well advised to evaluate for histories of trauma and post-traumatic stress symptoms and those treating PTSD to evaluate for sleep problems including insomnia, sleep-disordered breathing, and complex sleep-related behaviors. There is little in the literature to guide treatment of parasomnia phenomena that occur with PTSD. The notion that the occurrence of parasomnias is influenced by concurrent stress is widespread in the literature. Therefore alleviating symptoms of PTSD and general distress which would usually involve psychotherapy and sometimes medication could serve to reduce the likelihood of undesirable behaviors emerging from sleep. The parasomnia literature refers to the use of the high potency benzodiazepine, clonazepam as a treatment. However, this category of medication is not recommended for the treatment of PTSD and can be associated with negative outcomes [1]. Due to the hypothesized role for excessive noradrenergic activity in mediating sleep aspects of PTSD, the alpha-1 adrenergic antagonist prazosin was applied to treating nightmares and sleep disruption in the disorder. Its efficacy in this regard has now been supported by two modest-sized controlled clinical trials of male combat veterans [36,37]. In these trials, the medication was dosed aggressively and used at mean doses of 9.5 and 13 mg at bedtime, respectively. Adverse blood pressure effects were infrequent and not severe. While ratings for nightmares and insomnia were significantly improved, outcomes related to complex sleep behaviors were not reported.

While much is to be learned regarding the co-occurrence of specific parasomnias with PTSD, it does appear that PTSD and parasomnia disorders can both feature phenomena that are manifestations of breakdowns of the barriers between the normally discreet states of sleep and wake. Elucidation of how trauma and the process of PTSD development can lead to such disruptions will benefit our knowledge of PTSD and primary sleep disorders.

References

1. American Psychiatric Association. *Diagnostic and Statistical Manual of Mental Disorders*, 4th Edition. Washington, D.C., American Psychiatric Press, 1994.
2. Kessler R, Sonnega A, Bromet E, *et al.* Posttraumatic stress disorder in the National Comorbidity Survey. *Arch Gen Psychiatry* 1995; **52**: 1048–60.
3. Mellman T, Pigeon W. Dreams and nightmares in posttraumatic stress disorder. In Kryger M, Roth T, Dement W (Eds), Stickgold R (section ed.), *Principles and Practices of Sleep Medicine*, 4th Edition. Phildelphia: Elsevier, 2005.
4. Green B. Disasters and posttraumatic stress disorder. In Davidson JRT, Foa EB (Eds), *Posttraumatic Stress Disorder DSM-IV and Beyond*. Washington, D.C., American Psychiatric Press, 1993; 75–97.
5. Neylan T, Marmar C, Metzler T, *et al.* Sleep disturbances in the Vietnam generation: findings from a nationally representative sample of male Vietnam veterans. *American Journal of Psychiatry* 1998; **155**: 929–33.
6. Ohayon M, Shapiro C. Sleep disturbances and psychiatric disorders associated with posttraumatic

7. Kobayashi H, Boarts J, Delahanty D. Polysomnographically measured sleep abnormalities in PTSD: a meta-analytic review. *Psychophysiology* 2007; **44**: 660–9.

8. Germain A, Hall M, Katherine Shear M, *et al.* Ecological study of sleep disruption in PTSD: a pilot study. *Ann NY Acad Sci.* 2006; **1071**: 438–41.

9. Calhoun P, Wiley M, Dennis M, *et al.* Objective evidence of sleep disturbance in women with posttraumatic stress disorder. *J Traumatic Stress* 2007; **20**: 1009–18.

10. Krakow B, Melendrez D, Johnston L, *et al.* Sleep-disordered breathing, psychiatric distress, and quality of life impairment in sexual assault survivors. *J Nerv & Ment Dis* 2002; **190**: 442–52.

11. Breslau N, Roth T, Burduvali E, *et al.* Sleep in lifetime posttraumatic stress disorder, a community-based polysomnographic study. *Arch Gen Psychiatry* 2004; **61**: 508–16.

12. Pillar G, Malhotra A, Lavie P. Post-traumatic stress disorder and sleep – what a nightmare! *Sleep Med Rev* 2000; **4**: 183–200.

13. Cartwright R, Lloyd S. Early REM sleep: a compensatory change in depression? *Psychiatry Res* 1994; **51**: 245–52.

14. DeFazio V, Rustin S, Diamond A. Symptom development in Vietnam era veterans. *Am J Orthopsychiatry* 1975; **45**: 158–63.

15. Belicki K, Belicki D. Predisposition for nightmares: a study of hypnotic ability, vividness of imagery, and absorption. *J Clin Psychol* 1986; **42**: 714–8.

16. Ross R, Ball W, Sullivan K, *et al.* Sleep disturbance as the hallmark of posttraumatic stress disorder. *Am J Psychiatry* 1989; **146**: 697–707.

17. Mellman T, Kulick-Bell R, Ashlock L, *et al.* Sleep events in combat-related post-traumatic stress disorder. *Am J Psychiatry* 1995; **152**: 110–15.

18. Schreuder B, van Egmond M, Kleijn W, *et al.* Nocturnal re-experiencing more than forty years after war trauma. *J Traumatic Stress* 2000; **13**: 453–63.

19. Van Der Kolk B, Blitz R, Burr W, *et al.* Nightmares and trauma: a comparison of nightmares after combat with lifelong nightmares in veterans. *Am J Psychiatry* 1984; **141**: 187–90.

20. Kramer M, Schoen L, Kinney L. Nightmares in Vietnam veterans. *J Am Acad Psychoanal* 1987; **15**: 67–81.

21. Esposito K, Benitez A, Barza L, Mellman T. Evaluation of dream reports in combat-related PTSD. *J Traumatic Stress* 1999; **12**: 681–7.

22. Mellman T, David D, Bustamante V, *et al.* Dreams in the acute aftermath of trauma and their relationship to PTSD. *J Traumatic Stress* 2001; **14**: 1526–30.

23. Ross R, Ball W, Dinges D, *et al.* Rapid eye movement sleep disturbance in posttraumatic stress disorder. *Biol Psychiatry* 1994; **35**: 195–202.

24. Hefez A, Metz L, Lavie P. Long term effects of extreme situational stress on sleep and dreaming. *Am J Psychiatry* 1987; **144**: 344–7.

25. Woodward S, Arsenault N, Santerre C, *et al.* Polysomnographic characteristics of trauma-related nightmares. Presented at Annual Meeting of Association of Professional Sleep Societies, Las Vegas, Nevada, June, 2000.

26. Habukawa M, Uchimura N, Maeda M, *et al.* Sleep findings in young adult patients with posttraumatic stress disorder. *Biol Psychiatry* 2007; **62**: 1179–82.

27. Mellman T, Bustamante V, Fins A, *et al.* REM sleep and the early development of posttraumatic stress disorder. *Am J Psychiatry* 2002; **159**: 1696–701.

28. Inman D, Silver S, Doghramji K. Sleep disturbance in post-traumatic stress disorder: a comparison with non-PTSD insomnia. *J Traumatic Stress* 1990; **3**: 429–37.

29. Lavie P, Hertz G. Increased sleep motility and respiration rates in combat neurotic patients. *Biol Psychiatry* 1979; **14**: 983–7.

30. Brown T, Boudewyns A. Periodic limb movements of sleep in combat veterans with posttraumatic stress disorder. *J Traumatic Stress* 1996; **9**: 129–36.

31. Humphreys C, Lowe P, Williams S. Sleep disruption and domestic violence: exploring the interconnections between mothers and children. *Child Family Soc Work* 2009; **14**: 6–14.

32. Schenck C, Hurwitz T, Mahowald, M. REM sleep behavior disorder. *Am J Psychiatry* 1988; **145**: 652.

33. Husain A, Miller P, Carwile S. REM sleep behavior disorder: potential relationship to post-traumatic stress disorder. *J Clin Neurophysiol* 2001; **18**: 148–57.

34. Hinton D, Pich V, Chhean D, *et al.* Sleep paralysis among Cambodian refugees: association with PTSD diagnosis and severity. *Depression & Anxiety* 2005; **22**: 47–51.

35. Mellman T, Aigbogun N, Graves R, *et al.* Sleep paralysis and trauma, psychiatric symptoms and disorders in an adult African American population attending primary medical care. *Depression & Anxiety* 2008; **25**: 435–40.

36. Raskind M, Peskind E, Kanter E, *et al*. Reduction of nightmares and other PTSD symptoms in combat veterans by prazosin: a placebo-controlled study. *Am J Psychiatry* 2003; **160**: 371–3.

37. Raskind M, Peskind E, Hoff D, *et al*. A parallel group placebo controlled study of prazosin for trauma nightmares and sleep disturbances in combat veterans with posttraumatic stress disorder. *Biol Psychiatry* 2007; **61**: 928–34.

Section 1 Chapter 9

Introduction

Sexsomnias

Nikola N. Trajanovic and Colin M. Shapiro

Introduction and historical overview

Sexual arousal and sleep have never been at odds. Some of the well-known physiological phenomena associated with sleep were described centuries ago, most notably "wet dreams", nocturnal emissions in males, and nocturnal orgasms in females. Yet, a review of scientific literature suggests that until fairly recently, there has been only a low level of interest in sleep-related sexual phenomena. The first mention of sexual behavior associated with sleep in the scientific literature was in 1955 by Albrecht Langeluddeke [1] who, as a forensic psychiatrist, had an opportunity to see patients charged with sleep-related offences. He described a case of an 18-year-old worker who slept in a dormitory with another 15 workers. On one occasion, this young worker apparently during the night crossed the passage between beds and climbed into another person's bunk bed, touched his genitals and thrust, mimicking a sexual act. When confronted, he was unresponsive, showed confusion and was amnesic about the event in the morning. Langeluddeke described an archetypical sexsomnia patient – a young person with a history of sleepwalking, who exhibited behavior out of his character, sexual interests and patterns, and presumably precipitated by at least one factor (some degree of sleep deprivation – late retiring), with a notation of minor and non-specific psychopathology and concomitant with another parasomnia (sleep talking). Worthy of note is that the patient was exculpated based on the clinical presentation and expert witness' testimony.

Afterward, it appears that any mention of sleep-related sexual behavior lay dormant until a description of a single case suggesting sleep-related masturbation emerged in 1986 [2]. Sporadically thereafter, scarce reports about unusual sexually oriented behaviors that appeared to have arisen from sleep began to be reported as case studies at sleep conferences or in academic journals [3–8]. Based on previous work [4], the first conceptualization of sexual behaviors during sleep was published in 2003 [9], and proposed that sexual behavior in sleep (SBS), or "sexsomnia" as it was termed, should be considered to be a new (sub)type of NREM arousal parasomnia. Since then, an increasing academic interest in this topic and (often unwanted) public and media attention have produced a number of papers and descriptions dealing with this issue. A leading authority in the field of sleep medicine, the American Academy of Sleep Medicine, quickly realized the need to include the newly described parasomnic variant in the updated classification of sleep disorders (ICSD 2, 2005) [10], and classify it as a distinct variant of NREM arousal parasomnias.

Scientific studies suggest that SBS covers almost all aspects of human sexual behavior: from masturbation and fondling, to heterosexual and homosexual intercourse, to anal and oral sex. Partners of those acting sexually in sleep were either willing or unwilling, and sometimes included minors below the age of consent.

Different terms have emerged to describe this behavior. In clinical settings, the preferred term is "sexual behavior in sleep", which is an umbrella construct that covers all types of underlying (sleep) pathology. It appears that the term "sleepsex" is accepted for public/lay use. The term "sexsomnia" is our preferred term that is mostly used as a clinical colloquialism, and specifically covers parasomnic SBS (often only NREM parasomnic SBS). In our opinion, terms such as "abnormal" and "atypical" that are sometimes used in conjunction with SBS add an unnecessary level of stigmatization on the already frustrated and bewildered individuals who suffer from sexsomnia.

The Parasomnias and Other Sleep-Related Movement Disorders, ed. M. J. Thorpy and G. Plazzi. Published by Cambridge University Press. © Cambridge University Press 2010.

Furthermore, by not correctly qualifying every type of behavior, these terms may worsen matters in patients' everyday lives and thus should be avoided. Two adjectives are currently in use to describe this specific type of parasomnic activity: "sexual" and "sexualized". The latter adjective pertains to simple automatisms that do not have true behavioral quality, lack an affective component and suggest a high level of stereotypy without true sexual context. This would include, for example, touching the groin in sleep and pelvic thrusting. For all other more complex and clearly sexually oriented behaviors, we recommend using the adjective "sexual".

Clinical features

NREM parasomnias

Parasomnias featuring disorders of arousal are well described, if not well understood, phenomena. Some of them, such as sleepwalking, have been known for centuries, with abundant references in classic literature and scientific publications alike. Two other major arousal parasomnias are sleep terrors (pavor nocturnus) and confusional arousals. The essence of this group of parasomnias lies in phenomena of incomplete awakening and uncoordinated sleep–wake mechanisms [11]. A major discrepancy between the level of motoric activation and level of consciousness exists, resulting in inappropriate, bizarre and often (self-)injurious behavior. The spectrum of the impairment of consciousness spans from mild, as seen in confusional arousals, to significant and profound, as seen in some forms of sleepwalking. At the same time, motor activity ranges from the seemingly purposeful actions seen in confusional arousals to clear automatism seen in sleepwalking and its variants.

Simple confusional arousals may present in the form of a person who sits up in bed partly awakened, being unable to orient himself to his whereabouts for minutes, to more complex behavior such as a person grabbing a lamp instead of a phone that rings in the middle of the night or someone running to work without putting his pants on. Described variants of sleepwalking are even more impressive – from simple flailing of a hand in sleep, to a complex behavior that may involve driving a vehicle or using a weapon [12–14].

While it is a common belief that a parasomniac is actually fully asleep while performing these actions, this is usually not the case. In most cases, parasomnic behavior, in particular hypnopompic paroxysmal

Table 9.1 Medical/psychiatric automatisms that may be sleep-related.

- Epileptic automatisms
- Sleep automatisms (e.g. sleepwalking, sleep terrors, sleep-related eating, sleep-related sexual behaviors)
- Alcohol and drug-induced automatisms
- Metabolic automatisms (e.g. resulting from hypoglycemia)
- Organic CNS automatisms (e.g. transient global amnesia)
- Psychogenic automatisms (e.g. dissociative disorders, such as psychogenic fugue)

behavior that features in disorders of arousal, does not occur in sleep, but instead arises from sleep. Corresponding brain activity shows a run of (usually) dominant delta wave sleep abruptly interrupted by either light sleep, or more often, brain activity typical for awakening obscured by movement artifacts.

There are factors that may precipitate parasomnic activity, the most common being sleep deprivation, stress, fever, medications and alcohol/substance abuse. There is also a significant familial pattern with further increase in incidence if both parents have a history of parasomnia (Table 9.1).

One interesting sleep disorder that includes complex parasomnia behavior is sleep-related eating. Individuals who exhibit this unusual behavior find themselves in a situation where they get up in sleep, walk to the fridge, and indiscriminately eat whatever food they are able to reach, having no recollection of the event in the morning. It is important to recognize that an individual who suffers from this sleep disorder exhibits highly specific and stereotypic automatism [15,16].

In the continuum of aberrant nocturnal behavior, parasomnias fall between neurological disorders, such as, for example, frontal lobe seizures without a clear EEG substrate, and psychiatric disorders of the dissociative type. Some seizure disorders (e.g. complex partial seizures and frontal lobe seizures) can feature behavior suggestive of parasomnia. At the other end of the continuum, the dissociative states, such as fugue, do not stem from sleep pathology. Their incidence is rare and the connection to pre-sleep, post-sleep or intervening wakefulness is relatively easy to establish, even in the case of nocturnal events. There is also a specific psychopathology and pattern that may include similar daytime episodes.

In the case of overlapping symptoms, it is not always easy to establish a correct diagnosis, even after extensive testing and examination. It is possible that an individual may suffer from two parasomnias at the same time, or have a parasomnia and concomitant non-parasomnic sleep disorder [7,17,18].

Sexsomnia

Over the past decade, a large body of evidence has emerged confirming that sexual behavior can be associated with sleep pathology. A significant number of case reports and first epidemiological [19] and meta studies [20,21] suggest that sexual behavior in sleep primarily represents a distinctive variation of known types of NREM arousal parasomnias. Varieties of sexual behaviors in sleep range from simple automatisms, such as a brief episode of masturbation, fondling or sleep talking, to more complex behaviors that may involve both partners, include sleepwalking, and/or result in complete intercourse. Both heterosexual and homosexual contacts are reported. Often, there is an alteration of sexual behavior characteristics for the patient, exhibiting behavior that is atypical during wakefulness. A relatively prim individual will "talk dirty" during sexsomnia experiences and, conversely, some are described to be particularly amorous in the context of sexsomnia but not so in their regular lovemaking. There are examples of a sexsomnia patient initiating sexual intercourse while asleep and then abruptly, to the dismay of his partner, terminating the tryst with what appears to be an unlikely and disconnected comment such as "That's enough of that" prior to climaxing. Simple vocalization aside from the sexual moaning may also be present. The duration is typically the same as in other parasomnias, lasting from less than a minute to up to 30 minutes and rarely any longer. In a clinical setting, a gender bias was evident (more men were seen); however, a recent Internet survey [19] suggested that females may exhibit this behavior considerably more than previously thought (31% of the survey sample were females). Also, in the clinical setting, the age bias resulted in more patients being in their 30s and 40s, whereas the survey showed a high number of adolescent and post-adolescent respondents (age ranging from 15 to 67, more than 80% being younger than 35).

Sexsomnia causes significant physical and psychological negative consequences in a majority of clinically assessed patients [22]. This is less so when taking a non-clinical sample into consideration. This could be explained by the fact that many individuals who exhibit some form of sexsomnia (and their partners) do not find the condition disturbing, while some even appreciate a break in their usual sexual routines. This is one of the reasons why the condition remained unrecognized for so long. Another reason lies in the very nature of the problem: not many clinicians would ask relevant questions and few patients would volunteer such delicate information.

A common concern regarding sexsomnia is that it may result in complete intercourse, which raises a question whether such behavior can truly arise from sleep. Sceptics posit that, in men, the adequate penile erection resulting in an emission requires sexual desire and sexual arousal, which is accentuated by external stimuli and requires a certain level of cognition. Keeping this in mind, some of the fundamentals of human physiology need to be revisited in order to better understand the incidence of sexsomnia.

The existence of sleep-related penile erections (SRE) was first described seven decades ago and constitutes a common sleep phenomenon. As observed by Karacan *et al.* [23], SREs primarily occur in REM sleep but may, in a minority of events, occur in NREM sleep. Another common sleep phenomenon, albeit typically associated with puberty and adolescence, are "wet dreams", and they include both the SREs and sexual context through imagery internally generated during REM sleep. However, dream mentation is not necessarily associated only with REM sleep and can appear in a number of NREM parasomnias and sleep talking [11,24]. There is some evidence that approximately one-quarter of apparent "dream mentations" occur in NREM sleep. Thus, both the SREs and dream mentation could be seen in association with NREM sleep. This may be more so during an incomplete awakening seen in NREM parasomnias.

A prerequisite for motor aspects of sexsomnia is a propensity towards dissociation between higher cortical and motor centers typically seen in all of the NREM arousal parasomnias. Additional factors precipitating and perpetuating sexual behavior could be different types of contact stimulation (touching, rubbing) [19], often initiated by a bed partner that may, to some degree, replace or complement rudimentary sexual imagery. These points may explain how, in the absence of a clear sexual motivation guided by higher cortical structures, complex sexual behavior may emerge and run its course out of sleep. In the case of simpler sexual behaviors, one can appreciate that in the absence of sexual arousal (lack of penile erections or vaginal lubrication), sexual automatisms such as groping, fondling or sexualized moaning could be easily understood. In fact, a compellingly large number of sexsomnia patients engage in behaviors that do not reach climax (orgasm or ejaculations) in sleep.

In addition, one should also keep in mind that the normal sleep-related physiological phenomena of the sexual type, like morning penile erections that come with sexual arousal (stemming from a REM episode immediately preceding awakening), nocturnal vaginal lubrication, and "wet dreams" (nocturnal emission) may happen not only in sleep but also immediately after awakening. A similar pattern of post-sleep behaviors occurs in confusional arousals, a type of NREM arousal parasomnia, which is one of the reasons for the current classification of sexsomnia as a distinct variant of parasomnia.

Diagnosis of sexsomnia

Different factors may lead to complex sexual behavior in sleep. As in other NREM arousal parasomnias, there is usually a precipitating factor. A common conception is that sleep deprivation, alcohol or substance abuse and stress are the major precipitators of parasomnias [25]. An Internet survey [19] showed that, at least in the non-clinical setting, leading precipitators are physical contact, stress and fatigue, while substance abuse and use of alcohol remained reported by considerably fewer respondents (4 to 1 in favor of body contact). The issue of aberrant sexual drive remains unanswered in the absence of structured research addressing this issue.

Parasomnia behavior may be described during office visits, reported by a family member (a spouse or parent), a referring physician, a bed partner, or revealed during polysomnographic studies. Schenk et al. [20] make a very important point regarding the inclusion of specific questions into the standard sleep questionnaire that is given to patients during the office visits. Their proposal to include at least two questions is well-founded ("Has your libido or sexual activity changed, either while you are awake, or falling asleep, or during your sleep?" and "Has your bed partner observed any sexual vocalizations or sexual behaviors on your part while you are asleep?"). One of the most important aspects of clinical assessment is heteroanamnestic information from a bed partner (both past and present) or a witness, which could be extremely valuable in determining the nature of nocturnal sexual behavior. The physical examination often reveals physical injury to the patient or bed partner (bruises, lacerations, ecchymoses), often in relation to violent masturbation, aggressive fondling, holding of wrists, etc. Psychological testing may reveal thrill-seeking personality traits, negative emotions (guilt, shame, confusion, denial, anger, embarrassment), as well as ideas of infidelity, inadequacy, suspicion or rejection of partners.

Information about medication use does not provide any conclusive "tipping point" regarding diagnostic patterns. A small number of patients have been reported to be on selective serotonin re-uptake inhibitor (SSRI) medication (3% of one sample) at the time of their sexsomnia. In fewer instances, prompting some caution, patients were on anti-histamines, hormonal contraceptives [26], and zolpidem [27]. The latter medication was associated with sexsomnia in two patients and both the concomitant sleep-eating and sexsomnia episodes in one of the studied patients [20]. Use of SSRIs in patients who exhibit some form of sexsomnia merits caution, as it was also reported to be associated with *de novo* sexsomnia in a 30-year-old patient who had repeated episodes after starting treatment with escitalopram for his newly diagnosed depression [28]. Caution should be extended also to other serotonergic or non-serotonergic [29–31] antidepressant medications which could be connected to NREM parasomnia.

The family history is often positive for parasomnias and/or other sleep disorders. Personal history typically reveals other types of parasomnic behaviors aside from sexual or other concomitant sleep disorders (up to 50% of the queried sample [19], with disorders such as sleep-disordered breathing, insomnia, etc.) or concomitant mental disorder (up to 30% of the queried sample, with the highest incidence of depression and anxiety disorders).

The polysomnographic investigation may reveal some type of parasomnic activity most often related to SWS and sleep–wake or inter-sleep stage transitions. Sharp, abrupt, well-delineated SWS/NREM arousals are often seen, and they are typically disassociated from other sleep pathology, such as respiratory events or limb movements. In a small number of patients who suffer from concomitant sleep apnoea, causality between sleep disruption and onset of a parasomnic episode has been established, leading to an appropriate treatment. Abrupt SWS/NREM arousal itself is a moderately pathognomonic PSG finding, and confirms rather than establishes a diagnosis of parasomnia [32]. Patients who suffer from an NREM parasomnia typically have, on average, up to 50% more slow-wave sleep than their peers; such a finding in a patient with sexsomnia could be expected [33]. A hypersynchronous delta activity during the pre-paroxysmal periods has been reported by researchers in association to sexsomnia, but its true diagnostic value remains to be confirmed.

Standard PSG recording with the usual set of 6–8 EEG leads is certainly better than no PSG recording. However, for proper diagnosis, a full-EEG video PSG monitoring together with an extensive EMG monitoring that includes both legs and arms should be carried out. The PSG assessment should be scheduled for a minimum of two nights and should replicate a patient's home sleep pattern in as many elements as possible, including the bed-sharing that will involve the patient's partner in order to induce body contact and force arousals. In addition, anything obscuring the view should be removed if the patient is agreeable. A frank parasomnic activity in the form of the sexual behavior in sleep is rarely seen, even with a bed partner present (parasomnic behavior is typically less frequent in the clinical setting versus the patient's home); however, confusional arousals without sexual content could be expected. If possible, PSG investigation should be scheduled to include both a baseline and a sleep-deprivation night [34]. When the bed partner is not available, parasomnic behavior could be induced (precipitated) by another external arousing stimuli, such as a loud sound [35], administered during the early NREM SWS, or early NREM stage 2 sleep, if the baseline study showed little or no SWS (it could be expected, though, that there will be more SWS present during the recovery night following sleep deprivation). There is usually complete amnesia for the parasomnic event, while loose recollection of events or non-essential recall is present in a small number of cases. The events may be associated with some form of dream mentation with or without sexual context. To an onlooker, patients may act out of character, look "glassy-eyed", "mentally absent", "removed", or, in general, different in appearance and affect than during the "regular" sexual encounters.

In association with overnight PSG assessments, ancillary tests could be performed when necessary. These include urine drug tests, tests to measure blood levels of medications and alcohol, the Multiple Sleep Latency Test and psychological tests (Box B). A full evaluation should also include detailed psychiatric and neurological assessments.

The sleep studies can be performed in either a sleep laboratory or, when necessary, in a patient's home. These patients are often highly motivated and are keen to go to any lengths in order to find an answer to their problem. For some patients, they may be further motivated by the necessity of having clarity about their condition stemming from a pending legal process. Fears of intrusion of privacy or embarrassment, or cultural, educational, or religious predisposition rarely interfere with procedures and assessments. At the same time, clinical sensitivity and decorum are paramount.

Clinical course and forensic implications

Sexsomnia treatment has two objectives. First is to educate patients concerning their disorder. This includes steps to ensure better understanding of precipitating factors and sleep hygiene measures which are required for further sexsomnia management. This also involves learning how to provide a safe sleep environment, which is the key for preventing unwanted sexual contact. The majority of sexsomnia patients who find themselves sleeping in a new environment and sharing the premises with someone who is not their regular bed partner have probably already had previous sexsomnia experiences, which should help them to realize the potential dangers of failing to ensure safe sleeping arrangements. In addition, most sexsomnia patients also know what precipitates their parasomnia. Avoidance of such precipitators should also help in prevention of unwanted sexual contacts. Further steps are aimed at providing psychological counseling and support both to patients and to their families.

The second treatment objective is to provide pharmacological intervention when necessary, most often in the form of clonazepam, a common medication that is easily administered and titrated. Treatment outcome when using clonazepam or an alternative common benzodiazepine is comparable to that of other NREM arousal parasomnias [4,20,36,37]. Use of SSRIs should be considered with care, keeping in mind the potential adverse effect of this group of medication on sexsomnia.

Treating an underlying medical disorder, such as sleep apnea, can also improve or eliminate symptoms of sexsomnia [4,20,35]. Conversely, discontinuation of treatment (e.g. CPAP) can also lead to the relapse of parasomnias in general and sexsomnia in particular [4].

The level of recidivism in our clinical population is very low, but this needs to be confirmed in a larger-scale longitudinal study. The incidence of sexsomnia is unknown – based on the comparison between sexsomnia cases and cases of other NREM parasomnias in the clinical setting, the incidence of sexsomnia is estimated at less than 10% of all NREM arousal parasomnias and perhaps closer to 1–2%.

In general, patients with SBS are at risk of being charged of sexual offending or having other legal implications (close to 8% of the Internet sample [19]), particularly when minors are participants in their parasomnic activity. As studies have shown, some sexsomnia patients exhibited sexual behavior in sleep that is exclusively or partly oriented towards minors. This was typically opportunistic behavior in a situation where the patient was not sleeping with a regular sleep partner, or when the minor came into the sexsomniac's bed. It is not completely clear whether some undiagnosed paraphilia (paraphilias, such as pedophilia, are psychosexual disorders consisting of deviance from what is considered normal sexuality) played a role in these cases or whether their actions were mere coincidence. In our practice, we have seen predominantly selected and complex cases, while the Internet survey [19] provided for a better understanding of the non-clinical sample. In this survey, only 6% of the total sample engaged in a sexual contact with minors which, if not viewed as opportunistic and coincidental, is at least comparable to similar paraphilic preferences in the general population [38,39]. However, until we have descriptions of more cases, the issue of paraphilia as it relates to sexsomnia will not be answered satisfactorily.

The pressure to tease out malingering is often very high in conditions such as sexsomnia. It is relatively easy to establish a case of malingering if one has sufficient time and appropriate means to evaluate the patient longitudinally. It is a completely different situation when it comes to retrospectively establishing malingering in a highly scrutinized medico-legal situation, which requires a different kind of material evidence. A prudent course of action is for a non-biased scientist called to serve as an expert witness to conduct research with due diligence and, ideally, to provide objective evidence that serves no side in particular and that could be used by either side without modifications, adjustments or skewing [40,41]. A general guide to the process of forming a forensic opinion with the mnemonic CHESS may be helpful for clinicians dealing with legal aspects of sexsomnia and is given in Box A.

Box A: Forensic opinion formulation
C: formulating the *claim*
H: establishing a *hierarchy* of supporting evidence
E: *examining* the evidence for disclosure
S: *studying* the evidence
S: *synthesizing* a revised opinion

Lastly, the issue of an underlying psychiatric condition is only partially answered by the available data. It is not possible to recognize a common thread or any psychiatric condition that repeats more often in this group of patients as compared to other types of parasomnia [16,42–44]. However, some of the data suggest common features among patients, including risk-taking or "stimulation-seeking" personality traits.

Differential diagnosis

When it comes to considerations about diagnostic possibilities in the case of suspected sexsomnia, one's list inevitably begins with malingering. This is particularly true in highly publicized or legal cases, generating the need for highly sensitive and specific diagnostic procedures. Box B gives an overview of the initial assessment procedures in evaluating a patient with purported sexsomnia.

Box B: Investigation of a case of sexual activity when the individual claims to be asleep
- Interview the client, taking an exhaustive psychiatric and medical history
- Obtain independent accounts from collateral sources
- Arrange for a thorough physical examination along with a full biochemical and hematological screening
- Obtain past medical and psychiatric records
- Arrange for an electroencephalogram and neuroimaging
- Interview relatives of the client
- Obtain the victim's account
- Arrange for polysomnography
- Consider erotic preference testing
- Consider a blood or urine screen for drug abuse

Section 1: Introduction

- Psychological testing with a special emphasis on personality testing
- Psychodiagnostics
- Evaluate for psychopathy
- Generate a differential diagnosis and rule out malingering

Tools that we have today are those utilized in most of the specialized sleep clinics and include thorough and methodical anamnestic evaluation, and appropriate PSG testing. In the absence of a "silver bullet" – a simple and reliable test that would unmistakably diagnose sexsomnia – a structured stepwise process needs to be considered. A good example are the well-structured diagnostic guidelines devised by Mahowald *et al.* in relation to sleep-related violence. With some modifications, these guidelines could be applied to the diagnostics of sexsomnia (see Box C). The very key ingredient is to recognize that no single feature is likely to definitely "rule in" or "rule out" sexsomnia. Almost certainly the evaluation was not present and the client/patient/subject was not undergoing a PSG study at the time of the event. It therefore rests on the confluence of clinical factors discerned and the results of tests carried out that would allow one to come to an informed opinion both for clinical and medico-legal purposes.

Box C: Assessment guidelines for diagnosing sexsomnia (defined as NREM arousal parasomnia in accordance to ICSD 2)

(1) There should be a reason (by history of former polysomnographic evaluation, or assessment performed by an expert sleep physician) to suspect a bona fide sleep disorder. Similar episodes with benign or morbid outcome should have occurred previously.

(2) The duration of the action is usually brief (<30 min).

(3) The behavior is usually abrupt, immediate, impulsive and senseless without apparent motivation.

(4) In the case of an unwanted contact, although ostensibly purposeful, it is inappropriate to the total situation, out of (waking) character for the individual, and without evidence of premeditation.

(5) In the case of an unwanted contact, the victim is someone who merely happened to be present and who may have been the stimulus for the arousal.

(6) Immediately following the return to consciousness, there is perplexity or horror upon realization, without an attempt to escape or conceal or cover up the action.

(7) The witness to the event testifies of an apparent lack of awareness on the part of the individual during the sexsomnia episode.

(8) There is usually some degree of amnesia of the event; however, this amnesia need not be complete.

(9) The sexsomnia act may:
  (a) occur upon awakening (rarely immediately upon falling asleep) – but usually at least one hour after sleep onset;
  (b) occur upon physical/body contact in bed, or attempts to awaken the subject;
  (c) have been potentiated/precipitated by known factors.

(10) Post-hoc polysomnographic tests show essential features of NREM arousal parasomnia.

Derived from [40].

Again, a prudent course of action in the case of suspected malingering is to show due diligence and to concentrate on available scientific information, and not on conjectures.

Sexual behavior in sleep, considering the evidence that we have insofar, is primarily related to the disorder of NREM arousal mechanisms. In a minority of cases (<10% approximately), such a relation could not be established. A significant number of these cases pertain to different types of (nocturnal) seizures with sexual behaviors ranging from somatosensory phenomena to simple sexual automatisms. In the case of temporal lobe seizures, ictal activity originating, typically, in the dextral limbic section can produce orgasmic feelings ("epileptic orgasm", "orgasmic aura"), either during an aura or an ictal event. The electrical or chemical stimulation of the septal section of the limbic system can produce some form of the sexual pleasure or arousal. These findings could be juxtaposed to the findings of Bassetti *et al.*, who conducted a SPECT study on a patient with known NREM parasomnia of the sleepwalking type [45]. Their study showed that, aside from the increased blood flow in the area of the anterior cerebellum, immediately after the parasomnic episode areas of posterior cingulated cortex also show an increase in blood flow, while the large areas of the cortex remain metabolically quiet. This suggests the intricate disassociation of cortical and lower structures. In the case of sexsomnia, the assumption is that activation may involve limbic regions adjacent to the cingular cortex which are the regions that regulate sexual arousal. Baird et al. [46] recently identified six key brain regions that control sexual behavior: three subcortical (septal region, hypothalamus, ansa lenticularis/pallidus) and three cortical (frontal lobes, parietal lobes/paracentral lobule and temporal lobes/amygdala).

The SPECT study of Bassetti et al. showed that the associative cortical regions remain largely metabolically quiet and this may provide insight as to why patients with parasomnia/sexsomnia show changes in their behaviors, as opposed to the daytime patterns when cognitive functions remain preserved [45]. Those metabolically quiet structures also include centers controlling higher-order functions, such as learning, putting events in sequence and context, distinguishing between objective reality and intrinsic experiences and memorizing events, resulting in an impairment of consciousness during the parasomnic episode. This is why a person having parasomnia episodes lacks the cognitive functions to appreciate the seriousness and appropriateness of his acts, lacks awareness and has poor recollection of events (and, for that matter, cannot learn new skills during the parasomnic episode). On the other hand, some of the subcortical structures of the limbic system adjacent to the metabolically active region (posterior cingulate gyrus), as mentioned above, may sustain a similar increase in activity in predisposed individuals, resulting in a specific parasomnic behavior with a sexual component (Figure 9.1). Such a hypothesis, however, needs to be tested through corresponding functional neuroimaging studies. Worthy of note is the role of the hypothalamus in controlling both the aspects of sexual behavior and of the sleep–wake system.

Typically for temporal lobe epilepsies, ictal phenomena include sexual emotions (and in the case of seizures affecting the amygdala, experiential sensory phenomena), which is usually not the case in "sexual" seizures limited to other parts of the brain. A small number of often poorly documented reports describe cortical seizures that involve different sexual automatisms (groin touching, masturbation, sexual moaning) or agitated rudimentary sexual behaviors. At the far end of the sexual behavioral spectrum are frontal and temporal lobe seizures featuring pelvic thrusting and similar sexualized movements that are usually eas-

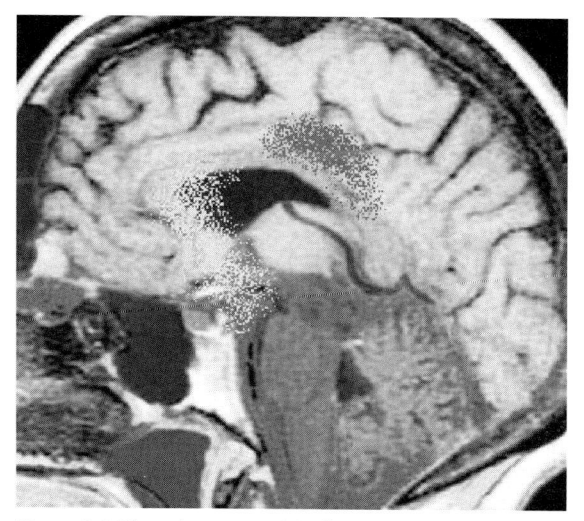

Figure 9.1 The color version of this figure can be found in the color plate section. Posterior cingulate gyrus (red), active during sleepwalking, in relation to portion of the limbic system (yellow) controlling a large segment of sexual behavior.

ily distinguishable from typical sexual behaviors. The characteristic diurnal distribution of sexual behaviors and automatisms, and lack thereof, could help differentiate seizure from parasomnia. This should be in conjunction with an extensive 24-h full-EEG and video monitoring. Nocturnal seizures also have a significantly higher rate of anamnestic recall. In regard to sleep-related frontal lobe seizures, the SPECT studies showed activation of the anterior cingulated gyrus associated with ictal activity.

It is useful to have in mind the features of NREM parasomnias and these are listed in Box D.

Box D: Diagnostic features of NREM parasomnias

Disorientation on awakening
Confusional behavior
Amnesia for the event
Trigger or precipitating event
Modulating or priming factors
Lack of concealment
Out-of-character behavior
Absence of factors suggesting intent
Substantiated clinic history
Absence of EEG abnormalities or PSG markers that could suggest a non-parasomnic pathology

---

A second type of sleep-related sexual behavior is not akin to NREM arousals, but to a different type of parasomnia: that of REM sleep behavior disorder

(RBD). Equivocal evidence suggests that a small number of the patients who exhibit sexual or sexualized behaviors in sleep either suffer from an overlap of NREM and REM parasomnia but with sexual behaviors associated solely with NREM sleep, or the existence of a mix of sexual behaviors and defensive motor behaviors typically associated with RBD but without an EEG/EMG substrate correlating to a clear case of RBD (perhaps in the form of a sleep-state dissociation) [8,20,47]. A report describing two patients [20] indicates that they were older males with a neurodegenerative disease (Parkinson's disease), using dopaminergic medication. Anecdotal evidence also suggests more frequent sexualized phenomena during REM sleep in the form of brief and stereotypical groin touching, unrelated to phasic loss of atonia, dream enactment or other excessive movements during REM sleep. A similar REM paroxysm was reported in connection to brief state-dependent head jerks, which are presently considered to be a physiological phenomenon [48].

A comprehensive review of conditions featuring sexual or sexualized behaviors done by Schenck et al. [20] identified several conditions that are not sexual sleep paroxysms in a true sense, but do have various levels of association of sexual contents with sleep and sleep pathology. A non-exclusive list of conditions starts with Kleine–Levin Syndrome, which features periodic hypersomnolence, hypersexuality and sexual disinhibition amongst other symptoms, restless legs syndrome (masturbation, rhythmic thrusting movements), narcolepsy (sexual hallucinations, cataplectic orgasm), sleep-related painful erections (increased sexual behaviors), sleep-related dissociative disorders (various sexual behaviors including attempts to re-enact past traumatic experiences), and nocturnal psychotic disorders (sexual delusions/hallucinations after awakenings), all of which have respective specific clinical features that make them distinguishable from the true sexsomnia.

Patients who suffer from sexsomnia are at higher risk of being charged for sexual offences [9,7,14,20,36,49–51]. The legislatures across the world differ considerably when dealing with this issue, and those jurisprudent differences are present even at national levels. It is to be expected that the outcome of future legal proceedings will depend not only on fundamentals of the medical science, but also on political, cultural and social considerations [52,53]. Legal aspects of parasomnias and sexsomnia in particular will remain an area of debate for many years to come.

Another form of sexual behavior related to sleep with forensic implications is sex with the sleeping victim. Since this problem does not have a sleep disorder in its origin, it will not be further discussed.

Conclusion

As we learn more about parasomnias and about sleep in general, we understand that sleep and wakefulness do not necessarily exclude each other. Sleep is not a passive process that involves complete suppression of mentation, drives, and motoric activity, and wakefulness does not always correspond to a full level of consciousness. Instead, the two states may co-exist at different neural levels. Sexsomnia brings another variable into the parasomnia equation: that is, of heightened sexual and autonomic arousal resulting in specific behaviors. This condition can take an emotional and social toll that is not always easy to bear.

By asking specific and appropriate questions we may learn of problems that concern the patient. Eliciting such information is particularly important as many patients may be too embarrassed to volunteer details of this nature – feeling that there is something bizarre and "unnatural" about their behavior and not realizing that it falls in the medical domain. This is particularly true for the conditions that we have described in this chapter.

References

1. Langeluddeke A. Delikte in Schlafzustanden. *Nervenarzt* 1955; **26**: 28–30.
2. Wong KE. Masturbation during sleep – a somnambulistic variant? *Singapore Med J* 1986; **27**: 542–3.
3. Hurwitz TD, Mahowald MW, Schluter JL. Sleep-related sexual abuse of children. *Sleep Res* 1989; **18**: 246.
4. Shapiro CM, Fedoroff JP, Trajanovic NN. Sexual behavior in sleep: a newly described parasomnia. *Sleep Res* 1996; **25**: 367.
5. Versonnen, F. Seksuele handelingen als bijzondere vorm van parasomnie? *Tijdschr Psychiatr* 1997; **39**: 409–14.
6. Schenck CH, Mahowald MW. An analysis of a recent criminal trial involving sexual misconduct with a child, alcohol abuse and a successful sleepwalking defence: arguments supporting two proposed new forensic categories. *Med Sci Law* 1998; **38**: 147–52.

7. Rosenfeld DS, Elhajjar AJ. Sleepsex: a variant of sleepwalking. *Arch Sex Behav* 1998; **27**: 269–78.

8. Alves R, Aloe F, Tavares S, *et al*. Sexual behavior in sleep, sleepwalking and possible REM behavior disorder: a case report. *Sleep Res Online* 1999; **2**: 71–2.

9. Shapiro CM, Trajanovic NN, Fedoroff JP. Sexsomnia – a new parasomnia? *Can J Psychiatry* 2003; **48**: 311–7.

10. American Academy of Sleep Medicine. *International Classification of Sleep Disorders – Second Edition (Diagnostic and Coding Manual)*. Westchester, IL: American Academy of Sleep Medicine, 2005.

11. Mahowald MW. NREM parasomnias. In Kryger MH, Roth T, Dement WC (Eds), *Principles and Practice of Sleep Medicine*. Philadelphia: W.B. Saunders Co., 2005.

12. Oswald I, Evans J. On serious violence during sleep-walking. *Br J Psychiatry* 1985; **147**: 688–91.

13. Schenck CH, Mahowald MW. A polysomnographically documented case of adult somnambulism with long-distance automobile driving and frequent nocturnal violence: parasomnia with continuing danger as a noninsane automatism? *Sleep* 1995; **18**: 765–72.

14. Bornemann MA, Mahowald MW, Schenck CH. Parasomnias: clinical features and forensic implications. *Chest* 2006; **130**: 605–10.

15. Schenck CH, Hurwitz TD, Bundlie SR, Mahowald MW. Sleep-related eating disorders: polysomnographic correlates of a heterogeneous syndrome distinct from daytime eating disorders. *Sleep* 1991; **14**: 419–31.

16. Winkelman JW. Clinical and polysomnographic features of sleep-related eating disorder. *J Clin Psychiatry* 1998; **59**: 14–9.

17. Ohayon MM, Guilleminault C, Priest RG. Night terrors, sleepwalking, and confusional arousals in the general population: their frequency and relationship to other sleep and mental disorders. *J Clin Psychiatry* 1999; **60**: 268–76.

18. Schenck CH, Boyd JL, Mahowald MW. A parasomnia overlap disorder involving sleepwalking, sleep terrors and REM sleep behavior disorder in 33 polysomnographically confirmed cases. *Sleep* 1997; **20**: 972–81.

19. Trajanovic NN, Mangan M, Shapiro CM. Sexual behavior in sleep: an internet survey. *Soc Psychiatry Psychiatr Epidemiol* 2007; **42**: 1024–31. Epub 2007 Oct 11.

20. Schenck CH, Arnulf I, Mahowald MW. Sleep and sex: what can go wrong? A review of the literature on sleep related disorders and abnormal sexual behaviors and experiences. *Sleep* 2007; **30**: 683–702.

21. Andersen ML, Poyares D, Alves RS, Skomro R, Tufik S. Sexsomnia: abnormal sexual behavior during sleep. *Brain Res Rev* 2007; **56**: 271–82. Epub 2007 Jul 13.

22. Mangan, MA. A phenomenology of problematic sexual behavior occurring in sleep. *Arch Sex Behav* 2004; **33**: 287–93.

23. Karacan I, Goodenough DR, Shapiro A. Erection cycle during sleep in relation to dream anxiety. *Arch Gen Psychiatry* 1966; **15**: 183–9.

24. Hartman D, Crisp AH, Sedgwick P, Borrow S. Is there a dissociative process in sleepwalking and night terrors? *Postgrad Med J* 2001; **77**: 244–9.

25. Pressman MR. Factors that predispose, prime and precipitate NREM parasomnias in adults: clinical and forensic implications. *Sleep Med Rev* 2007; **11**: 5–30; discussion 31–3.

26. Schenck CH, Mahowald MW. Two cases of premenstrual sleep terrors and injurious sleepwalking. *J Psychosom Obstet Gynecol* 1995; **16**: 79–84.

27. Mendelson WB. Sleepwalking associated with zolpidem. *J Clin Psychopharmacol* 1994; **14**: 150.

28. Krol DGH. Sekssomnia tijdens behandeling met een selectieve serotonineheropnameremmer. *Tijdschr Psychiatr* 2008; **50**: 735–9.

29. Kawashima T, Yamada S. Paroxetine-induced somnambulism. *J Clin Psychiatry* 2003; **64**: 483.

30. Khazaal Y, Krenz S, Zullino DF. Bupropion-induced somnambulism. *Addict Biol* 2003; **8**: 359–62.

31. Kunzel HE, Schuld A, Pollmacher T. Sleepwalking associated with reboxetine in a young female patient with major depression – a case report. *Pharmacopsychiatry* 2004; **37**: 307–08.

32. Pressman MR. Hypersynchronous delta sleep EEG activity and sudden arousals from slow-wave sleep in adults without a history of parasomnias: clinical and forensic implications. *Sleep* 2004; **27**: 706–10.

33. Blatt I, Peled R, Gadoth N, Lavie P. The value of sleep recording in evaluating somnambulism in young adults. *Electroencephalogr Clin Neurophysiol* 1991; **78**: 407–12.

34. Joncas S, Zadra A, Paquet J, Montplaisir J. The value of sleep deprivation as a diagnostic tool in adult sleepwalkers. *Neurology* 2002; **58**: 936–40.

35. Pilon M, Montplaisir J, Zadra A. Precipitating factors of somnambulism: impact of sleep deprivation and forced arousals. *Neurology* 2008; **70**: 2284–90. Epub 2008 May 7.

36. Guilleminault C, Moscovitch A, Yuen K, Poares D. Atypical sexual behavior during sleep. *Psychosom Med* 2002; **64**: 328–36.

37. Penas-Martinez ML, Guerrero-Peral AL, Toledano-Barrero AM, *et al.* Sexsomnia: descripción de un nuevo caso. *Rev Neurol* 2008; **47**: 331–2.

38. McConaghy N. Paedophilia: a review of the evidence. *Austral NZ J Psychiatry* 1998; **32**: 252–65.

39. Cohen LJ, Galynker II. Clinical features of pedophilia and implications for treatment. *J Psychiatr Pract* 2002; **8**: 276–89.

40. Mahowald MW, Bundlie SR, Hurwitz TD, Schenck CH. Sleep violence – forensic science implications: polygraphic and video documentation. *J Forensic Sci* 1990; **35**: 413–32.

41. Mahowald MW, Schenck CH. Parasomnias: sleepwalking and the law. *Sleep Med Rev* 2000; **4**: 321–39.

42. Kales A, Soldatos CR, Caldwell AB, *et al.* Somnambulism. Clinical characteristics and personality patterns. *Arch Gen Psychiatry* 1980; **37**: 1406–10.

43. Llorente MD, Currier MB, Norman S, *et al.* Night terrors in adults: phenomenology and relationship to psychopathology. *J Clin Psychiatry* 1992; **53**: 392–4.

44. Haba-Rubio J. Psychiatric aspects of organic sleep disorders. *Dialogues Clin Neurosci* 2005; **7**: 335–46.

45. Bassetti C, Vella S, Donati F, Wielepp P, Weder B. SPECT during sleepwalking. *Lancet* 2000; **356**: 484–5.

46. Baird AD, Wilson SJ, Bladin PF, Saling MM, Reutens DC. Neurological control of human sexual behavior: insights from lesion studies. *J Neurol Neurosurg Psychiatry* 2007; **78**: 1042–9. Epub 2006 Dec 22.

47. Oudiette D, De Cock VC, Lavault S, Leu S, Vidailhet M, Arnulf I. Nonviolent elaborate behaviors may also occur in REM sleep behavior disorder. *Neurology* 2009; **72**: 551–7.

48. Hogl B, Gschliesser W, Gasser S, Ulmer H, Poewe W, Brandauer E. Myoclonic head jerks in REM sleep: a common and age dependent feature in a sleep laboratory patient population. *SLEEP* 2006; **29**: A282–3.

49. Buchanan A. Sleepwalking and indecent exposure. *Med Sci Law* 1991; **31**: 38–40.

50. Fenwick, P. Sleep and sexual offending. *Med Sci Law* 1996; **36**: 122–34.

51. Ebrahim IO. Somnambulistic sexual behavior (sexsomnia). *J Clin Forensic Med* 2006; **13**: 219–24. Epub 2006 Mar 27.

52. Thomas TN. Sleepwalking disorder and mens rea: a review and case report. *Maricopa County Superior Court J Forensic Sci* 1997; **42**: 17–24.

53. Denno DW. A mind to blame: new views on involuntary acts. *Behav Sci Law* 2003; **21**: 601–18.

Section 1 Chapter 10

Introduction

Medico-legal consequences of parasomnias

Irshaad O. Ebrahim and Colin M. Shapiro

Introduction

And I see men become mad and demented from no manifest cause and at the same time doing many things out of place, and I have known many persons in sleep groaning and crying out, some in a state of suffocation, some jumping up and fleeing out of doors, and deprived of their reason till they awaken and afterwards becoming well and rational as before, although they be pale and weak.
Hippocrates, 400 BC

The parasomnias most frequently associated with forensic consequences are the disorders of arousal – confusional arousals, sleepwalking/sleep terrors – and their variant sexsomnia, parasomnia due to drug or substance and REM sleep behavior disorder (RBD). Most of these come to the attention of the courts because of a violent act resulting in injury, disability or death for which the accused claims amnesia. The violence may take the form of verbal, physical or sexual acts, or alternatively, the individual may be charged with acts of endangerment, e.g. dangerous driving, reckless endangerment, driving under the influence of drugs and/or alcohol, etc.

Violent behaviors arising from the sleep period are reported by about 2% of the adult population [1]. Chapter 2 provides a thorough review of the epidemiology of parasomnias. The first systematic literature review on sleepwalking violence was published in 1974 by Alexander Bonkalo, an eminent forensic psychiatrist who reviewed 50 historical reports of adult sleepwalking violence, 20 cases of murder and 30 related to other criminal acts. In this landmark article, the author pointed out several common characteristics of this group: a predominance of men, who were in the younger age range with a strong childhood and/or family history of sleepwalking, nocturnal enuresis, nightmares, and agitation on awakening. He was also the first to propose guidelines for the clinical and forensic evaluation of these cases [2]. Since then, there has emerged a significant medical literature on the relationship between violence and sleepwalking. Severe violence is less common, but there are a number of cases in which attacks of extreme ferocity have been recorded resulting in death. The Canadian case of *R. v Parks* indicates how complex and prolonged a violent sleepwalking episode can be [3,4]. More recently in the UK, the case of *R v. Lowe* demonstrated the degree of force possible through sleep-related violence [5]. Complex cases such as these are rare occurrences and more than 100 cases of sleep-related killing have been reported [6–18].

Sleep-related violence

There are numerous historical cases documenting sleep-related crimes dating back to the seventeenth century. In 1600, the knight J. v. Gutlingen was awakened from deep sleep by his friend, and in the confusion of awakening stabbed him to death. Gutlingen was tried by the court of Württenberg, found guilty of murder and sentenced to death. In 1686, Colonel Culpeper shot a guardsman and his horse on night patrol, and was tried at the Old Bailey, where he successfully argued that he was still asleep while committing the crime. The verdict was *manslaughter while insane* [2].

The first fully recorded case of a sleep-related murder occurred in Silesia in 1791. A 32-year-old laborer, Bernard Sehidmaizig, was aroused from deep sleep by some noise around midnight. Seeing the dim outline of a human shape and in a state of terror, he grabbed an axe and hit the terrifying figure, and by doing so killed his wife. In his defense, a professor of law, J. F. Meister, argued that there was *no rational motive* for this act, and that the accused was not fully awake at the time of the murder. He also stated that this homicide was committed in a condition called "sleep drunkenness" (*Schlaftrunkenheit*). He pointed out that *a person still sleeping had no free will* ("*In somno voluntas non erat libera*") [2].

In 1878, Simon Fraser, a 28-year-old laborer, aroused from sleep "saw a wild beast...jump on the bed to attack his child." In great excitement he seized the object he thought was the animal and dashed it to the wall; in reality, he killed his 18-month-old son. He was tried for murder and found not guilty after a statement by Lord Justice Clerk that the child was killed when the defendant was unconscious of the nature of the act "by reason of somnambulism" [7].

In 1933, a 31-year-old firefighter "woke to find he was battering his wife's head with a shovel". He reported no memory of getting out of bed or fetching the shovel, and there was an entire lack of motive as "he lived amicably with his wife" [13].

The causes and the differential diagnosis of violence arising within the sleep period are wide and varied, and some of the more commonly implicated disorders are listed in Table 10.1.

It is important to systematically investigate for all these possibilities and to always bear a high index of suspicion for malingering in the assessment of a person charged with violence that may be sleep-related or who is claiming amnesia for the episode.

A behavior is not a diagnosis – it is a presenting symptom of one of several possible diagnoses. Physical violence, sexual violence, dangerous driving, and self-injury may all occur from a single diagnosis, e.g. sleepwalking, epilepsy, etc., and rarely from multiple causes, and there may be several possible explanations for a single type of behavior.

The law and forensic parasomnias

The legal view on the violent and other criminal actions arising out of sleep can be traced back to the middle ages. In 1313 the Council of Vienne (France) stated that if a sleeper killed or wounded someone, he was not held culpable. A sixteenth-century Spanish canonist, Covarrubias, pointed out that acts during sleep cannot be sinful, except if the person arranges matters while still awake in a way that he will commit a particular act during sleep. A seventeenth-century Dutch jurist, Matthaeus, suggested that those who kill

Table 10.1 The differential diagnosis of sleep-related violence.

Organic medical and neurologic disorders

A. Vascular
   - Transient global amnesia (including migraine)
B. Mass lesions
   - Increased intracranial pressure
   - Deep midline structural lesions
C. Toxic/metabolic
   - Endocrine – thyrotoxicosis
   - Hypoxia/carbon monoxide poisoning
   - Drugs/alcohol (intoxication/withdrawal/alcoholic blackouts)
   - Thiamine deficiency (Wernicke–Korsakoff syndrome)
D. Infectious (limbic encephalitis)
E. Central nervous system (CNS) trauma
F. Seizures
   - Siezure disorders, e.g. complex partial seizures.
   - Nocturnal siezure disorder, e.g. nocturnal frontal lobe epilepsy

Sleep disorders

A. Disorders of arousal (confusional arousals, sleepwalking, sleep terrors)
B. Rapid eye movement (REM) sleep behavior disorder (RBD)
C. Nocturnal seizures
D. Automatic behavior
E. Narcolepsy and idiopathic CNS hypersomnia
F. Sleep apnea
G. Sleep deprivation
H. Sleep schedule/circadian rhythm disorder (including jetlag)

Psychogenic disorders

A. Dissociative states that may arise directly from sleep
   - Fugues
   - Multiple personality disorder
   - Psychogenic amnesia
B. Post-traumatic stress disorder
C. Malingering
D. Munchausen by proxy

while sleepwalking should be punished only if they harbored enmity toward their victim while awake. Mackenzie (1636–91), in his *Discourse Upon the Laws of Scotland*, agreed that those who "commit any crime whilst they sleep, are compared to infants... and therefore are not punisht...," except if there is enmity or fraud [2].

In the UK and common law jurisdictions, a person cannot be found guilty of an offence unless it is proved that the defendant has committed a criminal act (*actus reus*) *and* that he had a knowing intent to commit that act (*mens rea*). For a person to be convicted, both these elements – i.e. the physical part of the offence (*actus reus*) and the state of mind aspects (*mens rea*) – need to be present. "*Actus non fecit reus mens sit rea*": the deed does not make a man guilty unless his mind is guilty [22,23,24].

Unless the offence is a statutory one which carries an absolute liability (e.g. driving with a raised blood alcohol level), the doctrine of *mens rea*, or the presence of a guilty mind, can only be negated by three considerations:

1. the mind is not guilty because it is innocent (as in the case of mental retardation),
2. the mind is diseased,
3. at the time of the act there was an absence of mind (automatism).

In the USA, in order to secure a conviction in a criminal trial under The American Law Institute's Model Penal Code (MPC), the prosecution must prove all elements in the definition of the offense. Most importantly, for each offense element, the prosecution needs to establish:

1. that the conduct was *voluntary*; and
2. that the defendant acted with *culpability*, i.e. purposely (i.e. with intent), knowingly, recklessly or negligently.

These objective elements therefore include the conduct required for the offense as well as the circumstances and results of that conduct [19].

Voluntary conduct (also called the voluntary act requirement)

Under Section 2.01 of the MPC, the Requirement of Voluntary Act, the code states that:

1. A person is not guilty of an offense unless his liability is based on conduct which includes a voluntary act or the omission to perform an act of which he is physically capable.
2. The following are not voluntary acts within the meaning of this section: a reflex or convulsion; a bodily movement during unconsciousness or sleep; conduct during hypnosis or resulting from hypnotic suggestion; or, a bodily movement that otherwise is not a product of the effort or determination of the actor, either conscious or habitual.

The MPC's voluntary act requirement states that the "conduct that constitutes the offence must include a voluntary act" – if it does the requirement is fulfilled, if it does not, there is no offense (apart from omissions). This definition of "voluntariness" has been challenged, and a more comprehensive definition of the voluntary act requirement was proposed by the eminent academic Joel Feinberg: "an act is fully voluntary when it is a product of the actor's rational capacities without undue ignorance or impairment on the part of the actor or excessive pressure from the environment." Thus voluntariness should be viewed as a matter of degree rather than a threshold concept [20].

Culpability

In addition to proving that a criminal act was voluntary, the state has to prove that the defendant acted with culpability, i.e. it has to establish that the defendant acted purposely (i.e. with intent), knowingly, recklessly, or negligently regarding each material element of the offense.

When the state has satisfied both the voluntary act and culpability requirements, the defendant may avoid liability by providing a general defense.

In the USA, there are two broad categories of defense.

1. *Failure-of-proof defenses*: including the Voluntary Act and Culpability requirements (above).
2. *General Defenses* (including the *defense of specific excuses* involving an excusing condition such as epilepsy, somnambulism) regarding particular conduct. Legal scholars contend that *the excuse must involve a disability that the actor has that causes the excusing condition*. This disability must be confirmed on the basis of *observable indicators* (excluding the conduct from which the actor is seeking to be excused). The present scientific and medical knowledge base in forensic sleep medicine often cannot fully satisfy the legal community's demand for concrete confirmation and objective evidence of the excusing condition.

The insanity defense and automatism (i.e. the sleepwalking defense) remain relevant to criminal liability today, but the MPC definitions still rely on ideas that have not kept up to date with developments in neuroscience. This, combined with the inability to adequately define "consciousness," or for that matter even "voluntariness," has led to a theoretical foundation of defenses within the legal context that remains contentious. There is a need for the legal and medical view to coalesce as the current definitions lead inevitably to confusion and may at times lead to compromises in the delivery of justice [19,21].

The McNaghten Rules and the insanity defense

The McNaghten Rules (pronounced, and sometimes spelled, McNaughton) arose from the attempted assassination of the British Prime Minister, Robert Peel, in 1843 by Daniel McNaghten who instead killed Peel's private secretary. McNaghten was clearly mentally ill and suffered from paranoid delusions. A panel of judges formulated the rules or tests for juries to consider in cases where a defendant pleads insanity. The rules so formulated as McNaghten's Case 1843 10 C & F 200 have formed the basis for criminal liability in relation to mentally disordered defendants in common law jurisdictions ever since.

The most important of these rules states that:

the jurors ought to be told that in all cases every man is presumed to be sane, and to possess a sufficient degree of reason to be responsible for his crimes, until the contrary be proved to their satisfaction; and that to establish a defence on the ground of insanity, it must be clearly proved that, at the time of committing the act, the party accused was labouring under such a defect of reason, from disease of the mind, as not to know the nature and quality of the act he was doing; or, if he did know it, that he did not know he was doing what was wrong.

When these rules are satisfied, the accused may be found *not guilty by reason of insanity* (NGRI), and the sentence may be a mandatory or discretionary period of treatment in a secure hospital, or otherwise at the discretion of the court.

The insanity defense is recognized in Australia, Canada, England and Wales, Scotland, South Africa, the European Union (EU), New Zealand, the Republic of Ireland, and most US states with the exception of Montana, Idaho, and Utah. These three states have abolished the insanity defense entirely without abandoning the culpability requirement, and evidence of psychological/psychiatric dysfunction is only admissible when it is relevant to failure-of-proof defenses. Somnambulism (sleepwalking) has been treated by some states in the US as a form of insanity, and defendant(s) have succeeded in being found NGRI through the use of the McNaghten Rules [21–24].

The insanity defense in the USA

The MPC defines the criteria for NGRI thus:

[a] person is not responsible for criminal conduct if at the time of such conduct as a result of mental disease or defect he lacks substantial capacity either to appreciate the criminality [wrongfulness] of his conduct or to conform his conduct to the requirements of the law.

This set of tests is used in most jurisdictions in the US, as it addresses volitional impairment and requires that the defendant lacks *substantial* (rather than complete) capacity. It also substitutes "know" from the McNaghten Rules with "appreciate", providing a broader and more contextualised evaluation of the defendant's actions [19].

In 1982, some US states changed the criteria for the NGRI defense. The California electorate passed Proposition 8 and within Section 25(b) of the California Penal Code, a defendant is exculpated under the NGRI defense only when

he or she was incapable of knowing or understanding the nature and quality of his or her act **and** of distinguishing right from wrong at the time of the commission of the offense. [21]

In 1986, the US Federal Government adopted its first NGRI statute authorizing the NGRI finding only when "the defendant, as a result of severe mental disease or defect, was unable to appreciate the nature and quality or the wrongfulness of his acts." Current federal law has eliminated the second prong of the MPC insanity statutes – the control of conduct element; one may therefore be innocent in a state court and guilty in a federal court, with exactly the same facts.

The insanity defense in the UK and common law jurisdictions

In the UK, the NGRI defense is included within the rubric of automatism where it is classed as *insane automatism*, which utilises the McNaghten tests. The defendant is exculpated if the McNaghten criteria are fulfilled, i.e. that he or she was:

1. suffering from a disorder of reason,
2. caused by a disease of the mind, such that,
3. s/he did not know the nature and quality of his/her act or that it was wrongful.

Automatism

The seminal legal definition is that of Lord Denning in *Bratty v. A-G for Northern Ireland*:

an act which is done by the muscles without any control by the mind, such as a spasm, a reflex action, or a convulsion; or an act done by a person who is not conscious of what he is doing, such as an act done while suffering from concussion or while sleepwalking.

Fenwick provides a comprehensive medical definition of automatism:

An automatism is an involuntary piece of behaviour over which an individual has no control. The behaviour is usually inappropriate to the circumstances, and may be out of character for the individual. It can be complex, co-ordinated and apparently purposeful and directed, though lacking in judgment. Afterwards the individual may have no recollection or only a partial and confused memory for his actions. In organic automatisms there must be some disturbance of brain function sufficient to give rise to the above features. [22]

Automatism in the USA

Legally, automatism has been defined by the courts in the USA as "a defense against criminal liability for those defendants who perform illegal conduct in a state of unconsciousness or semi-consciousness." It may also apply to "behavior performed in a state of mental unconsciousness or dissociation without full awareness, i.e. somnambulism, fugue." Although the automatism defense classically involves conditions such as convulsions, reflexes and other acts that are performed without any conscious direction, the defense also applies to those who perform complex actions in a coordinated, directed fashion, but with substantially reduced awareness – hence courts have recognized this defense in cases in which the defendant's impaired consciousness was associated with epilepsy, somnambulism, concussion, physical or emotional trauma [21].

There is a lack of general consensus on the automatism defense in the USA. Some courts have held that automatism is a variation of the general defense of excuses interpreting the disorder as a defect of reason that prevented the defendant from knowing the nature and quality of his actions (*People v. Higgins*), other courts have accepted automatism as a form of insanity (*Tibbs v. Commonwealth*). Still others have accepted automatism as a separate defense specifically excluding insanity as part of the description (*People v. Martin, Fulcher v. State*). In *Jones v. State*, the court addressed automatism as a failure-of-proof defense that goes to the voluntary act requirement of the MPC stating that "automatism applies to involuntary acts totally beyond the control and knowledge of the defendant". The MPC includes somnambulism and convulsions as conditions that fail to meet the voluntary act requirements that can give rise to an automatism defense [21].

The British and common law view

The British courts divide automatism into two types – *non-insane* and *insane* automatism. Non-insane automatisms (sometimes called *sane*) are legally defined as arising from an *external cause*, e.g. a blow to the head or a bee sting, whereas insane automatisms are defined as arising from *an internal factor* (such as a brain disorder, for example a stroke or epilepsy). In Canada, automatism is classed as either *mental disorder automatism* (equivalent to insane in the UK) or *non-mental disorder automatism* (equivalent to non-insane in the UK). In Canada, *sleepwalking* is held to be a non-mental disorder (sane) automatism, and in the UK it is held to be insanity.

The history of the automatism defense and the sane vs. insane paradigms is best illustrated by examining the key legal cases. In 1955, in the case of *R v. Charlson*, the defendant assaulted his son and threw him out of a window. He was found to have a brain tumor and epilepsy, and the court accepted that his actions were a result of these conditions which were then legally defined as *sane* automatisms. The defendant was acquitted, as it was held at the time that a brain tumor and epilepsy could not be classed as insanity.

However, two years later, in the case of *R v. Kemp*, where the defendant, who suffered from cerebrovascular disease, assaulted his wife with a hammer, the court found that the most likely explanation for his behavior was an automatic act carried out due to a "disease of the mind", and therefore this was an *insane* automatism. This was contrary to the conclusion reached in the Charlson case where a disease of the mind was judged sane. As a result of the Kemp case, organic brain disease was classed as *insane* automatism, as the behavior arose from an *internal* cause. This was confirmed for sleepwalking in the case of *R v. Burgess*, as it was held on the medical evidence in this case that sleepwalking was a disease of mind and hence *an insane automatism*; and again in 1983, for epilepsy in the case of *R v. Sullivan*.

Section 1: Introduction

In the case of *Bratty v. A-G for N. Ireland* in 1963, Bratty, charged with killing a girl who was a passenger in his car by strangulation, claimed he was epileptic and in an automatic state as a defense. Lord Denning of the appeal court ruled that any mental disorder which had manifested itself in violence *and was prone to recur* was a disease of the mind and an insane automatism. Furthermore, Lord Denning wanted to make certain that those individuals who were habitually violent due to a medical condition would be detained in hospital. He said: "At any rate, it is the sort of disease for which a person should be detained in hospital rather than being given an unqualified acquittal." This view was reinforced again in the case of *R v. Sullivan*, where it was reasoned that the insanity defense in the UK was intended to protect the public from *recurrences of dangerous conduct*, and Sullivan, an epileptic, was detained in a mental hospital.

The 1973 case of *R v. Quick* has also contributed to the present definition of automatism. Quick, a psychiatric nurse, had insulin-dependent diabetes and had been charged with assaulting a patient whilst hypoglycemic following a small breakfast and after taking alcohol. Since this was a consequence of an insulin injection (an external factor), the plea of sane automatism was made. This was upheld in the court of appeal, since it was felt that diabetes per se did not cause a disease of the mind, but the *insulin* that was prescribed did (i.e. an *external* factor).

Importantly, the court in *R v. Quick* also stated that external factors *within the control of the individual* (alcohol/drugs) would *not* constitute a defense where the incapacity was self-induced, i.e. where *recklessness* can be shown. In Scotland, the case of *Finnegan v. Heywood* has reinforced this contention of recklessness, where it was held that as the sleepwalker knew that drinking alcohol precipitated his sleepwalking attacks, sleepwalking could not be used as a defense as he was responsible for taking the alcohol and was aware of the consequences of alcohol consumption [22–24].

The legal definition, however, does not contain any reference to an illness being acute or chronic. In *R v. Kemp*, in discussing the cerebral arteriosclerosis which was said to have caused the automatism at the time of the offence, Lord Justice Devlin said: "In my judgement the condition of the brain is irrelevant. So is the question of whether the condition of the mind is curable or incurable, transitory or permanent.... Temporary insanity is sufficient to satisfy them" (the McNaghten Rules) [22].

In Scotland, a landmark ruling in the 1991 case of *Ross v. HM Advocate* still forms the basis of the sane automatism defense. Ross had consumed beer that had been laced with LSD and subsequently assaulted another person. The defence was based on the *involuntary* ingestion of drugs resulting in automatism due to an external factor. The High Court found that the essential requirements needed for this type of defense were that the accused must have experienced a "total alienation of reason amounting to a complete absence of self control" due to "some external factor which was outwith the accused's control [and] which he was not bound to foresee" [25].

The 1989 Crimes Bill in New Zealand started moving the automatism debate from the *mens rea* test of automatism to the *actus reus* test, and states that "the real test is one of involuntariness. If the accused was not wholly unconscious but nevertheless acted involuntarily, he or she would be protected from criminal responsibility..." [26].

In Canada in 1971, the automatism defense was extended to include automatism induced by psychological trauma, a state of *dissociation* also referred to as *psychological blow automatism*. The first Supreme Court case dealing with psychological blow automatism was *R. v. Rabey*. In the Supreme Court of Canada case of *R. v. Stone*, a 42-year-old man accused of murdering his wife while apparently in a dissociative state raised the defenses of provocation and non-insane automatism based on a psychological blow. The jury ruled that the accused was not suffering from a disease of the mind and the accused was convicted of manslaughter. The law of automatism was rewritten in the *Stone* case. Before the case, unconsciousness was viewed as the predominant element in a state of automatism. The Stone case clarified that unconsciousness need not exist in a state of automatism; rather, the important element in automatism is whether criminal behavior is involuntary or not. Automatism was redefined as a state of *impaired* consciousness in which an individual, though capable of action, has *no voluntary control* over that action, and two types of automatism were delineated (insane and non-insane). It was also determined that a single approach to all cases involving claims of automatism should be taken, as automatism may arise in different contexts, i.e. psychological blow automatism, somnambulism, and extreme intoxication (e.g. alcoholic blackout) akin to a state of automatism.

The Canadian court in *Stone* made another fundamental shift in the law on automatism in terms of *the burden of proof*. In *R v. Parks*, it was the Crown who had the onus to prove all aspects of the act whereas in the *Stone* case the affirmative *onus was on the defense* to prove voluntariness, or lack thereof.

Commentators have also stressed a need for the triers of fact to consider whether the defendant poses a *continuing danger* to the community and the responsibility of the court to take a holistic approach, with the overarching concern being whether societal protection requires the defendant to undergo medical treatment and, if so, the finding should be one of mental disorder (insane) automatism. This was demonstrated in 2008 when the Canadian Court of Appeal ruled that a defendant previously acquitted due to non-mental disorder automatism and reclassified to a verdict of Not Criminally Responsible on Account of Mental Disorder should have regular monitoring by mental health professionals (*R v. Luedecke*).

In the UK, since the amendment of the Criminal Procedure (Insanity and Unfitness to Plead) Act (1991), by the Domestic Violence, Crime and Victims Act 2004, it matters less whether the classification is sane or insane automatism, except where there is a statutory sentence. The Act now allows the judge, in the case of insane automatism, to give an absolute discharge, a supervision order, or send the defendant to hospital with, if necessary, a restriction order (Section 41of the 1983 Mental Health Act), which can prevent the release of the defendant for life without the special permission of the Home Secretary. If the court finds the defendant not guilty due to sane automatism, then there can only be an absolute discharge. In these circumstances the only point is whether sleepwalkers should be classified as insane in the interests of public safety [27–30].

The role of the sleep expert

The discipline of forensic sleep medicine is at an embryonic stage. The majority of medical-scientific data exist in the form of small case series and case reports. The methodological and ethical difficulties in obtaining highly valid prospective data have been commented on by several experts. To provide an expert opinion, the expert must have detailed knowledge of the current developments in medicine, neuropsychology and neuroscience that explain how behaviors may occur without complete awareness, as well as an understanding of the limitations and controversies surrounding the legal demands made by prosecutors and/or defense attorneys. It is thus important that experts providing evidence for apparent sleep-related forensic cases be acutely aware of and follow guidelines laid down by their respective professional and regulatory bodies in their particular jurisdictions [4,8,11, 30–34].

The American view

The adversarial judicial system in the USA pits two parties – the defense and the prosecution – against each other. It is no surprise, then, that expert witnesses being retained by either the defense or the prosecution may be tempted to become a paid advocate for the party that engaged their services. The courtroom can thus become fertile ground for the appearance of "junk science", pitting expert witness advocates against each other with winning the case rather than revealing truth or delivering justice being the main motivation. The Federal Rules of Evidence describe standard procedures for expert testimony in federal courts. These rules, which were clarified by the United States Supreme Court in *Daubert v. Merrell Dow Pharmaceuticals*, Inc., and *Kumho Tire Co., Ltd. v. Carmichael*, restrict the intrusion of junk science, unreliable data, and inflammatory evidence into expert testimony. The *Daubert* ruling changed judicial analysis in the USA in that courts are duty bound to examine the scientific validity of the evidence and not merely the conclusions of the experts [35–38].

In response to the need for further clarity on these matters from a medical professional's perspective, the American Academy of Neurology (AAN) recently published updated guidelines on the qualifications and conduct of expert testimony [37].

Several commentators have recommended that sleep experts volunteer to serve as a court-appointed expert whose primary function is scientific education of lawyers, judges and juries, rather than one appointed by either the prosecution or defense. This role as *amicus curae* is to be encouraged and is a preferred route that would promote scientific objectivity [4,32,34].

The American Medical Association (AMA) has previously stated that expert witness testimony should be considered practice of medicine, and therefore subject to peer review. Good science must be determined by scientific consensus based on the best up-to-date and available data, and not only by the credentials of the expert witness [38,39].

A recent commentary recommends that "the best the medical expert can do is to provide an opinion that the condition is either 'highly unlikely,' 'likely,' or 'highly likely,' or that there are 'insufficient data to assess likelihood'" [34].

In the USA, it is within the judge's responsibility to determine the legitimacy of scientific evidence (and expertise) before admitting it. The gatekeeping power (and responsibility) of judges to exclude evidence based upon subjective belief or unsupported speculation is an important filtering effect that entitles trial judges to throw out "opinion evidence" from experts that is not backed by solid science [36–38].

The British and common law view

In the UK in the late 1990s, a thorough review was undertaken of the Civil Justice system by Lord Woolf. The result of this review was the introduction of The Civil Procedure Rules (CPR), the rules of civil procedure used by the courts in civil cases in England and Wales. Part of this review introduced and defined the specific roles and duties of expert witnesses under section CPR 35.3.

The most important requirement is one of *impartiality*. Experts must not regard themselves as advocates whose function is to promote the case of the instructing party. Their task is to assist *the Court* to deal with cases justly. So it matters not whether they have been instructed by the prosecution or the defense, the expert's report is for the Court and *not* for the party that instructed them. Furthermore, it is encouraged by the courts that experts provide a *single joint report* outlining all the facts of the case. This was illustrated by Lady Butler-Sloss: "As part of the attempt in the Civil Procedure Rules to move away from gladiatorial matches between partial witnesses, parties are increasingly encouraged to instruct a single joint expert. Such an expert can be appointed either by agreement or by order of the Court … this approach not only encourages a less adversarial approach to proceedings … and reduces delays" [38,40,41].

In 2005, the Civil Justice Council in England published the *Protocol for the Instruction of Experts to Give Evidence in Civil Claims* based on the CPR principles. Under section 4, Duties of Experts, it outlines the following test of independence of the expert: "a useful test of 'independence' is that the expert would express the same opinion if given the same instructions by an opposing party. Experts should not take it upon themselves to promote the point of view of the party instructing them or engage in the role of advocates." With regard to the expert's opinion, it states that experts should "indicate if an opinion is provisional, or qualified, or where they consider that further information is required or if, for any other reason, they are not satisfied that an opinion can be expressed finally and without qualification" [42].

This overriding duty to the court, the principle of impartiality and independence from the engaging party, was demonstrated in the sleep-related violence case of *R v. Lowe*, where the court requested a single joint report from the experts. More importantly, in the single joint report *all possible scenarios* were provided including the following:

1. The actions being conscious and motivated, i.e. that the defendant was lying or malingering.
2. The actions being part of an alcohol intoxicated state.
3. The actions were part of an automatism arising from a confusional arousal/sleepwalking episode.
4. The actions were part of an automatism arising from an epileptic episode.
5. A combination of the above.

The experts listed the factors for and the factors against each possibility, and left the decision on weighting each possibility to the judge and jury based purely on the facts presented and behaviors described. This avoided venturing into hypothetical issues of psychology or intent and encouraged a serious, factually based debate focused on educating the court and delivering justice [5].

Over the past decade, Australia, New Zealand, South Africa and Canada have also instituted similar rules to the CPR of England and Wales [43,44].

Canadian courts have gone a step further and cited the American *Daubert* case favorably, thus increasing judicial gatekeeping in assessing the validity of expert evidence. The Canadian Supreme Court has set four criteria for admissibility of expert testimony: relevance, necessity, absence of an exclusionary rule, and proper qualifications of the expert [36,38].

A recently published method to help experts maintain independence and provide unbiased testimony – the CHESS method for forensic opinion formulation – contains five steps: C, formulating the *claim* (preliminary opinion); H, establishing a *hierarchy* of supporting evidence; E, *examining* the evidence for exposure; S, *studying* the evidence; and S, *synthesizing* a revised opinion. The authors suggest that this method provides a framework for formulating, revising, and identifying limitations of opinions, which will allow experts to incorporate neutrality into forensic opinions [45].

The assessment of sleep-related violence

The assessment of a person accused of a violent act that may have arisen from sleep requires a systematic and thorough evaluation of all possible diagnoses. The core clinical presentation in purported sleep-related violence is one of *amnesia for a violent offense*. It follows then that the assessment and investigation of apparent sleep-related violence should include investigating for all possible causes of amnesic-related violence [46].

The common conditions implicated in apparent sleep-related violence are:

1. The Parasomnias
    a. Disorders of Arousal (DOA) – Confusional Arousal, Sleepwalking/Sleep Terror
    b. Parasomnia due to Drug or Substance
    c. REM Sleep Behavior Disorder
    d. Sexsomnia
2. Epilepsy
3. Alcohol- or Substance-Related Violence
4. Dissociation
5. Malingering

The parasomnias

The clinical assessment and investigation of the parasomnias are dealt with in Chapters 3–5. Specific parasomnias of relevance to the forensic context are described in Chapters 6–9, 11–14, 17 and 21, 29 and 30.

NREM parasomnias – disorders of arousal

For the diagnosis of NREM parasomnias in the forensic assessment of sleep-related violence, the following additional guidelines are useful.

1. There should be *disorientation on awakening*. A straight arousal into clear consciousness is unlikely to occur on awakening from a somnambulistic automatism.

2. *Confusional behavior* should occur. Any witness to the entire event should report inappropriate automatic behavior, preferably with an element of confusion.

3. There is usually complete *amnesia* for the event. Memories are poorly recorded during stage 3 and 4 sleep and equally poorly recalled. It is, however, possible for fragments of distorted memory to be retained.

4. *Trigger* or *precipitating factors* are important, such as the presence of an internal factor such as Sleep-Disordered Breathing (SDB) and Periodic Limb Movements (PLMs). The presence of external factors such as noise or physical contact or touch due to proximity may also trigger sleepwalking. Sleepwalking occurs usually due to something "going bump in the night" and hence the victim is frequently someone who just happened to be present and who may have been the stimulus, through touch, pressure, or noise for the violent episode [5,47,48].

5. *Modulating* or *Priming Factors* including the use of alcohol, drugs (prescribed and recreational), caffeine, prior sleep deprivation, disruption of the circadian sleep–wake pattern and the presence of a recent stressful life event(s) have been reported to be associated with an increase in sleepwalking episodes and sleep-related violence. Even in the presence of a modulating/priming factor, a trigger factor is still necessary for a sleepwalking episode to occur [49–51].

6. *Concealment*. There should be no attempt at concealment. Attempts to conceal the incident suggest the presence of consciousness and intent.

7. *Out of character behavior*. The behavior is almost always out of character for the individual. Thus sleep-related violence in a sleepwalker usually occurs in individuals who have never or rarely previously shown violent behavior during wakefulness and are usually "of good character" [2].

8. *Absence of any factors suggesting intent*. Evidence of pre-planning, motivation, and behaviors reported during the event that suggest conscious motivation all point a non-sleep-related cause of the violence.

In the forensic context, sleep laboratory studies (polysomnography, PSG) will add value by excluding or identifying possible trigger factors or other organic causes for the behavior, e.g. SDB, PLMs, etc. In addition, the PSG is essential to diagnose RBD and epilepsy (see below) [5,34,52].

It must be emphasized that as in the diagnosis of any medical condition, the diagnosis does not rest purely on the results of investigations, but rather on the analysis of all data including the history, physical examination of mental state, cognitive state, collateral information from family and professionals, and the results of tests and investigations. The facts of the case and the behavior during the "event" are very important, and all must fit that of a DOA. A normal PSG does not exclude the diagnosis of sleepwalking, nor can sleep studies provide confirmation or exclusion that a person was sleepwalking at the time of the alleged crime, but can only point to the likelihood of the diagnosis in combination with a substantiated clinical history and thorough clinical evaluation of the individual.

REM sleep behavior disorder (RBD)

The history, clinical features, investigation and treatment of RBD are dealt with in Chapter 14. The prior history of violent enactment of dreams, recall of the dreams, the history from the bed partner and the finding of the loss of REM atonia on the PSG will confirm the diagnosis. Where there are secondary causes such as medication, the medical history and sequence of symptoms will usually make clear the temporal relationship symptoms and commencement of offending substance.

The secondary causes of RBD that may be of relevance to the forensic context are alcohol withdrawal, stimulant abuse, psychotropic medication and the association with major stressful events. Issues that are likely to be brought to the fore in the medico-legal arena will be those to do with future risk of harmful behavior and prognosis. As idiopathic RBD is well controlled with medication and the risk of further neurological disease well-documented, the court is likely to recommend ongoing medical surveillance [33,53].

Epilepsy

Epilepsy is an important, although infrequent, cause of violence and an essential consideration in the differential diagnosis of apparent sleep-related violence. Chapter 30 deals with the clinical presentation, assessment and treatment of sleep-related epilepsy.

The neurophysiological relationship between epilepsy and DOA

In an attempt to provide a theoretical explanation for the complex motor symptoms characterizing nocturnal frontal seizures, Tassinari and coworkers hypothesized that the paroxysmal activity arising from the epileptogenic area acts as a trigger by the release of the central pattern generators (CPGs) that allow innate motor behaviors to emerge. Considering the similarity between epileptic events and some parasomnias (especially somnambulism), they speculate that the activation of the CPGs also plays a role in producing parasomnic behavior, stating that "irrespective of whether the trigger is an epileptic phenomenon or a sleep-related dysfunction, the resulting motor event is still the same and consists in the activation of repetitive motor patterns which represent innate motor behaviors" [54–56].

Clinical differentiation between epilepsy and DOA

Epilepsy and parasomnias not only share many common clinical presentations, but have also been treated in a similar manner by the law. Clinical differentiation between nocturnal frontal lobe epilepsy (NFLE) and the disorders of arousal (DOA) is difficult and sometimes impossible on clinical grounds alone for the following reasons.

Behavioral manifestations

The patterns are frequently similar, both in terms of the timing and the nature of the behavior. Epileptic interictal discharges are influenced by the state of arousal and seizures may be precipitated by sleep or occur primarily in certain sleep stages. Drowsiness and NREM sleep EEG activity facilitate the propagation and synchronization of epileptiform discharges, which in turn facilitate the clinical manifestation of seizures. Episodic nocturnal wanderings (ENW), a variant of NFLE, begin with a sudden awakening associated with movements followed by agitated somnambulism and violent motor behavior. This may be impossible to distinguish from a violent sleepwalking episode.

Witness description

A reliable description of motor events occurring during the night is often difficult to obtain from a witness or bed partner because observers may be lacking or, if present, not fully awake and reliable.

Reliability of diagnostic criteria

The available standard diagnostic criteria for nocturnal motor episodes lack reliability in the case of several parasomnias, and for NFLE are still in development [57].

Comorbidity, coexistence and natural history of DOA and NFLE

The possible coexistence of nocturnal parasomnic attacks in epileptic patients or their families and the finding that up to a third of the patients with NFLE have a history of sleep terrors, sleepwalking, sleep talking, rhythmic movement disorder and enuresis presents further difficulties in differentiating the two conditions. Parasomnic attacks have also been shown to be more common in patients with NFLE and in their family compared to controls [58–60].

DOA can usually be distinguished from seizures by their exclusive occurrence in sleep combined with the low rate of same-night recurrence and the non-stereotypical pattern of movements. The history of NREM parasomnias (early age of onset, decrease in frequency or disappearance after puberty, and rare episodes of long duration) differs from that of NFLE. NFLE, which first occurs between the ages of 10 and 20 years and often persists into adulthood, manifests frequently with complex and repetitive behavior of short duration and has a tendency for multiple same-night recurrences that occur in a stereotyped fashion with tremor, dystonia, ballism or abnormal movements present during the attack. The recent description of a possible variant of DOA, *status parasomnicus*, may make this clinical differentiation even more difficult [61,62].

Video-polysomnography (V-PSG) monitoring together with careful history-taking may thus represent the only tool to distinguish NFLE from other non-epileptic paroxysmal motor disorders of sleep. It is recommended that V-PSG and a full bipolar EEG montage (according to the International 10–20 System) be mandatory in all subjects with a complex motor presentation arising within the sleep period and some authors suggest a minimum 72-h observation period [60–63].

Alcohol- or substance-related violence

Violence due to alcohol and substance use is far more common than violence due to parasomnia and epileptic violent behaviors. Violence due to alcohol and/or substance use can occur during the intoxication or withdrawal.

Alcohol-related violence

Alcohol-related violence is usually the result of intoxication and less frequently due to withdrawal or seizures. Violent or criminal behavior may also accompany alcohol-seeking behavior, e.g. robbery to obtain alcohol. Alcohol-related violence is far more prevalent than that of violence due to parasomnia or seizures, and this should be an important consideration in the assessment of a purported sleep-related crime. Appropriate emphasis to this should be provided when alcohol is a cofactor in forensic cases of apparent sleep-related violence.

Alcohol and seizures

Alcohol is directly toxic to the brain and an epileptogenic compound. Alcohol intoxication can cause seizures in people without a history of epilepsy. Withdrawal from alcohol in alcohol-dependent individuals is an established cause of seizures, and alcohol can precipitate seizures in patients with epilepsy either due to its direct toxic effect and/or due to interactions with anti-epileptic medication. Alcohol-related seizures may occur spontaneously in individuals without a history of seizures or alcohol dependence. Concurrent risk factors include pre-existing epilepsy, structural brain lesions and the concomitant use of illicit drugs.

In the forensic context, Marinacci's landmark study on alcohol administration and EEG monitoring provides some insight into the complexities of the relationship between alcohol, violence and seizures. The same amount and type of alcoholic beverage that had precipitated the abnormal state was administered during EEG monitoring. Of the 402 individuals referred for evaluation of "amnestic destructive behavior" leading to confrontation with the law, or when alcohol had been the cause of temporary loss of consciousness, confusion, trance-like states, destructive rage, or "even major convulsions", 14% had temporal lobe spiking after the first dose of alcohol and 4.4% had definite automatic episodes, presumably complex partial seizures. Maletzky administered ethanol intravenously under EEG monitoring to 22 individuals with a history of alcohol-related violent behavior. All had normal baseline EEGs. With alcohol administration, EEG slowing occurred in 50% of subjects, and sharp waves were identified in 22%. Violent behavior or psychosis occurred with intoxication in 68% [64–66].

Section 1: Introduction

A recent review of all epilepsy NGRI verdicts in England and Wales between 1975 and 2001 found that 92% of all cases had an association with alcohol. Alcohol intoxication was a cofactor in 62% of cases and alcohol withdrawal in about 30%. The authors also make special note that only 7.3% of all NGRI verdicts over this 26-year study period were due to epileptic automatism making the finding of an epileptic automatism a very rare occurrence [67].

Alcoholic blackout

Alcoholic blackout is defined as "memory loss, without accompanying loss of consciousness, for events that occur during drinking". In the differential diagnosis of sleep-related violence, alcoholic blackouts are often difficult to distinguish from a parasomnia, as both present with complex coordinated behavior associated with amnesia for the events of the episode.

Blackouts are divided into two categories, "en bloc" blackouts, and "fragmentary" blackouts. En bloc blackouts are classified by the inability to later recall any memories from the intoxicated period, even when prompted. Fragmentary blackouts are characterized by the ability to recall certain events from an intoxicated period, yet be unaware that other memories are missing until reminded of the existence of these "gaps" in memory. Research indicates that fragmentary blackouts are far more common than en bloc blackouts. Two biological mechanisms may underlie the amnesia of alcoholic blackout. Ethanol is known to temporarily inhibit the biochemical brain processes that are necessary to form new memory traces, thus causing an encoding deficit. The other mechanism emphasizes state-dependent retrieval deficits. Information stored in memory during an intoxicated state would be inaccessible when sober.

With the increase in the binge-drinking culture, particularly amongst the adolescent and university age groups, recent studies have shown a surprisingly high prevalence of such blackouts amongst this group associated with a higher than expected degree of risk-taking behaviors including sexual activity, vandalism, and fighting. A recent study comparing the risk of violence with alcohol found a 13.2-fold increase of risk of criminal violence within 24 h of alcohol consumption. Furthermore, the prevalence of alcoholic blackouts is much more common among social drinkers than previously assumed. It is noteworthy that large amounts of alcohol – particularly if consumed rapidly – can produce either fragmentary or en bloc blackouts. It is now thought that the rate of increase of blood alcohol concentration (BAC) levels is more significant than the absolute BAC level, which is more significant in the genesis of an alcoholic blackout [68–73].

Alcohol and the law

There seems to be relative consistency in the legal view in the UK that the *voluntary* use of alcohol should not be considered a valid defense for criminal behavior (*R v. Quick, Finnegan v. Heywood*). In the Canadian court case *R v. Daviault*, however, the Supreme Court decided to acquit the defendant based on expert testimony that linked automatism to a blackout. In the EU, such an acquittal would be inconceivable because of the *culpa in causa* doctrine – the suspect is expected to know the consequences of excessive alcohol use and thus is held fully responsible for his or her behavior while under the influence. In the USA in *Wilson v. U.S.*, the trial court found the accused to be competent, pointing out that despite his organic amnesia, he had the capacity to understand the details of the case by relying on other sources of information. The U.S. Court of Appeals accepted the trial court's analysis of what was required for competence, based on the Dusky standard. Judge Leventhal pointed out that it is a common occurrence for a person to be convicted of *negligent* homicide, even though his memory is impaired by intoxication at the time of the crime. There is at present some debate within the medico-legal community regarding the nature and validity of a relationship between automatism and alcoholic blackout. The nexus of the debate revolves around whether someone in an alcoholic blackout possesses the requisite *mens rea* and on the degree of "voluntariness" exercised by the individual during a blackout [74–76].

Drug-related violence

The use and abuse of recreational and prescription medication and their forensic inter-relationships is well documented in Chapter 6, which provides a comprehensive overview of parasomnia due to drug or substance use.

Dissociation

Chapter 8 provides an overview of trauma, PTSD and parasomnias, and Chapter 17 on sleep-related dissociative disorders covers the clinical presentation, diagnosis, treatment and management aspects of the relevant dissociative disorders. The following references provide a comprehensive overview of dissociation and amnesia in the forensic context [77–79].

Malingering

The DSM-IV-TR defines malingering as "the intentional production of false or grossly exaggerated physical or psychological symptoms, motivated by external incentives such as avoiding military duty, avoiding work, obtaining financial compensation, evading criminal prosecution, or obtaining drugs."

An early study reported that 20% of the offenders claiming amnesia for an offence were fabricating the memory. More recently, it has been suggested that this may be much higher. The likelihood of malingered amnesia may be greater in offenders with anti-social personality disorder. In a survey of forensic practitioners, Rogers found 16% of malingerers in forensic cases and about 8% in non-forensic cases. In a further study, 15–17% of malingerers were found in forensic examinees and 7–8% in non-forensic. Pollock, using the MMPI-2 and the SIRS Interview Schedules, in 60 consecutive referrals from prison to a regional secure unit, found 32% to be either fabricating or exaggerating their symptoms. More interesting, malingering in civil cases of head injury showed rates as high as 40%.

A thorough clinical evaluation following the basic principles of history-taking, clinical examination, and repeated history-taking are important tools. It is also essential to study the defendant's first account, given to the police, as this often reveals a much greater knowledge of the offense than is subsequently claimed. Suspicion of malingering should be raised if the defendant claims to have sleepwalked for the first time during the offense, there is patchy recall of events, and this recall changes with repeated evaluations.

An in-patient assessment with 24-h observation by a multidisciplinary team may be necessary sometimes – here in the prison or secure hospital setting, it may be possible to observe the defendant over a number of days or weeks, carefully recording all interactions and behaviors. Under these circumstances, the individual is under significant pressure to produce sleepwalking episodes to bolster his defense, and a multidisciplinary assessment of any "sleepwalking" episode should be able to delineate a true episode from that which was "optimistically dreamed up" by the individual. The exclusion of a malingered defense is one that should take the highest priority where an expert is tasked with assessing a case of an apparent sleep-related crime [80–83].

Conclusion

The medico-legal consequences of the parasomnias embrace the areas of sleep disorders, neurology, psychiatry and forensic medicine. The expert involved in the forensic evaluation of an apparent sleep-related crime has to, of necessity, have the requisite clinical skills and qualifications to straddle all these disciplines, and more importantly be able to provide an unbiased and scientifically valid viewpoint when presenting in the courtroom.

It is not the role of the sleep expert to make a case for or against a particular defense; rather, the primary role of the expert should be to provide all possible scenarios based on valid, substantiated and current medical and scientific data in the field. It is essential that s/he take a holistic, non-partisan view of the case after a thorough examination of all the information and full examination of the accused/defendant. A multidisciplinary team approach to the evaluation of the individual involved in these actions is to be recommended combined with an impartial, ethical and scientifically valid approach to expert testimony.

References

1. Ohayon M, Caulet M, Priest R. Violent behavior during sleep. *J Clin Psychiatry* 1997; **58**: 369–76.
2. Bonkalo A. Impulsive acts and confusional states during incomplete arousal from sleep: Criminological and forensic implications. *Psychiatr Q* 1974; **48**: 400–09.
3. Broughton R. NREM arousal parasomnias. In Kryger MH, Roth T, Dement WC (Eds), *Principles and Practice of Sleep Medicine*. 3rd ed. Philadelphia, PA: W.B. Saunders 2000; 693–706.
4. Cartwright R. Sleepwalking violence: A sleep disorder, a legal dilemma, and a psychological challenge. *Am J Psychiatry* 2004; **161**: 1149–58.
5. Ebrahim IO, Fenwick P. Sleep related automatism and the law. *Med Sci Law* 2008; **48**: 124–36.
6. Yellowless D. Homicide by a somnambulist. *J Ment Sci* 1878; **24**: 451–8.
7. Podolsky E. Somnambulistic homicide. *Dis Nerv Syst* 1959; **20**: 534–6.
8. Mahowald M, Cramer Bornemann MA. NREM sleep-arousal parasomnias. In Kryger MH, Roth T, Dement WC (Eds), *Principles and Practice of Sleep*

Medicine. 4th edition. Philadelphia, PA: Elsevier Saunders, 2005: 892–925.
9. Broughton RJ, Shimizu T. Dangerous behaviour at night. In Shapiro C, McCall Smith A (Eds), *Forensic Aspects of Sleep*. Chichester: Wiley, 1997: 65–83.
10. Moldofsky H, Gilbert R, Lue FA, et al. Forensic sleep medicine: Violence, sleep, nocturnal wandering: Sleep-related violence. *SLEEP* 1995; **18**: 731–9.
11. Ebrahim IO, Wilson W, Marks R, Peacock KW, Fenwick P. Violence, sleepwalking and the criminal law: (1) The medical aspects. *Criminal Law Rev* 2005; 601–13.
12. Fenwick P. Murdering while asleep. *Br Med J* 1986; **293**: 574–5.
13. Hopwood JS, Snell HK. Amnesia in relation to crime. *J Ment Sci* 1933; **79**: 27–41.
14. Broughton RJ, Shimizu T. Sleep-related violence: A medical and forensic challenge. *Sleep* 1995; **18**: 727–30.
15. Guilleminault C, Moscovitch A, Leger D. Forensic sleep medicine: Nocturnal wandering and violence. *Sleep* 1995; **18**: 740–8.
16. Schenck CH, Arnulf I. Sleep and sex: What can go wrong? A review of the literature on sleep related disorders and abnormal sexual behaviors and experiences. *SLEEP* 2007; **30**: 683–702.
17. Howard C, d'Orban PT. Violence in sleep: Medico-legal issues and two case reports. *Psychol Med* 1987; **17**: 915–25.
18. Oswald I, Evans J. On serious violence during sleep walking. *Br J Psychiatry* 1985; **147**: 688–91.
19. The American Law Institute. Model Penal Code and Commentaries (Official Draft and Revised Comments), Part I – General Provisions §§1.01 to 2.13, Philadelphia: The American Law Institute, 1985, liii, 420 p., see §2.01, "Requirement of Voluntary Act; Omission as Basis of Liability; Possession as an Act" at pp. 212–24.
20. Feinberg J. *The Moral Limits of the Criminal Law*. Vol. 3, *Harm to Self*. New York: Oxford University Press, 1986.
21. Schopp RF. *Automatism, Insanity, and the Psychology of Criminal Responsibility: A Philosophical Inquiry*. New York, NY: Cambridge University Press, 1991.
22. Fenwick P. Somnambulism and the law: A review. *Behav Sci Law* 1987; **5**: 343–57.
23. Fenwick P. Automatism and the law. *Lancet* 1989; **2**: 753–4.
24. Fenwick P. Automatism, medicine and the law. *Psychol Med Monogr* 1990; Suppl. **17**; 1–27.
25. Beaumont G. Automatism and hypoglycaemia. *J Forensic Legal Med* 2007; **14**: 103–07.
26. Government, Crimes Bill 1989, introduced in May 1989, xxvii, 156p. See on Clause 19, "Involuntary acts" pp. iv–v and 14.
27. Yeo S. Clarifying automatism. *Int J Law Psychiatry* 2002; **25**: 445–58.
28. Bourget D, Whitehurst L. Amnesia and crime. *J Am Acad Psychiatry Law* 2007; **35**: 469–80.
29. Glancy GD, Bradford JM, Fedak L. A comparison of R. v. Stone with R. v. Parks: two cases of automatism. *J Am Acad Psychiatry Law* 2002; **30**: 541–7.
30. McCall Smith A, Shapiro CM (Eds). *Forensic Aspects of Sleep*. Chichester: John Wiley and Sons, 1997.
31. Wilson W, Ebrahim IO, Fenwick P, Marks R. Violence, sleepwalking and the criminal law: (2) The legal aspects. *Criminal Law Rev* 2005; **8**: 614–23.
32. Mahowald MW, Schenck CH. Parasomnias: Sleepwalking and the law. *Sleep Med Rev* 2004; **4**: 321–39.
33. Cramer Bornemann MA, Mahowald MW, Schenck CH. Parasomnias: Clinical features and forensic implications. *Chest* 2006; **130**: 605–10.
34. Cramer Bornemann MA. Role of the expert witness in sleep-related violence trials. Virtual mentor. *Am Med Assoc J Ethics* 2008, **10**: 571–7.
35. Federal Rules of Evidence. Available at http://www.law.cornell.edu/rules/fre. Accessed December 31, 2008.
36. *Daubert v. Merrell Dow Pharmaceuticals*, 509 U.S. 579 (1993).
37. American Academy of Neurology. Qualifications and guidelines for the physician expert witness. Available at http://www.aan.com/globals/axon/assets/2687.pdf. Accessed January 20, 2009.
38. Beecher-Monas E. *Evaluating Scientific Evidence: An Interdisciplinary Framework for Intellectual Due Process*. New York, NY: Cambridge University Press, 2007.
39. Weintraub MI. Expert witness testimony. An update. *Neurologic Clinics* 1999; **17**: 363–9.
40. *Access to Justice: Final report by the Rt. Hon the Lord Woolf, Master of the Rolls*. London: HM Stationery Office, 1996.
41. Butler-Sloss E. Expert witnesses, courts and the law. *J R Soc Med* 2002; **95**: 431–4.
42. Civil Justice Council. *Protocol for the instruction of Experts to give Evidence in Civil Claims*. Available at: http://www.justice.gov.uk/civil/procrules_fin/contents/form_section_images/practice_directions/pd35_pdf_eps/pd35_prot.pdf. Last accessed January 7, 2009.
43. Guidelines for Expert Witnesses in Proceedings in the Federal Court of Australia: Practice Direction.

Part 3.3 – *Opinion of the Evidence Act* 1995 (Cth), May 2008.

44. South African Law Commission, Discussion Paper 96. Available at http://www.law.wits.ac.za/salc/salc.html. Last accessed January 6, 2009.

45. Willis CS. The CHESS method of forensic opinion formulation: Striving to checkmate bias. *J Am Acad Psychiatry Law* 2008; **36**: 535–40.

46. Bourget D, Whitehurst L. Amnesia and crime. *J Am Acad Psychiatry Law* 2007; **35**: 469–80.

47. Guilleminault C, Leger D, Philip P, Ohayon MM. Nocturnal wandering and violence: Review of sleep clinic population. *J Forensic Sci* 1998; **43**: 158–63.

48. Pressman MR. Disorders of arousal from sleep and violent behavior: The role of physical contact and proximity. *SLEEP* 2007; **30**: 1039–47.

49. Pressman MR. Factors that predispose, prime and precipitate NREM parasomnias in adults: Clinical and forensic implications. *Sleep Med Rev* 2007; **11**: 5–30.

50. Ebrahim IO, Fenwick PB. Response to Pressman: "Factors that predispose, prime and precipitate NREM parasomnias in adults: Clinical and forensic implications": *Sleep Med Rev* 2007; 11: 5–9. *Sleep Med Rev* 2007; **11**: 241–3.

51. Cartwright R. Re: Pressman, M. Factors that predispose, prime and precipitate NREM parasomnias in adults: Clinical and forensic implications. *Sleep Med Rev* 2007; 11: 5–30. *Sleep Med Rev* 2007; **11**: 327–9.

52. Cartwright R. Sleep-related violence: Does the polysomnogram help establish the diagnosis? *Sleep Med* 2000; **1**: 331–5.

53. Mahowald MW, Schenck CH. REM sleep parasomnias. In Kryger MH, Roth T, Dement WC (Eds), *Principles and Practice of Sleep Medicine*. 3rd ed. Philadelphia, PA: W.B. Saunders, 2005: 724–41.

54. Parrino L, Halasz P, Tassinari CA, Terzano MG. CAP, epilepsy and motor events during sleep: The unifying role of arousal. *Sleep Med Rev* 2006; **10**: 267–85.

55. Tassinari CA, Gardella E, Meletti S, Rubboli G. The neuroethological interpretation of motor behaviours in "nocturnal-hyperkynetic-frontal-seizures": Emergence of "innate" motor behaviours and role of central pattern generators. In Beaumanoir A, Andermann F, Chauvel P, Mira L, Zifkin B (Eds), *Frontal Lobe Seizures and Epilepsies in Children*. France: John Libbey; 2003, 43–5.

56. Tassinari CA, Rubboli G, Gardella E, et al. Central pattern generators for a common semeiology in fronto-limbic seizures and in parasomnias. A neuroethologic approach. *Neurol Sci* 2005; **26**(Suppl 3): s225–32.

57. Vignatelli L, Bisulli F, Zaniboni A, *et al*. Interobserver reliability of ICSD-R minimal diagnostic criteria for the parasomnias. *J Neurol* 2005; **252**: 712–7.

58. Tinuper P, Lugaresi E. The concept of paroxysmal nocturnal dystonia. In Bazil CW, Malow BA, Sammaritano MR (Eds), *Sleep and Epilepsy: The Clinical Spectrum*. Amsterdam: Elsevier Science; 2002: 277–82.

59. Bisulli F, Naldi I, Vignatelli L, *et al*. Paroxysmal motor phenomena during sleep: Study of the frequency of parasomnias in patients with nocturnal frontal lobe epilepsy and their relatives. *Epilepsia* 2005; **46**(Suppl 6): 284.

60. Tinuper P, *et al*. Movement disorders in sleep: Guidelines for differentiating epileptic from non-epileptic motor phenomena arising from sleep. *Sleep Med Rev* 2007; **11**: 251–4.

61. Trajanovic NN, Shapiro CM, Ong A. Atypical presentation of NREM arousal parasomnia with repetitive episodes. *Eur J Neurol* 2007; **14**: 947–50.

62. Provini F, Plazzi G, Lugaresi E. From nocturnal paroxysmal dystonia to nocturnal frontal lobe epilepsy. *Clin Neurophysiol* 2000; **111**(Suppl. 2).

63. Hughes JR. A review of sleepwalking (somnambulism): The enigma of neurophysiology and polysomnography with differential diagnosis of complex partial seizures. *Epilepsy & Behavior* 2007; **11**: 483–91.

64. Marinacci AA. A special type of temporal lobe (psychomotor) seizures following ingestion of alcohol. *Bull LA Neurol Soc* 1963; **28**: 241–50.

65. Mattson RH. Seizures associated with alcohol use and alcohol withdrawal. In Browne TR (Ed), *Epilepsy, Diagnosis and Management*. Boston: Little, Brown and Co., 1983: 325–32.

66. Hauser WA, Ng SKC, Brust JCM. Alcohol, seizures, and epilepsy. *Epilepsia* 1988; **29**(Suppl. 2): S66–78.

67. Reuber M, Mackay RD. Epileptic automatisms in the criminal courts: 13 cases tried in England and Wales between 1975 and 2001. *Epilepsia* 2008; **49**: 138–45.

68. Lishman SA. Alcoholic blackout: State-dependant learning. *Arch Gen Psychiatry* 1974; **30**: 46–53.

69. White AM, Matthews DB, Best PJ. Ethanol, memory, and hippocampal function: A review of recent findings. *Hippocampus* 2000; **10**: 88–93.

70. Wechsler H, Lee JE, Kuo M, Seibring M, Nelson TF, Lee H. Trends in college binge drinking during a period of increased prevention efforts. Findings from 4 Harvard School of Public Health College Alcohol Study surveys: 1993–2001. *J Am Coll Health* 2002; **50**: 203–17.

71. White AM, Jamieson-Drake DW, Swartzwelder HS. Prevalence and correlates of alcohol-induced blackouts among college students: Results of an e-mail survey. *J Am Coll Health* 2002; **51**: 117–31.

72. Weissenborn R, Duka T. Acute alcohol effects on cognitive function in social drinkers: Their relationship to drinking habits. *Psychopharmacology (Berl)* 2003; **165**: 306–12.

73. White AM. What happened? Alcohol, memory blackouts, and the brain. *Alcohol Res Health* 2003; **27**: 186–96.

74. van Oorsouw, Merckelbach H, Ravelli D, Nijman H, Mekking-Pompen I. Alcoholic blackout for criminally relevant behavior. *J Am Acad Psychiatry Law* 2004; **32**: 364–70.

75. Granarcher Jnr RP. Commentary: Alcoholic blackout and allegation of amnesia during criminal acts. *J Am Acad Psychiatry Law* 2004; **32**: 371–4.

76. Merikangas J. Commentary: Alcoholic blackout – does it remove *mens rea*? *J Am Acad Psychiatry Law* 2004; **32**: 375–7.

77. Markowitsch HJ. Psychogenic amnesia. *NeuroImage* 2003; **20**: S132–8.

78. Yasuno F, Nishikawa T, Nakagawa Y, *et al.* Functional anatomical study of psychogenic amnesia. *Psychiatry Res* 2000; **99**: 43–57.

79. Stone JH. Memory disorder in offenders and victims. *Crim Behav Ment Health* 1992; **2**: 342–56.

80. Rogers R, Sewell K, Morey LC, Ustad KL. Detection of feigned mental disorders on the personality assessment inventory: A discriminant analysis. *J Pers Assess* 1996; **67**: 629–40.

81. Bagby RM, Rogers R, Buis T, *et al.* Detecting feigned depression and schizophrenia on the MMPI-2. *J Pers Assess* 1968; **3**: 650–64.

82. Pollock PH, Quigley B, Worley KO. Feigned mental disorder in prisoners referred to forensic mental health services. *Journal of Psychiatric and Mental Health Nursing* 1997; **4**: 9–15.

83. Mittenberg W, Patton C, Canyock EM, Condit DC. Base rates of malingering and symptom exaggeration. *J Clin Exp Neuropsychol* 2002; **24**: 1094–102.

Section 2
Disorders of arousal

Section 2 Chapter 11

Disorders of arousal

Confusional arousals

Gregory Stores

It might be said that the use of the term "confusional arousals" can itself be confusing in that it refers to somewhat separable sleep disorder entities which, largely depending on the age of the patients under consideration, are often merged or subject to different emphasis. Indeed, some accounts dwell exclusively on one age group or the other.

Although they have features in common, childhood confusional arousals tend to be different from those in adults regarding such aspects as etiology, precipitants, associations with other sleep disorders, complications and significance, differential diagnosis, treatment requirements, and prognosis. For the sake of clarity, therefore, in this chapter, based on the information in the available literature, the topic will be considered separately according to whether they occur in children or in adults. This separation should not be considered absolute, if only because early-onset confusional arousals sometimes persist into adult life.

Definition

According to the 2005 edition of the International Classification of Sleep Disorders or ICSD-2 [1], the essential features of confusional arousals are mental confusion or confusional behavior during or following arousals from sleep, typically from deep non-rapid eye movement (NREM) or slow-wave sleep (SWS) in the first part of the night, but also upon attempted awakening from sleep in the morning. More specific aspects are disorientation in time and space, slowing of mental processes and speech, diminished responsiveness, anterograde and retrograde impairment of memory, and inappropriate behavior.

History

One of the alternate names given in ICSD-2, *Elpenor syndrome*, is derived from the story in Homer's Odyssey in which Elpenor, a companion of Odysseus, having become intoxicated with alcohol before going to sleep, was suddenly woken by a noise and, in a confusional state, fell and broke his neck [2].

In his splendid 1974 historical account, Bonkalo quotes a series of apparent instances of confusional arousal cases in the English and other European literature from 1600 through subsequent centuries [3]. Broughton [4] refers to confusional episodes being induced experimentally in man as early as 1897.

In many of Bonkelo's examples, offences, including homicide, were considered to have been attributable to automatic behavior during arousal from sleep. This and other forensic aspects, about which there has been increasing interest in recent years, will be discussed later.

Terminology

In addition to Elpenor syndrome, other ICSD-2 alternate terms for confusional arousals also have quite early origins: "l'ivresse du sommeil" by 1840 [5], and "sleep drunkenness" or "Schlaftrunkenheit" by 1905 [6]. "Excessive sleep inertia" is another alternate name in ICSD-2. Since the 1979 Diagnostic Classification of Sleep and Arousal Disorders [7], "confusional arousal" has been included as a disorder of arousal, grouped with sleepwalking and sleep terrors.

For the purposes of this review, it is helpful to make certain distinctions (not always clear in the literature) between some of the terms mentioned above.

- *Confusional arousals* are defined as already suggested, including the basic feature of occurrence in SWS in the early part of sleep.
- *Sleepwalking* implies similar physiological and clinical features, but, understandably, also involves walking.

The Parasomnias and Other Sleep-Related Movement Disorders, ed. M. J. Thorpy and G. Plazzi. Published by Cambridge University Press. © Cambridge University Press 2010.

- *Sleep terrors* involve a particularly high degree of autonomic arousal (more so than confusional arousals).
- *Sleep drunkenness* also has the basic arousal features, but this term refers to occurrence following partial arousal after awakening, with accompanying unsteadiness. It is used mainly in connection with states of excessive daytime sleepiness (hypersomnia).
- *Sleep inertia* is the feeling and appearance of "grogginess" for a while after waking up.
- Some accounts include reference to *automatic behavior*, a general term for actions in a state of diminished consciousness, with relative unresponsiveness to the environment, and consequent impaired recall.

As discussed shortly, confusional arousals, sleepwalking and sleep terrors (collectively called "arousal disorders") are considered to be on a continuum. Some accounts, including a number of those cited in the text of this chapter, tend to merge discussion of the first two of these types in particular.

Confusional arousals in childhood

The notion of confusional arousals in children has received less attention overall compared with that concerning adults, and distinctions according to age are not always made. Accounts usually combine adults and children and often contain a rather bland statement along the lines of "this disorder is quite frequent in childhood and decreases with age" (ICSD-2 only goes somewhat further than this), ignoring the various likely differences between adults and children that were mentioned earlier. This is but one of many examples of the incomplete emancipation of the field of children's sleep disorders medicine from that concerning adults [8].

However, some pediatrically inclined writers have reported their experience of confusional arousals, mainly in young children. In the absence of detailed epidemiological or clinical studies (and, indeed, formal evidence-based recommendations about treatment), the information is largely anecdotal or impressionistic in nature (a criticism, however, which also applies largely to adult reports).

It might be the case that some of the etiological and other comparative complexities of confusional arousals in adults would come to light with more refined investigation of those in children. However, at present, childhood confusional arousals are simply viewed as one of the three basic forms of one type of sleep disorder, namely 'arousal disorders', along with sleepwalking and sleep terrors (see Chapters 12 and 13 for detailed accounts), only rarely invoking involvement of other types of sleep disorders. Some overall points about childhood arousal disorders in general are initially appropriate in order to provide a background for more specific discussion of confusional arousals.

General points about childhood arousal disorders including confusional arousals [9]

Arousal disorders are common in childhood. In a minority, they persist into adult life, and in a few they begin in adolescence, or even adult life. Arousal does not mean that the child wakes up; the arousal is, in fact, a partial arousal usually from deep NREM sleep (slow-wave sleep or SWS) to another, lighter stage of sleep.

As mentioned, three main forms of arousal disorder are described. These are best seen as forming a continuum of basically the same type of sleep disorder. Indeed, episodes sometimes combine elements of all three, and a child might display a sequence of confusional arousals in early childhood, sleepwalking later, followed by sleep terrors in late childhood and adolescence. Alternatively, features of all three forms can occur at any one stage of development. Similarly, the family history of arousal disorder can take a variety of forms.

Sleepwalking and sleep terrors are well known; confusional arousals are generally less well recognized. Clinically, all share a curious combination of features suggestive of being simultaneously awake and asleep. Despite seeming to be alert (indeed, sometimes highly aroused), the child appears confused and disoriented and relatively unresponsive to environmental events, including parents' attempts to communicate. There is little or (usually) no recall of events during each episode of disturbed behavior.

In such arousals, various behaviors can occur, either simple in nature (for example, sitting up in bed and mumbling) or complicated, such as rushing out of the house in a highly agitated state, as happens in some sleepwalking episodes and sleep terrors. Other, more complex behaviors occasionally described in young people include aggressive acts and sleep-related eating disorders. The child remains asleep during the episode itself, failing to recognize his parents or be comforted by them, although waking sometimes occurs at the end of it, particularly in later childhood or adolescence.

Usually only one episode occurs during the night, within the first 2 h or so after going to sleep when SWS is most abundant. However, some children predisposed to arousal disorders also have such arousals arising from light NREM and REM sleep, giving rise to multiple episodes throughout the night. Such repeated episodes are usually less dramatic each time. Partial arousals are possible during daytime naps.

The main predisposing factor is genetic: a first-degree family history of partial arousals has been reported in the vast majority of cases, the fundamental pathophysiological feature appearing to be instability of deep NREM sleep [10].

There are many possible precipitating factors in constitutionally predisposed individuals. These include fever, systemic illness, increase of SWS from sleep loss, irregular sleep schedules or CNS-depressant medication, internal or external sleep-interrupting stimuli (such as a full bladder, sleeping in an unfamiliar environment, or the child being woken forcefully by a sudden noise or pain, for example), and stressful psychological experiences which may precipitate or maintain the occurrence of the episodes and also influence their severity. Sleep-disordered breathing and, to a lesser extent, restless legs syndrome and periodic limb movements have also been implicated as possible triggers [11].

The more dramatic forms of arousal disorder may well be interpreted by parents as a sign of medical or psychiatric disorder, which is rarely correct. However, arousal disorders can be socially disadvantageous, especially when they occur away from home, and this can give rise to emotional upset. Also, accidental injury often occurs when the child moves about the house or further afield, only partially aware of the surroundings.

If a detailed description is obtained, special investigations are not usually necessary for the recognition of arousal disorders. However, polysomnography (PSG) (extended to include additional physiological parameters beyond basic measures together with audiovisual monitoring) during episodes might be helpful if, despite careful clinical evaluation, the distinction still cannot be made between partial arousals and the other predominantly childhood parasomnias which involve complicated behavior at night. Such disorders include rhythmic movement disorders (e.g. headbanging or body rolling), nightmares, or sleep-related seizures such as those in benign centrotemporal epilepsy of childhood, in all of which detailed assessment will usually distinguish them from arousal disorders [12].

There are a number of important principles regarding the management of childhood arousal disorders.

- Parental anxiety is usually lessened by explanation with reassurance (where justified) that these often dramatic and frightening events do not mean that the child is ill or disordered, and that the events can usually be expected to stop spontaneously by later childhood or adolescence.
- Regular and adequate sleep routines to prevent loss or disruption of sleep resulting in an increased amount of SWS are important, as well as avoidance of other known precipitating factors.
- The environment should be as safe as possible to reduce the risk of injury, e.g. removal of obstructions in the bedroom, secure windows, install locks or alarms on outside doors, or cover windows with heavy curtains.
- Parents should be encouraged to refrain from trying to waken or restrain the child during an episode. Understandably, seeing their child apparently distressed, parents may feel the need to comfort their child and try by various means (perhaps including shaking).

  Apart from being difficult to achieve, this is counterproductive because, if successful, the child will be confused and frightened, probably making the episode more severe and violent. It is also unnecessary because, being asleep during the episode, the child will not have been distressed in the way they supposed. It is much better to remain calm, ensure that the child does not come to harm, and wait until the episode subsides and then help the child back to restful sleep.
- If, as is usually the case, the child has no recall of the episodes, there is little point in relating the episodes, as this may become a source of anxiety.
- "Scheduled awakening" has been recommended at least for sleepwalking or sleep terror episodes which are frequent and consistent in the time at which they occur. This consists of the child being gently and briefly woken 15–30 min before the episode is due. The procedure is repeated nightly for up to a month. Preliminary reports suggest that where there is improvement it can be maintained for at least several months.

- Medication should be reserved for particularly worrying, embarrassing or dangerous arousals where other measures have failed [13]. Benzodiazepines (such as low-dose clonazepam) and tricyclic drugs (e.g. imipramine), both of which reduce SWS, have been used but with mixed results. Use of benzodiazepines is best restricted to short-acting forms continued for several weeks at most to avoid possible hazards of long-term use. Rebound effects can occur when medication is discontinued, resulting in an increase of arousal episodes.
- If there is evidence of an underlying psychological problem, appropriate enquiries and help are indicated.

Clinical features of confusional arousals in children

These share the general characteristics of the other arousal disorders, but without the child walking or displaying the intense autonomic arousal seen in agitated sleepwalking and especially in sleep terrors. They occur mainly in infants and toddlers (probably most of whom have such episodes to some extent, at least in mild form) and almost invariably before the age of 5. Exact prevalence is uncertain from the limited information available. They become less frequent as adolescence approaches, during which time they may be the only type of arousal episode, or give way to sleepwalking or sleep terrors.

An episode may begin with mumbling, moaning or whimpering, gradually increasing movements which then progress to agitated and confused behavior with marked perspiration, crying (perhaps intense, but not screaming), calling out, or thrashing about. Sometimes this causes the child to fall out of bed, although injuries are less likely than in the other arousal disorders. The child's eyes may be open or closed. Typically, although appearing to be awake, the child does not respond when spoken to and may seem to "stare right through" his parents. Any forceful attempts to intervene may meet with severe resistance and even aggression.

Parents are often very alarmed, some are said to fear that their child appears "possessed" [14], and, wanting to console the child, they may make vigorous attempts to waken him, without success or only with much trying. However, such efforts may actually prolong the arousal and, if the child is woken to some extent, cause confusion and fear.

Each episode usually lasts 5–15 min (sometimes much longer) before the child calms down spontaneously and returns to restful sleep. Enuresis may occur during or after an episode.

The differential diagnosis at this age includes the other arousal disorders and sleep-related seizures of which there are several varieties [15]. Identification of the distinctive clinical characteristics of these conditions (by means of audiovisual recordings, if necessary) should aid correct diagnosis but physiological recording may be required in diagnostically difficult cases. Often, confusional arousals are referred to as "nightmares" or "bad dreams"' in the loose, inaccurate use of these terms for any dramatic parasomnia.

Many of the general points about arousal disorders discussed above apply to confusional arousals, although some are not relevant at this early stage of development. In addition, for the precipitating factors that are relevant, some accounts of childhood confusional arousals also implicate certain hypersomnia-causing sleep disorders, namely obstructive sleep apnea, narcolepsy and idiopathic hypersomnia. However, it is unclear to what extent this is actually based on observations in the young age group, and how far it is simply extrapolation from older patients with confusional arousals.

Typical confusional arousals rarely require specific treatment which, however, may be appropriate, in the ways outlined earlier, if they are combined with other types of partial arousal. As mentioned, spontaneous remission can be expected.

Confusional arousals in adults

The same basic definition of confusional arousals applies to both children and adults. Their polysomnographic features are also basically equivalent and, as in young patients, they can constitute part of the triad of types of arousal disorders where they have persisted from childhood.

However, as mentioned at the start of this review, differences exist regarding prevalence, some of the clinical manifestations, the other etiological and clinical settings in which they can occur (i.e. their relationships with other sleep disorders), precipitating factors, other associated features according to the admittedly limited information available on this point, their diagnostic features and differential diagnosis, the complications (including legal) to which they can give rise, treatment requirements, and also prognosis. Each of these aspects will be considered in turn.

Prevalence

There are uncertainties about the prevalence of confusional arousals at any age, but it is generally agreed that they are much less common in adults than in children. ICSD-2 quotes figures of 17.3% between 3 and 13 years of age, and 2.9–4.2% in patients over 15, with no gender differences [1].

Clinical manifestations

The impression gained is that, especially in response to forced awakenings, the behavioral disturbance in adult episodes is more forceful, vigorous and resistive, sometimes leading to violent behavior (see later). Bruxism might be an additional feature (although possibly also in children). If a confusional arousal is induced in people whose occupation calls for skilled performance, they may well perform less than skilfully when woken.

ICSD-2 refers to two variants of confusional arousals in adolescents and adults.

- One is *severe morning sleep inertia* (or sleep drunkenness) after waking up rather suddenly from SWS in the first part of the night.
- The other is *sleep-related sexual behavior* (or "atypical sexual behavior during sleep", "sexsomnia", or "sleepsex"), which is thought to occur during both confusional arousals and sleepwalking. This condition will be considered later.

To these can be added *sleep-related violence* [16], although it is not clear how often this is a feature of confusional arousals rather than other arousal disorders.

Predisposing and precipitating factors including associations with other sleep disorders

This aspect is more complex and varied than in children's confusional arousals. Although genetic factors are also prominent in adults, a range of other types of sleep disturbance are acknowledged as additional predisposing influences.

As in children, anything that deepens sleep or impairs the process of waking up can act this way, although the profile of such influences is somewhat different in adults. For example, it is usually said to include medication with a CNS-depressant effect, such as hypnotics or tranquilizers and metabolic, toxic and other illnesses which deepen or disturb sleep. However, it has been suggested that many reported cases supposedly illustrating the influence of such factors do not fully conform to ICSD-2 criteria of arousal disorders [10].

Other sleep disorders which predispose to confusional arousals are additional hypersomnias of central origin, such as narcolepsy and idiopathic hypersomnia; circadian sleep–wake cycle disorders (especially those due to shift work, particularly at night); and sleep-disordered breathing disorders such as obstructive sleep apnea (OSA). Occasionally, confusional arousals have been associated with certain CNS lesions, especially those likely to affect arousal systems.

Similarly, some of the precipitating factors in adult arousal disorders would be generally less likely in children, such as alcohol consumption or substance abuse, periodic limb movement disorder, and some psychotropic medications including those used for affective disorders. In their different ways, these factors disturb sleep and, in predisposed individuals, seemingly enhance the abnormal effect of forced awakening.

Other associations with confusional arousals in adults

The point has already been made that systematic, thorough research on arousal disorders is difficult to identify. The international, large-scale population study of adult confusional arousals by Ohayon and his colleagues is the exception [17].

Between 1994 and 1997, all members of a representative sample of 13,057 subjects, over the age of 14 years, from the UK, Germany and Italy (79.6% of all subjects initially contacted), were systematically interviewed by telephone about their sleep habits and disorders, as well as their circumstances and general health.

Confusional arousals, defined according to ICSD-90 criteria [18], occurring at least once a month, were identified in 2.9% of the overall sample, reducing from 6.1% in the 15–24 age group to 1.4% in those over 64. No gender differences were seen. Of the overall number, 1% of those with confusional arousals also often reported memory deficits, being disorientated, or slowing of thought and speech.

Many of the other findings concerning associated features were in keeping with published clinical impressions. Night shift or other shift workers reported higher rates than those working days. Other apparent associations were anxiety, bipolar and depressive disorders, and a range of possible sleep disorders or behaviors (as far as could be judged from the limited questioning involved in the survey), OSA, insomnia, hypersomnia, hypnagogic and hypnopompic hallucinations, sleep talking, and sleep bruxism. Violent or injurious behavior was a further associated feature.

Commendable though this apparently unique epidemiological investigation has been, its complicated findings need to be replicated and clarified. Also, confusional arousals might be more common than even the results of this survey suggest because some people may not be aware that they suffer from them, especially if there is no independent observer.

As mentioned, many of the results are compatible with previous clinical reports, but the relationships between the presence of confusional arousals and associated conditions, including other sleep disorders, calls for further study.

Possibly most attention has been paid to adult confusional states occurring in the context of hypersomnia, including *idiopathic hypersomnia*. This relatively recently described condition, and, it is thought, often confused in the past with other causes of hypersomnia, remains the subject of debate regarding its suggested different forms [19].

The essential features of its "polysymptomatic" form are prolonged nocturnal sleep, great difficulty waking up, and excessive daytime sleepiness with repeated sleep episodes, often prolonged and (in contrast to the sleep attacks in narcolepsy) unrefreshing. Sleep drunkenness is common [20] and can be difficult to treat. Various socio-economic consequences of idiopathic hypersomnia, presumably in part because of sleep drunkenness, have been reported, such as poor occupational performance, accidents (including sleeping at the wheel), impotence and sensitivity to alcohol [19,21]. In contrast to arousal disorders, idiopathic hypersomnia is rare in children. The prospect of eventual improvement seems generally poor.

Confusional arousals can occur in association with *other causes of hypersomnia* encountered mainly (although by no means exclusively) in adults. These are narcolepsy with or without cataplexy (especially after prolonged daytime naps containing SWS), OSA, and on rebound from sleep deprivation (whatever the cause out of the many possibilities) resulting in an increase in SWS. Although often listed, periodic leg movement in sleep remains debatable as a cause of hypersomnia [22].

Confusional arousals might occur in the additional (less usual) causes of hypersomnia [19], such as hypothyroidism and other endocrine disorders, CNS lesions (e.g. head trauma), post-viral infection (for instance, infectious mononucleosis), and also heavy sedation. Hypersomnia can also be a feature of psychiatric disorder, notably severe depression, alcoholism or substance abuse.

Diagnosis and differential diagnosis of confusional arousals

Regarding the various conditions just listed as possible causes of hypersomnia and, therefore, confusional arousals, it should be emphasized that some of these conditions (and others) may themselves have confusional elements in common with confusional arousals. Differentiation of true confusional arousals from these other disorders is based on the recognition of the distinctive features of each of them.

The characteristic features of confusional arousals were described earlier. Ideally, PSG evidence would be obtained that these arousals arise from SWS. Some support for a clinical diagnosis of confusional arousals can be provided by the demonstration of multiple arousals from SWS unaccompanied by confusional behaviors [1], but a normal PSG does not exclude the diagnosis.

This distinctive combination of clinical and PSG features does not characterize the other conditions that enter into the differential diagnosis of confusional arousals. In addition to those already mentioned, these other conditions include sleepwalking and sleep terrors and also other parasomnias, especially those of a dramatic type, including some sleep-related epileptic seizures and REM sleep behavior disorder (RBD).

Some sleep-related seizures are seen mainly in children and, although partial in type, they rarely indicate structural brain pathology and run a benign course, usually resolving spontaneously before adulthood [15]. An exception is *nocturnal frontal lobe epilepsy* (NFLE), which can take a variety of forms [23], including some with a pronounced confusional element.

However, the many other clinical characteristics of these seizures, including particularly dramatic motor automatisms and vocalizations, and their timing, usually mark them as different from confusional arousals. That said, because differentiation from arousal disorders in general is not always easy (if only because EEG findings in this form of epilepsy, even during seizures, is often unhelpful), guidelines have been suggested as an aid to correct diagnosis [24].

Unlike arousal disorders, RBD [25] arises from REM sleep, mainly later in the night. It has very distinctive clinical features and associations with other disorders. Because of a pathological preservation of muscle tone during REM sleep, people with this condition are able to act out their dreams and can behave disruptively while asleep before waking up and (ideally) describing the corresponding content of their dream. If this has been violent, it can have led to damage, or injury to the patient or anyone nearby, including the bed partner. Once thought to occur only in elderly men, RBD has now been described at other ages, in women and also (rarely) in children [26].

The condition is closely associated with neurodegenerative disorders (notably Lewy body disease, multiple system atrophy and Parkinson's disease) of which it can be the harbinger, and certain medications including anti-depressants, as well as various other organic factors. Fortunately, RBD is readily treatable, especially with clonazepam. Occasionally, it co-exists with arousal disorders including confusional arousals ("parasomnia overlap disorder") [27].

Complications

Serious misconduct during childhood arousal disorders is rarely described [28], but those in adults are increasingly said to give rise to anti-social behavior, and its consequences including legal sanctions. However, how often this happens is difficult to judge.

As mentioned earlier, *acts of violence* have been reported. Bonkalo [3] describes possible examples from ancient times onwards, although the limited details available make the diagnosis somewhat uncertain, as the author admits. Many instances are presented ranging from Elpenor in Ancient Greece, through the Middle Ages up to near the time of writing. There is interesting reference to debates in the medieval and post-medieval periods whether someone committing such crimes should be judged sinful or legally responsible for his actions.

Bonkalo goes on to suggest guidelines for the clinical and forensic evaluation of cases. These mainly include identifying the characteristic clinical features of confusional arousals as described previously in the present chapter. His guidelines have much in common with more recent formulations concerning arousal disorders for forensic purposes [29]. Coming more up to date, in their review of violent parasomnias in general, Mahowald and Schenck [30] have discussed arousal disorders and human violence. In addition to reports of homicide and other acts of violence in sleepwalking and sleep terrors (including drug-induced examples), they refer to murders and other crimes (such as Bonkalo's "cases") attributed to sleep drunkenness related to obstructive sleep apnea and narcolepsy.

It was mentioned earlier that ICSD-2 now includes in its confusional arousals section *sleep-related sexual behavior* ("*sleepsex*" or "*sexsomnia*"). This increasingly publicized condition has been the subject of an extensive recent review, based mainly on a computerized literature search of cases, and proposed classification [31]. A wide range of sleep-related disorders associated with abnormal sexual behaviors and experiences was identified, in which parasomnias featured prominently, especially confusional arousals. Forensic consequences were common.

The condition had been reported mainly in males who commonly engaged in sexual fondling and sexual intercourse with females, whereas females mainly engaged in masturbation and sexual vocalizations. Several cases of sleepsex with minors were noted. In all arousal disorder cases, there was no recall of the sleepsex episodes. Sometimes, there was also a history of other parasomnias, such as sleepwalking or sleep-related eating disorder, or OSA, which itself was considered to have promoted sleepsex.

Bed partners often incurred physical injury from the sexual assaults, the patients less so. Commonly, both partners suffered psychological upset such as embarrassment, shock, alarm, annoyance, shame or guilt, and sometimes marital estrangement as a result. Only occasionally did the bed partner find the episodes pleasurable.

It was emphasized that it was uncommon for perpetrators of the sleepsex acts to have personal experience of sexual deprivation or frustration, a history of psychiatric disturbance, or previous history of sexual misconduct. A positive note was sounded about response when treatment had been given. This usually took the form of clonazepam, with continuous positive airway pressure (CPAP) used in the few cases of OSA. The review quotes a web-based survey (subject to limitations because of lack of detail in particular) in which respondents reported similar psychosocial reactions to their experience of sleepsex encounters [32].

Finally, the review discussed medico-legal issues connected with sleepsex, particularly where arousal disorder is proposed as a defense, and also the evaluation and management of sleep-related sexual complaints. As a parting shot, intriguing possible examples from the literature of confusional arousals and sleepsex are quoted, including one from Thomas Hardy's *Tess of the d'Urbervilles*, first published in 1891 [33]. Briefly, the heroine, Tess (probably in her early teens), was sexually assaulted by a man whom she had repeatedly rebuffed in the past. Exhausted, she had rapidly fallen deeply asleep in a forest late at night. The villain of the piece forced himself on her, raped her and made her pregnant. Hardy referred to this occurrence in which Tess "had been stirred to confused surrender..." and had acted with "inadvertence".

From various details of the event and others around that time, the authors of the review considered that Tess had six factors that night which provoke confusional arousals: her youth, acute sleep deprivation, physical exhaustion, forced awakening by her assailant, acute distress from an upsetting confrontation with another woman earlier that evening, as well as longstanding distress at being pressurized to marry a man she did not love, namely, her assailant. Their "clinical" interpretation of the situation was that Tess had precipitously fallen into deep sleep from which she was forcefully partially aroused and then, in a confused state, she had not resisted her assailant's advances, in striking contrast to her feelings about him when awake. Interesting!

Recently, there have been vigorous exchanges in the literature about various aspects of arousal disorders and criminal acts. This followed an article by Pressman entitled "Factors that predispose, prime and precipitate NREM parasomnias in adults: clinical and forensic implications" [10]. Some of the debate was mainly about appropriate evidence by expert witnesses in court in helping to decide the likelihood that an alleged offense was committed in the course of an arousal disorder [34].

Other exchanges [35,36] were concerned with more technical matters (although relevant to forensic issues), such as the possibility of an objective physiological indicator of the propensity to have arousal disorder episodes (as yet undetermined), and whether (contrary to the traditional view) in people genetically predisposed to arousal disorders, NREM is lighter than normal and the sleeper more easily aroused into a confusional mixed state of sleep and wakefulness. Also at variance with usual contentions is that opinions are divided whether or not alcohol acts as a predisposing factor or trigger to sleepwalking or related disorders [37,38].

In the course of these debates, it was suggested that it is the combination of (a) factors that lead to increased SWS, and (b) stimuli or substances that have the opposite effect of triggering arousals from SWS (such as loud noise, respiratory events as in OSA, or caffeine) that provokes the abnormal behavior of confusional arousals or sleepwalking [36]. Based on a review of cases from the medical and legal literature, it has been said that provocations by and close proximity to the victim seems common in violent arousal disorder behaviors, especially confusional arousals [39].

The contestants in the above disputes acknowledged the need for further research to clarify these largely unresolved issues.

Treatment and prognosis

As mentioned earlier, childhood confusional arousals do not usually require treatment, only advice to parents that they can be considered to be a passing phase. The same cannot necessarily be said of confusional arousals in adult life when they have more of a tendency to persist, depending on their etiology and relationship to other sleep disorders, as already discussed. However, if frequent and severe, apart from the relatively specific treatment for (say) an accompanying and responsible sleep disorder, e.g. CPAP for OSA, pharmacological treatment may be beneficial: for example, in the form of clonazepam (to which reference has already been made in relation to sleepsex occurring in the course of confusional arousals) or anti-depressants such as imipramine and possibly paroxetine or trazodone [40].

Conclusions

Confusional arousals are an interesting and important form of sleep disorder. In a number of respects they have different associations and implications according to the age at which they occur. Childhood confusional arousals are generally benign in that they are self-limiting and can be expected to remit spontaneously by adult life at the latest. They are not particularly associated with other conditions, including other sleep disorders, nor do they have significant psychosocial consequences. In contrast, adult confusional arousals are often linked to other disorders and can give rise to antisocial acts with serious medico-legal implications.

Although, at any age, confusional arousals are known to be associated with an abnormal arousal response during SWS, in the absence of a readily demonstrable objective aid to diagnosis, their recognition rests essentially on clinical grounds. It is clear from current accounts and the debates to which reference was made earlier about various aspects of arousal disorders, that the field is ripe with research possibilities of both a basic scientific and clinical nature.

References

1. American Academy of Sleep Medicine. *International Classification of Sleep Disorders, 2nd ed: Diagnostic and Coding Manual*. Westchester, IL: American Academy of Sleep Medicine, 2005.
2. Homer. *The Odyssey*, Book 10. Revised edition. Harmondsworth: Penguin Classics, 2003.
3. Bonkalo A. Impulsive acts and confusional states during incomplete arousal from sleep: Criminological and forensic implications. *Psychiatr Q* 1974; **48**: 400–09.
4. Broughton RJ. Sleep disorders: Disorders of arousal? *Science* 1968; **159**: 1070–8.
5. Marc C. *De La Folie*. Paris: Bailliere, 1840.
6. von Gudden H. Die physiologische und pathologische Schlaftrunkenheit. *Arch Psychiat* 1905; **40**: 989–1015.
7. Association of Sleep Disorders Centers: Diagnostic Classification of Sleep and Arousal Disorders, prepared by the Sleep Disorders Classification Committee, Roffwarg HP, Chairman. *Sleep* 1979; **2**: 1–137.
8. Stores G. Aspects of sleep disorders in children and adolescents. *Dialog Clin Neurosci* 2009; **11**: 81–90.
9. Stores G. The parasomnias. In Stores G (Ed), *A Clinical Guide to Sleep Disorders in Children and Adolescents*. Cambridge: Cambridge University Press, 2001; 117–42.
10. Pressman MR. Factors that predispose, prime and precipitate NREM parasomnias in adults: Clinical and forensic implications. *Sleep Med Rev* 2007; **11**: 5–30.
11. Guilleminault C, Palombini L, Pelayo R, et al. Sleepwalking and sleep terrors in prepubertal children: What triggers them? *Pediatrics* 2003; **111**: e17–25.
12. Stores G. Parasomnias of childhood and adolescence. In Jenni O, Carscadon M (Eds), Sleep in Children and Adolescents. *Sleep Med Clin* 2007; **2**: 405–17.
13. Dahl RE. The pharmacologic treatment of sleep disorders. *Psychiatr Clin North Am* 1992; **15**: 161–78.
14. Rosen G, Mahowald MW, Ferber R. Sleepwalking, confusional arousals, and sleep terrors in the child. In Ferber R, Kryger M (Eds), *Principles and Practice of Sleep Medicine in the Child*. Philadelphia: Saunders, 1995; 99–106.
15. Stores G. Aspects of parasomnias in childhood and adolescence. *Arch Dis Child* 2009; **94**: 63–9.
16. Broughton RJ, Shimizu T. Sleep-related violence: A medical and forensic challenge. *Sleep* 1995; **18**: 727–30.
17. Ohayon M, Priest R, Zulley J, et al. The place of confusional arousals in sleep and mental disorders: Findings in a general population sample of 13,057 subjects. *J Nerv Ment Dis* 2000; **188**: 340–8.
18. Diagnostic Classification Steering Committee, Thorpy MJ, Chairman. *International Classification of Sleep Disorders: Diagnostic and Coding Manual*. Rochester, MN: American Sleep Disorders Association, 1990.
19. Billiard M, Dauvilliers Y. Idiopathic hypersomnia. *Sleep Med Rev* 2001; **5**: 351–60.
20. Roth B, Nevsimalova S, Rechtschaffen A. Hypersomnia with "sleep drunkenness". *Arch Gen Psychiatry* 1972; **26**: 456–62.
21. Broughton R, Nevsimalova S, Roth B. The socio-economic effects of idiopathic hypersomnia. In *Sleep 1978* (Tirgu-Mures), 1980: 229–33.
22. Mendelson WB. Are periodic leg movements associated with clinical sleep disturbance? *Sleep* 1996; **19**: 219–23.
23. Provini F, Plazzi G, Montagna P, et al. The wide clinical spectrum of nocturnal frontal lobe epilepsy. *Sleep Med Rev* 2000; **4**: 375–86.
24. Tinuper P, Provini F, Bisulli F, et al. Movement disorders in sleep: Guidelines for differentiating epileptic from non-epileptic motor phenomena arising from sleep. *Sleep Med Rev* 2007; **11**: 255–67.
25. Mahowald MW, Schenck CH. REM sleep parasomnias. In Kryger MH, Roth T, Dement WC (Eds), *Principles and Practice of Sleep Medicine*, 4th ed. Philadelphia, PA: Elsevier Saunders, 2005; 897–916.
26. Stores G. Rapid eye movement sleep behaviour disorder in children and adolescents. *Dev Med Child Neurol* 2008; **50**: 728–32.
27. Schenck CH, Boyd JL, Mahowald MW. A parasomnia overlap disorder involving sleepwalking, sleep terrors, and REM sleep behaviour disorder in 33 polysomnographically confirmed cases. *Sleep* 1997; **20**: 972–81.

28. Oswald I, Evans J. On serious violence during sleepwalking. *Br J Psychiatry* 1985; **147**: 688–91.
29. Mahowald MW, Schenck CH. Medical–legal aspects of sleep medicine. *Neurologic Clin* 1999; **17**: 215–34.
30. Mahowald MW, Schenck CH. Violent parasomnias: Forensic medicine issues. In Kryger MH, Roth T, Dement WC (Eds), *Principles and Practice of Sleep Medicine*, 4th ed. Philadelphia, PA: Elsevier Saunders, 2005; 960–8.
31. Schenck CH, Arnulf I, Mahowald MW. Sleep and sex: what can go wrong? A review of the literature on sleep related disorders and abnormal sexual behaviors and experiences. *Sleep* 2007; **30**: 683–702.
32. Mangan MA. A phenomenology of problematic sexual behavior occurring in sleep. *Arch Sex Behav* 2004; **33**: 287–93.
33. Hardy T. *Tess of the d'Urbervilles* (first published 1891). New edition. London, Penguin Popular Classics, 2007.
34. Ebrahim I, Fenwick P. Response to Pressman: "Factors that predispose, prime and precipitate NREM parasomnias in adults: Clinical and forensic implications". *Sleep Med Rev* 2007; **11**: 5–30. *Sleep Med Rev* 2007; **11**: 241–7 (including reply and response by Pressman MR, Mahowald MK, Schenck CH).
35. Cartwright R. Letter to the Editor re. Pressman M. Factors that predispose, prime and precipitate NREM parasomnias in adults: Clinical and forensic implications. *Sleep Med Rev* 2007; **11**: 5–30. *Sleep Med Rev* 2007; **11**: 327–33 (including response by Pressman MR).
36. Cartwright R. Letter to the Editor re. Pressman M. Response to Rosalind Cartwright's Letter to the Editor. *Sleep Medicine Reviews* 2007; **11**(4): 329–333. *Sleep Med Rev* 2008; **12**: 77–82 (including response by Pressman MR).
37. Pressman MR, Mahowald MW, Schenck CH, *et al.* Alcohol-induced sleepwalking or confusional arousal as a defence to criminal behavior: A review of scientific evidence, methods and forensic considerations. *J Sleep Res* 2007; **16**: 198–212.
38. Ebrahim I, Fenwick P. Letter to the Editor re: Pressman *et al.* Alcohol-induced sleepwalking or confusional arousal as a defence to criminal behavior: A review of scientific evidence, methods and forensic considerations. *J Sleep Res* (2007) **16**: 198–212. *J Sleep Res* 2008; **17**: 470–2.
39. Pressman MR. Disorders of arousal from sleep and violent behavior: The role of physical contact and proximity. *Sleep* 2007; **30**: 1039–47.
40. Mahowald MW, Bornemann MAC. NREM sleep – arousal parasomnias. In Kryger MH, Roth T, Dement WC (Eds), *Principles and Practice of Sleep Medicine*, 4th ed. Philadelphia, PA: Elsevier Saunders, 2005; 889–96.

Section 2 Chapter 12

Disorders of arousal

Sleepwalking

Antonio Zadra and Jacques Montplaisir

The focus of this chapter is sleepwalking, also known as somnambulism. That people sometimes engage in complex ambulatory behaviors during sleep has been known for centuries. Shakespeare, for instance, described in *Macbeth* a now famous sleepwalking episode during which a guilt-ridden Lady Macbeth tries to wash imaginary blood stains from her hands while speaking of the crimes she and her husband have committed. Until the early to mid 1960s, sleepwalkers were generally thought to be in a dissociative state related to dreaming, possibly enacting repressed traumatic experiences. Following Broughton's landmark contribution [1] and the early work of Kales and his collaborators [2], sleepwalking was conceptualized as a "disorder of arousal." Together with confusional arousals and sleep terrors, sleepwalking constitutes one of the key non-rapid-eye-movement (NREM) sleep parasomnias.

The clinical presentation, PSG characteristics, prevalence, associated factors, pathophysiology and treatment of this parasomnia will be reviewed. Two variants of somnambulism, namely sleep-related abnormal sexual behaviors (sexsomnia) and sleep-related eating disorder, are not discussed here as they are covered elsewhere in this volume (see Chapters 9 and 21).

Clinical findings

Clinical presentation

The symptoms and manifestations that characterize sleepwalking can show great variations both within and across predisposed patients. The sleepwalker's emotional expression can range from calm to extremely agitated, while the actual behavioral manifestations can range from simple and isolated actions (e.g. sitting up in bed, pointing at a wall, fingering bed sheets) to complex organized behaviors (e.g. re-arranging furniture, cooking or eating, getting dressed, driving a vehicle). Given the heterogeneous nature of sleepwalking episodes, their duration can vary from a few seconds to dozens of minutes. Associated mental activity often includes misperception and relative unresponsiveness to external stimuli, confusion, perceived threat and variable retrograde amnesia. The number of legal cases of sleep-related violence involving sleepwalking is on the rise and fundamental questions have been raised as to the medico-forensic implications of these acts [3,4]. A review of medico-legal consequences of parasomnias is presented Chapter 10.

Although sleepwalking is often characterized in terms of its automatic behaviors, ongoing work into the phenomenology of somnambulism indicates that perceptual, cognitive and affective dimensions can play an important role in the subjective experience of adult sleepwalking [5]. Furthermore, some patients report that their somnambulistic behaviors are motivated by an intrinsic sense of urgency or underlying logic that explains (albeit not always logically) their behaviors during episodes.

Whereas the occurrence of sleepwalking in children is frequently viewed as a relatively benign condition, somnambulism in adults can result in serious injury to the sleeper or others. Indeed, it is adult patients' experiences of aggressive and/or injurious behavior during sleep that typically lead them to seek professional help. In many cases, patients report having suffered serious injuries (e.g. contusions, fractures to limbs, rib cage, multiple lacerations) and/or having attacked a bed partner during an episode [6]. In one polysomnographic investigation of 100 consecutive patients consulting for repeated nocturnal injury [7], 54 received a diagnosis of sleepwalking/night

Table 12.1 Clinical criteria for sleepwalking disorder.

DSM-IV Diagnostic Criteria for Sleepwalking Disorder (307.46)

A. Repeated episodes of rising from bed during sleep and walking about, usually occurring during the first third of the major sleep episode.
B. While sleepwalking, the person has a blank, staring face, is relatively unresponsive to the efforts of others to communicate with him or her, and can be awakened only with great difficulty.
C. On awakening (either from the sleepwalking episode or the next morning), the person has amnesia for the episode.
D. Within several minutes after awakening from the sleepwalking episode, there is no impairment of mental activity or behavior (although there may initially be a short period of confusion or disorientation).
E. The sleepwalking causes clinically significant distress or impairment in social, occupational, or other important areas of functioning.
F. The disturbance is not due to the direct physiological effects of a substance (e.g. a drug of abuse, a medication) or a general medical condition.

ICSD-II Diagnostic Criteria for Sleepwalking Disorder

A. Ambulation occurs during sleep.
B. Persistence of sleep, an altered state of consciousness or impaired judgment during ambulation demonstrated by at least one of the following:
   i. Difficulty in arousing the person.
   ii. Mental confusion when awakened from an episode.
   iii. Amnesia (complete or partial) for the episode.
   iv. Routine behaviors that occur at inappropriate times.
   v. Inappropriate or nonsensical behaviors.
   vi. Dangerous or potentially dangerous behaviors.
C. The disturbance is not better explained by another sleep disorder, medical or neurological disorder, mental disorder, medication use, or substance use disorder.

terrors. Of these 54 patients, over half had repeatedly run into walls and furniture while almost 20% had jumped out of windows, left the house and driven automobiles, wandered around streets, walked into lakes, or climbed ladders. Furthermore, 4 of the 54 patients (7.4%) had wielded weapons such as loaded shotguns. A second laboratory investigation of 64 consecutive adult patients with sleepwalking or sleep terrors found that a significant proportion reported a history of sleep-related violence leading to the destruction of property (e.g. breaking of walls, doors, windows, plumbing) or serious self-injury [8]. Similarly, one study of 50 chronic sleepwalkers found that 30% had injured themselves or others in the course of at least one episode [9].

Diagnostic considerations

Table 12.1 presents the diagnostic criteria for sleepwalking in the American Psychiatric Association's DSM-IV [10] and the American Academy of Sleep Medicine's ICSD-II [11]. Episodes typically develop from incomplete arousals from slow-wave sleep (stages 3 and 4 sleep) and sometimes from stage 2 sleep. As a consequence, sleepwalking tends to take place in the first third of the night when slow-wave sleep is predominant.

Diagnosis of sleepwalking can often be made based on a detailed clinical history, including complete description of the time course and content of sleep-related behaviors. Given that variable retrograde amnesia characterizes many somnambulistic episodes, descriptive information from family members or a bed partner can be particularly valuable. Similarly, home video recording can also be helpful in characterizing behavioral manifestations. It should be noted, however, that sleepwalking and sleep terrors can co-occur [6,7,12], and that the two conditions are sometimes difficult to differentiate [13].

Sleep laboratory investigations can be useful in ruling out other disorders (e.g. nocturnal seizures, episodic nocturnal wandering, REM sleep behavior disorder), but no validated sleep protocol exists to confirm the diagnosis. The principal difficulty in diagnosing sleepwalking directly with polysomnography is that behavioral events rarely occur in the laboratory [2,14,14]. In addition, when partial episodes do develop, they are usually less complex than what is described for the patient's home environment and the presence of bed rails typically raised on either side of the patient's bed can also dissuade or impede patients from actually leaving their beds. Several polysomnographic features including frequent arousals from slow-wave sleep, the presence of hypersynchronous delta waves, and diminished slow-wave activity have been proposed as indirect evidence supporting the diagnosis, but these variables show poor sensitivity and specificity [3,16].

Sleepwalking can be secondary to sleep respiratory events, including obstructive sleep apnea (OSA) and upper airway resistance syndrome, or other sleep disorders such as periodic limb movement disorder. An association between sleepwalking/sleep terrors and sleep-disordered breathing (SDB) has been described in several studies [17–19], including one population-based cohort study of pre-adolescent school-aged children [20]. Treatment of the precipitating sleep disorder may result in a disappearance of the disorder of arousal [19]. Similarly, one investigation of 50 adults with chronic somnambulism found that many patients presented with SDB and that treatment of the SDB with continuous positive airway pressure (CPAP) or surgery controlled sleepwalking [9]. However, some studies find that a majority of adult sleepwalkers referred to a sleep disorders clinic by their treating physician for suspected somnambulism do not suffer from comorbid sleep disorders [21].

Rarely, sleepwalking may develop as a result of medical or neurological conditions. *De novo* somnambulism has been described in patients presenting with thyrotoxicosis caused by diffuse toxic goiter or Graves' disease. Disorders of arousal can also be triggered by medication including sedatives/hypnotics, neuroleptics, lithium, minor tranquilizers, stimulants, and antihistamines.

Use of sleep deprivation and forced arousals

As previously noted, diagnosing somnambulism with objective instruments such as polysomnography can be difficult, as even partial episodes rarely occur in the sleep laboratory. Two techniques that may increase the probability of recording more complex behavioral manifestations are sleep deprivation and the presentation of auditory stimuli during SWS. When compared to baseline recordings, one study found that 40 h of sleep deprivation significantly increased the number of somnambulistic episodes recorded in the sleep laboratory [15]. Forty hours of sleep deprivation, however, is very demanding for most patients and clinical laboratories. A less-demanding protocol involves 25 h of sleep deprivation with recovery sleep being initiated in the morning. A recent investigation of 40 consecutive sleepwalkers (including 10 with either PLMS or mild sleep apnea syndrome) revealed that 25 h of sleep deprivation was also effective in increasing both the frequency and complexity of somnambulistic events recorded in the sleep laboratory [21]. Combining data from all 40 patients shows that recovery sleep resulted in one or more episodes being recorded from 36 (90%) of the sleepwalkers.

Thus, a relatively short period of sleep deprivation resulting in daytime recovery sleep can effectively facilitate the emergence of somnambulistic behaviors. The fact that none of the control subjects investigated in these studies experienced nocturnal behavioral manifestations in the laboratory demonstrates that sleep deprivation alone does not lead to somnambulistic episodes, but rather that it increases the probability of somnambulistic behaviors in predisposed individuals. When compared to baseline sleep recordings, both the 40 and 25 h sleep deprivation protocols resulted in marked decreases in the number of awakenings from stage 1 sleep, from stage 2 sleep and from REM sleep. However, only the 25 h sleep deprivation protocol significantly increased the number of awakenings from SWS. This indicates that sleepwalkers are particularly vulnerable to increased homeostatic sleep pressure following sleep deprivation when recovery sleep is initiated at a circadian time of increasing wake propensity.

It had been suggested that the simultaneous combination of factors that deepen sleep (e.g. sleep deprivation) with those that fragment sleep (e.g. environmental or endogenous stimuli) increases the chances of sleepwalkers experiencing an episode. This hypothesis was recently tested in a study that investigated the effects of forced arousals from experimental auditory stimuli in ten adult sleepwalkers and ten control subjects during normal sleep and following post-sleep deprivation recovery sleep [22]. The characteristics of the induced somnambulistic behaviors are presented in Table 12.2. Forced arousals during SWS were successful in experimentally inducing somnambulistic episodes in the adult sleepwalkers and, as predicted, sleep deprivation significantly increased the forced arousals' efficacy. In fact, while no

Table 12.2 Characteristics of induced somnambulistic events in sleepwalkers during normal and recovery sleep with auditory stimuli (AS).

	Normal sleep with AS	Recovery sleep with AS	P value
Total number of induced episodes during SWS	7	23	–
Number of patients experiencing at least one induced episode during SWS	3/10 (30%)	10/10 (100%)	0.005
Mean (SD) frequency of induced episodes during SWS	0.7 (1.3)	2.3 (1.2)	0.040
Mean percentage of AS trials that induced an episode during SWS	19.8 (37.1)	57.3 (31.7)	0.035
Mean (SD) intensity in dB of the AS that induced episodes	48.6 (12.1)	53.5 (11.5)	ns

AS, auditory stimuli; SWS, slow-wave sleep (stage 3 and 4 sleep); ns = not significant.

somnambulistic episodes were induced in controls, the presentation of auditory stimuli during daytime recovery sleep resulted in all ten patients experiencing one or more induced episodes. These results support the hypothesis that via its homeostatic pressure for increased SWS, sleep deprivation facilitates the occurrence of sleepwalking in predisposed individuals and that this effect can be augmented by incorporating forced arousals.

Natural history

Sleepwalking is more common in childhood than in adulthood, as most children will experience, at least temporarily, one or more of the NREM sleep parasomnias during childhood or early adolescence. The peak incidence of sleepwalking (approximately 17%) is around 12 years of age [23]. Children with sleepwalking tend to outgrow the disorder during mid to late adolescence, but somnambulism can persist into adulthood in up to 25% of cases [24]. In addition, children with sleep terrors can develop sleepwalking at a later age, and the two parasomnias can occur within the same episode (e.g. sleep terror followed by sleepwalking). Sleepwalking occurs in approximately 2–4% of adults with no significant gender differences [17,24,25]. However, there is some evidence to suggest that given comparable histories, males are more likely than females to experience somnambulistic behaviors in the sleep laboratory [21]. As previously described, adult sleepwalking can lead to sleep-related injuries.

Several factors have been reported as facilitating or precipitating somnambulistic episodes in predisposed individuals, and some researchers have grouped them into factors that deepen sleep and factors that fragment sleep [26]. Factors that deepen sleep and which are capable of facilitating or triggering sleepwalking include intense physical activity, hyperthyroidism, fever, sleep deprivation, and neuroleptics or medications with depressive CNS effects. Factors that fragment sleep and are capable of facilitating or triggering sleepwalking include the presence of other sleep disorders such as SDB, stress and environmental or endogenous stimuli.

Finally, hormonal factors may also influence the frequency with which women experience sleep terrors and injurious sleepwalking, as these can emerge premenstrually [27], while sleepwalking can decrease during pregnancy, particularly in primiparas [28].

Laboratory investigations

Polysomnography

Sleep laboratory investigations have yielded considerable information on the polysomnographic characteristics of sleepwalkers. No consistently robust differences exist between adult somnambulistic patients and control subjects in terms of their overall sleep architecture and normal cycling among sleep stages. However, some unusual sleep-related processes have been described as characterizing the sleep of patients suffering from somnambulism. These include NREM sleep instability, hypersynchronous delta waves, irregular build-up of slow-wave activity, and unique EEG characteristics prior to and during somnambulistic episodes.

NREM sleep instability

When compared to controls, adults and children with sleepwalking/sleep terrors show increases in the cyclic alternating pattern rate [29], a measure of NREM

Chapter 12: Sleepwalking

Figure 12.1 Slow-wave activity (SWA) over four consecutive NREM-REM cycles in 15 sleepwalkers and 15 healthy paired controls. Power is significantly reduced in the second half of the first NREM period. Awakenings from SWS are indicated on the two horizontal lines below the graph (from [32]).

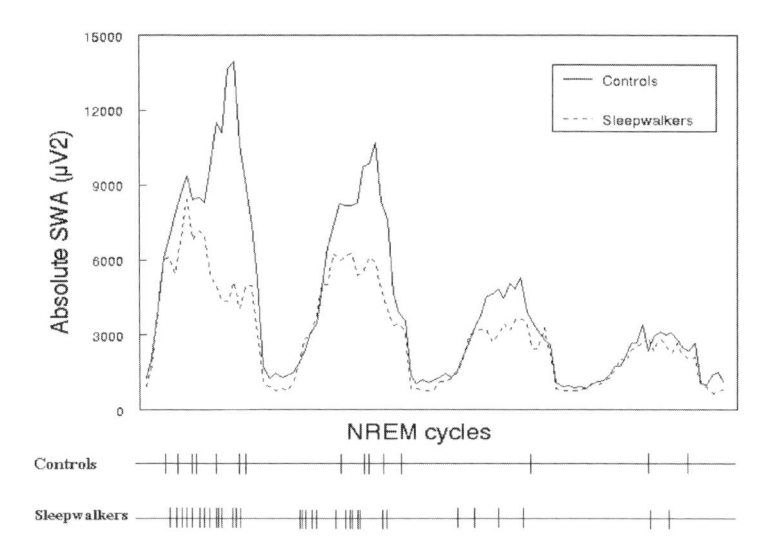

instability which expresses the organized complexity of arousal-related phasic events. Sleepwalkers also experience a greater number of arousals and brief microarousals out of SWS than do controls [14,30]. NREM sleep instability and arousal oscillation may thus represent a typical microstructural feature of parasomniacs' NREM sleep and may play a role in triggering sleepwalkers' abnormal motor episodes.

Hypersynchronous delta waves

Although not always clearly operationalized, hypersynchronous delta activity (HSD) is usually described as continuous high voltage (>150 uV) delta waves occurring during SWS or immediately prior to an episode. Some texts present HSD as a well-established feature of sleepwalker's sleep EEG. However, careful studies of HSD and other forms of delta activity prior to sleepwalking episodes have yielded mixed to poor results [13,16,31]. For example, one study [13] found that most behavioral and non-behavioral arousals from SWS in adult patients were not preceded by a delta wave build-up, and that only 15.5% were preceded by delta wave clusters.

The occurrence of HSD was recently assessed by our group [16]: the data showed that (a) HSD was present in 80% of controls during baseline recording, but HSD occurred more frequently during sleepwalkers' sleep EEG; (b) sleep deprivation increased HSD during stage 4 sleep in both groups; and (c) there was no evidence that somnambulistic episodes are immediately preceded by a build-up in HSD. Taken together, these findings indicate that HSD, which represents an increased activity of the neural structures involved in the regulation of delta activity during NREM sleep, occurs in the SWS of normal controls, and that it has a low specificity for the diagnosis of somnambulism.

Slow-wave activity

EEG slow-wave activity (SWA: spectral power in the 0.75–4.5 Hz band) is a quantitative measure of SWS dynamics and is considered an indicator of sleep depth or sleep intensity. Gaudreau et al. investigated the power and dynamics of SWA in adult sleepwalkers and controls and showed that sleepwalkers had significantly less overall SWA power, with the greatest difference occurring during the first NREM cycle (see Figure 12.1) [32]. A similar reduction in SWA was also reported in two other studies of sleepwalkers/sleep terror patients [30,33]. These data indicate that normal SWA build-up is impeded by sleepwalkers' frequent awakenings from SWS.

Post-arousal EEG activity

Early studies reported that the EEG recorded during somnambulistic episodes was characterized by continuous and diffuse non-reactive alpha rhythms or by patterns of low-voltage delta and beta activity without evidence of clear wakefulness. Schenck and coworkers described three post-arousal EEG patterns that characterized the first 10 s of most SWS arousals in adults with sleepwalking/sleep terrors: (I) diffuse rhythmic and synchronous delta activity, most prominent in bilateral anterior regions and with a typical frequency of 2.2 Hz, a typical amplitude of 85 uV, and a typical

Section 2: Disorders of arousal

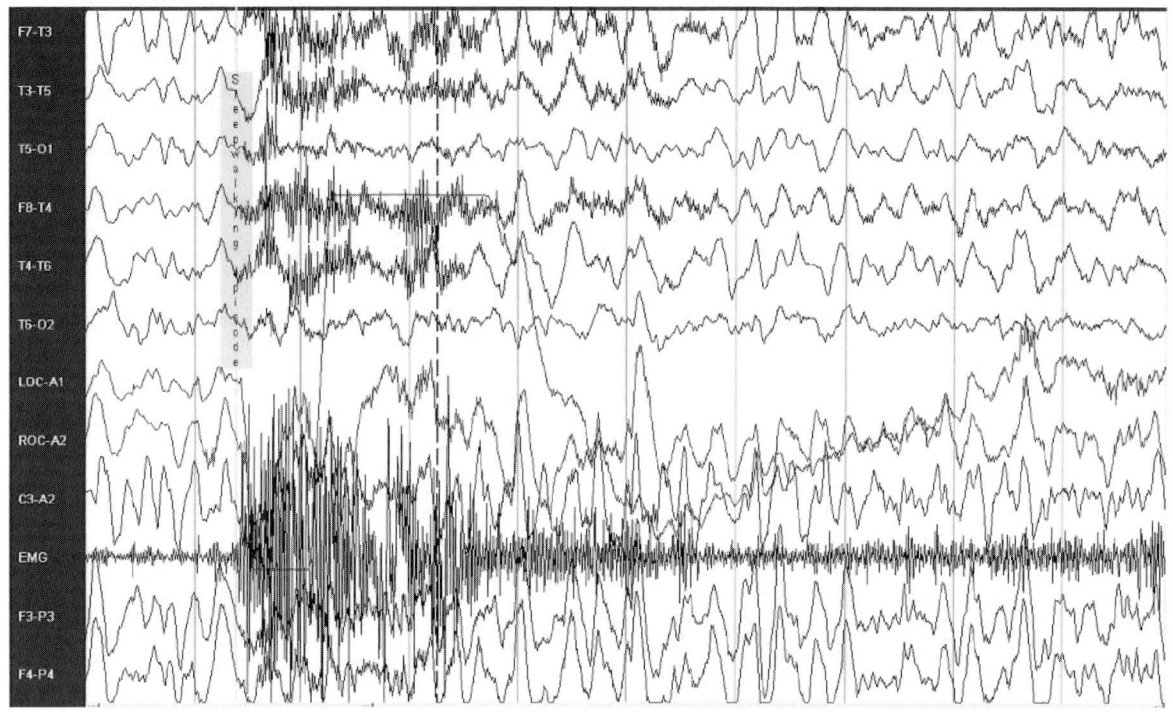

Figure 12.2 The color version of this figure can be found in the color plate section. Example of post-arousal EEG pattern I during a behavioral episode from stage 4 sleep in a 19-year-old man. The EEG shows diffuse and rhythmic delta activity and is most predominant in the anterior regions.

duration of 20 s; (II) diffuse and irregular moderate-to-high voltage delta and theta activity intermixed with alpha and beta activity; and (III) prominent alpha and beta activity [13]. Irrespective of specific EEG patterns, delta activity was present in 44% of the post-arousal EEGs.

More recently, these patterns were assessed during behavioral arousals in adult sleepwalkers [34]. The two more frequently observed forms of post-arousal activity were patterns II and III. These patterns were also the only two that occurred during stage 2 episodes. Delta activity was present in almost 50% of all episodes from SWS and 20% of those from stage 2 sleep. Pattern I (diffuse rhythmic and synchronous delta activity), which only occurred during events emerging from SWS, was more likely to accompany simple somnambulistic episodes than complex ones. Examples of patterns I and II are presented in Figures 12.2 and 12.3.

Other experimental investigations

A transcranial magnetic stimulation study examined motor cortex excitability during wakefulness in 8 sleepwalkers and 18 controls [35]. Sleepwalkers showed significant hypo-excitability of some inhibitory circuits as revealed by reduced short interval intracortical inhibition, cortical silent period duration, and short latency afferent inhibition.

One SPECT study was performed during a sleepwalking episode recorded from a 16-year-old man with a history of somnambulism [36]. An increase of 25% in rCBF was found in the posterior cingulate and anterior cerebellum compared to SWS without episodes. The authors suggest that variations in the motor and emotional manifestations of sleepwalking may be related to different activation patterns of the cingulate cortex, as it modulates behavior in response to emotional processes. A decrease in rCBF in frontoparietal associative cortices was also noted in comparison to the wakefulness pattern of normal subjects. Since this pattern occurs in normal SWS, this finding suggests that the brain is indeed sleeping during somnambulism. These pilot findings thus support the notion that sleepwalking is a dissociated state consisting of motor arousal and persisting mind sleep.

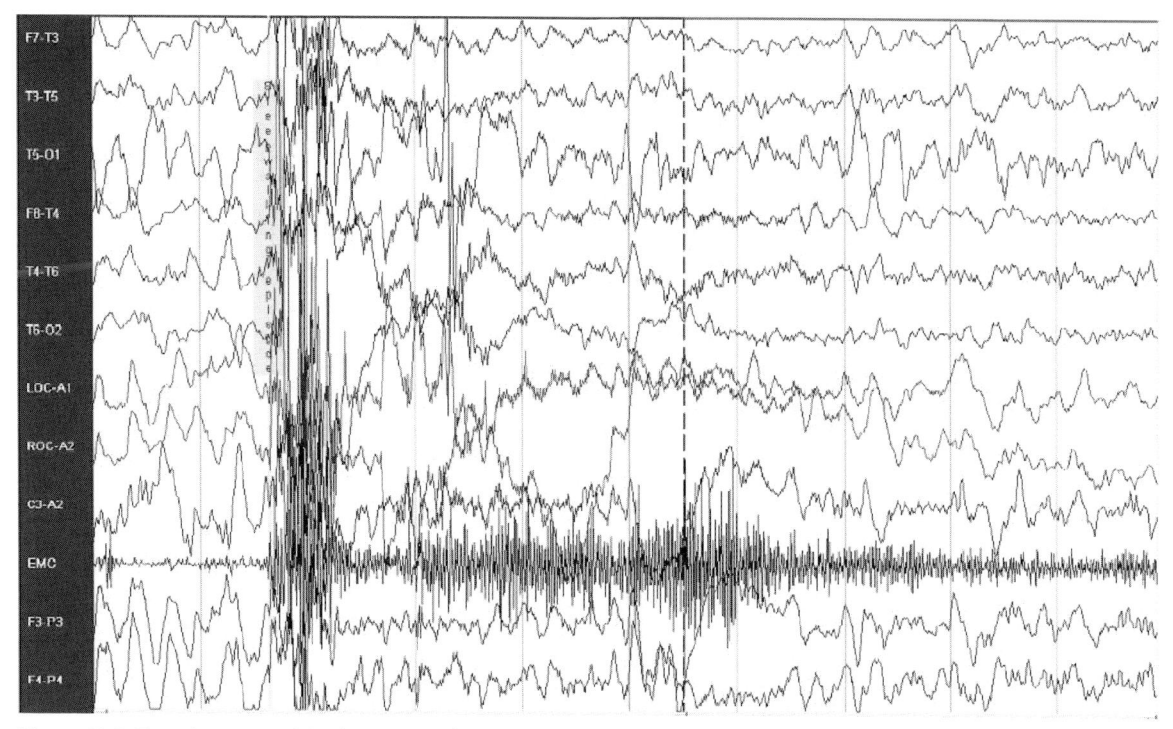

Figure 12.3 The color version of this figure can be found in the color plate section. Example of post-arousal EEG pattern II during a behavioral episode from stage 4 sleep in a 23–year-old woman. The EEG shows irregular delta and theta activity intermixed with faster activity.

Genetics

There is a strong genetic component to somnambulism. About 80% of somnambulistic patients have at least one family member affected by this parasomnia, and the prevalence of somnambulism is higher in children of parents with a history of sleepwalking. A population-based twin study [24] of 1045 MZ and 1899 DZ pairs showed a considerable genetic effect in adulthood sleepwalking (probandwise concordance five times higher in MZ than DZ pairs), although the effect in childhood sleepwalking was not as pronounced (1.5 times higher in MZ than DZ pairs). In fact, HLA-DQB1 typing in sleepwalkers and their families indicates that somnambulism may be associated with excessive transmission of the HLA-DQB1*05 and *04 alleles [37].

It has been suggested that the clinical similarities between sleepwalking and sleep terrors indicate a common genetic predisposition. Sleepwalking may be a more prevalent and less severe manifestation of the same substrate that underlies sleep terrors [38].

Associated factors and pathology

The exact pathophysiological mechanisms of somnambulism remain unclear. In addition to the atypical sleep parameters and genetic component reviewed above, other factors have been proposed, including psychopathology and deregulation of serotonergic systems.

Older studies have held that the presence of somnambulism (with or without concomitant sleep terrors) in adulthood is associated with major psychopathology [39,40]. Epidemiologic evidence suggests a higher prevalence of psychopathology among adult patients with arousal disorders [17], and psychopathology has been reported in subgroups of adolescents with sleep terrors and/or sleepwalking [41]. However, many adult patients do not present with a DSM-based [10] psychiatric disorder, nor do they necessarily have highly disturbed personality traits [7,9,42,43].

Serotonin has been hypothesized to be involved in the pathophysiology of sleepwalking on the basis that certain factors implicating the serotonergic system (e.g. certain drugs, fever) can precipitate sleepwalking [44]. In addition, sleepwalking episodes are four to nine times more commonly associated with abnormalities in the metabolism of serotonin, such as Tourette syndrome or migraine headaches.

Management

Treatment is often unnecessary when episodes are benign and not associated with potential injury. In this case, reassuring the patient/family about the benign nature of the episodes and demystifying the events is often sufficient. However, attention should be paid to potential precipitating factors, such as sleep deprivation, stress and environmental disturbances, so that such factors can be avoided. When patients present with a history of agitated somnambulism, precautions should be taken to ensure a safe sleep environment (e.g. removing obstructions in the bedroom, securing windows, installing locks or alarms on outside doors, placing barriers in stairways, removing sharp or otherwise dangerous objects).

As highlighted in a recent review article [45], controlled clinical trials for the treatment of somnambulism are lacking. Hypnosis (including self-hypnosis) has been found to be effective in both children and adults presenting with chronic sleepwalking [46–48]. In children, the preferred treatment for somnambulism consists of a behavioral technique called anticipatory or scheduled awakening. Parents keep a diary of their child's episodes and determine the approximate time at which the episodes typically occur. They will then awaken their child about 15–20 min before the episode's typical time of occurrence for a period of one month. This simple intervention can yield rapid results and benefits are maintained for several months after the end of the treatment [49].

When sleepwalking is secondary to sleep respiratory events or other sleep disorders, treatment of the precipitating sleep disorder may result in a disappearance of somnambulism [19].

Pharmacological treatment should be considered only if the behaviors are hazardous or extremely disruptive to the bed partner or other household members. Benzodiazepines (clonazepam or diazepam) and tricyclic anti-depressants (imipramine) can be effective [50]. However, pharmacotherapy does not always result in adequate control of sleepwalking [9]. Treatment should always include instructions on sleep hygiene, avoidance of sleep deprivation, and stress management.

Conclusions

Despite numerous clinical and empirical investigations, the exact mechanisms which give rise to somnambulism remain unclear. Of the factors suggested as being operant, those involving genetics and abnormal sleep parameters appear the most promising in elucidating our understanding of this sleep disorder. Although the precise mode of inheritance for sleepwalking is not fully understood, a genetic contribution has been well documented. Strong support also exists for the idea that sleepwalkers experience difficulties in maintaining stable and consolidated NREM sleep. Furthermore, sleepwalkers appear to be particularly vulnerable to increased homeostatic sleep pressure following sleep deprivation when recovery sleep is initiated at a circadian time of increasing wake propensity. Considerable progress has also been made in the study of EEG activity prior to and during somnambulistic episodes. The limited data collected on neuroimaging and transcranial magnetic stimulation in sleepwalkers suggest that, although methodologically challenging, these investigative tools may pave the way towards a better understanding of disorders of arousal.

Unlike most sleep disorders, the diagnosis of sleepwalking is still primarily based on the patient's clinical history. The development of an investigative protocol that would allow researchers and clinicians to establish a polysomnographically based diagnosis for sleepwalking remains central. This issue is especially important given the growing number of medico-legal cases of sleep-related violence. A recent series of studies have shown that sleep deprivation significantly increases the frequency of somnambulistic events recorded in the laboratory. Moreover, the probability of recording an episode in predisposed individuals can be further increased by combining sleep deprivation with experimental forced awakenings. Although the results obtained thus far appear promising, additional work on larger and more varied clinical samples is needed.

A variety of non-pharmacological as well as pharmacological treatments have been recommended for long-term management of somnambulism. However, well-designed controlled clinical trials are needed to guide and support treatment decisions.

References

1. Broughton RJ. Sleep disorders: disorders of arousal? *Science* 1968; **159**: 1070–8.
2. Kales A, Jacobson A, Paulson MJ, et al. Somnambulism: Psychophysiological correlates. I. All-night EEG studies. *Arch Gen Psychiat* 1966; **14**: 586–94.
3. Pressman M. Factors that predispose, prime and precipitate NREM parasomnias in adults: Clinical and forensic implications. *Sleep Med Rev* 2007; **11**: 5–30.
4. Pressman MR, Mahowald MW, Schenck CH, et al. Alcohol-induced sleepwalking or confusional arousal as a defense to criminal behavior: A review of scientific evidence, methods and forensic considerations. *J Sleep Res* 2007; **16**: 198–212.
5. Zadra A, Pilon M, Montplaisir J. Phenomenology of somnambulism. *Sleep* 2006; **29**: A269.
6. Kavey NB, Whyte J, Resor SR, et al. Somnambulism in adults. *Neurology* 1990; **40**: 749–52.
7. Schenck CH, Milner DM, Hurwitz TD, et al. A polysomnographic and clinical report on sleep-related injury in 100 adult patients. *Am J Psychiatry* 1989; **146**: 1166–73.
8. Moldofsky H, Gilbert R, Lue FA, et al. Forensic sleep medicine: Violence, sleep, nocturnal wandering: Sleep-related violence. *Sleep* 1995; **18**: 731–9.
9. Guilleminault C, Kirisoglu C, Bao G, et al. Adult chronic sleepwalking and its treatment based on polysomnography. *Brain* 2005; **128**: 1062–9.
10. American Psychiatric Association. *Diagnostic and Statistical Manual of Mental Disorders: DSM-IV*. 4th ed. Washington, DC: APA, 1994.
11. American Academy of Sleep Medicine. *ICSD-2: International Classification of Sleep Disorders: Diagnostic and Coding Manual*. 2nd ed. Westchester, IL: American Academy of Sleep Medicine, 2005.
12. Hublin C, Kaprio J, Partinen M, et al. Parasomnias: Co-occurrence and genetics. *Psychiatr Genet* 2001; **11**: 65–70.
13. Schenck CH, Pareja JA, Patterson AL, et al. Analysis of polysomnographic events surrounding 252 slow-wave sleep arousals in thirty-eight adults with injurious sleepwalking and sleep terrors. *J Clin Neurophysiol* 1998; **15**: 159–66.
14. Blatt I, Peled R, Gadoth N, et al. The value of sleep recording in evaluating somnambulism in young adults. *Electroencephalogr Clin Neurophysiol* 1991; **78**: 407–12.
15. Joncas S, Zadra A, Paquet J, et al. The value of sleep deprivation as a diagnostic tool in adult sleepwalkers. *Neurology* 2002; **58**: 936–40.
16. Pilon M, Zadra A, Joncas S, et al. Hypersynchronous delta waves and somnambulism: Brain topography and effect of sleep deprivation. *Sleep* 2006; **29**: 77–84.
17. Ohayon MM, Guilleminault C, Priest RG. Night terrors, sleepwalking, and confusional arousals in the general population: Their frequency and relationship to other sleep and mental disorders. *J Clin Psychiatry* 1999; **60**: 268–76.
18. Espa F, Dauvilliers Y, Ondze B, et al. Arousal reactions in sleepwalking and night terrors in adults: The role of respiratory events. *Sleep* 2002; **25**: 871–5.
19. Guilleminault C, Palombini L, Pelayo R, et al. Sleepwalking and sleep terrors in prepubertal children: What triggers them? *Pediatrics* 2003; **111**: e17–25.
20. Goodwin J, Kaemingh K, Fregosi R, et al. Parasomnias and sleep disordered breathing in Caucasian and Hispanic children – the Tucson children's assessment of sleep apnea study. *BMC Med* 2004; 2. Available at http://www.biomedcentral.com/1741-7015/2/14. Accessed January 15, 2005.
21. Zadra A, Pilon M, Montplaisir J. Polysomnographic diagnosis of sleepwalking: Effects of sleep deprivation. *Ann Neurol* 2008; **63**: 513–9.
22. Pilon M, Montplaisir J, Zadra A. Precipitating factors of somnambulism: Impact of sleep deprivation and forced arousals. *Neurology* 2008; **70**: 2284–90.
23. Klackenberg G. Somnambulism in childhood: Prevalence, course and behavioral correlations. *Acta Paed Scand* 1982; **71**: 495–9.
24. Hublin C, Kaprio J, Partinen M, et al. Prevalence and genetics of sleepwalking: A population-based twin study. *Neurology* 1997; **48**: 177–81.
25. Goldin PR. Epidemiology of nine parasomnias in young adults. *Sleep Res Online* 1997; **26**: 367.
26. Broughton R. NREM arousal parasomnias. In Kryger MH, Roth T, Dement WC (Eds), *Principles and Practice of Sleep Medicine*. 3rd ed. Philadelphia, WB Saunders, 2000; 693–706.
27. Schenck CH, Mahowald MW. Two cases of premenstrual sleep terrors and injurious sleep-walking. *J Psychosom Obst Gyn* 1995; **16**: 79–84.
28. Hedman C, Pohjasvaara T, Tolonen U, et al. Parasomnias decline during pregnancy. *Acta Neurol Scand* 2002; **105**: 209–14.
29. Zucconi M, Oldani A, Ferini-Strambi L, et al. Arousal fluctuations in non-rapid eye movement parasomnias: The role of cyclic alternating pattern as a measure of sleep instability. *J Clin Neurophysiol* 1995; **12**: 147–54.
30. Espa F, Ondze B, Deglise P, et al. Sleep architecture, slow wave activity, and sleep spindles in adult patients

with sleepwalking and sleep terrors. *Clin Neurophysiol* 2000; **111**: 929–39.

31. Pressman MR. Hypersynchronous delta sleep EEG activity and sudden arousals from slow-wave sleep in adults without a history of parasomnias: Clinical and forensic implications. *Sleep* 2004; **27**: 706–10.

32. Gaudreau H, Joncas S, Zadra A, *et al*. Dynamics of slow-wave activity during the NREM sleep of sleepwalkers and control subjects. *Sleep* 2000; **23**: 755–60.

33. Guilleminault C, Poyares D, Aftab FA, *et al*. Sleep and wakefulness in somnambulism: A spectral analysis study. *J Psychosom Res* 2001; **51**: 411–6.

34. Zadra A, Pilon M, Joncas S, *et al*. Analysis of postarousal EEG activity during somnambulistic episodes. *J Sleep Res* 2004; **13**: 279–84.

35. Oliviero A, Della Marca G, Tonali PA, *et al*. Functional involvement of cerebral cortex in adult sleepwalking. *J Neurol* 2007; **254**: 1066–72.

36. Bassetti C, Vella S, Donati F, *et al*. SPECT during sleepwalking. *Lancet* 2000; **356**: 484–5.

37. Lecendreux M, Bassetti C, Dauvilliers Y, *et al*. HLA and genetic susceptibility to sleepwalking. *Mol Psychiatry* 2003; **8**: 114–7.

38. Kales A, Soldatos CR, Bixler EO, *et al*. Hereditary factors in sleepwalking and night terrors. *Br J Psychiatr* 1980; **137**: 111–8.

39. Pai MN. Sleep-walking and sleep activities. *J Ment Sci* 1946; **92**: 756–65.

40. Kales A, Soldatos CR, Caldwell AB, *et al*. Somnambulism. Clinical characteristics and personality patterns. *Arch Gen Psychiat* 1980; **37**: 1406–10.

41. Gau S-F, Soong W-T. Psychiatric comorbidity of adolescents with sleep terrors or sleepwalking: A case-control study. *Aust NZ J Psychiat* 1999; **33**: 734–9.

42. Mahowald MW, Schenck CH. Dissociated states of wakefulness and sleep. In Lydic R, Baghdoyan HA (Eds), *Handbook of Behavioural State Control: Cellular and Molecular Mechanisms*. New York: CRC Press, 1999; 143–58.

43. Schenck CH, Boyd JL, Mahowald MW. A parasomnia overlap disorder involving sleepwalking, sleep terrors, and REM sleep behavior disorder in 33 polysomnographically confirmed cases. *Sleep* 1997; **20**: 972–81.

44. Juszczak GR, Swiergiel AH. Serotonergic hypothesis of sleepwalking. *Med Hypotheses* 2005; **64**: 28–32.

45. Harris M, Grunstein RR. Treatments for somnambulism in adults: Assessing the evidence. *Sleep Med Rev* 2009; **13**: 295–7.

46. Reid WH, Ahmed I, Levie CA. Treatment of sleepwalking: A controlled study. *Am J Psychother* 1981; **35**: 27–37.

47. Hauri PJ, Silber MH, Boeve BF. The treatment of parasomnias with hypnosis: A 5-year follow-up study. *J Clin Sleep Med* 2007; **3**: 369–73.

48. Hurwitz T, Mahowald M, Schenck C, *et al*. A retrospective outcome study and review of hypnosis as treatment of adults with sleepwalking and sleep terror. *J Nerv Ment Dis* 1991; **179**: 228–33.

49. Tobin JD, Jr. Treatment of somnambulism with anticipatory awakening. *J Pediatr* 1993; **122**: 426–7.

50. Remulla A, Guilleminault C. Somnambulism (sleepwalking). *Expert Opin Pharmacother* 2004; **5**: 2069–74.

Section 2 Chapter 13

Disorders of arousal

Sleep terrors

Meredith Broderick and Christian Guilleminault

History

The first known report of night terrors may have been in Latin translations of Rhazes' *Practica Puerorum*, which was described as "mater puerorum," meaning hysterical fits in children or mother of the children [1]. In this 910 AD Latin version, Rhazes' description is translated:

> now follows about a certain affliction which is called mater puerorum. This infirmity happens to children in the first period of life frequently. The sign of it is great wailing or much fear during sleep, and fever increased by the sleeplessness and from the child's mouth a foul odor issues forth. The cause of this ailment is the taking of more milk that the child can digest. The cure of it is in correcting the milk. The child, therefore, is given the sixth part of a dram of dyapliris and diasmuscum with the milk daily. The sovereign remedy in this condition is the great theriac.

During Rhazes' time, research shows that mater puerorum may have been used to describe both epileptic attacks and night terrors. In antiquity, night terrors and epileptic episodes were frequently attributed to demons. The term mater puerorum was no longer used after the Renaissance, but in modern day, pavor nocturnus is generally accepted as synonymous with night terrors or sleep terrors in children and incubus attacks in adults. Historically, night terrors have been reported in association with scary stories before bedtime, breathing abnormalities during sleep such as that which occurs with adenotonsillar hypertrophy, digestive disorders, vascular disease, or epilepsy. In Freud's time, with the advent of psychoanalysis and dream analysis, night terrors were postulated as being a type of anxiety attack related to unconscious mental conflicts. This theory was strengthened by the association between the occurrence of night terrors in childhood which coincided with the anal and oedipal periods of psychological development. Until the link between slow wave sleep and night terrors was recognized, the Freudian influence on theories of night terrors was prominent.

In a case report published in 1953, Sullivan described night terrors as an indication of an emotional problem arising out of certain stages in a child's development [2]. He wrote that the root of the problem was a basic fear of being hurt which came from the child's increasing awareness of being separate from his mother. He wrote, "prevention and treatment of night terrors was dependent on attention to parental attitudes about sexual and aggressive activity, as well as to the precipitating factors." In the case, he described a 4 years- and 5-months-old white girl with awakenings of inconsolable screaming that bugs were in the room. After describing a thorough evaluation of the parents and the child, he concluded the episodes were due to a conflict between the child's wishes and her fears of retaliation by a parent. He recommended methods to help the child express her feelings during daytime play as well as moving the other child into separate bedrooms. He recommended barbiturate sedation to help suppress the episodes in addition to nursery school during the day to allow the child a forum for more aggressive expression. With these suggestions and after four months, the night terror episodes ceased. These historical accounts of night terrors highlight the importance of culture on some of the current investigations and attempts at conceptualization of night terrors.

With the development of sleep laboratories, more objective findings such as electroencephalography and physiological parameters have and are being studied.

In 1965, Gastaut and Broughton published work demonstrating the important association of night terrors as arousals from stage 4 sleep, which was around the same time that sleepwalking and enuresis were also described as arising from stage 4 sleep [3]. This discovery was in contrast to the known association of dreams with REM sleep, and accordingly was an important breakthrough distinction in the classification of night terrors. After this, interest shifted towards identifying triggers of the night terrors, which at the time was thought to be an expression of emotional conflicts in NREM sleep, a time when inhibitory barriers are lowered. In 1973, Fisher *et al.* described four types of anxious arousals from sleep: stage 4 night terrors, REM nightmares, stage 2 awakenings, and hypnagogic nightmares [3]. They wrote that the distinguishing feature of night terrors was the severity. They emphasized the concept that night terrors did not occur during sleep, but as part of an arousal response associated with autonomic discharges and behavioral responses. To be considered a night terror, the patient had to have autonomic activation. In their case series they elicited episodes by using a buzzer and described key features of night terrors: a near doubling of the resting heart rate estimated at around 108 beats per minute, increases in amplitude and respiratory rate initiated with a gasp, anxiety, and decreases in skin resistance. They noted a direct relationship between the amount of delta sleep preceding a night terror and the intensity of the spell, as well as the fact that two-thirds of night terrors occur in the first non-REM (NREM) period. In their investigations, night terrors were also always associated with sleep talking. Their hypothesis was that night terrors represented a heightened tendency in certain individuals to trigger a fight or flight response based on the capability to elicit episodes with a buzzer. At the same time, because of the mental content contained in the episodes, they also postulated a relationship between prior traumatic experiences. In 1974, Taboada wrote that the causative factor in night terrors was fear of death [4]. He described a case report of a 7-year-old boy who was otherwise healthy who developed night terrors after attending summer camp. With hypnosis, he was able to uncover the boy's fear of big waves and of the boat at camp capsizing with children in it. By asking the boy to imagine he was slightly older and able to turn the boat, the night terrors subsequently abated. Taboada also reiterated previous observations of the thin line between nightmares and night terrors, with the distinction being the fragmentary or absent dream recall in patients with nightmares. In examining the historical medical literature on night terrors, sleep terrors, pavor nocturnus, or incubus attacks it is important to note that there is significant overlap with reports of sleep paralysis, anxiety dreams, nightmares, confusional arousals, and sleepwalking [5]. Historically, the distinction has not always been clear, and to a certain extent there is a still an overlap in these disorders. Night terrors, sleepwalking, and confusional arousals are often still grouped in the medical literature.

Clinical findings

Classically, night terrors arise during the first sleep cycle, usually within 1–3 h of sleep (Table 13.1). In her analysis of 40 patients with night terrors, Joyce Kales reported an average time of occurrence of 106.6 min after sleep onset [3]. The episode begins suddenly with vocalization, which can be screaming or crying, sometimes associated with sitting up in bed, thrashing, agitation, confusion, a facial expression of fear and sympathetic activation. Patients are only partially responsive to the environment during episodes, which usually last a few minutes but can range anywhere from 30 s to 30 min. Typically, the episodes last from 1 to 10 min. Joyce Kales' study reported an average duration of 6 min [6]. They rarely occur more than once per night. In this same group of patients, 75% reported a real, potential or actual injury during the episodes, and 18% had walked out of their house. Night terrors

Table 13.1 Night terrors.

Timing	15–90 min after sleep onset
Characteristics	Extreme autonomic discharge Tachycardia Perspiration Vocalization Distress Staring Inconsolable Amnesia
Differential diagnosis	Nightmares, REM behavioral disorder, nocturnal panic attacks, epilepsy, sundowning syndrome
Treatment	Psychotherapy Hypnosis Cognitive behavioral therapy Valium, imipramine, melatonin, paroxetine Waking therapy

can occur more than once a night and up to several times per week. There is little or no recall of the event the morning after the event.

Night terrors can be distinguished from other paroxysmal events during sleep by two essential features: the characteristic autonomic activation during the event, and retrograde amnesia following it. Night terrors are associated with vocalizations and autonomic activation with more behavioral expression of fear and anxiety compared to nightmares. During night terrors, patients are difficult to arouse and have less recall of the spells compared to patients with nightmares.

In a classic description of a night terror, the episode begins with a vocalization, which may manifest with a blood curdling or animal-like scream followed by a fight or flight response consisting of tachycardia, tachypnea, tremulousness, mydriasis, sweating, and increased respiratory rate [7]. The clinical manifestation of night terrors is generally agreed upon and consistently described as an "arousal response," characterized by autonomic activation and behavioral manifestations because the EEG pattern is consistent with a waking, alpha pattern with a clinical state of disorientation. Researchers have postulated different theories characterizing the state of an individual having a night terror, including automatisms or dissociation within wakefulness.

Night terrors share many similar clinical characteristics to sleepwalking and confusional arousals such as confusion, timing of occurrence, association to slow-wave sleep, age, physiological changes, and genetics. Because of these associations, night terrors, confusional arousals, and sleepwalking are often considered part of the same pathophysiological spectrum with any true distinction in a gray area, as there is often an overlap where both conditions co-exist in the same patient. Night terrors have been considered on the same pathophysiological spectrum as sleepwalking in that they are both disorders of arousal, originate in NREM sleep, and are a sign of CNS immaturity. On this spectrum, night terrors would be on the more severe end of the spectrum.

A few studies have focused on whether mental content during NREM sleep is the trigger of the night terrors. In one of these studies, the most common reports of dream content by subjects with night terrors were: fear of aggression by a person or persons, things closing in or being trapped in a small area, fear of falling, fear of aggression by sleep lab staff, and fear of being left alone [8]. Fisher et al. reported a mean of 58% recall of mental content from night terrors [8]. The content originated from both the pre-arousal and post-arousal states.

Night terrors often occur in patients with psychopathology, especially in adults with post-traumatic stress syndrome. Researchers have postulated that situations heightening anxiety may have an impact on hormones that causes arousal of the reticular system, which in turn heightens arousal and causes sleep disturbances [9]. Personality characteristics have also been examined in patients with night terrors using the Minnesota Multiphasic Personality Inventory (MMPI). Their profiles were consistent with inhibition of outward expression of aggression, lowered self-esteem, anxiety, depression, and phobicness. In this study, patients with night terrors had psychiatric evaluations with a psychiatric diagnosis in 85% consisting of anxiety, depression, phobias, obsessions, and personality disorders. Crisp et al. studied six patients with night terrors and compared them to sleepwalkers and normal patients. Patients with night terrors scored higher on the hysteria scale of the Crown–Crisp experiential index, while all other psychological characteristics were comparable, suggesting a tendency for dissociation [10]. Llorente reported six patients with night terrors, all of whom had a previously diagnosed psychiatric disorder. Despite the co-existence of psychiatric disorders in patients with night terrors, they did not appear to be related in clinical course or exacerbations.

Night terrors must be distinguished from nocturnal panic attacks, which are also associated with arousal from sleep with autonomic activation. The main distinguishing characteristic is the lack of confusion and amnesia in patients with nocturnal panic attacks.

Night terrors have also been reported as a side effect of patients being treated with sedative hypnotics, stimulants, anti-histamines, tricyclic anti-depressants and neuroleptics such as risperdone [7,11–13]. Strayhorn et al. reported frightening dreams in 50% of patients on a single daytime dose of tricyclic anti-depressants and 25% of patients on a single dose of neuroleptics. The mechanism is thought to be a result of an increase in NREM sleep by these medications, although there is some controversy to this claim, as there have also been reports of successful treatment of night terrors with imipramine [14]. Other precipitants of night terrors suggesting an organic component are febrile illnesses, head injury, and brainstem pathology.

The International Classification of Sleep Disorders second edition classifies sleep terrors in the same category as confusional arousals and sleepwalking, which are both also classified as parasomnias and disorders of arousal from NREM sleep. The diagnostic criteria of sleep terrors includes: a sudden episode of terror occurring during sleep, initiated by a cry or loud scream that is accompanied by autonomic nervous system and behavioral manifestations of intense fear. There must be associated difficulty in arousing the person, mental confusion when awakened from an episode, complete or partial amnesia for the episode, or dangerous or potentially dangerous behaviors. Lastly, the disturbance should not be better explained by another sleep disorder, medical, or neurological disorder, mental disorder, medication use, or substance use disorder [15].

Natural history

A combination of genetic, maturational, organic, and psychological factors are thought to play a role in the development and natural history of night terrors. In general, night terrors can be classified into two subtypes based on the age of onset. Patients with an earlier onset form of night terrors with a normal psychological profile typically have a benign course with resolution into adolescence, and are thought to be attributed to a maturation process in development. This can be conceptualized as an idiopathic form of night terrors. The later onset type is associated with an abnormal psychological profile, persistence into adulthood, and a greater likelihood of treatment.

Prevalence studies of night terrors vary in the literature, especially because of discrepancies in the definition of a night terror. In 1968 Kales et al. reported an incidence of night terrors in 1–3% of children 5–12 years of age [16]. A population study in the UK of 4972 subjects reported night terrors in 2.2% of the population with comparable rates between men and women [17]. This study found predominance in younger people and a decrease with age. Laberge et al. reported a prevalence of 17.3% in 1353 Canadian children between 6 and 16 years of age [18]. Ages of onset reported range from 3 to 74 years [19]. It is estimated that 30% of children will experience at least one night terror in their lives [20].

Night terrors are less frequent than nightmares in any age group [21]. Early-onset night terrors often begin before 10 years of age and are outgrown by adolescence [21]. Many children with sleep terrors will go on to sleepwalk, and vice versa. The common features of sleepwalking and night terrors suggest they may be linked by genetic or environmental factors, although psychological factors cannot be ruled out as contributory causes.

DiMario et al. studied 19 patients with early-onset night terrors to characterize the natural history [22]. Of 19 patients, 13 had EEGs performed, which were all negative for epileptic activity. The age of onset in 10 subjects was between 1.5 and 3.5 years. The median age of onset for all 19 subjects was 3.5 years. Questionnaires revealed an initial frequency from once per week to several times per year. In 11 children (70%), the initial frequency at the time of onset was the same as the peak frequency. In the remainder of the sample, the peak frequency was not reached for 2–9 years. Also, 63% reached a peak frequency of one or more night terror per week. Only one child had more than one episode per night. The mean duration of night terrors was 3.9 years, ranging from 6 months to 13 years. In this study, parents identified the following as precipitants: overtiredness, fever, separation, loss, moving, divorce, change of school, death in the family, return to school from vacation, or change of school. They also looked at possible familial patterns and found that 11 of 18 children with available family histories had a first-, second-, or third-degree relative with another parasomnia. Their data suggested a positive correlation between a longer duration of night terrors in patients with a positive family history of sleepwalking.

Some evidence suggests that development of night terrors after the age of 10 years is a positive predictor of persistence into adulthood; these patients are predicted to have a more chronic course and are more likely to require intervention [23]. In the later-onset form of night terrors, episodes may persist for up to 43 years [4]. Some evidence suggests that night terrors persisting into adulthood may have increased psychopathology.

Joyce Kales et al. published data looking at the clinical characteristics and personality patterns in patients with night terrors [6]. She found the mean age of onset of 40 patients examined was 12.5 years, 55% of whom reported occurrence of a major life event prior to the onset. The mean duration was 15.6 years. Patients reported seven night terrors per month, and 92% reported increasing frequency with mental stress. Fatigue increased frequency in 25% of patients, and a change of environment in 45%. Nightmares were reported in 72%, sleepwalking in 75%, insomnia in 52%, and enuresis in 40%. Interestingly, 72% of patients reported at least one prior episode of sleepwalking.

Although night terrors typically follow a benign clinical course, because of the association of violence during the attacks, they can occasionally be dangerous, especially if exacerbated by alcohol [24]. In severe cases, night terrors can result in injurious behavior. Schenck *et al.* described three patients with characteristics of night terrors/sleepwalking during intensive care unit admissions possibly due to precipitation by stress, medications, metabolic abnormalities and changes in sleep–wake patterns [25]. In another extreme case, the wife of a patient with dramatic night terrors developed post-traumatic stress disorder [26]. A case series of 54 patients reported injurious night terrors/sleepwalking in one-third of patients with onset after 16 years of age [27]. One patient began having episodes at age 58. Schenck *et al.* reported 33 cases of a "parasomnia overlap syndrome" involving sleepwalking, night terrors, and REM behavior disorder [28].

Ohayon *et al.* identified the following as independent risk factors positively associated with night terrors: sleep talking, subjective sense of choking, alcohol intake at bedtime, violent or injurious behaviors during sleep, hypnagogic hallucinations, obstructive sleep apnea (OSA) syndrome, and nightmares [17]. Community-based studies have also shown a relationship between night terrors and higher rates of bedtime resistance, sleep onset delay, night awakenings, and reduced sleep duration [29].

One of the key features of night terrors is the dramatic autonomic discharge during sleep with an increase in sympathetic tone associated with pupil dilation, increased heart rate, and decreased galvanic skin resistance. With this, suggestion has been made for an association of night terrors with sudden unexplained nocturnal death syndrome (SUNDS) in patients with underlying cardiac conduction abnormalities [30].

Night terrors can have a significant impact in a patient's personal life as they can affect or even endanger a bed partner. Injury during episodes is an important consideration, especially in individuals with certain roles such as military personnel.

Clinical evaluation and laboratory investigations

The first challenge in clearly conceptualizing and studying night terrors is to establish a firm description so that they can be distinguished from other paroxysmal episodes occurring during sleep, such as nightmares, epilepsy, cluster headaches, or other parasomnias. A comprehensive history and physical examination should be conducted to characterize age of onset, timing of associated stressful life events, frequency of episodes, duration, content, precipitants, family history, a history of febrile illnesses, other sleep disorders, and global development. Temporal and frontal lobe epilepsy are important considerations in the differential diagnosis of night terrors. Epilepsy can be differentiated from night terrors by the presence of daytime episodes, stereotypical activities, or focal motor abnormalities. Rarely, hysterical and dissociative conditions can masquerade as night terrors. However, in these conditions the patient maintains alertness and the episodes are longer in duration [31]. Elderly patients with organic cognitive impairment or chronically ill patients may have a "sundowning" syndrome with nocturnal wandering that should be distinguished from night terrors and sleepwalking.

In a landmark paper in *Science* in 1968, Broughton described the association of night terrors as a sudden phenomenon arising out of SWS with a pattern similar to a waking pattern during the spell itself. Patients may have hypersynchronous high-voltage slow-wave activity lasting 10–30 s prior to muscular activation during a night terror [32]. When comparing the sleep architecture of patients with parasomnias to normal patients, patients with parasomnias are observed as having more sleep fragmentation reflected by increased wake after sleep onset (WASO), number of awakenings greater than 1 min, and arousal indices [33]. Sleep fragmentation is concentrated in SWS, representing instability of SWS in patients with night terrors and sleepwalking. Studies comparing resting EEGs of patients with night terrors have not been shown to differ from age-matched controls [34].

In 1995, Pressman *et al.* reported a case of a 35-year-old man who experienced night terrors triggered by a rebound of SWS with initiation of continuous positive airway pressure (CPAP) therapy for OSA [35]. This association led researchers to examine whether respiratory events could lead to fragmentation of sleep and parasomnias using esophageal manometry. Espa *et al.* found that respiratory events leading to arousals occur more frequently in patients with parasomnias compared to normal subjects, suggesting a role for abnormal breathing events in precipitation of the parasomnias themselves [36]. Furthermore, these researchers postulated an elevated arousal threshold in these patients as a result of abnormal sleep density, contributing to the confused state that is characteristic of parasomnias.

Recent studies have also demonstrated a relationship between night terrors and other sleep disorders, such as sleep-disordered breathing (SDB) or restless legs syndrome (RLS) [37]. Therefore, evaluation for other sleep disorders including clinical evaluation and polysomnography is often indicated.

Night terrors beginning in middle age are infrequent, and these patients should have neuroimaging to rule out a brain tumor, especially if associated with neurological complaints. There are several cases in the literature citing an association of neurological disease with night terrors. There is one case report in the literature of a 48-year-old woman with new onset of night terrors after treatment for a right thalamic brain tumor [38]. Somatoform disorders should be considered in patients with later onset, a negative family history for night terrors, and a major life stressor.

Genetics

There are several papers reporting night terrors in up to three generations of families, suggesting a familial pattern of inheritance. In 1980, Kales *et al.* described a "two threshold" multifactorial model of inheritance of sleepwalking and night terrors [39]. In this model, they suggested a genetic predisposition to sleepwalking and night terrors that must be evoked by an environmental cue in addition to a genetic component. In this cohort, 27 family pedigrees of a patient with night terrors were investigated, and 26 had one or more family members with either sleepwalking, night terrors, or a combination of both. The prevalence of sleepwalking and night terrors in first-degree relatives was estimated as being ten times greater than in the general population.

Management

Treatment of night terrors can be divided into two categories: behavioral and medical strategies. In terms of behavioral treatments, several have been examined for night terrors, including psychotherapy, medications, safety precautions and wake therapy. However, not all cases of night terrors require treatment, as the most disturbing characteristics may sometimes be limited to what is experienced by an observing parent or bed partner. In these cases, reassurance that there is not a severe underlying health condition is all that is necessary. Parents or bed partners should be advised against attempting to awaken or intervene during the episode, as doing this may increase confusion and precipitate a dramatic or even violent reaction. In addition, many cases in children resolve with development as they reach adolescence. Modifications of the environment may be necessary depending on the characteristics of the episodes. Recommendations such as placing bells on doors, using gates to block stairways and kitchens, heavy drapery, recommending sleeping on the ground floor, and eliminating any potentially dangerous objects may be necessary depending on the clinical presentation to ensure safety.

Waking treatment has also been recommended as an effective therapy which consists of waking a child immediately before onset of the night terror based on autonomic arousal [40]. Lask *et al.* instructed parents of 19 children with night terrors, ranging from ages 5 to 13 years, to wake the child fully 10–15 min prior to the time of onset, or if that was not possible, at the earliest time of autonomic onset [41]. The child was allowed to return to sleep after approximately 5 min. The night terrors ceased within 1 week of beginning therapy in all cases, although in three cases, episodes returned after 4–7 weeks and responded to repeated therapy. One year follow-up confirmed cessation of spells. Subsequent reports of wake therapy quoted an 80% success rate, although other researchers have reported no success with this method [7,40]. The mechanism of action was presumed to be related to an interruption of "faulty slow wave sleep" with a restoration of normal sleep patterns.

Insight-oriented psychotherapy has been recommended as a behavioral treatment for patients with night terrors when an underlying psychological disturbance is suspected. This is suggested when the clinician suspects that night terrors are manifesting as difficulty coping with frustration, conflict, and inwardly directed aggression and stress. Psychotherapy allows individuals to learn to react more constructively in response to conflicts and stressors [31]. Psychotherapy, hypnosis, or cognitive behavioral therapy for night terrors may include exploring fear of failure and hostility [42]. If the patient has phobias, desensitization may also play a role in effective therapy. Case reports of successful treatment of night terrors with psychotherapy were reported in the 1980s [23]. In these cases, therapy was conducted in weekly sessions over 20–23 months with the idea that internalization of emotions precipitates night terrors, and with psychotherapy the patients were able to develop insight into expressing emotions in an adaptive way so that episodes were significantly reduced or eliminated. In successful cases of treatment of night terrors with psychotherapy, a direct, flexible, and active therapist was proposed as the most successful component [23]. The patient can also learn to become more tuned in with night terrors as a gauge of their stress levels. Hypnosis has also been reported as a treatment for night terrors, although hypnosis in children is difficult, and individuals have varying degrees of susceptibility for hypnosis. Some clinicians have also recommended using the mental content of the night terror with rehearsal of alternate endings during the daytime as a therapeutic strategy [43].

In general, medical treatment is not recommended for children with night terrors because of the benign nature and clinical course of this type of night terror [44]. There are several different approaches to identifying when medical treatment should be initiated. Keith et al. suggested treatment when serious pathology is suggested by the frequency of the events without remission over time, especially in the setting of daytime anxiety or obvious family psychopathology [45]. Very frequent episodes that disrupt the quality of sleep, endanger the individual, or cause psychosocial dysfunction are indications for medical treatment. The earliest reports of pharmacological treatment of night terrors was done by Pesikoff and Davis, who treated sleep walking and night terrors in seven children with imipramine 10–50 mg at bedtime [46]. Of these patients, two had night terrors and both had resolution with treatment. Burstein et al. reported successfully treating five patients, three women and two men with a mean age of 29.9 years who developed night terrors after traumatic motor vehicle accidents with post-traumatic stress syndrome and post-concussive syndrome [47]. These patients were treated with imipramine 200–300 mg at bedtime with a therapeutic effect within 5 days of treatment. Deepening of sleep was the proposed clinical impact, which resulted in less apprehension associated with sleep, decreased frequency of night terrors, less awakenings, and easier return to sleep after arousals. All of the patients previously failed treatment with lorazepam. Marshall et al. also recommended treatment of night terrors with imipramine in patients with night terrors in the setting of post-traumatic stress syndrome [9]. In his paper, he postulated that the mechanism of action was through lowering arousals. At the time of publication, there was ongoing debate about whether suppressing the night terrors was a good thing because some thought they would inevitably manifest in some other dysfunctional way. The mechanism was questioned, since imipramine is known not to decrease stage 4 sleep. Fisher et al. and Glick et al. each treated one patient with imipramine, and in all cases it was ineffective. In contrast, others have postulated that the mechanism of action may be due to an increase in drug-induced arousals. Therefore, some critics thought the mechanism was due to a placebo response, but the fact that these patients did not respond to other medications suggested against this.

Fisher et al. reported suppression of 80% of episodes with diazepam 5–20 mg with a corresponding 90% decrease in stage 4 sleep in six adults [3]. The effect took place after two weeks and lasted even for a short time after discontinuation of therapy. Another study performed by Glick et al. also suggested a response to diazepam [48]. Taboada et al. reported use of diazepam and flurazepam [4]. Vela et al. published a case series of six patients treated with bromazepam 1.5 mg 30 min prior to bedtime with inconclusive results of its effectiveness in treating night terrors, but a statistically significant reduction in SWS [49]. The efficacy of midazolam has been attributed to its rapid onset of action, hypnotic effect with a suppression of arousals, and reduction in SWS. Allen et al. reported two patients on psychotropic medications with night terrors treated effectively with clorazepate 7.5–15 mg [50]. Both drugs are metabolized to desmethyldiazepam, which has an anxiolytic effect which also may account for its clinical effectiveness. Suppression of SWS, anxiolytic properties, and sedation may be the mechanism of benzodiazepines as effective pharmacotherapy for night terrors. They should be administered in the lowest possible doses necessary to minimize side effects and generally 90 min prior to bedtime [7]. Often after three to four weeks of therapy and resolution of night terrors, medication can be tapered. In 2004, L-5-hydroxytryptophan 2 mg/kg at bedtime was reported as a successful treatment of night terrors in 29 of 31 patients at one month follow-up [51].

Recent reports have also described successful treatment of night terrors with paroxetine 20–40 mg daily [52,53]. The mechanism is thought to be the direct result of increasing 5-hydroxytryptamine concentrations in the brainstem and indirectly through an antidepressant effect. Paroxetine has several advantages over the benzodiazepines. Those advantages are that it is not a drug of abuse and patients do not develop tolerance to it.

There is one case report in the literature of successful treatment of night terrors in a 12-year-old boy with coinciding Asperger's syndrome, sleep phase delay, and sleepwalking, with melatonin 5 mg dispensed 30 min before bedtime [54]. The authors postulated a relationship between treating sleep deprivation and successfully treating parasomnias.

Lastly, some cases of night terrors may be related to other sleep disorders. Guilleminault *et al.* evaluated 84 patients with either night terrors or a combination of night terrors and sleepwalking [37]. In this sample, 49 children were found to have coinciding SDB and 43 were subsequently treated with tonsillectomy with or without adenoidectomy and with or without turbinate reduction. In follow-up polysomnography 3–4 months post-operatively parents and sleep logs indicated a disappearance of parasomnias. Therefore, treatment of an underlying sleep disorder should not be overlooked as a potential treatment of night terrors.

Conclusions

Night terrors are fascinating entities that share many of the same characteristics of the other parasomnias occurring as arousals from NREM sleep. Further research examining the distinction between early onset, later onset, and familial patterns of night terrors may help to reveal the underlying pathophysiology of night terrors as they relate to sleep architecture, arousal thresholds, and genetics. An interesting question that remains to be determined is if night terrors, sleepwalking, and confusional arousals truly are part of the same pathophysiological spectrum or rather are distinct entities. In future research, a clear distinction should be made to allow analysis of these questions.

References

1. Kottek SS. "Mater puerorum". A medieval naming for an enigmatic children's disease. *Eur J Pediatr* 1981; **137**: 75–9.
2. Sullivan RB. Night terrors in childhood: Case report No. 268. *Clin Proc Child Hosp Dist Columbia* 1953; **9**: 157–61.
3. Fisher C, Kahn E, Edwards A, Davis DM. A psychophysiological study of nightmares and night terrors. I. Physiological aspects of the stage 4 night terror. *J Nerv Ment Dis* 1973; **157**: 75–98.
4. Taboada EL. Night terrors in children: Causes and treatment. *Tex Med* 1974; **70**: 70–2.
5. Stern MM. Pavor nocturnus. *Int J Psychoanal* 1951; **32**: 302–09.
6. Kales JD, Kales A, Soldatos CR, Caldwell AB, Charney DS, Martin ED. Night terrors. Clinical characteristics and personality patterns. *Arch Gen Psychiatry* 1980; **37**: 1413–7.
7. Mason TB, 2nd, Pack AI. Sleep terrors in childhood. *J Pediatr* 2005; **147**: 388–92.
8. Fisher C, Kahn E, Edwards A, Davis DM, Fine J. A psychophysiological study of nightmares and night terrors. 3. Mental content and recall of stage 4 night terrors. *J Nerv Ment Dis* 1974; **158**: 174–88.
9. Marshall JR. The treatment of night terrors associated with the posttraumatic syndrome. *Am J Psychiatry* 1975; **132**: 293–5.
10. Crisp AH, Matthews BM, Oakey M, Crutchfield M. Sleepwalking, night terrors, and consciousness. *Br Med J* 1990; **300**: 360–2.
11. Flemenbaum A. Pavor nocturnus: A complication of single daily tricyclic or neuroleptic dosage. *Am J Psychiatry* 1976; **133**: 570–2.
12. Strayhorn JM, Nash JL. Frightening dreams and dosage schedule of tricyclic and neuroleptic drugs. *J Nerv Ment Dis* 1978; **166**: 878–80.
13. Prueter C, Luecke FG, Hoff P. Pavor nocturnus as a side effect of a single daily risperidone dose. *Gen Hosp Psychiatry* 2005; **27**: 300–01.
14. Beitman BD, Carlin AS. Night terrors treated with imipramine. *Am J Psychiatry* 1979; **136**: 1087–8.
15. Sateia MJ. *The International Classification of Sleep Disorders, Second Edition: Diagnostic and Coding Manual.* Westchester, IL: American Academy of Sleep Medicine, 2005.
16. Kales A, Beall GN, Berger RJ, *et al.* Sleep and dreams. Recent research on clinical aspects. *Ann Intern Med* 1968; **68**: 1078–104.
17. Ohayon MM, Guilleminault C, Priest RG. Night terrors, sleepwalking, and confusional arousals in the general population: Their frequency and relationship to other sleep and mental disorders. *J Clin Psychiatry* 1999; **60**: 268–76; quiz 77.

18. Laberge L, Tremblay RE, Vitaro F, Montplaisir J. Development of parasomnias from childhood to early adolescence. *Pediatrics* 2000; **106**: 67–74.

19. Llorente MD, Currier MB, Norman SE, Mellman TA. Night terrors in adults: Phenomenology and relationship to psychopathology. *J Clin Psychiatry* 1992; **53**: 392–4.

20. Ferber R. Sleep, sleeplessness, and sleep disruptions in infants and young children. *Ann Clin Res* 1985; **17**: 227–34.

21. Murray JB. Psychophysiological aspects of nightmares, night terrors, and sleepwalking. *J Gen Psychol* 1991; **118**: 113–27.

22. DiMario FJ, Jr., Emery ES, 3rd. The natural history of night terrors. *Clin Pediatr (Phila)* 1987; **26**: 505–11.

23. Kales JC, Cadieux RJ, Soldatos CR, Kales A. Psychotherapy with night-terror patients. *Am J Psychother* 1982; **36**: 399–407.

24. Hartmann E. Two case reports: Night terrors with sleepwalking – A potentially lethal disorder. *J Nerv Ment Dis* 1983; **171**: 503–05.

25. Schenck CH, Mahowald MW. Injurious sleep behavior disorders (parasomnias) affecting patients on intensive care units. *Intensive Care Med* 1991; **17**: 219–24.

26. Baran AS, Richert AC, Goldberg R, Fry JM. Posttraumatic stress disorder in the spouse of a patient with sleep terrors. *Sleep Med* 2003; **4**: 73–5.

27. Schenck CH, Milner DM, Hurwitz TD, Bundlie SR, Mahowald MW. A polysomnographic and clinical report on sleep-related injury in 100 adult patients. *Am J Psychiatry* 1989; **146**: 1166–73.

28. Schenck CH, Boyd JL, Mahowald MW. A parasomnia overlap disorder involving sleepwalking, sleep terrors, and REM sleep behavior disorder in 33 polysomnographically confirmed cases. *Sleep* 1997; **20**: 972–81.

29. Mehlenbeck R, Spirito A, Owens J, Boergers J. The clinical presentation of childhood partial arousal parasomnias. *Sleep Med* 2000; **1**: 307–12.

30. Melles RB, Katz B. Sudden, unexplained nocturnal death syndrome and night terrors. *J Am Med Assoc* 1987; **257**: 2918–9.

31. Kales JD, Soldatos CR, Kales A. Treatment of sleep disorders I: Insomnia. *Ration Drug Ther* 1983; **17**: 1–7.

32. Jacobson A, Kales A, Lehmann D, Zweizig JR. Somnambulism: All-night electroencephalographic studies. *Science* 1965; **148**: 975–7.

33. Espa F, Ondze B, Deglise P, Billiard M, Besset A. Sleep architecture, slow wave activity, and sleep spindles in adult patients with sleepwalking and sleep terrors. *Clin Neurophysiol* 2000; **111**: 929–39.

34. Soldatos CR, Vela-Bueno A, Bixler EO, Schweitzer PK, Kales A. Sleepwalking and night terrors in adulthood: Clinical EEG findings. *Clin Electroencephalogr* 1980; **11**: 136–9.

35. Pressman MR, Meyer TJ, Kendrick-Mohamed J, Figueroa WG, Greenspon LW, Peterson DD. Night terrors in an adult precipitated by sleep apnea. *Sleep* 1995; **18**: 773–5.

36. Espa F, Dauvilliers Y, Ondze B, Billiard M, Besset A. Arousal reactions in sleepwalking and night terrors in adults: The role of respiratory events. *Sleep* 2002; **25**: 871–5.

37. Guilleminault C, Palombini L, Pelayo R, Chervin RD. Sleepwalking and sleep terrors in prepubertal children: What triggers them? *Pediatrics* 2003; **111**: e17–25.

38. Di Gennaro G, Autret A, Mascia A, Onorati P, Sebastiano F, Paolo Quarato P. Night terrors associated with thalamic lesion. *Clin Neurophysiol* 2004; **115**: 2489–92.

39. Kales A, Soldatos CR, Bixler EO, et al. Hereditary factors in sleepwalking and night terrors. *Br J Psychiatry* 1980; **137**: 111–8.

40. Lask B. Sleep disorders. "Working treatment" best for night terrors. *Br Med J* 1993; **306**: 1477.

41. Lask B. Novel and non-toxic treatment for night terrors. *Br Med J* 1988; **297**: 592.

42. Soldatos CR, Kales A. Sleep disorders: Research in psychopathology and its practical implications. *Acta Psychiatr Scand* 1982; **65**: 381–7.

43. Maskey S. Sleep disorders. Simple treatment for night terrors. *Br Med J* 1993; **306**: 1477.

44. Kales A, Soldatos CR, Kales JD. Sleep disorders: Insomnia, sleepwalking, night terrors, nightmares, and enuresis. *Ann Intern Med* 1987; **106**: 582–92.

45. Keith PR. Night terrors. A review of the psychology, neurophysiology, and therapy. *J Am Acad Child Psychiatry* 1975; **14**: 477–89.

46. Pesikoff RB, Davis PC. Treatment of pavor nocturnus and somnambulism in children. *Am J Psychiatry* 1971; **128**: 778–81.

47. Burstein A. Treatment of night terrors with imipramine. *J Clin Psychiatry* 1983; **44**: 82.

48. Glick BS, Schulman D, Turecki S. Diazepam (Valium) treatment in childhood sleep disorders. A preliminary investigation. *Dis Nerv Syst* 1971; **32**: 565–6.

49. Vela A, Dobladez B, Rubio ME, et al. Action of bromazepam on sleep of children with night terrors. I. Sleep organization and heart rate. *Pharmatherapeutica* 1982; **3**: 247–58.

50. Allen RM. Attenuation of drug-induced anxiety dreams and pavor nocturnus by benzodiazepines. *J Clin Psychiatry* 1983; **44**: 106–08.

51. Bruni O, Ferri R, Miano S, Verrillo E. L-5-Hydroxytryptophan treatment of sleep terrors in children. *Eur J Pediatr* 2004; **163**: 402–07.

52. Lillywhite AR, Wilson SJ, Nutt DJ. Successful treatment of night terrors and somnambulism with paroxetine. *Br J Psychiatry* 1994; **164**: 551–4.

53. Wilson SJ, Lillywhite AR, Potokar JP, Bell CJ, Nutt DJ. Adult night terrors and paroxetine. *Lancet* 1997; **350**: 185.

54. Jan JE, Freeman RD, Wasdell MB, Bomben MM. A child with severe night terrors and sleep-walking responds to melatonin therapy. *Dev Med Child Neurol* 2004; **46**: 789.

Section 3
Parasomnias usually associated with REM sleep

Section 3 Chapter 14

Parasomnias usually associated with REM sleep

REM sleep behavior disorder

Raffaele Manni and Michele Terzaghi

History

REM sleep behavior disorder (RBD) was first formally identified in 1986 by Schenck and Mahowald in five elderly subjects presenting similar motor behavioral patterns during REM sleep consisting of violent dream-enacting behaviors [1].

Although there already existed anecdotal reports of similar episodes arising from REM sleep during tricyclic anti-depressant treatment and in the context of acute psychosis related to alcohol and drug abuse, Schenck and Mahowald were the first to recognize RBD as a distinct parasomnia with a clinical and polysomnographic (PSG) pattern similar to that seen 20 years earlier in animal models of RBD. In a review of their personal data and of the literature over the 16 years following the formal identification of RBD, these same authors highlighted the existence of acute and chronic, idiopathic and symptomatic forms of RBD, and also the idea that RBD may herald the onset of synucleinopathies [2].

REM sleep behavior disorder first appeared, with clear diagnostic criteria, in the International Classification of Sleep Disorders (ICSD) in 1990. These criteria have recently been updated in the ICSD-2 2005 version [3], and in the American Academy of Sleep Medicine (AASM) atlas of sleep scoring [4].

Even though RBD may occur in childhood, it generally has onset after the age of 50 years and shows a strong male prevalence. The frequency of occurrence of RBD in the general population is unknown. A prevalence of 0.38% in a community sample of elderly in Hong Kong [5] and of 0.5% in a large general population sample in the UK [6] were estimated on the basis of the finding of dream-enactment behaviors in sleep-related violent episodes.

Early descriptions of RBD have been identified by Schenck and Mahowald in Cervantes' *Don Quixote* (1605) and by Pierre Schultz and Francois Curtin in a monk appearing in Brillant Savarin's *The Physiology of Taste* (1825) [2].

Alternative names for RBD, mentioned in ICSD-2, are: oneirism, stage 1 REM (these two terms, now abandoned, were used prior to the formal identification of the condition and may be considered its "historic" names), REM sleep without atonia (used by basic scientists), paradoxical sleep without atonia, and REM sleep motor parasomnia. RBD is the internationally recognized acronym.

Clinical findings

The clinical manifestations of RBD are typically dream-related motor-behavioral manifestations that appear to be the enactment of a fight. These manifestations range from simple, primitive, purposeless jerky movements of the head, face, neck, trunk, arms/legs, hands/feet, or whole body, to complex movements, such as gesturing, pointing, punching, and kicking (Figure 14.1). The movements may be accompanied by shouting, yelling, crying, laughing or more or less structured and comprehensible sleep talking. Patients rarely get out of bed and walk during RBD episodes.

The jerky, violent movements that sometimes cause patients to fall out of bed can (in up to approximately 79% of cases) result in injury to the patient and their bed partner. Personal injuries such as bruises, lacerations, bone fractures and even subdural hematomas and spleen ruptures have been observed. The episodes tend to occur during the second part of the night, although RBD episodes occurring shortly after falling asleep have been reported in subjects with short REM latency, and RBD episodes during daytime sleep in narcoleptic patients. Different episodes varying in severity (from minimal to very intense) may occur

The Parasomnias and Other Sleep-Related Movement Disorders, ed. M. J. Thorpy and G. Plazzi. Published by Cambridge University Press. © Cambridge University Press 2010.

Section 3: REM sleep parasomnias

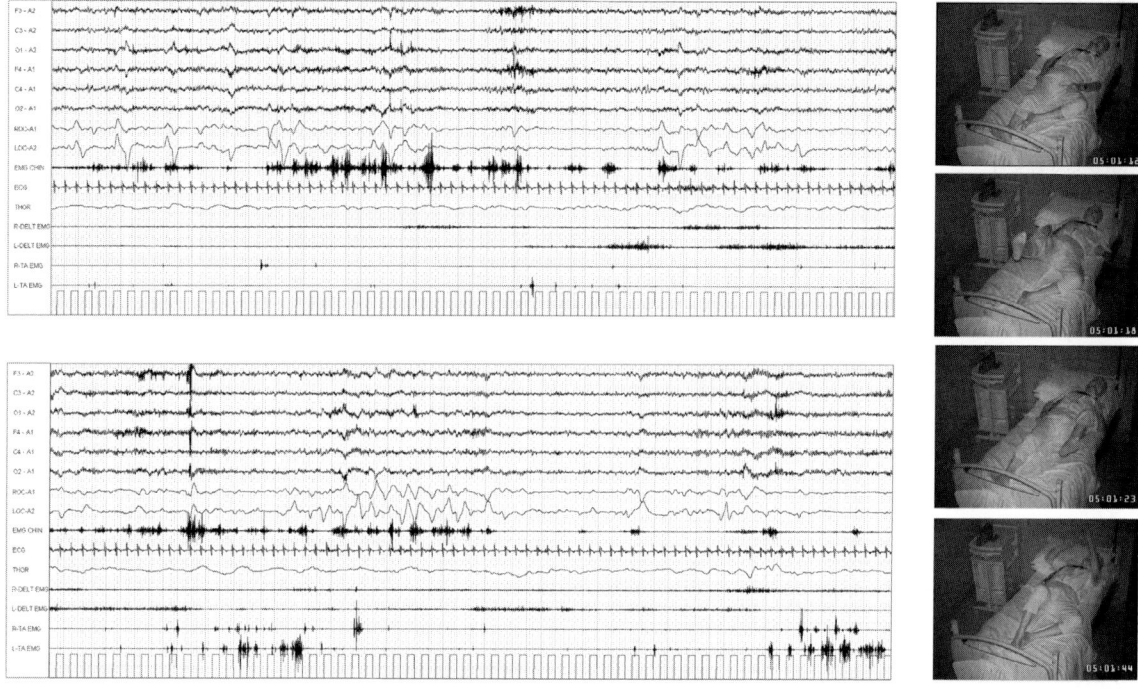

Figure 14.1 Ictal PSG tracing during a RBD episode. Full-blown RBD episode is illustrated (right column) by pictures showing kicking and punching. R-DELT EMG: right deltoid; L-DELT EMG: left deltoid; R-TA: right anterior tibialis; L-TA: left anterior tibialis.

in the course of a single night. On awakening, patients report having dreamed of being attacked or subjected to aggression, these reports being consistent with the motor-behavioral pattern observed during the RBD episode. In contrast with the aggressive behaviors displayed during episodes, RBD patients are reportedly very quiet and mild-mannered people. Low scores on an aggressivity scale have been recorded in subjects affected by idiopathic RBD, and RBD patients do not usually show psychiatric morbidity [7].

Compared with the movements observed in idiopathic RBD, those occurring in Parkinson's disease (PD) and parkinsonian syndromes are reportedly less pronounced and less frequently violent, but equally jerky [8].

The diagnostic criteria for RBD, as set out in ICSD-2, combine clinical and PSG features:

A. Presence of REM sleep without atonia (RSWA) on PSG.
B. At least one of the following:

   (1) sleep-related, injurious, potentially injurious or disruptive behaviors by history (i.e. dream enactment behavior), and/or

   (2) abnormal REM sleep behavior documented during polysomnographic monitoring.

C. Absence of EEG epileptiform activity during REM sleep unless RBD can be clearly distinguished from any concurrent REM sleep-related seizure disorder.
D. The sleep disorder is not better explained by another sleep disorder, medical or neurological disorder, mental disorder, medication use or substance use disorder.

Even though the need for "presence of REM sleep without atonia", meaning either sustained muscle activity (tonic activity) or excessive transient muscle activity (phasic activity), or both, is clearly stated as a necessary criterion for RBD diagnosis in ICSD-2, no indications are given about how REM without atonia should be quantified; furthermore, there is no mention of a cut-off above which the loss of atonia should be considered of pathological significance. However, in the recently published AASM *Manual for the Scoring of Sleep and Associated Events* [4], the recommended PSG features for scoring RBD are as follows:

- For "tonic activity": "an epoch of REM sleep with at least 50% of the duration of the epoch having a

chin EMG amplitude greater than the minimum amplitude in NREM."
- For phasic activity: "In a 30-second epoch of REM sleep divided into ten sequential 3-second mini-epochs, at least five (50%) of the mini-epochs contain bursts of transient muscle activity. In RBD, excessive transient muscle activity bursts are 0.1–5.0 seconds in duration and at least four times as high in amplitude as the background EMG activity".

However, several different approaches to the quantification of REM without atonia in RBD, involving both visual and spectral analysis [9–11], are currently under way, and further criteria are likely to be forthcoming.

Clinical–pathophysiological subtypes

Subclinical or preclinical RBD, status dissociatus and parasomnia overlap syndrome are the clinical–pathophysiological subtypes of RBD, according to ICSD-2.

Subclinical RBD is characterized by a PSG pattern of muscular tone dyscontrol during REM sleep in the absence of a clinical history of RBD or of complex behaviors (although minimal, subtle motor behavioral manifestations may be captured on video). Subclinical RBD is also called preclinical RBD, on the basis of the assumption that it is an early, clinically silent manifestation of REM with muscular tone dyscontrol destined to evolve into clinical RBD. However, since this evolution manifests itself in only a quarter of subclinical RBD cases [3], further longitudinal studies are needed to demonstrate a strong association between subclinical RBD and the eventual emergence of clinical forms of RBD.

First described by Schenck *et al.* in 33 subjects in 1997, *parasomnia overlap disorder* is the co-occurrence, in the same subject, of RBD with a disorder of arousal (sleepwalking, night terrors, confusional arousals) [12]. The complexity of the clinical picture can present a diagnostic challenge. Parasomnia overlap disorder generally has onset in childhood and a male prevalence, but it may occur in all age groups, either as an idiopathic or as a symptomatic form (post-traumatic, tumoral, demyelinating, neurodegenerative or iatrogenic diseases).

Status dissociatus is characterized by a complex clinical picture consisting of dream-related behaviors ("dream enactments") strongly reminiscent of RBD, alternating or overlapping with wakefulness and other sleep behaviors [13].

Accordingly, PSG recordings show a mixture of NREM sleep, wakefulness and REM sleep, with a pattern that does not fully correspond to the standard markers of any of these states.

There exist experimentally induced animal models of status dissociatus, resulting from lesions or manipulation at the thalamic, hypothalamic and brain stem level [14]. However, dissociation of states also occurs in animals as a spontaneous state, as in the concurrence of swimming or flight with sleep in birds and the phenomenon of unihemispheric sleep in bottle-nosed dolphin.

After the initial descriptions by Mahowald and Schenck in 1991, other cases of status dissociatus have been reported in humans, in the context of various medical conditions: narcolepsy, PD, multiple system atrophy (MSA), alcohol withdrawal, recent cardiac surgery, severe sleep apnea, brain stem lesions and fatal familial insomnia [2,14–16].

Co-existing pathologies
Narcolepsy

The literature contains anecdotal reports of co-existing RBD and narcolepsy in both adults [17,18] and children [19], in some cases with the RBD episodes as the presenting symptoms [20]. With the exception of one case in which the association was with an isolated mediotegmental lesion, the narcolepsy is idiopathic. Systematic investigations of the occurrence of RBD episodes in idiopathic narcolepsy have shown a frequency of 7–36%, no gender preference, and an earlier age at onset compared with idiopathic RBD; they are also more likely to occur in forms of narcolepsy with cataplexy. Furthermore, an increased frequency of both REM sleep without atonia and phasic EMG events in REM sleep has been reported in narcoleptic subjects without overt RBD manifestations compared with controls [11]. Accordingly, it has been hypothesized that hypocretin/dopaminergic system dysfunctions may lead to motor dyscontrol during REM sleep in narcolepsy.

On the basis of the current body of literature, it appears that the association between RBD and narcolepsy is clinically significant and warrants further investigation in order to clarify the pathophysiology of these two sleep disorders.

Post-traumatic stress disorder

A strong association between RBD and post-traumatic stress disorder has been reported. It was suggested that similar neuropathological processes involving loss of peri-locus coeruleus neurons with subsequent disinhibition of tegmental pontine nuclei may explain the frequent co-existence of these two disorders [21].

Neurodegenerative diseases

Full-blown as well as subclinical RBD has been reported in association with many neurodegenerative disorders, especially with α-synucleinopathies [22]: PD, dementia with Lewy bodies (RBD is included as a suggestive feature for diagnosis), MSA, and pure autonomic failure [23]. RBD may precede, even by years, the onset of synucleinopathies [24–28]. One of the most fascinating questions is whether it is possible to identify these susceptible patients in advance. On the assumption that it is possible, research aiming to clarify the clinical picture that might allow early identification of these cases is under way. This research should lead to the identification of early markers of impending neurodegenerative disease, and thus of individuals warranting particularly careful follow-up and, possibly, early treatment.

In rare cases, RBD has been reported in non-synucleinopathies (mostly tauopathies and amyloidopathy); cases occurring in Progressive Supranuclear Palsy, spinocerebellar ataxia (SCA-3), and Alzheimer's disease (AD) are also documented [23,28]. However, in most of these cases a Lewy body disease variant could not be ruled out.

Differential diagnosis

Several factors make it difficult to arrive at a definite diagnosis of RBD based on clinical findings alone, and definite diagnosis should not be reached in the absence of confirmatory overnight video-PSG data. In fact, the clinical manifestations of RBD overlap with those of quite a few other conditions.

The following parasomnia and non-parasomnia disorders should be taken into account in the differential diagnosis of RBD.

NREM arousal-related parasomnias (sleepwalking, sleep terrors)

The clinical features of NREM parasomnias that help to distinguish them from RBD are a young age at onset, a lack of gender prevalence, occurrence of episodes during the first part of the night, and a lack of clear recall of a dream sequence. Furthermore, walking and running are rarely observed in RBD.

Rhythmic movement disorder (RMD)

The onset or relapse, in adulthood, of RMD, especially when the disorder occurs during REM sleep, may lead to a misdiagnosis of RBD. Furthermore, the fact that rhythmic movements have been known to occur in the context of RBD episodes, both phenomena being documented on video-PSG, means that, in some cases, the differential diagnosis between these two conditions may be difficult [29]. However, such cases are very rare, and given that RMD is typically seen in childhood, often manifesting itself both during wakefulness and during sleep, the need to differentiate between the RMD and RBD arises very infrequently.

Epileptic nocturnal seizures

Problems of differential diagnosis may also arise between RBD and nocturnal epileptic seizures, given that there is a certain similarity between the motor and behavioral pattern observed in RBD and the ictal and post-ictal phenomena of nocturnal epileptic seizures, namely temporal and frontal lobe seizures [30].

The hyperkinetic manifestations of nocturnal frontal lobe epilepsy (NFLE) can mimic the brisk, violent, arm and/or leg movements seen in RBD, even though tonic and dystonic movements, typical of NFLE, have never been documented in RBD. Motor and verbal automatisms during temporal lobe seizures may mimic the semi-purposeful gesturing, utterances and sleep talking found in RBD. Furthermore, the occurrence, during nocturnal temporal lobe seizures in both NREM and REM sleep, of abrupt movements, wandering, shouting, aggressive behaviors or vivid dream-like enactments may be reminiscent of the aggressive behavior seen in RBD. However, unlike most nocturnal forms of temporal lobe epilepsy and some forms of frontal lobe epilepsy, RBD cannot, by definition, also occur during wakefulness.

A scale was proposed for frontal lobe epilepsy and parasomnia (FLEP) as a tool to distinguish NFLE from NREM parasomnias and RBD [31]. However, the scale recently proved rather unreliable in distinguishing NFLE from RBD in a series of 71 subjects referred to a tertiary sleep and epilepsy unit for diagnosis of nocturnal motor-behavioral episodes [32].

The risk of misdiagnosis is reportedly even greater in cases of comorbidity between RBD and epileptic phenomena, which can signify either the presence of interictal epileptiform abnormalities in awake and sleep EEG tracings of RBD or the co-occurrence of RBD and epileptic seizures in the same subject (estimated to be present in up to 12.5% of a series of 80 elderly subjects with epilepsy) [33,34]. Synchronized video-PSG is thus mandatory to establish the nature (RBD or epileptic) of a patient's motor-behavioral episodes and thus whether he is affected by both disorders. It is advisable to use extended EEG montages in these cases, as it has been shown that the use of standard sleep EEG montages (used for sleep scoring) may fail to capture epileptic discharges.

Obstructive sleep apnea with agitated arousals (pseudo-RBD)

Complex, sometimes violent, motor-behavioral episodes can occur on arousal after an apneic event or in the post-arousal period during REM or NREM sleep. Such episodes remit after continuous positive airway pressure (CPAP) treatment for obstructive sleep apnea (OSA).

In subjects with OSA, these RBD-like episodes may be misdiagnosed as RBD [16]. Yet RBD and OSA, both disorders showing a strong prevalence in males and in middle age, can also co-exist in the same patient, making it extremely difficult to reach a definite differential diagnosis between RBD and pseudo-RBD episodes.

Nocturnal psychogenic dissociative disorders

Even though dissociative states resulting in violent behaviors generally occur in the daytime, cases of dissociative disorders arising exclusively or predominantly during the night have been reported, and this subgroup of disorders is now coded in ICSD-2 under the heading Parasomnias ("sleep-related dissociative disorders") [3]. Psychological testing together with a past, generally childhood, history of (usually sexual) abuse may make it easier to distinguish sleep-related dissociative disorders from RBD. Polysomnography helps in difficult cases and in cases with forensic implications, demonstrating that "sleep-related dissociative" episodes actually occur in a clear pattern of wakefulness after an awakening from sleep [35].

Malingering

It may be difficult to distinguish between cases of malingering and genuine RBD episodes. Video-PSG can help in these cases, documenting the occurrence of malingering episodes while the subject is awake or, in the absence of overt clinical manifestations during the monitored night, the lack of the characteristic picture of REM sleep without atonia [35].

Natural history

Cases of idiopathic or symptomatic RBD in childhood and adolescence are very infrequent. Because of the rarity of these forms and the lack of long-term follow-up data, little is known about the natural history of early-onset RBD [2]. Symptomatic forms of RBD early in life may be iatrogenic or due to inflammatory or demyelinating CNS disease. Available data seem to indicate that idiopathic RBD in childhood, which could be interpreted as abnormal tonic and phasic muscle activity during REM sleep caused by poor inhibition of spinal and brain stem motor networks due to immaturity of cortical and subcortical CNS inhibitory systems, is probably transitory and self-limiting [2].

Classical forms of RBD typically have onset in men aged over 50 years. In most cases, RBD is brought to the physician's attention several years after its onset making it difficult to establish its possible prodromes.

Schenck and Mahowald reported prodromes (persistent sleeptalking, yelling, limb twitching and limb and body jerking) in the absence of a picture of complex behaviors and lasting a mean of 22 years (range 2–48 years) in 25% of 96 cases of RBD [36]. From a clinical and neurophysiopathological perspective, it could be interesting to explore prodromes in RBD, as their existence may indicate a lifelong continuum of motor dyscontrol during REM sleep whose clinical manifestations differ in type and intensity at different times in the patient's life. Interestingly, forms of RBD evolving into status dissociatus have recently been reported in two cases of MSA [15]. The authors suggested that status dissociatus may be an extreme manifestation of RBD in neurodegenerative diseases.

Around a third of patients with PD and parkinsonian syndromes have full-blown RBD and the proportion is even higher (up to 50%) if subclinical forms are also included [21]. Instead, RBD is found in 80–95% of patients with MSA [25] and in 50–80% of those with dementia with Lewy bodies [28]. PD associated with RBD reportedly differs from PD-only, patients with PD+RBD being more likely to show an akinetic-rigid pattern, autonomic alterations and the development of cognitive deficits [22,37]. According to evidence in the literature, the onset of RBD that initially appears to be idiopathic can be followed by the onset of neurodegenerative diseases, namely of an alpha-synucleinopathy.

Schenck and Mahowald reported subsequent emergence of a parkinsonian disorder (4 years after diagnosis of RBD and 13 years after its onset) in 38% of a series of initially apparently idiopathic RBD cases. The proportion of patients who developed a parkinsonian disorder rose to 65% when the follow-up was extended to 7 years after the initial diagnosis [24].

Iranzo et al. found that 45% of patients initially diagnosed with idiopathic RBD at a tertiary sleep center developed a neurological disorder within 11.5 years of the reported onset of RBD and 5.1 years of the diagnosis of idiopathic RBD (mean values). These disorders were PD in nine patients, dementia with Lewy bodies in six, MSA with predominant cerebellar syndrome in one, and mild cognitive impairment in four patients with prominent visuo-spatial dysfunction [26].

Recently, Postuma et al., in a long-term follow-up study of idiopathic RBD patients, found that 26 out of 93 patients (28%) developed a neurodegenerative disorder (PD in 14, dementia with Lewy bodies in 7, AD in 4 and MSA in 1), with the estimated risk of neurodegenerative disease development rising from 17.7% at 5 years to 52.4% at 12 years [27].

These data, together with others documenting the existence in otherwise idiopathic RBD of alterations similar to the neuropsychological, autonomic and sensory abnormalities seen in synucleinopathies (so-called early markers of neurodegenerative diseases in RBD) raise questions over the existence of true forms of idiopathic RBD [38]. Indeed, some authors have suggested that the more cautious term "cryptogenic RBD" might be more appropriate [39].

On the other hand, adult-onset idiopathic RBD can spontaneously remit, just as it can persist without the subsequent emergence of a neurological disorder. The evolution of subclinical RBD into a full-blown clinical form of RBD has not yet been shown to be an invariable pattern, even though subclinical RBD may be associated with the eventual emergence of clinical RBD in at least 25% of cases [3]. Furthermore, remissions were recently reported in about a quarter of patients whose RBD had had onset within a full clinical picture of PD [40].

Taken together, these data indicate that non-progressive forms of RBD do exist. Longitudinal studies are needed to better define the natural history of RBD, which is unlikely to prove unequivocal.

Laboratory investigations

Polysomnography

A single full-nighttime-synchronized video-PSG recording is usually adequate to establish a definite diagnosis of RBD, providing that at least one RBD episode, coinciding with a REM phase, is captured, or, should there be no clinical manifestations, providing that there emerges a clear pattern of REM without atonia or REM with exaggerated phasic EMG activity.

Standard polysomnographic montages should be used [2] (Figures 14.2 and 14.3). The chin and leg muscles are usually monitored by means of surface EMG. However, upper limb muscle activity should also be monitored since RBD motor manifestations can, in a few subjects, consist mainly of arm and hand movements. Simultaneous recording of the mentalis, flexor digitorum superficialis, and extensor digitorum brevis muscles has recently proved to be the best muscle combination for capturing REM sleep phasic EMG activity in subjects with RBD [41].

Extended EEG montages are recommended for differential diagnosis versus epileptic seizures (Figure 14.4).

Other investigations

Conventional neuroimaging investigations, such as brain CT and MRI, are not mandatory. However, they should be performed when a neurological dysfunction is suspected on the basis of the clinical history and results of the neurological examination. Obviously, conventional neuroimaging is crucial in distinguishing idiopathic from symptomatic forms of RBD. The potential usefulness of cardiac (123)I-metaiodobenzylguanidine (MIBG) scintigraphic assessment as a supportive diagnostic indicator for idiopathic RBD is currently being evaluated [42].

There are a few other laboratory investigations that, while not strictly necessary in order to diagnose RBD, may help in the assessment of affected subjects. As the clinical significance of the alterations they can detect becomes clearer, these examinations, currently used mainly for research purposes at tertiary sleep centers,

Figure 14.2 Exaggerated twitching during REM sleep in a case of RBD R-BR: right brachio radialis; L-BR: left brachio radialis; R-TA: right anterior tibialis; L-TA: left anterior tibialis.

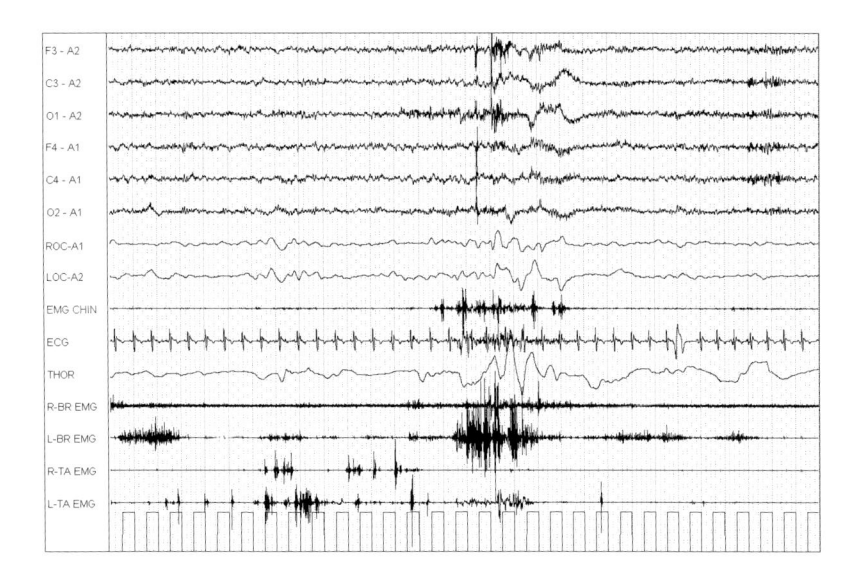

Figure 14.3 REM sleep without atonia and exaggerated twitching in a case of RBD R-BR: right brachio radialis; L-BR: left brachio radialis; R-TA: right anterior tibialis; L-TA: left anterior tibialis.

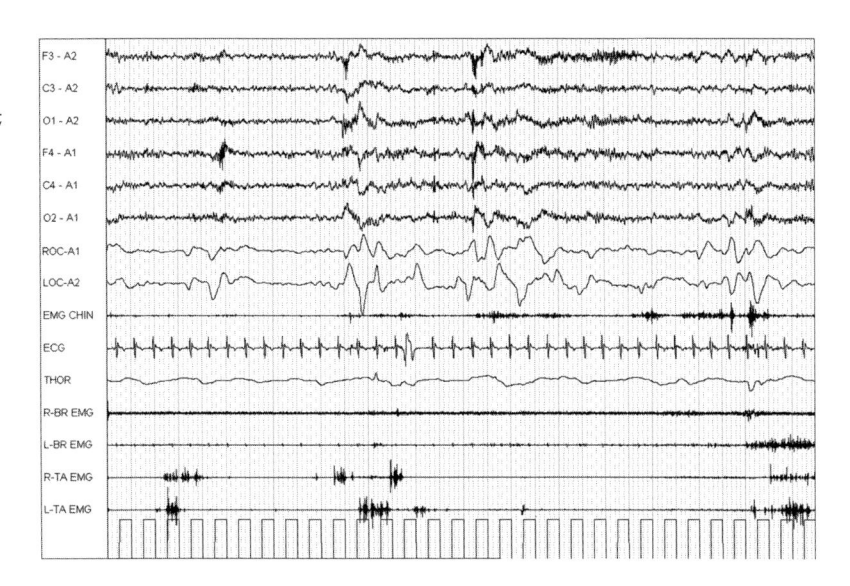

Figure 14.4 RBD in a patient investigated by extended EEG montages.

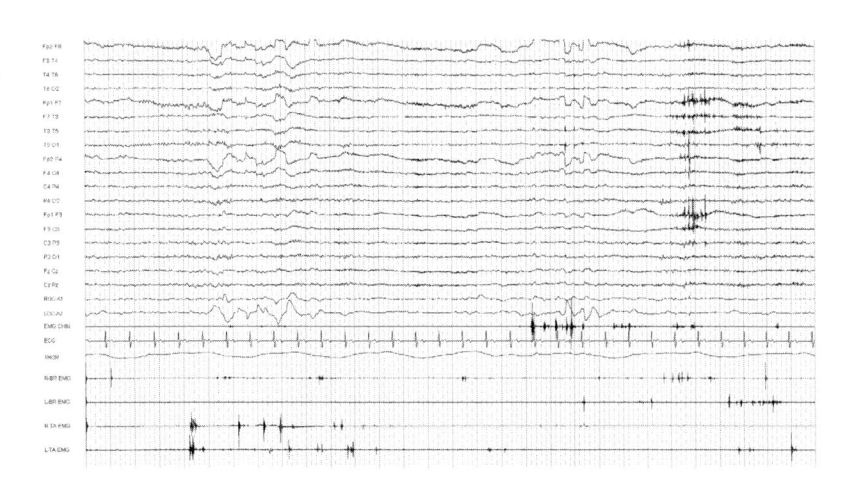

might become valuable investigations in the comprehensive work up of RBD.

PET and SPECT studies have shown decreased presynaptic dopamine transporter binding in the nigrostriatal system in subjects with idiopathic RBD. However, the ultimate neurobiological significance of this alteration, with regard to the possible subsequent development of PD or parkinsonisms in these subjects, is unclear. The same applies to abnormalities of visual–constructional function and visual–spatial memory on neuropsychological testing, olfactory alterations, and evidence of EEG slowing on spectral analysis of waking EEG in idiopathic RBD.

Genetics

Very little is known about the role of genetic factors in RBD. Familial patterns of the disorder are rarely encountered and are, in any case, difficult to identify. Since RBD is a late-onset parasomnia, affected subjects are rarely able to report symptoms suggestive of RBD in parents or ancestors. There is no evidence suggesting that prevalence rates of RBD differ in white and black people.

A strong association (significantly higher than in controls) of HLA DQwI with RBD without narcolepsy was reported in a single study of white men [2].

Pathology

In animal models the structures involved in the genesis of RSWA and RBD are fairly well delineated. Lesions of the sublaterodorsal nucleus (in rats) and/or magnocellular reticular formation/subcoeruleus/peri coeruleus nuclei (in cats) are strongly implicated in the genesis of RSWA, while pons lesioning induces enacting behaviors, whose complexity is dependent on the site and size of the lesion, in cats. All in all, experimental animal models of RBD suggest that the neuronal networks whose dysfunction underlies the genesis of RBD are located mainly in the brain stem. By contrast, the critical networks involved in human RBD pathogenesis are yet to be fully identified [28].

In humans, RBD has been associated with several etiologies and abnormalities.

Structural and functional abnormalities – loss of neuroanatomical integrity due to vascular, neoplastic or demyelinating lesions of the pontine tegmentum has been associated with RBD, unilateral lesions being sufficient to induce non-lateralized RBD. Combined functional MRI and SPECT documented reduced blood flow in the pons and frontal regions in RBD. Ictal neuroimaging revealed lesions in the dorsal and right pontine tegmentum, left upper pons, pontine white matter, and pontomesencephalic junction.

Furthermore, RBD, albeit in few cases, has been reported to occur in neurological disorders primarily involving the limbic system, without apparent pontine damage (e.g. limbic encephalitis [43]).

Neurotransmission abnormalities – as mentioned, PET and SPECT studies have shown decreased presynaptic dopamine transporter binding in RBD in the framework of a continuum of striatal presynaptic dopaminergic dysfunction (from subclinical RBD to clinical RBD and PD) [44]. However, it is not known whether these changes are causative or secondary functional adaptations.

GABAergic (clonazepam) and dopaminergic (L-dopa, dopamine agonists) treatments, as well as melatonin, have been reported to improve RBD, whereas tricyclic anti-depressants, SSRIs, and SNRIs may aggravate/induce it; thus, a complex interplay of neurotransmitters is likely to be involved in the genesis of the condition [28].

Neuropathological studies – brainstem-predominant Lewy body disease lesions have been reported in two autopsy studies of idiopathic RBD patients [45,46]. Data on the involvement of nigral degeneration (unlikely) and pontine cholinergic neuron depletion (possible) in RBD genesis are inconsistent.

The association of RBD with neurodegenerative disorders, in particular synucleinopathies, fits in with Braak's proposed neuropathological staging system for PD, which describes a temporal sequence of synuclein deposition from the medulla to more rostral structures [47]. Indeed, according to this model, dysfunction of the pons (stage 2) predates parkinsonism and cognitive dysfunction. However, variable inter-individual vulnerability of brainstem nuclei can be postulated, since RBD is not a universal finding in extrapyramidal disorders, and stable cases (in which the progression of the degeneration is hypothesized to stop at stage 2) do exist.

Physiopathogenesis

Consensus is lacking as regards the physiopathogenesis of RBD in humans. Most of the data indicate that brainstem networks play a fundamental role in the genesis of RBD motor manifestations, and it has been speculated that motor dyscontrol might in turn influence the oneiric component, thereby making RBD, as a whole, a brainstem-related phenomenon [2,28]. In fact, it has been proposed that the aggressive dream-related behavior displayed in RBD could be motor activity triggered by motor pontine dyscontrol, in accordance with the hypothesis that propioception/esteroception afferents of moving limbs are processed by the sleeping brain and interpreted as dangerous experience according to the "activation-synthesis" model of dream generation by Hobson and McCarley [48].

However, movements and expressed emotions, including pleasant ones, vary widely during RBD episodes, and a simple dysfunction of the pontine nuclei does not appear to be an adequate explanation for all the features that are observed.

The wide range of observed movements includes primitive and more complex (gestures, actions) ones [49]. While the gross, jerky, sometimes apparently archaic movements, including rhythmic movements, of the whole body or of one of its parts, probably arise from activation of the central pattern generators in the brainstem-spinal cord [29], the more complex, elaborate movements (pointing, gesturing, punching, etc.) may originate from the motor cortex, with activation of other brain areas giving rise to patterns of varying complexity [49,50]. To date, there is no evidence that focal cortical stimulations can give rise to RBD episodes, although electrical stimulation of the cingulate gyrus triggers movements similar to those commonly seen in RBD episodes.

We recently advanced the more complex, but highly speculative, hypothesis that the dreaming experience activates the complex visuo-motor loop that includes the mirror neurons; this would lead the dreamer to mimic and thus reproduce ("enact") the actions unfolding before him in his dream (usually frightening dreams in the case of patients affected by RBD) [49]. The presence of RSWA would allow the movements (i.e. "the enactment") to occur.

Management

To date, no randomized, double-blinded, prospective, placebo-controlled study has been conducted to test the efficacy and tolerability of pharmacological treatment of RBD. Effective and satisfactory in most idiopathic and symptomatic cases (up to 90%), pharmacological therapy of RBD consists of low doses, at bedtime, of clonazepam [2,28,51], which can, however, produce excessive sedation in the elderly and a worsening of sleep-disordered breathing. Melatonin may be beneficial as an adjunctive treatment, making it possible to reduce clonazepam doses [51].

Anecdotal reports and uncontrolled, retrospective studies of small patient series suggest that levodopa and pramipexole (D3 agonist) reduce RBD manifestations. Recently a prospective clinical and PSG study of the efficacy of pramipexole in controlling RBD manifestations in 11 consecutive patients failed to demonstrate any significant positive effect [52].

As yet, there is no adequate evidence of the potential efficacy of benzodiazepines other than clonazepam (triazolam, alprazolam), acetylcholinesterase inhibitors (donepezil, galantamine) or neuroleptics (clozapine, quetiapine) in reducing the frequency and severity of RBD manifestations.

Conclusions and future directions

The formal identification of RBD in 1986 widened the spectrum of differential diagnosis in nocturnal sudden-onset motor behavioral episodes, offering a fascinating interpretation of sleep disorders as symptoms potentially heralding neurodegenerative diseases and further expanding our notion of "the state of being".

The development of several lines of clinical and basic research may uncover the true neurobiological meaning and importance of RBD. General population prevalence and incidence rates of RBD, defined according to standardized criteria, are still awaited, as is the identification of risk factors (environmental, genetic) for RBD and for the development of neurodegenerative diseases in subjects affected by RBD. Existing and new therapeutic options should be tested in multicenter clinical trials. In particular, there is a need to identify new drugs that may be submitted to the relevant public health authorities for approval. The impact of RBD on the quality of life of patients and their families also needs to be explored so that appropriate help can be offered.

References

1. Schenck CH, Bundlie SR, Ettinger MG, Mahowald MW. Chronic behavioral disorders of human REM sleep: A new category of parasomnia. *Sleep* 1986; **9**: 293–308.
2. Schenck CH, Mahowald MW. REM sleep behavior disorder: Clinical, developmental, and neuroscience

perspectives 16 years after its formal identification in SLEEP. *Sleep* 2002; **25**: 120–38.

3. American Academy of Sleep Medicine. *The International Classification of Sleep Disorders: Diagnostic and Coding Manual*, 2nd ed. Westchester, IL: American Academy of Sleep Medicine, 2005.

4. Iber C, Ancoli-Israel S, Chesson A, Quan SF for the American Academy of Sleep Medicine. *The AASM Manual for the Scoring of Sleep and Associated Events: Rules, Terminology and Technical Specifications*, 1st ed. Westchester, IL: American Academy of Sleep Medicine, 2007.

5. Chiu HF, Wing YK, Lam LC, *et al.* Sleep-related injury in the elderly – An epidemiological study in Hong Kong. *Sleep* 2000; **23**: 513–17.

6. Ohayon MM, Caulet M, Priest RG. Violent behavior during sleep. *J Clin Psychiatry* 1997; **58**: 369–76.

7. Fantini ML, Corona A, Clerici S, Ferini-Strambi L. Aggressive dream content without daytime aggressiveness in REM sleep behavior disorder. *Neurology* 2005; **65**: 1010–15.

8. Iranzo A, Santamaría J, Rye DB, *et al.* Characteristics of idiopathic REM sleep behavior disorder and that associated with MSA and PD. *Neurology* 2005; **65**: 247–52.

9. Lapierre O, Montplaisir J. Polysomnographic features of REM sleep behavior disorder: Development of a scoring method. *Neurology* 1992; **42**: 1371–4.

10. Consens FB, Chervin RD, Koeppe RA, *et al.* Validation of a polysomnographic score for REM sleep behavior disorder. *Sleep* 2005; **28**: 993–7.

11. Ferri R, Franceschini C, Zucconi M, *et al.* Searching for a marker of REM sleep behavior disorder: Submentalis muscle EMG amplitude analysis during sleep in patients with narcolepsy/cataplexy. *Sleep* 2008; **31**: 1409–17.

12. Schenck CH, Boyd JL, Mahowald MW. A parasomnia overlap disorder involving sleepwalking, sleep terrors, and REM sleep behavior disorder in 33 polysomnographically confirmed cases. *Sleep* 1997; **20**: 972–8.

13. Mahowald MW, Schenck CH. Insights from studying human sleep disorders. *Nature* 2005; **437**: 1279–85.

14. Lugaresi E, Tobler I, Gambetti P, Montagna P. The pathophysiology of fatal familial insomnia. *Brain Pathol* 1998; **8**: 521–6.

15. Vetrugno R, Alessandria M, D'Angelo R, *et al.* Status dissociatus evolving from REM sleep behavior disorder in multiple system atrophy. *Sleep Med* 2009; **10**: 247–52.

16. Iranzo A, Santamaría J. Severe obstructive sleep apnea/hypopnea mimicking REM sleep behavior disorder. *Sleep* 2005; **28**: 203–06.

17. Nightingale S, Orgill JC, Ebrahim IO, *et al.* The association between narcolepsy and REM behavior disorder (RBD). *Sleep Med* 2005; **6**: 253.

18. Mattarozzi K, Bellucci C, Campi C, *et al.* Clinical, behavioural and polysomnographic correlates of cataplexy in patients with narcolepsy/cataplexy. *Sleep Med* 2008; **9**: 425–33.

19. Bonakis A, Howard RS, Ebrahim IO, *et al.* REM sleep behaviour disorder (RBD) and its associations in young patients. *Sleep Med* 2009; **10**: 641–5.

20. Nevsimalova S, Prihodova I, Kemlink D, *et al.* REM behavior disorder (RBD) can be one of the first symptoms of childhood narcolepsy. *Sleep Med* 2007; **8**: 784–6.

21. Husain AM, Miller PP, Carwile ST. REM sleep behavior disorder: Potential relationship to post-traumatic stress disorder. *J Clin Neurophysiol* 2001; **18**: 148–57.

22. Postuma RB, Gagnon JF, Vendette M, *et al.* REM sleep behaviour disorder in Parkinson's disease is associated with specific motor features. *J Neurol Neurosurg Psychiatry* 2008; **79**: 1117–21.

23. Gagnon JF, Postuma RB, Mazza S, *et al.* Rapid-eye-movement sleep behaviour disorder and neurodegenerative diseases. *Lancet Neurol* 2006; **5**: 424–32.

24. Schenck CH, Bundlie SR, Mahowald MW. REM behavior disorder (RBD): Delayed emergence of parkinsonism and/or dementia in 65% of older men initially diagnosed with idiopathic RBD, and analysis of the minimum and maximum tonic and/or phasic electromyographic abnormalities found during REM sleep. *Sleep* 2003; **26**: A318.

25. Plazzi G, Corsini R, Provini F, *et al.* REM sleep behavior disorders in multiple system atrophy. *Neurology* 1997; **48**: 1094–7.

26. Iranzo A, Molinuevo JL, Santamaria J, *et al.* Rapid-eye-movement sleep behaviour disorder as an early marker for a neurodegenerative disorder: A descriptive study. *Lancet Neurol* 2006; **5**: 572–7.

27. Postuma RB, Gagnon JF, Vendette M, *et al.* Quantifying the risk of neurodegenerative disease in idiopathic REM sleep behavior disorder. *Neurology* 2009; **72**: 1296–300.

28. Boeve BF, Silber MH, Saper CB, *et al.* Pathophysiology of REM sleep behaviour disorder and relevance to neurodegenerative disease. *Brain* 2007; **130**: 2770–88.

29. Manni R, Terzaghi M. Rhythmic movements in idiopathic REM sleep behavior disorder. *Mov Disord* 2007; **22**: 1797–800.

30. Bazil CW. Nocturnal seizures. *Semin Neurol* 2004; **24**: 293–300.

31. Derry CP, Dvey M, Johns M, et al. Distinguishing sleep disorders from seizures: Diagnosing bumps in the night. *Arch Neurol* 2006; **63**: 705–09.

32. Manni R, Terzaghi M, Repetto A. The FLEP scale in diagnosing nocturnal frontal lobe epilepsy, NREM and REM parasomnias: Data from a tertiary sleep and epilepsy unit. *Epilepsia* 2008; **49**: 1581–5.

33. Manni R, Terzaghi M, Zambrelli E. REM sleep behavior disorder and epileptic phenomena: Clinical aspects of the comorbidity. *Epilepsia* 2006; **47**: 78–81.

34. Manni R, Terzaghi M. REM behavior disorder associated with epileptic seizures. *Neurology* 2005; **64**: 883–4.

35. Bornemann MA, Mahowald MW, Schenck CH. Parasomnias: Clinical features and forensic implications. *Chest* 2006; **130**: 605–10.

36. Schenck CH, Hurwitz TD, Mahowald MW. Symposium: Normal and abnormal REM sleep regulation: REM sleep behaviour disorder: An update on a series of 96 patients and a review of the world literature. *J Sleep Res* 1993; **2**: 224–31.

37. Vendette M, Gagnon JF, Décary A, et al. REM sleep behavior disorder predicts cognitive impairment in Parkinson disease without dementia. *Neurology* 2007; **69**: 1843–9.

38. Postuma RB, Lang AE, Massicotte-Marquez J, Montplaisir J. Potential early markers of Parkinson disease in idiopathic REM sleep behaviour disorder. *Lancet Neurol* 2006; **5**: 552–3.

39. Ferini-Strambi L, Di Gioia MR, Castronovo V, et al. Neuropsychological assessment in idiopathic REM sleep behavior disorder (RBD): Does the idiopathic form of RBD really exist? *Neurology* 2004; **62**: 41–5.

40. Gjerstad MD, Boeve B, Wentzel-Larsen T, et al. Occurrence and clinical correlates of REM sleep behaviour disorder in patients with Parkinson's disease over time. *J Neurol Neurosurg Psychiatry* 2008; **79**: 387–91.

41. Frauscher B, Gschliesser V, Brandauer E, et al. Video analysis of motor events in REM sleep behavior disorder. *Mov Disord* 2007; **22**: 1464–70.

42. Miyamoto T, Miyamoto M, Inoue Y, et al. Reduced cardiac 123I-MIBG scintigraphy in idiopathic REM sleep behavior disorder. *Neurology* 2006; **67**: 2236–8.

43. Iranzo A, Graus F, Clover L, et al. Rapid eye movement sleep behavior disorder and potassium channel antibody-associated limbic encephalitis. *Ann Neurol* 2006; **59**: 178–81.

44. Eisensehr I, Linke R, Noachtar S, et al. Reduced striatal dopamine transporters in idiopathic rapid eye movement sleep behavior disorder. Comparison with Parkinson's disease and controls. *Brain* 2000; **123**: 1155–60.

45. Uchiyama M, Isse K, Tanaka K, et al. Incidental Lewy body disease in a patient with REM sleep behavior disorder. *Neurology* 1995; **45**: 709–12.

46. Boeve BF, Dickson DW, Olson EJ, et al. Insights into REM sleep behavior disorder pathophysiology in brainstem-predominant Lewy body disease. *Sleep Med* 2007; **8**: 60–4.

47. Braak H, Bohl JR, Muller CM, et al. Stanley Fahn Lecture 2005: The staging procedure for the inclusion body pathology associated with sporadic Parkinson's disease reconsidered. *Mov Disord* 2006; **21**: 2042–51.

48. Hobson JA, McCarley RW. The brain as a dream state generator: An activation-synthesis hypothesis of the dream process. *Am J Psychiatry* 1977; **134**: 1335–48.

49. Manni R, Terzaghi M, Glorioso M. Motor-behavioral episodes in REM sleep behavior disorder and phasic events during REM sleep. *Sleep* 2009; **32**: 241–5.

50. De Cock VC, Vidailhet M, Leu S, et al. Restoration of normal motor control in Parkinson's disease during REM sleep. *Brain* 2007; **130**: 450–6.

51. Gugger JJ, Wagner ML. Rapid eye movement sleep behavior disorder. *Ann Pharmacother* 2007; **41**: 1833–41.

52. Kumru H, Iranzo A, Carrasco E, et al. Lack of effects of pramipexole on REM sleep behavior disorder in Parkinson disease. *Sleep* 2008; **31**: 1418–21.

Section 3 Chapter 15

Parasomnias usually associated with REM sleep

Recurrent isolated sleep paralysis

James Allan Cheyne

Introduction

Sleep paralysis is a transient, conscious state of involuntary immobility occurring in transitions between sleeping and waking and is classified as a parasomnia associated with rapid-eye-movement periods (REMPs) [1]. The paralysis is consistent with atonia observed during normal REMPs produced by hyperpolarization of the spinal motoneurons originating in cholinoceptive neurons in dorsolateral regions of the pontine reticular formation [2]. Although individuals are unable to make gross bodily movements during sleep paralysis, they are often able to open their eyes and are aware of their surroundings, being capable of later providing veridical reports on events that occurred during the episode [2]. During paralysis individuals may attempt to cry out and sometimes produce moaning sounds. Frightening hypnagogic hallucinoid experiences often accompany sleep paralysis.

Terminology

Sleep paralysis has traditionally been linked with narcolepsy as part of the "narcoleptic tetrad," of excessive daytime sleepiness, cataplexy, sleep paralysis and hypnagogic hallucinations. With incidence rates at least an order of magnitude greater than narcolepsy, sleep paralysis is, however, far more common as an isolated phenomenon. Although both sleep paralysis and hypnagogic hallucinations have been reported to be common among narcoleptics, the association of nightmares, dreams, and nocturnal awakenings with narcolepsy all yield effect sizes at least as large as those for sleep paralysis and hypnagogic hallucinations, but considerably smaller than for cataplexy and daytime sleepiness [3]. Hence, the association of both sleep paralysis and hypnagogic hallucinations with narcolepsy is considerably weaker than for daytime sleepiness and cataplexy.

Sleep paralysis without narcolepsy is often referred to as Isolated Sleep Paralysis (ISP). When it occurs repeatedly, the term Recurrent Isolated Sleep Paralysis (RISP) is employed. The present chapter focuses on RISP, although there appear to be few differences between the presentation of sleep paralysis with and without narcolepsy, or related to frequency or chronicity of RISP episodes.

Prevalence

Estimates of RISP prevalence vary dramatically, yielding estimates between 6% and 40% [4–8]. These discrepancies likely result from a combination of differences in sampling methods, populations surveyed – student samples yield especially high prevalence estimates – wording of questions, and RISP criteria. For example, wording of questions sometimes refers only to paralysis and sometimes to paralysis plus one or more hypnagogic experiences. Prevalence studies often include people reporting once-in-a-lifetime occurrences and hence have limited utility for RISP.

There are a few studies reporting the prevalence of differing severity levels (i.e. frequency) of RISP across individuals. It is evident from Table 15.1 that, despite differing scaling between studies, there appears to be a continuum of severity with no clear break between the incidence of "mild" and "severe" cases. Although the estimates vary, the number of people reporting weekly episodes is non-trivial. Moreover, some individuals report multiple episodes in the course of a single night. A further problem in obtaining accurate estimates of frequency is that RISP episodes can occur in bouts, with long intervals of remission rendering it difficult for people to make accurate estimates of frequency.

The Parasomnias and Other Sleep-Related Movement Disorders, ed. M. J. Thorpy and G. Plazzi. Published by Cambridge University Press. © Cambridge University Press 2010.

Table 15.1 Prevalence rates as a function of RISP frequency.

Frequency of sleep paralysis episodes	Percentage reporting
Student survey [4] (N = 870)	
Once/lifetime	8.0
2–5 times/lifetime	12.5
5 or more times/lifetime	8.6
Phone survey [7] (N = 4115)	
<Once/month	4.0
Once/month	1.4
At least once/week	0.8
Web survey [10] (N = 264)	
<5 times	10.2
1–5 times/year	14.0
5–4 times/month	10.2
>Once/week	5.9

SOREMPS and timing

Sleep paralysis is often considered a sleep-onset problem under the assumption that episodes occur at the beginning of the sleep period during a Sleep Onset REM Period (SOREMP) [e.g. 9]. RISP episodes do, however, occur throughout the normal sleep period, although with increased concentration at the beginning and end of sleep [10–12]. However, such findings do not necessarily contradict the hypothesis that sleep paralysis is a sleep onset phenomenon. One needs to distinguish between initial sleep onset at the beginning of the sleep period and sleep onset following brief nocturnal awakenings. If one wakes during a REMP, it is possible, when falling asleep again, to experience a SOREMP. On the other hand, individuals sometimes report episodes when waking from a conventional dream [11,12]. Thus, it is possible that RISP episodes also sometimes occur as a consequence of REM persistence during transitions from sleep to waking.

In a prospective study of the timing of RISP episodes, approximately half were found to occur within 2 h of bedtime [12]. Episode frequency declined sharply after the first hour, with a slight increase 6–7 h later (i.e. as the time of waking approached). Thus, although episodes were found to cluster around bedtimes, many episodes occurred well into the sleep period and may have been sleep offset events. Therefore, it is possible that RISP reflects a more general problem of state transitions. People reporting RISP are more likely than controls to report more early morning awakenings and more disrupted sleep [7]. In addition, RISP may also betray a low tolerance for disrupted sleep–wake rhythms. People reporting a RISP episode following sleep disruption reported greater fatigue and more napping, and performed poorly on a vigilance task during sleep interruption [9].

Although the timing of episode onset varies considerably between individuals, they report similar onset latencies across occasions [12]. Thus, it is reasonable to consider people as having relatively consistent early, middle, or late post-bedtime episodes, potentially reflecting either anomalous circadian patterns or homeostatic effects of consistencies in routines, bedtimes, or activity patterns prior to sleep.

Cognitive arousal and sleep pressure

RISP may indicate poor state boundary control and, like narcolepsy, reveals a dysfunction in the maintenance of, and transitions between, different states [13]. As in narcolepsy, all states appear to be fragmented with high transition frequencies, short durations, and disturbed rhythmicity with resulting disruption of nocturnal sleep–wake periodicity and a failure of inhibition of REM during such transitions. Such failures may be exacerbated or precipitated by conditions of high arousal. Consistent with this hypothesis, an effective procedure for inducing sleep paralysis in the laboratory employs a disrupted wake–sleep schedule, the multiphase sleep–wake schedule (MPS) [9]. The procedure involves waking subjects prior to anticipated REMPs (based on polysomnography), administering cognitively demanding tasks, and then allowing them to attempt to regain sleep. MPS regimes likely produce high levels of cognitive arousal precipitating episodes by increasing the potential for waking during immediate postinterruption REMPs. The MPS schedule provides direct evidence for the REM basis for RISP. The procedure may, however, artifactually create a SOREMP–sleep paralysis association because later REMPs will occur after task-induced arousal levels have diminished. The foregoing may offer clues about why sleep-onset episodes are common. Pre-sleep arousal in more naturalistic situations (e.g. late night work) could merely *contingently* produce sleep-onset RISP episodes. A version of RISP, night shift paralysis, observed among shift workers may be a striking example [14]. Night shift paralysis has been noted to occur rarely before midnight and

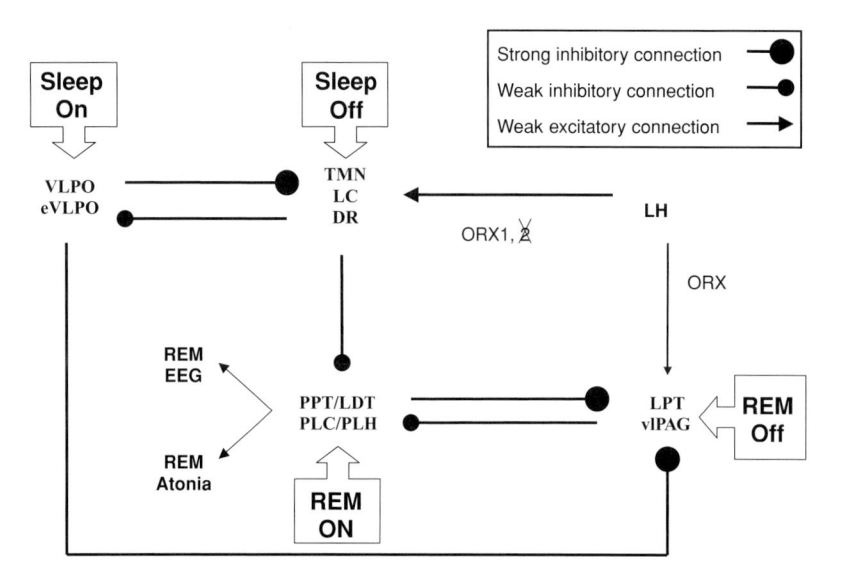

Figure 15.1 Flip-flop model of RISP. Upper-right block represents the sleep–wake flip-flop switch. Lower left block represents REM-on–REM-off flip-flop. Reduction in availability of ORX2 creates imbalance between both sleep–wake and REM–NREM states, leading to increases in sleep and REM pressure as well as an increase in sleep–wake and REM–NREM transitions and their coordination. VLPO, ventrolateral preoptic area; eVLPO, extended VLOP; TMN, tuberomamillary nuclei; LC, locus coeruleus; DR, dorsal raphé; PPT, pedunculopontine tegmentum; LDT, laterodorsal tegmentum; LPT, lateral pontine tegmentum; PLC, perilocus coeruleus; vlPAG, ventrolateral periaqueductal gray; PLH, posterior lateral hypothalamus.

to increase steeply thereafter to peak around 05:00 am. This may occur because sleep onset occurs after individuals have struggled through the night to maintain wakefulness. In addition, chronic cases of RISP may be exacerbated when individuals become frightened or anxious about recurrent episodes when trying to fall asleep during high-frequency bouts, essentially creating a positive feedback loop (see below).

RISP neurophysiology

RISP has typically been thought to reflect anomalies of the functioning of monoaminergic and/or cholinergic neural systems. Specifically, RISP episodes have been hypothesized to be produced by either cholinoceptive or cholinergic sleep-on hyperactivation, or of noradrenergic or serotonergic sleep-off hypoactivation [2]. Recently, however, the role of these neuromodulators in state transitions has been questioned. Although experimental cholinergic stimulation has been reported to promote, and monoamine reuptake inhibition to inhibit REM, lesions of cholinergic and monoaminergic nuclei have limited effects on transitions to and from REM suggesting that the sources of control and disruption of state transitions may lie elsewhere [15].

A possible flip-flop switch anomaly

Recent proposals have suggested physiologically plausible interacting flip-flop switches for regulating sleep–waking and REM–NREM transitions, respectively [15,16]. The flip-flop switch hypothesis is based on evidence of mutual GABAergic inhibition of sleep-on/sleep-off and REM-on/REM-off neural populations. Interaction between two mutually inhibitory centers generates a flip-flop switch. When one side inhibits the other, it thereby disinhibits itself. Such arrangements are stable at only one extreme or the other, avoiding intermediate states and producing abrupt changes between two periodically stable states. In addition, linkage of wake–sleep and REM–NREM switches prevents REM during waking as the sleep-off neural populations also inhibit REM-on neurons during waking (see Figure 15.1). Importantly, however, if one side of a flip-flop switch is chronically weakened, both sides of the mutually inhibitory divide ride closer to their switch point. Relatively small perturbations of the system can then activate the flip-flop switch leading to more frequent transitions and yielding the surprising outcome that, although the system will spend less time in the state governed by the weakened side, there will be many more transitions between states and hence the frequency of episodes of even the compromised state will increase.

Orexin (hypocretin) neurons in the posterior and lateral hypothalamus are active during waking and cease firing during REM with excitatory inputs to both sleep-off and REM-off neural populations in the pons (see Figure 15.1). Lesions of orexin neurons increase sleep and it has been proposed that the loss of orexin-producing neurons selectively weakens the sleep-off side of the sleep-on/sleep-off switch and the REM-off side of the REM-on/REM-off switch through diminished excitatory stimulation of both sleep-off

Chapter 15: Recurrent isolated sleep paralysis

and REM-off neurons, leading to a disruption of both sleep–wake and REM–NREM periodicity [15].

It is well established that loss of orexin neurons is associated with narcolepsy [13]. Thus it has been hypothesized that, in the case of narcolepsy for example, a weakening of the sleep-off state then produces both increased bouts of sleep during day and night waking characteristic of narcolepsy [16]. More modest compromising of orexin availability and/or selective reduction in the number of orexin 2 receptors might have similar but more subtle effects relevant for RISP. Partial loss of orexin 2 receptors, for example, would likely affect REM-off to a greater extent than sleep-off neurons leading to an imbalance in the mutual inhibition of the sleep-on/sleep-off neurons and a somewhat greater imbalance between REM-on and REM-off neurons (see Figure 15.1). This, in turn would have the effect of disrupting the REM–NREM flip-flop switch more than the sleep-on/sleep-off switch, resulting in modest increases of daytime sleepiness and night waking and somewhat weaker inhibition of REM-on during waking. Finally, there would be relatively greater disruption of the REM-on/REM-off switch, potentially permitting REM atonia with or without hypnagogic hallucinations (REM EEG) during sleep–wake transitions.

The nature of RISP hallucinoid experiences

RISP-related hallucinations have been found to fall into three categories or thematic groups labeled intruder, incubus, and vestibular-motor (V-M) experiences [5,17,18]. Intruder hallucinations include a sense of a threatening presence with visual, auditory, and tactile hallucinations, including footsteps, voices, and apparitions. Incubus experiences include feelings of suffocation, pressure or weight on the chest, pain, and thoughts of impending death. Intruder and incubus factors are correlated with one another and with rated fear and, when sufficiently vivid, are interpretable as threat and assault experiences, respectively.

V-M hallucinations constitute a distinct set different from intruder or incubus experiences and include sensations of linear and angular acceleration described as floating, flying, spinning, and falling. Also reported are out-of-body experiences (OBEs), autoscopy (seeing oneself from an external station-point) and fictive motor movements (e.g. illusory walking across the room in an attempt to switch on a light). V-M halluci-

Table 15.2 Major groupings of hallucinations associated with RISP. Percentage of individuals reporting each type of hallucination for a single episode in parentheses. $N = 383$ [18].

Major categories of hallucinations		
Intruder	**Incubus**	**Vestibular-motor**
Sensed presence (58)	**Breathing (47)**	**Vestibular (31)**
Threatening (37)	Smothering (24)	Floating (21)
Watching (42)	Choking (8)	Flying (4)
Visual (43)	**Pressure (53)**	Falling (8)
Human (18)		
Animal (3)	**Death thoughts (37)**	
Auditory (45)		**Out-of-body experiences (22)**
Noise (16)	**Pain (22)**	
Speech (14)		Autoscopy (13)
Human movement (13)		
Environmental (8)		**Illusory motor movements (24)**
Animal sounds (3)		
Tactile (30)		
Grasping (17)		
Touching (10)		
Bedcover movement (13)		

nations are less frightening and, indeed, are somewhat positively correlated with blissful feelings. Percentages of individuals reporting specific experiences are provided in Table 15.2.

The three-factor structure has been replicated in several large studies of subjects varying in age, RISP frequency, and a variety of demographic variables [5,17,18]. It should be noted that the meaningful patterning among the multiple modalities revealed by statistical analyses is not necessarily detected by the experients. Many individuals will report only disconnected and incoherent sensations, although elements within factors still tend to co-occur across individuals and within episodes [18].

Psychophysiology of intruder and incubus experiences

A model of intruder and incubus experiences, based on the structural properties of the experiences and known REM physiology (Figure 15.2, right), focuses

Section 3: REM sleep parasomnias

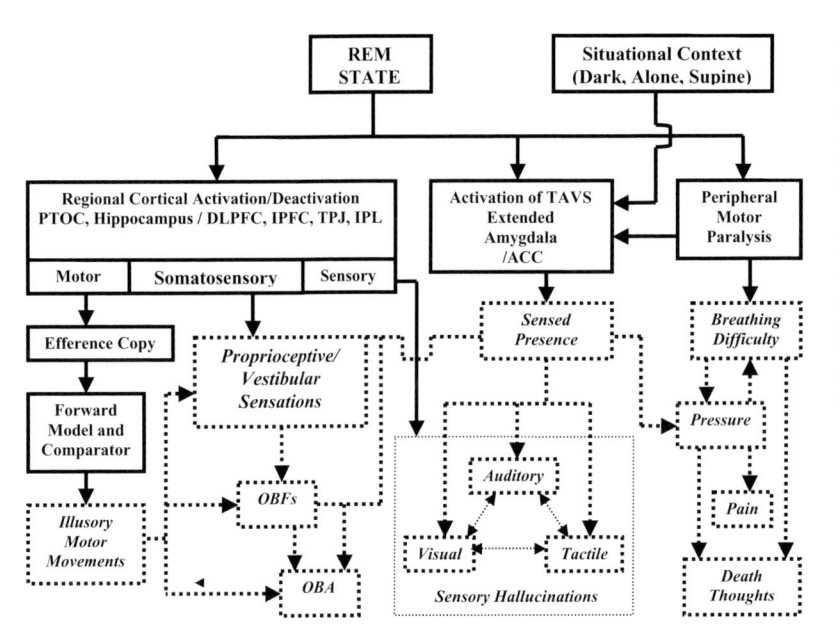

Figure 15.2 Model of sequence of events and major causal pathways for RISP hallucinations: theoretical neural components and connections are represented by solid boxes and arrows. Reported events (labeled in italics) and empirical associations are represented by dashed boxes and arrows. REM, rapid eye movement; PTOC, posterior temporo-occipital cortex; DLPFC, dorso-lateral prefrontal cortex; TPJ, temporo-parietal junction; IPL, inferior parietal lobule; TAVS, threat-activated vigilance system; ACC, anterior cingulate cortex; OBFs, out-of-body feelings; OBA, out-of-body autoscopy.

on REM-induced amygdalar activation hypothesized to be responsible for the sense of a threatening presence. Under this hypothesis such activation biases patterns of cortical activity to generate imagery consistent with perceived threat. Simultaneously, the concurrent paralysis creates breathing difficulties that are often described as feeling like a weight on the chest, and the threatening presence experience causes this weight to be interpreted as a person or creature sitting on the chest (Figure 15.2, lower left).

The foregoing hypotheses are consistent with observations that the amygdala and associated structures show increased activity during REMPs [19]. These structures are implicated in responses to threat and appear to be a substrate for a threat-activated vigilance system (TAVS; Figure 15.2) [20,21]. The TAVS is conjectured to facilitate the acquisition and disambiguation of information regarding incipient threats through lowered sensory thresholds and selective perceptual biases [21]. Not only are TAVS structures enhanced during REM, the prefrontal cortex, an area that modulates and inhibits the amygdala, is deactivated [19,22]. The combination of these features of REM during RISP while conscious, supine, paralyzed, and helpless, usually in the dark, likely amplifies REM-related TAVS activity, increasing the biased vigilance for threats, whether externally perceived or internally REM-generated.

Psychophysiology of vestibular-motor hallucinations

V-M hallucinations likely arise via interactions between subcortical and cortical vestibular centers (Figure 15.2, left). Of particular interest is evidence of compromised parietal functioning during REM periods with the potential of disrupting integration of vestibular, proprioceptive, and tactile sensory information [19]. In addition, pontine vestibular centers are closely associated with REM on–off centers [23]. Brain imaging studies report reduced activity in parietal areas, particularly the temporal–parietal junction (TPJ) during REM, as well as decreased activation of the intralaminar thalamus, which innervates frontal and parietal association areas [19,24]. Moreover, despite a general cerebellar deactivation during REM, the cerebellar vermis, an important component of the vestibular system, shows evidence of increased activity. These findings suggest the possibility that hypoactivation of cortical vestibular areas during RISP episodes may compromise the ability of these areas to integrate conflicting information from multiple cortical sources and enhanced subcortical vestibular activity. These speculations have been reinforced by reports of induced vestibular sensations, including OBEs, by direct electrical subdural stimulation in the region of the TPJ [25].

Figure 15.3 From the neuromatrix to OBEs. The neuromatrix is a distributed neural system processing and integrating bodily processes including vestibular sensations, motor plans and their efference copy, and proprioception. Anomalous bodily-self experiences (in italics) are postulated to arise from disruption of the components of the neuromatrix. Specifically, the model proposes that REM states produce conflicting somatosensory patterns of activation and/or deactivation of areas important for integration of such somatosensory information (e.g. TPJ). OBFs, out-of-body feelings; OBA, out-of-body autoscopy [26].

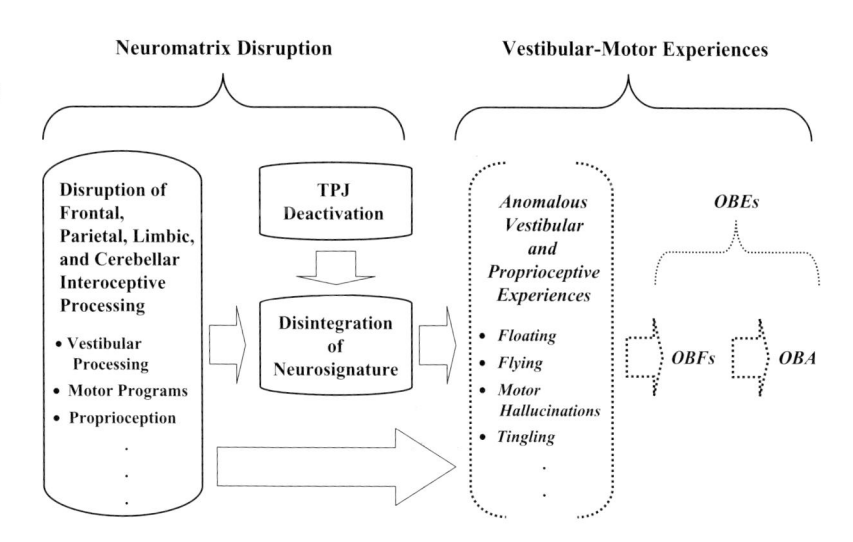

According to the V-M model, disruption of the integrating center of a distributed vestibular neuromatrix affects the processing a variety of bodily senses involving vestibular, motor, and proprioceptive systems. During RISP episodes, in contrast to conventional dreams, vestibular hallucinations are contradicted by conscious awareness that one is stationary and lying in bed. The experience of the bodily self requires coordination among kinesthetic, vestibular, and motor neural systems and resolving of apparently conflicting information. Failure of such integration can lead to anomalous bodily experiences such as those experienced during RISP episodes (Figure 15.3). When sufficiently severe, such disruption could also produce extreme anomalous experiences such as OBEs and autoscopy [26].

Effects of sleeping position

It has long been informally observed that RISP episodes occur most often in the supine position [27]. These informal observations have been corroborated by recent systematic studies [6,11,28,29]. In one investigation of four body positions – supine, prone, and left or right lateral decubitus – more respondents reported episodes to occur in the supine position than all other positions combined [11]. The supine position was also up to four times more common during RISP episodes than when normally falling asleep. RISP experients did not report lying in the supine position more than found for non-RISP samples. The supine position during RISP episodes was, however, reported to be more prevalent at the middle and end of sleep than at the beginning, suggesting that the RISP episodes at the later times might result from position changes associated with brief microarousals during REM consistent with the state fragmentation hypothesis discussed previously.

There are numerous grounds to suspect that restraint is more stressful in the supine than in the prone position [11]. Rats have been found to have a more elevated adrenocortical stress response to supine than prone restraint. Immobilized mental patients find supine restraint less tolerable than in the prone position. Human infants have been reported to be more than twice as likely to roll over from the supine to the prone position as from prone to supine. There is also a curious parallel with tonic immobility (TI), which occurs in certain animals, possibly including humans, in response to predation. TI is a state of profound but temporary paralysis found in many animals as a response to handling, inversion, and especially restraint in the supine position. Finally, both supine position and REM affect the incidence of obstructive sleep apnea (OSA). Reactions to the supine position might well contribute to an increase in microarousals during sleep and associated RISP as well as to distress during episodes.

Age of onset and episode frequency

RISP episodes have a marked bias to adolescent onset, with a mean onset age of 16–17 years of age, although first episodes have been reported across the life span [6,30]. Experiences reported are similar across ages, although earlier reported onset does

Section 3: REM sleep parasomnias

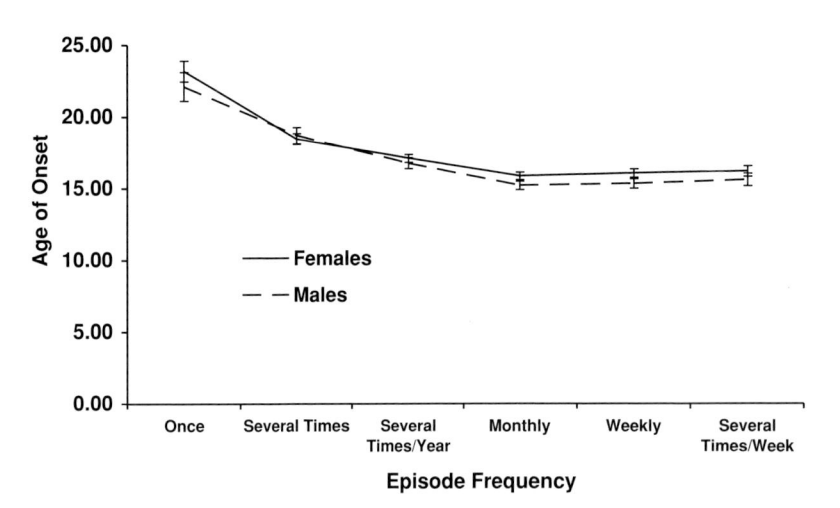

Figure 15.4 Age of onset of sleep paralysis episodes as a function of frequency of episodes and sex. N (female) = 3799. N (male) = 2019 [30].

seem to be associated with more frequent episodes (Figure 15.4). Intruder hallucinations are more common among novice experients than V-M hallucinations, with incubus experiences being intermediate. Subjects reporting frequent episodes reported a greater proportion of V-M hallucinations. Perhaps, as some individuals become more experienced, they begin to focus on less frightening V-M hallucinations. Indeed, a small minority of experients report that they find RISP episodes to be interesting spiritual and psychological experiences and may even make efforts to induce episodes.

Sex differences

Several recent surveys have reported much higher prevalence rates among women than men, although this may vary across cultures [6,26,30]. Females also report more intense incubus experiences and higher levels of fear than do men [11]. The sex ratios reported bear striking similarities to those for traumatic nightmares [31]. The sex differences for both RISP and traumatic nightmares may, of course, reflect reporting biases. Combinations of intruder and incubus hallucinations are occasionally experienced as compelling rape scenarios with sensations of vaginal and anal penetration, especially among women [5]. Otherwise, there appear to be few sex differences in RISP experiences.

Relation to affective disorders

Fear is the overwhelming emotion reported during RISP episodes, much higher than for dreams [17,32].

It has frequently been suggested that the intense fear associated with RISP episodes is evidence of hypersensitivity or hyperreactivity of fear systems [33,34]. In addition, RISP has been associated with a variety of affective disorders including depression [7,8, but see 35], panic disorder [35], PTSD [34], and social anxiety [36]. The association of depression and RISP is of particular interest given that depression is also associated with short REM latencies following sleep onset consistent with the SOREMP hypothesis [37]. The picture is confused, however, by a recent study reporting a robust association between depression and RISP, but also that severely depressed patients had significantly *longer* REM latencies following sleep onset [8].

Depressed patients are particularly likely to report difficulty falling asleep, night waking, and early waking [8]. Indeed, standard measures of depression frequently include items referring to sleep problems. Thus, it is possible that depression might contribute contingently to increased RISP episodes via increased sleep–wake transitions and hence increased opportunities for episodes in susceptible individuals. At least one study, however, reported that depression and sleep disruptions were independently associated with RISP [8]. It is also possible that frequent, intense bouts of RISP episodes might precipitate acute episodes of anxiety and depression [38].

Selective serotonin reuptake inhibitors (SSRI) are commonly used both for affective disorders and for management of RISP (see below). It has been suggested that serotonin deficiency might result in increased sensitivity to threat because of diminished inhibitory modulation of sensory input leading the amygdala to overreact to normally non-threatening stimuli [39]. Intruder and incubus experiences might therefore indicate a predisposition to endogenous amygdalar activation during REM.

People who experience RISP with a sense of threatening presence have been reported to score higher on a measure of social anxiety than those who report RISP without the felt presence [36]. When both groups were compared to a non-RISP group, however, those who reported a presence had social anxiety scores that were virtually identical to the control group. Surprisingly, people who experienced RISP without a sense of presence had lower levels of social anxiety than either of the other two groups. Perhaps the absence of the sense of presence during RISP requires a particularly non-reactive TAVS!

PTSD, nightmares, and RISP

RISP experiences can be found in the early dream literature described as prototypical *nightmares* [40]. During the first half of the twentieth century the term "nightmare" came to be used more generally to refer to any frightening dream. In the latter half of the century researchers tended either to exclude the earlier form of the nightmare in theoretical and empirical research, or to conflate the two. In any case, frightening dreams and RISP episodes can certainly co-occur. PTSD patients have reported that, upon waking from their frequent nightmares, they sometimes find themselves paralyzed. In one case, RISP episodes following traumatic nightmares were reported to be more terrifying than the preceding nightmares [41]. More generally, the role of stress and trauma is frequently implicated in sleep paralysis episodes and, consistent with the TAVS hypothesis, people reporting memories of childhood sexual abuse report frequent and distressing sleep paralysis episodes and more intense intruder and incubus, but not V-M, experiences [42].

Management of RISP

The management of RISP and hypnagogic hallucinations is most often discussed in the context of narcolepsy. Anti-depressants have long been used to treat RISP symptoms in the context of narcolepsy, presumably because of their REM-suppressing effects [2]. A recent update on recommendations for treatment of narcolepsy and parasomnias continued to recommend tricyclic anti-depressants, fluoxetine and sodium oxybate as effective treatments for sleep paralysis and hypnagogic hallucinations, although the committee noted the variable quality of published clinical supporting evidence [43]. The committee concluded that tricyclic anti-depressants, SSRIs, and venlafaxine are effective for management of both sleep paralysis and hypnagogic hallucinations. This recommendation was, however, described as largely based on "committee consensus" and "anecdotal experience of committee members." In addition, a problematic aspect of such medications results from the episodic nature of RISP. Individuals sometimes report that episodes often appear unpredictably and persist over a period of days or weeks, with long intervals of months or years without episodes. Such patterning suggests the use of anti-depressants for only the most chronic and persistent cases. In addition, patients sometimes report bouts of extremely intense RISP episodes when anti-depressant treatment ceases.

Those who experience RISP episodes only in the supine position might obtain relief simply by not sleeping on their backs. Unfortunately, episodes can occur when susceptible individuals inadvertently turn to the supine position when changing position during sleep state transitions to and from REM. The use of a soft obstructing object attached to bed clothes preventing spontaneous turning onto one's back during sleep, such as has been recommended for OSA, might prove beneficial for cases that uniquely or most often experience RISP in the supine position.

As many RISP experients in developed countries have no prior knowledge of sleep paralysis they often make worse-case interpretations of the meaning of the episodes. Over the years many experients have reported to the author concerns that they may find themselves permanently paralyzed in something akin to locked-in syndrome, or that the experiences signal incipient psychosis, stroke, or even demonic possession. Such beliefs likely contribute significantly to RISP-related distress. Participants in our own research spontaneously report experiencing considerable relief on discovering that their experiences have a name, are reasonably well understood scientifically and medically, and do not indicate serious pathology. Hence, sober, factual information about RISP may be one of the most important palliative strategies for very considerable numbers of sufferers (see also [29]).

RISP, a culture-bound syndrome

As noted, people place their experiences within a wide range of both natural and supernatural contexts raising the question: is RISP a culture-bound syndrome [44]? The notion of a culture-bound, or culture-limited, syndrome is beset by a range of conceptual, definitional, and ideological problems [45]. In addition, such "syndromes" are often not syndromes, but local explanations for a diverse set of misfortunes; or not culture-bound, or syndromes, but observable in many cultures [45]. RISP clearly falls within the latter group [44]. The basic RISP syndrome has been reported in numerous cultures under local names and with local explanations and folk treatments. None the less, different cultures, or even the same culture at different times, often focus on specific themes, such as the Popobawa nocturnal rape scenario in Zanzibar [46]. Thus, there appears to be local temporal and spatial modulation of RISP experiences and their interpretation. Folk explanations typically involve spirit possessions, old hag attacks, ghostly visitations, and alien abductions [47]. In these accounts, vampiric demons, spirits, witches or other alien creatures sit on the victim's chest and smother or choke their helpless victims. Thus, people from different ethnic groups or even local subcultures are likely to experience and/or to present their RISP experiences with different emphases colored by local interpretations. RISP episodes may mimic or even precipitate psychopathological behavior and/or lead to health professionals misdiagnosing patient-expressed beliefs, behavior, and resulting anxiety/depression as evidence of psychopathology [38]. Misdiagnosis seems especially likely for people who hold traditional views entailing persecutory demonic agents (conjured up by envious neighbors, in-laws, etc.), the nature of which is likely to increase anxiety and depression following episodes.

Genetic factors in RISP

RISP prevalence rates have frequently been reported to vary across different groups, with higher rates being reported among, for example, African-Americans and Japanese than among people of European descent [6]. Such differences may, however, reflect cultural differences in knowledge and availability of cultural labels. Genetic studies of RISP are very rare. Although RISP does appear to be familial [48], at least one study of familial RISP patients failed to find HLA DR2 or DQ1 association [49].

Concluding observations

RISP severity and distress

Many studies use frequency as the sole index of severity of RISP. However, individual episodes vary substantially in terms of the intensity of the experiences. Frequency and intensity may provide distinctive information about different aspects of RISP. Frequency variations, for example, may potentially reveal something about circadian and homeostatic anomalies. Intensity variations may reflect affective reactivity, relative engagement of subcortical and cortical subareas, and cholinergic and monoaminergic neuromodulators. The clinical significance of RISP will be a function of severity (frequency and intensity of episodes) and patient reactivity, pre-existing levels of anxiety, depression, etc., and other environmental and cultural sources of stress [31]. Each of these different dimensions of RISP experience warrant individual attention in both research and clinical practice.

Four questions, some clues and hypotheses

The questions are four that must always be asked about all biological phenomena [50]. How is a particular organism physically constituted as to be capable of, or prone to, performing particular actions or having particular kinds of sensitivities, whether pathological or normal? What are the situations that give rise to those actions and experiences? What are the developmental constraints on such phenomena? And, ultimately, how did those particular organisms evolve to respond in particular ways to particular situations, with particular developmental constraints?

Currently, the hypothesis of the role of orexin in modifying the functioning of the wake—sleep/REM–NREM flip-flop switches offers a potentially fruitful direction of research directed at the first question. The importance of the cognitive arousal plus sleep pressure hypothesis, relevant to the next two questions, is suggested by several observations: the effectiveness of the multiphase sleep–wake schedule in producing RISP episodes, nightshift paralysis, and RISP episodes following nightmares and dreams. In addition, with regard to the third question, adolescent onset and high rates of RISP in student populations might arise in conjunction with physiological changes, in part, because adolescents are increasingly working late "cramming" for tests, completing assignments, etc. Future laboratory investigations using variations of the MPS should pursue these questions. Finally, with regard to the final question, the pervasive associations with affective disorders and trauma are particularly suggestive, as are the intriguing parallels with tonic immobility. Both suggest engagement of evolved affective strategies closely anatomically and biochemically with REM mechanisms. Exploration of the amygdalar TAVS hypothesis, utilizing the MPS strategy to investigate the effects of induced affective as well as cognitive arousal on RISP episodes and the associated hypnagogic experiences would prove fruitful.

Education

RISP, despite the evidence for its ubiquity, remains a largely unknown phenomenon in Western society among both the general public and health professionals. People are typically at a loss to find terms of reference for RISP experiences. Popular interpretations vary wildly, from demon possession, to stroke, to unspecified neurological or psychiatric illness, potentially leading people to be reluctant to disclose fully and honestly their experiences or, conversely, to describe them in ways that encourage misdiagnosis. Participants in our research frequently express astonishment and relief when learning about RISP, having assumed that their own experiences were unique and indicative of serious underlying pathology. There seems little reason to doubt that broader public and professional education regarding RISP would prevent or reduce distress levels as well as leading people to seek and receive assistance.

References

1. Thorpy MJ. *International Classification of Sleep Disorders: Diagnostic and Coding Manual.* Rochester: American Sleep Disorders Association, 1990.
2. Hishikawa Y, Shimizu T. Physiology of REM sleep cataplexy and sleep paralysis. In Fahn S, Hallett H, Lüders M, *et al.* (Eds), *Advances in Neurology Vol 67.* Philadelphia: Lippencott-Raven, 1995; 245–71.
3. Ohayon MM, Priest RG, Zulley J, *et al.* Prevalence of narcolepsy symptomatology and diagnosis in the European general population. *Neurology* 2002; **58**: 1826–33.
4. Cheyne JA, Newby-Clark IR, Rueffer SD. Sleep paralysis and associated hypnagogic and hypnopompic experiences. *J Sleep Res* 1999; **8**: 313–7.
5. Cheyne JA, Rueffer SD, Newby-Clark IR. Hypnagogic and hypnopompic hallucinations during sleep paralysis: Neurological and cultural construction of the night-mare. *Consc Cogn* 1999; **8**: 319–37.
6. Fukuda K, Ogilvie RD, Chilcott L, *et al.* The prevalence of sleep paralysis among Canadian and Japanese college students. *Dreaming* 1998; **8**: 59–66.
7. Ohayon MM, Zulley J, Guilleminault C, *et al.* Prevalence and pathological associations of sleep paralysis in the general population. *Neurol* 1999; **52**: 1194–200.
8. Szklo-Coxe M, Young T, Finn L, *et al.* Depression: Relationships to sleep paralysis and other sleep disturbances in a community sample. *J Sleep Res* 2007; **16**: 297–312.
9. Takeuchi T, Fukuda, K, Sasaki Y, *et al.* Factors related to the occurrence of isolated sleep paralysis elicited during a multi-phasic sleep–wake schedule. *Sleep* 2002; **25**: 89–96.
10. Buzzi G, Cirignotta F. Isolated sleep paralysis: A web survey. *Sleep Res Online* 2000; **3**: 61–6.
11. Cheyne JA. Situational factors affecting sleep paralysis and associated hallucinations: Position and timing effects. *J Sleep Res* 2002; **11**: 169–77.
12. Girard TA, Cheyne JA. Timing of spontaneous sleep paralysis episodes. *J Sleep Res* 2006; **5**: 222–9.
13. Nishino S, Riehl J, Hong J, *et al.* Is narcolepsy a REM sleep disorder? Analysis of sleep abnormalities in narcoleptic Dobermans. *Neurosci Res* 2000; **38**: 437–46.
14. Folkard S, Condon R, Herbert M. Night shift paralysis. *Experiential* 1983; **40**: 510–2.
15. Lu J, Sherman D, Devor M, *et al.* A putative flip-flop switch for control of REM sleep. *Nature* 2006; **441**: 589–94.
16. Saper CB, Chou TC, Scammell TE. The sleep switch: Hypothalamic control of sleep and wakefulness. *Trends Neurosci* 2001; **24**: 726–31.
17. Cheyne JA. Sleep paralysis and the structure of waking-nightmare hallucinations. *Dreaming* 2003; **13**: 163–79.
18. Cheyne JA, Girard TA. Paranoid delusions and threatening hallucinations: A prospective study of hypnagogic/hypnopompic hallucinations during sleep paralysis. *Conscious Cogn* 2007; **16**: 959–74.
19. Maquet P, Ruby P, Maudoux A, *et al.* Human cognition during REM sleep and the activity profile within frontal and parietal cortices: A reappraisal of functional neuroimaging data. In Laureys S (Ed), *Progress in Brain Research*, Vol. **50**. Amsterdam: Elsevier, 2005; 219–27.
20. LeDoux JE. Emotion circuits in the brain. *Ann Rev Neurosci* 2000; **23**: 153–84.

21. Whalen PJ. Fear, vigilance, and ambiguity: Initial neuroimaging studies of the human amygdale. *Curr Dir Psychol Sci* 1998; **7**: 177–88.

22. Hariri AR, Mattay VS, Tessitori A, *et al*. Neurocortical modulation of the amygdala response to fearful stimuli. *Biol Psychiatr* 2003; **53**: 494–501.

23. Hobson JA, Stickgold R, Pace-Schott EF *et al*. Sleep and vestibular adaptation: Implications for function in microgravity. *J Vestib Res* 1998; **8**: 81–94.

24. Braun AR, Balkin TJ, Wesensten NJ, *et al*. Regional cerebral blood flow throughout the sleep–wake cycle. *Brain* 1997; **120**: 1173–97.

25. Blanke O, Landis T, Spinelli L, *et al*. Out-of-body experience and autoscopy of neurological origin. *Brain* 2004; **127**: 243–58.

26. Cheyne JA, Girard, TA. The body unbound: Vestibular-motor hallucinations and out-of-body experiences. *Cortex* 2009; **45**: 201–15.

27. Jones EM. *On the Nightmare*. London: Hogarth Press, 1931.

28. Cheyne JA, Girard TA. Spatial characteristics of hallucinations associated with sleep paralysis. *Cogn Neuropsychiat* 2004; **9**: 281–300.

29. Dahmen N, Kasten M, Müller, MJ, *et al*. Frequency and dependence on body posture of hallucinations and sleep paralysis in a community sample. *J Sleep Res* 2002; **11**: 179–80.

30. Cheyne JA. Sleep paralysis episode frequency and number, types and structure of associated hallucinations. *J Sleep Res* 2005; **14**: 319–24.

31. Levin R, Nielsen TA. Disturbed dreaming, post-traumatic stress disorder, and affect distress: A review and neurocognitive model. *Psychol Bull* 2007; **133**: 482–528.

32. Parker JD, Blackmore SJ. Comparing the content of sleep paralysis and dream reports. *Dreaming* 2002; **12**: 45–59.

33. Nielsen TA. Felt presence: Paranoid delusion or hallucinatory social imagery? *Conscious Cogn* 2007; **16**: 975–83.

34. Ohayon MM, Shapiro CM. Sleep disturbances and psychiatric disorders associated with posttraumatic stress disorder in the general population. *Compr Psychiat* 2000; **41**: 469–78.

35. Otto MW, Simon NM, Powers M, *et al*. Rates of isolated sleep paralysis in outpatients with anxiety disorders. *J Anx Dis* 2006; **20**: 687–93.

36. Simard V, Nielsen TA. Sleep paralysis-associated sensed presence as a possible manifestation of social anxiety. *Dreaming* 2005; **15**: 245–60.

37. Thase ME, Kupfer DJ, Spiker DG. Electroencephalographic sleep in secondary depression: A revisit. *Biol Psychiatry* 1984; **19**: 805–14.

38. Gangdev P. Relevance of sleep paralysis and hypnic hallucinations to psychiatry. *Austral Psychiat* 2004; **12**: 77–80.

39. Phelps EA. Emotion and cognition: Insights from the study of the human amygdala. *Ann Rev Psychol* 2006; **57**: 27–53.

40. MacNish R. *The Philosophy of Sleep*. New York: Appleton & Co, 1834.

41. Hogben GL, Cornfield RB. Treatment of traumatic war neurosis with phenelzine. *Arch Gen Psychiatry* 1981; **38**: 440–5.

42. Abrams MP, Mulligan AD, Carleton RN, *et al*. Prevalence and correlates of sleep paralysis in adults reporting childhood sexual abuse. *J Anx Dis* 2008; **22**: 1535–41.

43. Morgenthaler TI, Kapur VK, Brown T. Practice parameters for the treatment of narcolepsy and other hypersomnias of central origin: An American Academy of Sleep Medicine Report. *Sleep* 2007; **30**: 1705–11.

44. Hinton DC, Hufford DJ, Kirmayer LJ. Culture and sleep paralysis (Editorial). *Transcult Psychiat* 2005; **42**: 5–10.

45. Simons RC, Hughes CC (Eds), *The Culture-bound Syndromes: Folk Illnesses of Psychiatric and Anthropological Interest*. New York: Spectrum, 1985.

46. Walsh M. The politicization of Popobawa: Changing explanations of collective panic in Zanzibar. *J Hum* 2009; **1**: 23–33.

47. Hufford DJ. *The Terror that Comes in the Night: An Experience-centered Study of Supernatural Assault Traditions*. Philadelphia: University of Pennsylvania Press, 1982.

48. Roth B, Bruhova S, Berkova L. Familial sleep paralysis. *Schweiz Arch Neurol Neurochir Psychiatr* 1968; **102**; 321–30.

49. Dahlitz M, Parkes JD. Sleep paralysis. *The Lancet* 1993; **341**: 406–07.

50. Tinbergen N. *The Study of Instinct*. Oxford: Oxford University Press, 1951.

Section 3 Chapter 16

Parasomnias usually associated with REM sleep

Nightmare disorder

Michael Schredl

History

Nightmare reports can be found throughout history. It was assumed, for example, that demons or devils send nightmares to torment the more or less innocent sleeper. Sexual connotations like mythical creatures having intercourse with the dreamer ("succubus" for men, "incubus" for women) have been linked to nightmares. The picture of Johann Heinrich Füssli "Der Nachtmahr" painted in 1781 in different versions is widely known; a hairy beast is sitting on the chest of a beautiful woman causing the feeling of being choked.

Having occasional nightmares is a very common experience; 70–90% of young adults have reported that they experienced a nightmare at least once in their lifetime [1,2]. Nightmares are usually defined as frightening dreams that awaken the dreamer (DSM IV, [3]). There are two problems, though, with this restricted definition. First, several researchers have demonstrated that very negatively toned dreams that do not wake the dreamer can be as disturbing as nightmares and have coined the term "bad dreams" for this class of dreams [4]. On average, the emotional intensity of nightmares is higher than that of bad dreams, but there is a large overlap [5]. Whether or not the sleeper is able to judge if the dream emotion was really the cause for waking is still an open question [6]. Some characteristic dreams – like being chased and waking up just before the attacker grabs you, or falling dreams with waking up just before hitting the ground – are obvious examples of dreams that awaken the dreamer, but other dream themes may not be that clear. Secondly, detailed studies revealed that up to 30% of the nightmares are not dominated by fear but rather by other emotions like extreme sadness, anger, disgust, and confusion [7,8].

Clinical findings

Nightmares are REM sleep phenomena and often occur in the second half of the night. Upon awakening, the person is oriented about her/his surroundings and can give a detailed description of the dream action. Typical nightmare contents are being chased (50%), death or injury (20%), death or injury of close persons (15%), and falling (10%) [9].

Nightmares should be differentiated from night terrors, post-traumatic re-enactments, and nocturnal panic attacks. Night terrors are associated with slow-wave sleep and occur predominantly in the first part of the night (see Chapter 13). Post-traumatic re-enactments also differ from nightmares in that they can occur during REM sleep as well as NREM sleep [10]. About 50% of the nightmare topics are related to the trauma, but distressing nightmares without specific reference to the trauma can also occur (see Chapter 8). Nocturnal panic attacks can be triggered by nightmares [11], but the panic has its peak after awakening – usually accompanied by death anxiety and somatic symptoms of a panic attack – whereas the nightmare anxiety decreases upon awakening from the dream (see also Chapter 29).

Nightmare disorder

Relatively similar clinical diagnostic definitions are presented in the *Diagnostic and Statistical Manual of Mental Disorders* (text revision; DSM–IV–TR; [12]) and the *International Classification of Sleep Disorders* (ICSD-2; [13]). Nightmares are characterized by recurrent awakenings from sleep with recall of intensely disturbing dream mentation, usually involving fear or anxiety, but also anger, sadness, disgust, and other dysphoric emotions. On awakening, the person is quickly

---

The Parasomnias and Other Sleep-Related Movement Disorders, ed. M. J. Thorpy and G. Plazzi. Published by Cambridge University Press. © Cambridge University Press 2010.

alert with little to no confusion or disorientation. Since nightmares are experienced by many people, it would be helpful for diagnosing a specific patient to have a more specific definition of "recurrent (ICSD-2)" or "repeated (DSM–IV–TR)". The DSM–IV–TR explicitly states that nightmares must cause clinically significant distress or impairment in social, occupational, or other important areas of function [12]. In clinical practice, cut-offs around the frequency of one nightmare per week or more often have been used [14]. In children, the fear of nightmares at sleep onset is also an indicator for the distress caused by nightmares [15].

Nightmares and sleep quality

Several researchers conceptualize nightmares as a primary sleep disorder [16], because empirical evidence clearly demonstrated low subjective sleep quality in nightmare sufferers, presumably due to direct effects (waking up from the nightmares and prolonged periods of wakefulness after the nightmare before falling asleep again) and indirect effects (prolonged sleep latencies due to fear of falling asleep because of expecting the re-occurrence of nightmares) [17]. Nightmare frequency and the severity of insomnia complaints were associated even if the current stress level – which might cause nightmares as well as insomnia complaints – was statistically controlled [18]. The therapy studies also show that a reduction of nightmare frequency is paralleled by an increase in sleep quality [19].

Nightmare frequency vs. nightmare distress

The hypothesis has been put forward that poorly adjusted persons (i.e. persons with high neuroticism scores) are more distressed by their nightmares – regardless of their frequency – than are well-adapted persons [20]. This would explain the inhomogeneous findings regarding the relationship between waking-life psychopathology and nightmare frequency and the higher correlation coefficients for the relationship between nightmare distress and psychopathology as compared to the correlation coefficients between nightmare frequency and psychopathology [21]. However, most of the studies have relied on the Belicki scale for measuring nightmare distress, a measure that is strongly confounded with nightmare frequency (correlation coefficients ranging from $r = .24$ to $.47$). To avoid this methodological pitfall, a scale measuring the distressing effect of a single nightmare was developed [22]. As expected, neuroticism was correlated with nightmare frequency ($r = .39$), with the sum score of the Belicki scale ($r = .42$), but not with the single nightmare distress scale ($r = .19$) or nightmare intensity ($r = .04$). The hypothesis that persons with high neuroticism scores overestimated nightmare distress can be rejected; nightmare frequency seems to be the most important factor in determining distress attributed to nightmares.

Nightmares and sleep physiology

In the nineteenth century, several scientists held the view that nightmares are caused by a shortage of oxygen [23]. Using a cloth to block mouth and nose, Boerner [24] was able to induce nightmares in three different sleepers. In pilot studies, a few examples of breathing-related nightmares in patients with sleep apnea have been collected. For example, a sleep apnea patient reported having recurrent nightmares of the following type: he was lying in a coffin – dead. He cried: "My god, please don't let me die, I am still young and I have small children," and woke up, gasping for breath [25].

Despite the illustrative examples, a large-scale study [25] with 323 apnea patients did not reveal any correlation between nightmare frequency and respiratory parameters (respiratory disturbance index, nadir of oxygen desaturation). Overall, nightmare frequency was not elevated in comparison to healthy controls, i.e. the oxygen hypothesis is not supported by modern research findings.

Recently, Germain and Nielsen [26] carried out a polysomnographic study in 11 nightmare sufferers. They reported a nightmare frequency of one or more nightmares per week. Although they reported considerable nightmare distress, their sleep parameters recorded in the sleep laboratory did not differ from those of healthy controls, e.g. sleep efficiency (92.1% vs. 92.7%), sleep onset latency (14 min vs. 11 min), REM sleep percentage (21.2% vs. 21.5%). However, they found an elevated index of periodic limb movements during sleep, which might be an effect of intense negative dreaming. The sleep lab findings contrast with the subjective reports of the patients. This might be an effect of the laboratory surroundings: many sleep researchers reported that nightmares occur less often in the lab than at home [27]. This effect might be attributed to the "caring" environment, the presence of a sleep technician, someone interested in their history, listening to them empathically and taking them seriously.

Fisher *et al.* [28] carried out an extensive laboratory study to investigate the physiology of nightmares. They included 38 patients suffering from three or more nightmares per week and studied their sleep over 162 nights. Although they recorded a fair number of night terror attacks ($N = 50$), only 22 nightmares occurred in the laboratory. From the patients' evaluations, those in the lab were very much less severe than at home; supporting a strong effect of the laboratory setting. Only for three very intense nightmares were marked increases in heart rate (an increase of 20 beats per minute), respiration rate (an increase from 18 to 30 breaths per minute) and the number of eye movements measured in the 8 min prior to the awakening. This is in contrast with the dramatic findings (increases in heart rate from 64 to about 120–150 beats per minute) during night terror attacks. Despite the intense anxiety experienced during a nightmare, the autonomic reaction during nightmares is moderate.

Prevalence

The prevalence of children experiencing nightmares once a week or more often is estimated to be about 5% [29]. Although nightmare frequency decreases with age (peak prevalence rates at ages 6–10 years), large-scaled representative studies indicate that about 5% of the adult population suffers from nightmares [30–32]. Nightmare frequency is higher in girls and women [18], and decreases with age [33]. Regarding measurement of nightmare frequency, two methodological issues have to be taken into account. First, studies indicate that parental estimates of nightmare frequency are lower than self-estimates by the children [34], indicating that surveys based on parents' data might underestimate the nightmare disorder prevalence. Second, diary studies found higher frequencies of nightmares compared to retrospective measures, so that questionnaire surveys might also underestimate nightmare prevalence [4].

Etiology

The etiology of nightmares is best described by a disposition–stress model (see Table 16.1). A large-scale, Finnish twin study [35] clearly demonstrated that genetic factors play a role in the etiology of nightmares. Whereas trait anxiety was often not related to nightmare frequency in adults, studies in children and adolescents often found an association between the two [9]. Hartmann [36] has shown that the personality dimension called "thin boundaries" is associated with the occurrence of frequent nightmares. Persons who are creative, sensitive, and who have intense but problematic relationships, unusual sensory perceptions, and extraordinary occupations suffer from nightmares more often. With respect to the Big Five Factor model of personality, the neuroticism factor is strongly related to nightmare frequency [18].

Table 16.1 Etiology of nightmares.

Disposition–stress model
Genetic factors
Trait factors ("thin boundaries", trait anxiety, neuroticism)
State factors (stress)
Trauma
Drugs

Maintaining factors (cognitive avoidance)

Regarding state factors, the presence of current stressors increases nightmare frequency in children, in non-clinical student samples, and also in nightmare sufferers [37–39]. Interestingly, one study [18] was able to demonstrate that the effect of personality (neuroticism, thin boundaries) is mediated by the occurrence of stress, i.e. persons with high neuroticism scores experience more stress in their waking life and, therefore, experience nightmares more often. Experiencing a trauma (war experiences, sexual abuse, natural disasters, and severe accidents) can result in a full-blown post-traumatic stress disorder (PTSD) with nightmares as one of the core symptoms, but often nightmare frequency is elevated even if no other PTSD symptoms are present [10]. Within a detailed nightmare history the question about current medication should always be included, since quite a few compounds, such as anti-depressants (e.g. selective serotonin re-uptake inhibitors, SSRIs), acetylcholinesterase inhibitors or anti-hypertensive medication, can cause nightmares [40]. In their neurocognitive model of nightmare formation, Levin and Nielsen [41] postulated that specific brain areas like the amygdala, the medial prefrontal cortex, the hippocampus, and the anterior cingulated cortex play a role in the interaction of dispositional and situational factors in nightmare pathology. The cognitive model of Spoormaker [42] assumes that specific cues (dream contents) trigger nightmare scripts, resulting in a replay of the nightmare. This model parallels nightmares with other waking anxiety disorders where anxiety symptoms persist if the person avoids an active confrontation with the fear. Statements like "This was only a dream" can be considered as a cognitive strategy to avoid confronting the anxiety experienced within the dream. Most adolescents reported that trying to forget the nightmare is their primary coping strategy with nightmares [15]. So, avoidance behavior maintains the nightmares even if the original trigger (e.g. stressor) is no longer active.

Management

First, the question arises as to when nightmares should be treated (see the section on "Nightmare Disorder"). Similar to other mental disorders, it is important to evaluate whether the person suffers from her/his nightmares in a considerable way. Treatment should be offered to patients reporting negative effects on daytime mood and functioning, worries at sleep onset (fear that a nightmare might occur), and complaints of insomnia. If a cut-off is needed, for example for evaluating nightmares in children, a figure of one or more nightmares per week is reasonable [14].

Whereas drugs, e.g. REM sleep-suppressing tricyclic anti-depressants, are often ineffective in the treatment of nightmares, several different psychological interventions seem more promising. Although several case report series indicate that lucid dreaming is an effective tool in coping with nightmares, the major problem with this technique is the fact that induction of lucid dreams (learning to have dreams where you know you are dreaming) is highly expensive and protracted [43]. Systematic desensitization was shown to be effective in the treatment of nightmares [44]. The most effective and also the simplest treatment strategy was developed by Barry Krakow and coworkers [45] and is called Imagery Rehearsal Treatment (IRT).

Based on the clinical experience of the present author, the reduced form of IRT (as depicted in Table 16.2) includes the basic steps necessary for the effective treatment of nightmares. For most patients, it is helpful to point out the analogy of coping with fear and anxiety in the waking life.

The first step consists of confrontation, which is simply writing down the dream or – for children – the drawing of the most important dream scene. In the second step, the person is asked to imagine a new ending to the dream. Children were asked to draw

Table 16.2 Therapeutic principles.

Step 1: Confrontation
- Record or draw the dream

Step 2: Coping with the situation in the nightmare
- Construct a new dream ending or add something to the drawing that reduces the fear

Step 3: Training for the coping strategy
- About 5–10 min per day over a 2-week period

something into the picture which reduces anxiety. Ideally, the therapist should encourage the person to develop her/his own personal coping strategy for the nightmare situation and refrain from giving suggestions. The coping strategy should include active behavior. Flying away or hiding is often not helpful (because they still reflect avoidance), so one simply asks whether other strategies might be applicable as well. The "solution" of the dream must not be realistic; most psychologists advise not to increase violence (e.g. killing the opponent) while coping with the dream situation. The "new dream" should be written down. The last step consists of internalizing the new strategy by imagining the new ending 5–10 min every day over a 2-week period. The repetition during waking life affects subsequent dreams. Interestingly, the effect of the intervention often generalizes, i.e. nightmares with other topics are affected and include more adequate coping strategies.

For the IRT, several randomized controlled trials (RCT) have been carried out including lifelong nightmare sufferers [19,46,47] and sexually assaulted women with PTSD [48]. A single group session of 2.5 h duration was effective in reducing nightmare frequency in 39 patients with idiopathic nightmares from six nightmares per week to two nightmares per week [18]. In addition, sleep quality and daytime mood improved. To illustrate the procedure, two case reports from the present author's clinical practice will be given.

Case report – adult

A 22-year-old woman consulted our sleep center due to nightmares that started several months ago. The anamnesis also indicates that several night terror attacks also occurred. Two polysomnographic recordings (including breathing parameters and tibialis EMGs) were normal, with the exception of low sleep efficiency (first night: 67.8%, second night: 76.7%). Nightmares and night terrors did not occur in the sleep laboratory. The psychometric measurement of sleep behavior and sleep quality revealed that sleep quality and the feeling of being refreshed in the morning was not reduced, but daytime sleepiness score was elevated (1.6 standard deviations above the mean of a comparable student sample).

In the first session, the patient reported current stressors. A severe conflict in the core family resulted in a complete cessation of her relationship with her parents. The therapeutic principles, including confronting, coping and training, were explained to the patient. It was easy for her to get the idea of this approach because it was similar to the treatment of anxiety. Within the nightmare of the previous night, the patient was in the dressing room of a fitness club. At first her complete family was present. Then, her mother was in the center and verbally attacked and criticized the dreamer. She felt very helpless with respect to the accusations. Answering the question as to how the dream could be altered, she came up with several suggestions: ignoring the mother, active acting like saying something to her mother, expressing her needs. The "new dream" included the active confronting of the mother and the sentence: "I can manage my life myself."

In the second session two weeks later, the patient reported that she trained the new dream ending regularly the first week and that no new nightmares including her mother occurred. Several other negatively toned dreams, however, occurred. One of those was a recurring nightmare: The dreamer stays at the house of her grandmother and is now in the kitchen. At first, the overall emotional tone is positive. Then she senses that there is something threatening outside the house that might come inside and threaten her. The scene changes, the dreamer finds herself in a white room with several fantasy characters (pleasant characters). Two of the characters encourage her to step outside the house and confront the threatening something alone. At this point, she usually wakes up. The awakening from the last dream was at 5 a.m., the anxiety she felt in the dream was still present after waking up. After talking about the different dream elements (e.g. relationship to her grandmother to whom the patient has a positive connection), the patient was again asked to imagine a new ending to the dream. The patient visualized how she goes outside and confronts the unknown threat with the help of the friendly fantasy characters.

In the follow-up session two weeks later, the patient reported a complete cessation of nightmares and that the dreams she recalled incorporated new and active behavior patterns. The dreamer felt more confident in

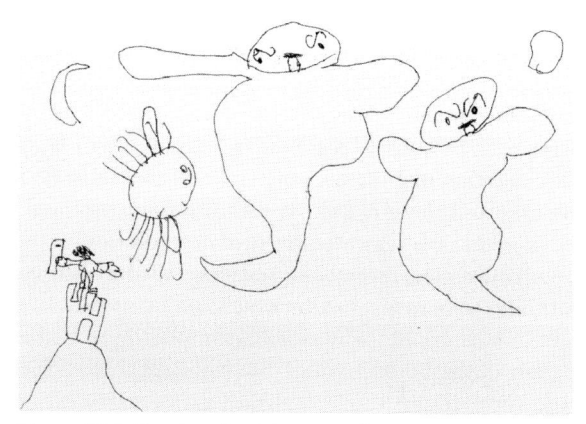

Figure 16.1 Drawing of a nightmare with a coping strategy included.

dealing with other dream characters and was able to express her needs. She also reported a marked lessening of daytime sleepiness. Even though the stressors did not change over the treatment period, the intervention did reduce nightmare frequency by strengthening the dream ego, i.e. the negative effect of the stressor on dreaming and sleep was significantly reduced.

Case report – child

A mother consulted our sleep center because her son (5 years old) had suffered from nightmares every night over the last month. Before that, nightmares rarely occurred. Common topics were ghosts, shadows and horrid monsters. At night, he called out for his mother and needed comfort for up to two hours because after the nightmare he could not fall asleep easily. The mother was not aware of any incidents triggering the period of intense nightmares. The boy was somewhat shy but free from any psychopathology or somatic problems.

After taking the nightmare history, the boy was asked to draw a recent nightmare (see Figure 16.1). The dreamer is walking within a castle (bottom, left) and carrying a book. He is very frightened by the sight of two enormous ghosts (the differences in sizes between the figures and himself clearly reflect the fear involved). After being asked what might help to reduce his anxiety, the boy drew a large spider between him and the ghosts, facing the ghosts and protecting him.

After this first session, the boy continued this work with the help of his mother by drawing several pictures of other nightmares and concentrated on one of them each day for about 10–15 min. Within two weeks, the nightmare frequency was drastically reduced. Although the topics of the dreams did not change very much, the fear around these pictures was almost completely gone. Sleep behavior and quality were back to normal. A follow-up session a year later revealed that nightmares were still rare (about once a month) and the boy did not feel distressed by them. For several nightmares he invented new solutions (one involving a magic spray). He has developed a positive attitude towards his dreams which can be seen in the fact that he occasionally asked his mother to record a dream in the booklet which she had kept during the study period.

Conclusions

Nightmares are common and about 5% of the population report that they suffer from nightmares. Fortunately, nightmares can be treated effectively with a brief and simple intervention method which can be classified as a cognitive technique [45]. The beneficial effect was demonstrated for idiopathic nightmares as well as post-traumatic nightmares, in children and in adults. The basic principle of confronting and coping with the nightmare situation is easily understandable for the patients and can be done without professional assistance and, thus, encourage self-help.

In addition to the clinical aspect, nightmares are also an interesting topic for basic sleep and dream researchers. First, the body–mind interaction can be studied; for example, the correlation between emotional intensity and brain networks related to emotions in waking life [41]. In the near future, techniques such as magnetic resonance imaging will be applicable to sleep if the scanner noise can be reduced markedly. Since nightmares occur quite rarely in the sleep laboratory, large-scaled studies with ambulatory measurement units should be conducted to shed light on the physiological parameters during REM sleep before awakening from a nightmare. The lack of consistent results from sleep laboratory studies might be solely attributable to the "lab effect" (reducing emotional dream intensity due to the "caring" environment). Since nightmares reflect stressors and PTSD-related nightmares often replay the trauma experienced by the person, they might help in elucidating the role of dreams in sleep-related memory consolidation.

References

1. Englehart RJ, Hale DB. Punishment, nail-biting and nightmares: A cross-cultural study. *J Multicultural Counsel Develop* 1990; **18**: 126–32.
2. Schredl M, Morlock M, Bozzer A. Kindheitserinnerungen und Träume Erwachsener. *Z Psychosom Med Psychoanal* 1996; **42**: 25–33.
3. American Psychiatric Association. *Diagnostisches und Statistisches Manual Psychischer Störungen (DSM IV)*. Göttingen: Beltz, 1996.
4. Zadra A, Donderi DC. Nightmares and bad dreams: Their prevalence and relationship to well-being. *J Abnorm Psychol* 2000; **109**: 273–81.
5. Zadra A, Pilon M, Donderi DC. Variety and intensity of emotions in nightmares and bad dreams. *J Nerv Ment Dis* 2006; **194**: 249–54.
6. Blagrove M, Haywood S. Evaluating the awakening criterion in the definition of nightmares: How certain are people in judging whether a nightmare woke them up? *J Sleep Res* 2006; **15**: 117–24.
7. Dunn KK, Barrett D. Characteristics of nightmare subjects and their nightmares. *Psychiatr J University Ottawa* 1988; **13**: 91–3.
8. Rose MW, Perlis ML, Kaszniak AW. Self-reported dream emotion: Nightmares and vivid dreams. *Sleep Res* 1992; **21**: 132.
9. Schredl M, Pallmer R, Montasser A. Anxiety dreams in school-aged children. *Dreaming* 1996; **6**: 265–70.
10. Wittmann L, Schredl M, Kramer M. The role of dreaming in posttraumatic stress disorder. *Psychother Psychosom* 2007; **76**: 25–39.
11. Schredl M, Kronenberg G, Nonell P, et al. Dream recall, nightmare frequency, and nocturnal panic attacks in patients with panic disorder: Their relationship to nocturnal panic attacks. *J Nerv Mental Dis* 2001; **189**: 559–62.
12. American Psychiatric Association. *Diagnostic and Statistical Manual of Mental Disorders (Text Revision)*. Washington, DC: APA, 2000.
13. American Academy of Sleep Medicine. *International Classification of Sleep Disorders, Version 2 (ICSD-2)*. Westchester, IL: AASM, 2005.
14. Schredl M. Behandlung von Alpträumen. *Prax Kinderpsychol Kinderpsychiatr* 2006; **55**: 132–40.
15. Schredl M, Pallmer R. Geschlechtsunterschiede in Angstträumen von SchülerInnen. *Prax Kinderpsychol Kinderpsychiatr* 1998; **47**: 463–76.
16. Spoormaker VI, Schredl M, Van Den Bout J. Nightmares: From anxiety symptom to sleep disorder. *Sleep Med Rev* 2006; **10**: 19–31.

17. Krakow B, Tandberg D, Scriggins L, et al. A controlled comparison of self-rated sleep complaints in acute and chronic nightmare sufferers. *J Nerv Ment Dis* 1995; **183**: 623–7.

18. Schredl M. Effects of state and trait factors on nightmare frequency. *Eur Arch Psychiatr Clin Neurosci* 2003; **253**: 241–7.

19. Krakow B, Kellner R, Pathak D, et al. Imagery rehearsal treatment for chronic nightmares. *Behav Res Ther* 199; **33**: 837–43.

20. Belicki K. Nightmare frequency versus nightmare distress: Relation to psychopathology and cognitive style. *J Abnorm Psychol* 1992; **101**: 592–7.

21. Levin R, Fireman G. Nightmare prevalence, nightmare distress, and self-reported psychological disturbance. *Sleep* 2002; **25**: 205–12.

22. Schredl M, Landgraf C, Zeiler O. Nightmare frequency, nightmare distress and neuroticism. *North Am J Psychol* 2003; **5**: 345–50.

23. Waller J. *Abhandlung über das Alpdrücken, den gestörten Schlaf, erschreckende Träume und nächtliche Erscheinungen*. Frankfurt: Philipp Heinrich Guilhauman, 1824.

24. Boerner J. *Das Alpdrücken: Seine Begründung und Verhütung*. Würzburg: Carl Joseph Becker, 1855.

25. Schredl M, Schmitt J, Hein G, et al. Nightmares and oxygen desaturations: is sleep apnea related to heightened nightmare frequency? *Sleep Breath* 2006; **10**: 203–09.

26. Germain A, Nielsen TA. Sleep pathophysiology in posttraumatic stress disorder and idiopathic nightmare sufferers. *Biol Psychiatr* 2003; **54**: 1092–8.

27. Hartmann E. *The Nightmare: The Psychology and Biology of Terrifying Dreams*. New York: Basic Books, 1984.

28. Fisher C, Byrne J, Edwards A, et al. A psychophysiological study of nightmares. *J Am Psychoanal Assoc* 1970; **18**: 747–82.

29. Schredl M, Pallmer R. Alpträume bei Kindern. *Prax Kinderpsychol Kinderpsychiatr* 1997; **46**: 36–56.

30. Bixler EO, Kales A, Soldatos CR, et al. Prevalence of sleep disorders in the Los Angeles metropolitan area. *Am J Psychiatr* 1979; **136**: 1257–62.

31. Janson C, Gislason T, De Backer W, et al. Prevalence of sleep disturbances among young adults in three European countries. *Sleep* 1995; **18**: 589–97.

32. Ohayon MM, Morselli PL, Guilleminault C. Prevalence of nightmares and their relationship to psychopathology and daytime functioning in insomnia subjects. *Sleep* 1997; **20**: 340–8.

33. Salvio MA, Wood JM, Schwartz J, et al. Nightmare prevalence in the healthy elderly. *Psychol Aging* 1992; **7**: 324–5.

34. Schredl M, Fricke-Oerkermann L, Mitschke A, et al. Factors affecting nightmares in children: parents' vs. children's ratings. *Eur Child Adol Psychiatr* 2009; **18**: 20–5.

35. Hublin C, Kaprio J, Partinen M, et al. Nightmares: Familial aggregation and association with psychiatric disorders in a nationwide twin cohort. *Am J Med Gen (Neuropsychiatr Gen)* 1999; **88**: 329–36.

36. Hartmann E. *Boundaries in the Mind*. New York: Basic Books, 1991.

37. Kales A, Soldatos CR, Caldwell A, et al. Nightmares: Clinical characteristics and personality pattern. *Am J Psychiatr* 1980; **137**: 1197–201.

38. Koulack D, Nesca M. Sleep parameters of type A and B scoring college students. *Percep Motor Skills* 1992; **74**: 723–6.

39. Schredl M, Biemelt J, Roos K, et al. Nightmares and stress in children. *Sleep Hypnosis* 2008; **10**: 19–25.

40. Pagel JF, Helfter P. Drug induced nightmares – An etiology based review. *Hum Psychopharm* 2003; **18**: 59–67.

41. Levin R, Nielson TA. Disturbed dreaming, posttraumatic stress disorder, and affect distress: A review and neurocognitive model. *Psychol Bull* 2007; **133**: 482–528.

42. Spoormaker VI. A cognitive model of recurrent nightmares. *Int J Dream Res* 2008; **1**: 15–22.

43. Spoormaker VI, Van Den Bout J. Lucid dreaming treatment for nightmares: A pilot study. *Psychother Psychosom* 2006; **75**: 389–94.

44. Miller WR, DiPilato M. Treatment of nightmares via relaxation and desensitization: A controlled evaluation. *J Consult Clin Psychiatr* 1983; **51**: 870–7.

45. Krakow B, Zadra A. Clinical management of chronic nightmares: Imagery Rehearsal Therapy. *Behav Sleep Med* 2006; **4**: 45–70.

46. Kellner R, Neidhardt J, Krakow B, et al. Changes in chronic nightmares after one session of desensitization or rehearsal instructions. *Am J Psychiatr* 1992; **149**: 659–63.

47. Neidhardt EJ, Krakow B, Kellner R, et al. The beneficial effects of one treatment session and recording of nightmares on chronic nightmare sufferers. *Sleep* 1992; **15**: 470–3.

48. Krakow B, Hollifield M, Johnston L, et al. Imagery rehearsal therapy for chronic nightmares in sexual assault survivors with posttraumatic stress disorder: A randomized controlled trial. *J Am Med Assoc* 2001; **286**: 537–45.

Section 4: Other parasomnias

Section 4 Chapter 17

Other parasomnias

Sleep-related dissociative disorder

Christina J. Calamaro and Thornton B. A. Mason

History

Dissociation is a separation of discrete mental processes from the mainstream of brain activity with disruptions in integrated functions of consciousness, memory, identity, or perception of the environment [1–4]. Sleep-related dissociative disorders, a variant of dissociative disorders, are parasomnias that can emerge at any point during the sleep period, either at transition from wakefulness to sleep or within several minutes after awakening from stages 1 or 2 non-rapid eye movement (NREM) sleep or REM sleep [5].

In the *Diagnostic Statistical Manual of Mental Disorders* (Fourth Edition, Text Revision; DSM IV-TR) there are five major types of dissociative categories diagnostic for dissociative disorder: dissociative amnesia, dissociative identity disorder, dissociative fugue, depersonalization disorder, and dissociative disorder not otherwise specified (NOS) [1,5]. Of the five categories, three categories of dissociative disorders (dissociative identity disorder, dissociative fugue, and dissociative disorder NOS) have been identified with sleep-related dissociative disorders [5–7]. This chapter will review dissociative disorders and their relationship with parasomnias, as well as demonstrating the link to significant trauma that may precipitate these sleep-related behaviors.

Most sleep-related dissociative disorders have corresponding daytime episodes of disturbed behavior, confusion, and associated amnesia. Additionally, patients with sleep-related dissociative disorder have predisposing or precipitating symptoms associated with traumatic life experiences, including child abuse [3], combat [8], adult interpersonal violence [9], and natural disasters [10]. Accordingly, dissociation is often associated with post-traumatic stress and is considered to be mainly a post-traumatic response [8,11].

Dissociation is a crude and primitive psychological defense initiated because of a failure or inadequacy of one or more mature and adaptive defenses in the face of overwhelming stress. The maladaptive characterization of dissociation comes from the fact that the distressing experience is encapsulated (set apart from typical consciousness) and resists integration with the individual's day-to-day experience. Intense or prolonged trauma may resist psychic integration at a narrative or linguistic level. These experiences may emerge as activity rather than narrative memory when environmental or internal cues prompt them. As such, previous trauma may be re-enacted [12].

Individuals who have experienced a traumatic event are more likely to dissociate than individuals who have not, and individuals who experience more dissociative phenomena are more likely to also experience higher levels of trauma-related distress [13]. It is theorized that dissociative phenomena and subsequent trauma-related distress may relate to fears about death and fears about loss or lack of control above and beyond the occurrence of the traumatic event itself. Such fears about death and loss/lack of control may also help differentiate traumatized individuals who suffer psychologically to varying degrees. This response to trauma and to forms of trauma-related distress may manifest in disrupted sleep and abnormal sleep behaviors [13,14]. A hierarchical model of dissociation by Putnam posits that primary dissociation (e.g. fragmentation, forgetfulness, emotional numbing) co-occurs with several symptom constellations (aggressive behavior, mood swings, substance abuse). These features are considered secondary or tertiary responses to dissociation, where dissociation serves as a mediator. Observable symptoms or risky behaviors may not be prominent until adolescence or early adulthood [15]. In children, many of these symptoms and behaviors are misdiagnosed as attention, learning or conduct problems, or even psychoses.

Clinical findings

Sleep-related dissociative disorders arise out of established wakefulness, but occur in the general setting of sleep (that is, in transition before sleep onset or after an awakening). As noted, most patients with sleep-related dissociative disorders also have daytime dissociative disorders and histories of trauma or abuse. Patients may also have past or current histories of major anxiety and mood disorders, post-traumatic stress disorder (PTSD), suicide attempts, mutilating behaviors, and psychiatric hospitalizations. During nocturnal dissociative episodes, patients can engage in a variety of behaviors that may be elaborate and bizarre, lasting minutes to an hour or longer. The patients may show marked agitation (e.g. screaming or running in a frenzy), with perceived dreaming that is actually a dissociated wakeful memory of past abuse. Other behaviors can include a nocturnal fugue state (where a patient leaves home) or bouts of abnormal eating (binges, consuming uncooked foods) [5].

A patient's clinical features may in turn support a specific dissociative disorder subtype diagnosis that has been associated with sleep-related episodes, specifically dissociative identity disorder, dissociative fugue, or dissociative disorder NOS. For example, the essential feature of dissociative identity disorder is the presence of two or more distinct identities or personality states that recurrently take control of behavior. There is an inability to recall important personal information, the extent of which is too great to be explained by ordinary forgetfulness. The disturbance is not due to the direct physiological effects of a substance or a general medical condition. Individuals with dissociative identity disorder frequently report having experienced severe physical and sexual abuse, especially during childhood [16].

Dissociative fugue involves sudden, unexpected travel away from home or one's customary place of daily activities, with inability to recall some or all of one's past. This is accompanied by confusion about personal identity or even the assumption of a new identity. The disturbance does not occur exclusively during the course of dissociative identity disorder, and is not due to the direct physiological effects of a substance or a general medical condition. Symptoms of dissociative fugue may cause clinically significant distress or impairment in social, occupational, or other important areas of functioning. Onset is usually related to traumatic, stressful, or overwhelming life events. Single episodes are most commonly reported and may last from hours to months [16].

Dissociative disorder NOS has as the predominant feature a dissociative symptom (i.e. a disruption in the usually integrated functions of consciousness, memory, identity, or perception of the environment) that does not meet the criteria for any specific dissociative disorder. Clinical presentation may be similar to dissociative identity disorder, but fails to meet those criteria fully. Examples of dissociative disorder NOS include: (1) presentations in which (a) there are not two or more distinct personality states, or (b) amnesia for important personal information does not occur; (2) derealization unaccompanied by depersonalization in adults; (3) states of dissociation that occur in individuals who have been subjected to periods of prolonged and intense coercive persuasion (e.g. brainwashing, thought reform, or indoctrination while captive); and (4) dissociative trance disorder, in which single or episodic disturbances in the state of consciousness, identity, or memory that are indigenous to particular locations and cultures occur, and involves narrowing of awareness of immediate surroundings or subjectively uncontrolled stereotyped behaviors/movements [16].

Patients with dissociative symptoms are thought to exist along a continuum of severity and can go undiagnosed, obscuring the potential for sleep-related dissociative disorders. Indeed, individuals diagnosed with dissociative disorders occupy the high end of the dissociative continuum [17]. For example, Sar et al. demonstrated that 64% of consecutive psychiatric patients with DSM-III-R borderline personality disorder also had a DSM-IV Axis-I dissociative disorder diagnosis concurrently [18]. For the health care provider, when treating the patient with a diagnosed psychiatric disorder, it is important to be cognizant of the potential for comorbid diagnoses of a dissociative disorder, and additionally the potential presence of a dissociative sleep-related disorder.

Natural history

With any form of sleep-related dissociative disorder, onset can be gradual and sporadic in nature. Females are reported to be affected predominantly, and onset can range from childhood to midlife. The course often remains chronic and severe. Events can occur several times weekly to multiple times nightly [5]. Complications include injuries to the patient and/or bed partner, including ecchymoses, lacerations, fractures, and burns [5].

To illustrate the breadth and range of sleep-related dissociative disorders, different clinical presentations of these disorders are considered next, followed by specific examples.

Dissociative behavior and sleep walking or sleep terrors

While not classified as sleep-related dissociative disorders, arousal parasomnias such as sleepwalking and sleep terrors have been hypothesized by some to be rooted in dissociative behavior; such potential associations are controversial, however. It has been suggested that sleepwalking and sleep terrors are symptomatic of a protective dissociative mechanism that is thought to be mobilized when intolerable impulses, feelings and memories escape within sleep, as a result of the diminished control of mental defense mechanisms [12]. Sleepwalking and sleep terrors are related parasomnias, both characterized by sudden arousals from NREM sleep, particularly deep NREM (slow-wave or N3) sleep, during which the individual may present with a constricted awareness of his/her surroundings. In the case of sleepwalking, this arousal is associated with motor activity, which may be elaborate and purposive. On the other hand, the arousal of sleep terrors manifests as an intense scream accompanied by prominent autonomic discharge, and often motor activity which is more agitated than sleepwalking [16,19]. It is also possible that some nocturnal episodes that resemble sleepwalking or sleep terrors are actually sleep-related dissociative episodes.

It has also been suggested that sleepwalking/sleep terrors are more likely when the patient has a history of major psychological trauma. In a group of 22 adult patients referred to a tertiary sleep disorders service with possible sleepwalking/sleep terrors, six patients reported a history of such trauma [12]. Subjects described sleepwalking/sleep terrors associated with vivid dream-like experiences or behavior related to flight from attack. In this study, when patients with a history of trauma were compared to those without, they were very similar with regard to age of onset, age of referral, sex, and diagnosis (that is sleepwalking or night terrors). The "trauma" group differed from the "no trauma" group with regard to the phenomenology of the parasomnia. Of those who had a history of trauma, 5 out of 6 (83%) reported vivid, dream-like mental content accompanying the event, as compared with 4 out of 16 (25%) of those without a history of trauma ($p = 0.049$ using Fisher's exact test). All the former reported attempting to flee from an attacker, compared with just 25% of the latter ($p = 0.003$, Fisher's exact test). Other themes reported by the "no trauma" group included searching for a lost object, searching for or consuming food, protecting a bed partner, or behavior or vocalization with no clear meaning [12]. Two of the six patients who had experienced a traumatic event described mental content during the sleepwalking/night terrors that was an exact re-experiencing of the original event, as cited in the first case example.

Case presentations: case one

Hartman and colleagues present an example as a case study: a middle-aged, unmarried woman who lived with her elderly parents, presented with complaints of a history of "nightmares" lasting five years in duration [12]. She reported getting up and sleepwalking after 60–90 min of sleep. On a number of occasions she had driven her car several miles in this condition, and had come to full awareness in an isolated place, to the sound of her car alarm some distance away. These events were accompanied by vivid, terrifying, and stereotyped mental content in which she was attempting to fight off a male attacker. This "nightmare" was a re-enactment of an incident which occurred when she was 10 years old. While out walking, she had been abducted, taken to a shed, and raped in a sadistic manner by a man not known to her. He threatened to maim her if she spoke of it, and when she returned home she concealed her internal injuries, and "put it to the back of my mind." She completed school and went on to train as a nurse. She remained heterosexually inactive, and was stable and successful in other respects. She had no psychiatric problems until the onset of her presenting symptom, five years earlier. The onset of these events was precipitated abruptly by the experience of caring for a young girl admitted to her hospital unit, who had also been raped and beaten. This case illustrates the occurrence of later onset sleepwalking/sleep terror-like episodes with fugue features, in the setting of post-traumatic symptoms during wakefulness [12].

The results of the Hartman *et al.* study indicate that scores on the dissociation questionnaire (DIS-Q) were normal, although generally higher in the small "trauma" subgroup [12]. These scores were similar to those characterizing individuals with PTSD. Their "trauma" group also scored particularly highly on the anxiety, phobic, and depression scales of the Crown–Crisp experiential index. In contrast, the "no trauma" group scored more specifically highly on the anxiety scale, along with major trends to high depression and hysteria scale scores. The authors concluded that a history of major psychological trauma existed in only a minority of adult patients presenting with sleepwalking/sleep terrors. In this subgroup, trauma appears to dictate the subsequent content of the attacks. However, the symptoms express themselves within the form of the sleepwalking/sleep terrors rather than as REM sleep-related nightmares. Importantly, the majority of subjects with sleepwalking/sleep terrors and with no history of major psychological trauma show no clinical or DIS-Q evidence of dissociation during wakefulness [12].

Case two

While the age of onset can vary up to middle adulthood, one case of a school-aged child with sleep-related dissociative disorder has been reported [20]. A previously healthy 6-year-old girl was evaluated for bizarre episodes of dramatic regressive behavior. These episodes began two months prior to presentation, and were first noted at home during the daytime, lasting only minutes. Two weeks after onset, the episodes increased in duration up to several hours and began to occur around the time of sleep several nights per week. Prominent features included sudden rolling back of the eyes, crawling on the ground, intermittent facial twitching and infantile speech with guttural noises throughout. Twenty-two days prior to her evaluation, an episode occurred during school hours; the patient's mother was notified of the event and told that the child could not return to school until her condition was stabilized. Social history revealed the patient was living with her mother, maternal uncle and grandmother; she visited her biological father several weekends each month. On one occasion at her father's apartment, the patient reported a hand "came in through the window to grab her". Without further details, her family was unsure if this event actually occurred. There had been no prior concern for developmental delays, although the patient was now failing first grade, and had few friends in first grade. Overnight polysomnography was performed with an expanded EEG montage. After approximately 2 min of stage 1 sleep the patient became combative and later attempted to bite the technician at the bedside (Figure 17.1A–C; Table 17.1). Vocalization throughout the episode consisted primarily of grunting, with minimal words spoken. She placed various objects (remote controls, blanket) in her mouth. In addition, she used polysomnography leads to tie a technician's hands. There was no abnormal EEG correlate during this episode, and specifically no seizure activity. The entire episode lasted 117 min, after which the patient returned to sleep. No further episodes were noted during the polysomnogram (Figure 17.2).

Table 17.1 Polysomnogram results.

Sleep distribution: TST % and total minutes	
Stage 1	12.8/50.5
Stage 2	37.4/147
Stage 3	4.4/17.5
Stage 4	22.9/90
REM	22.5/88.5
Sleep efficiency	70%
PLMI	Within normal limits
AHI	Within normal limits
EEG seizure montage	No seizure activity

ST, total sleep time; PLMI, Periodic Limb Movement Index; AHI, Apnea Hypopnea Index.

The cases described illustrate the potential relationships between sleepwalking/night terror phenomenology and symptoms of dissociative events. The external motor re-enactment of the circumstances of the trauma is suggestive of the repetition seen with PTSD and also seems to be a classical example of the dissociative process as originally described by Pierre Janet [12,21]. In the first case, Hartman *et al.* suggest these dissociative events were confined to the patient's sleeping hours, and she could tolerate her waking distress and depression. In the case of the school-aged child, a range of dissociative phenomena was experienced throughout the day and night, which may have reflected the severity of her deep-seated post-traumatic stress [12,20].

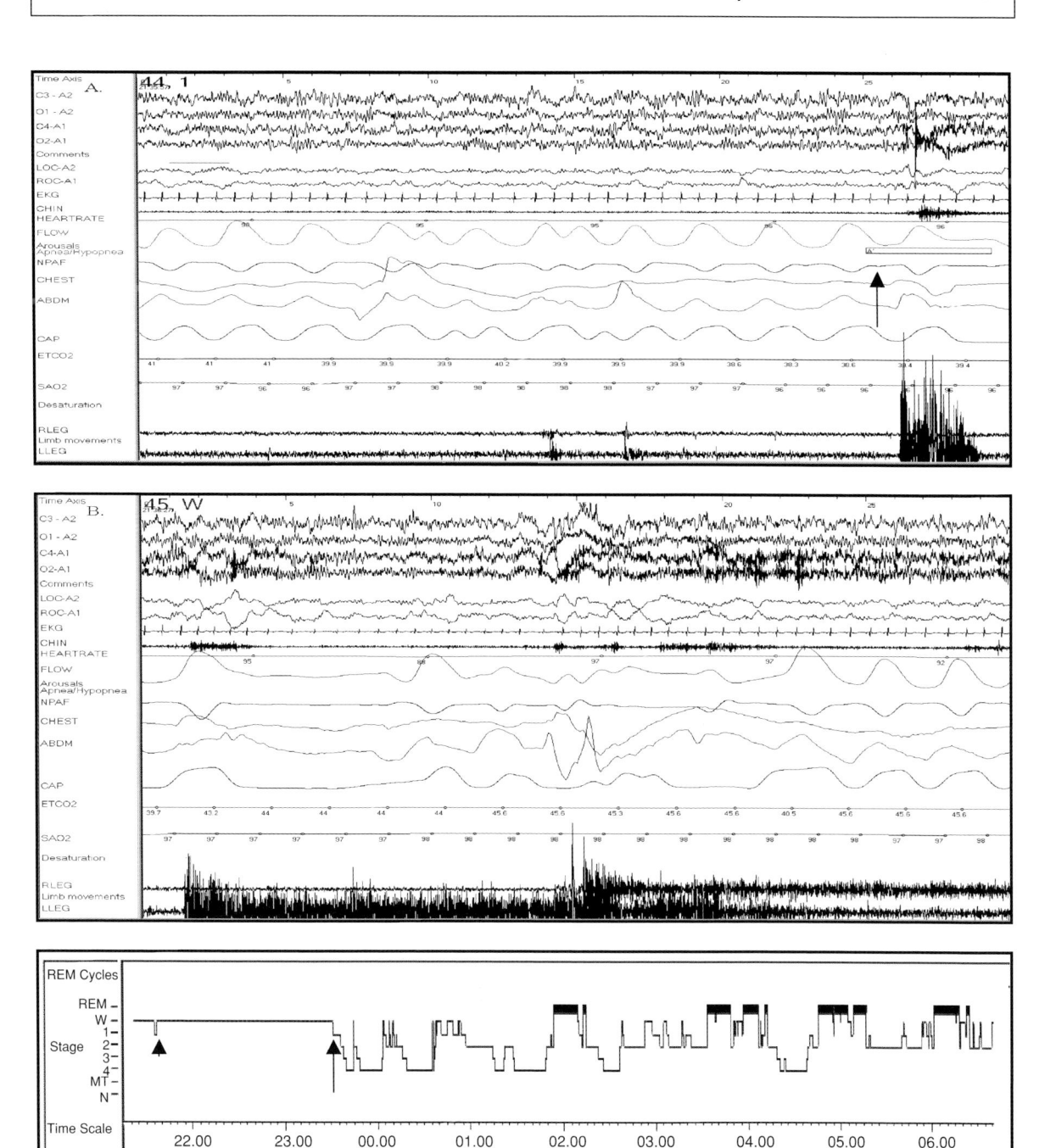

Figure 17.1 The color version of this figure can be found in the color plate section on page XX. Overnight polysomnogram graphics. Both (A) and (B) demonstrate two consecutive 30-s epochs near the beginning of the study (22 min after lights out). (A) The patient is in wake–sleep transition (stage 1 NREM sleep), with fragmented alpha rhythm in the EEG and slow rolling eye movements (horizontal line). In the final 4 s of this epoch, there is an arousal (A1) marked by an increase in EEG frequencies and increased muscle activity (in the chin and leg leads). (B) The patient is awake with prominent leg movement, eye blinking, and increased baseline EEG activity. From this epoch forward, for nearly 2 h the patient remains awake and engaged in the episode described in the text. (C) The hypnogram shows the start (arrowhead) and end of the episode (arrow), as well as normal sleep stage transitions thereafter, with no further episodes of prolonged awakening.

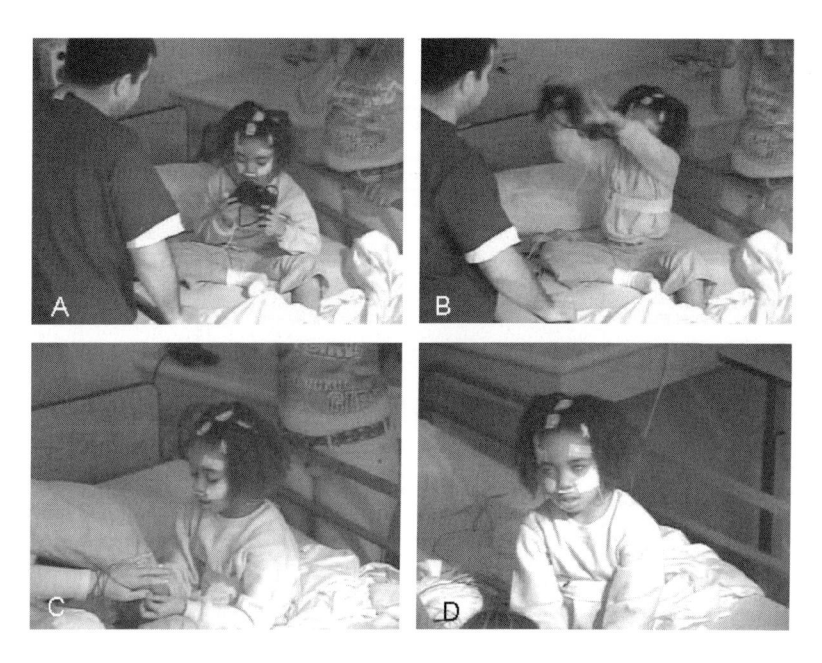

Figure 17.2 Still images from a digital video recording during polysomnography. (A) The patient places a video game control console in her mouth. (B) A few seconds later, she throws the console toward one of the technicians. (C) Using a monitoring lead, the patient ties the hand of a technician at the bedside. (D) In one of several similar episodes, the patient has fleeting upward eye deviation.

Dissociation and sexualized behavior during sleep

Compared to physical abuse, childhood sexual abuse may be related to more deleterious long-term outcomes. Features may include anxiety, depression, somatic and sexualized responses. Also noted are risk-taking behaviors such as self-mutilation, suicidality, physical and sexual aggression, sexual revictimization, and substance abuse. Nevertheless, no unique psychiatric profile or course of adjustment for the sexual abuse survivor has been identified. It remains unclear whether sexual versus physical abuse has the predominant effect on dissociation; however, the majority of studies suggest that severe sexual abuse in childhood has the strongest relationship with dissociation in adults. Variation in how abuse is defined or its severity assessed may contribute to this uncertainty [15].

Foote *et al.* assessed dissociative disorders in a sample of adults recruited from an outpatient psychiatric clinic, in the setting of a largely Hispanic inner city population. Of patients interviewed, 29% received a diagnosis of dissociative disorder, a prevalence much higher than those found in prior assessments of psychiatric inpatients (with an average prevalence of about 12%) [14]. Compared to patients without a dissociative disorder diagnosis, patients with dissociative disorder were significantly more likely to report childhood sexual abuse (74% vs. 29%) and childhood physical abuse (71% vs. 27%). There were no significant differences in this sample for demographic variables such as gender, age, ethnicity, education level, or income. Overall, the entire population had extremely high prevalences of physical abuse (40%) and sexual abuse (42%), which were seen as driving the connection with dissociation [14].

Schenck and colleagues published the first literature review and formal classification of a wide range of documented sleep-related disorders associated with abnormal sexual behaviors and experiences [22]. Sexualized (repetitive behavior without affect) and frankly sexual behaviors (with affect) can emerge with sleep-related dissociative disorders. Sexualized behaviors may be accompanied by defensive behaviors and moaning, and constitute re-enactment of a past abuse situation. The patient may report re-enactment as a "dream," which in fact is recall in an awake state. Nocturnal dissociated states of wakefulness can include thrashing behavior, pelvic thrusting, and animalistic prowling on all four limbs with growling; these represent attempted re-enactments of past abuse scenarios. Return to full contact with reality may be gradual as the patient "wakes up" from the dissociated state [22]. These abnormal sexual behaviors are classified under parasomnias and referred to as "sleepsex" or "sexsomnia" [5,22,23]. Patients with this category of sleep-related dissociative disorder may scream, demonstrate marked agitation, or engage in violent sexual acts [5,24]. Further manifestations may include sexualized or defensive behavior, typically as re-enactments of previous physical or sexual abuse situations [7,22].

Case presentation

Schenck and colleagues report a case of animalistic nocturnal personality involving a 19-year-old male who would prowl around the house on all four limbs while growling for approximately 30–60 min per episode twice weekly while occasionally chewing on a piece of uncooked bacon. A thinly disguised recurrent sexualized "dream" during his nocturnal dissociated states of wakefulness consisted of his being a large jungle cat approaching a female zookeeper who held a piece of raw meat in her hand which he wanted to pounce on and "snatch" from her hand and eat. However, "an invisible force field" prevented him from getting near to her, and he felt "frustrated" by being kept away and not having the raw meat. He would then "wake up" (i.e. snap out of his dissociated wakeful state) and be confused and groggy, and would only gradually re-establish contact with reality [22].

Dissociation and violent sexual behavior during sleep

Violence, during or out of sleep, related to abnormal alertness has been reported in greater detail in the literature over the last decade [23,25]. The absence of full alertness or impairment of brain function due to associated sleep disorders has been considered a legal defense in crimes and homicides [25].

The sleep-related violent behavior described below is associated with parasomnias, occurring as the result of a diathesis, and is precipitated by stressors and mediated by disturbed NREM sleep physiology [23]. A general population survey has indicated that sleep-related violence is much more common than known by physicians. Two percent of the general population report the occurrence of sleep-related violence [26]. Aggressive, harmful behavior during sleep can occur, ranging from harm to the bed partner to harm to self [6,23].

Case presentation

A 33-year-old man with no prior history of violent behavior grabbed his wife during the first third of the night, tore off her clothes, and forced intercourse. She pleaded and defended herself but was unable to "reach" him. The wife reported that he seemed "far away" and appeared "glassy-eyed." Once sexual intercourse occurred, the husband fell asleep. Cries and noises had awakened a teenage child, who called 911, which brought the police. The husband had no memory of or explanation for the behavior. The wife went to the police station the next day, as requested by the police officer at the scene, but then refused to pursue legal proceedings. She believed that her husband had a medical problem, and the couple sought medical help [23].

Differential diagnoses

There are several potential considerations for the differential diagnosis of sleep-related dissociative disorders, including an NREM arousal disorder parasomnia (such as agitated sleepwalking, confusional arousals or sleep terrors), a parasomnia associated with REM sleep (such as REM behavior disorder or nightmares), or nocturnal seizures.

Non-REM arousal parasomnias are part of a continuum that share overlapping features, include sleepwalking, confusional arousals, and sleep terrors. While most arousal parasomnias occur in slow-wave sleep (stages 3 and 4 of NREM sleep), they can also occur in stage 2 NREM sleep [7,27]. Characteristics of these disorders include incomplete transition from slow-wave sleep, automatic behavior, altered perception of the environment and some degree of amnesia for the event. These parasomnias classically occur in the first third of the night, when slow-wave sleep is most prominent. These disorders peak at 8–12 years; although no gender differences are observed, a positive family history is often noted [7,27]. The most effective treatment includes reassurance for parents, with focus on institution of safety measures for the child to prevent injury during these arousals, as well as maintaining routine sleep hygiene and monitoring caffeine intake before bedtime, so that sleep efficiency and duration are not compromised [7,27]. In sleep-related dissociative disorders, there may be no family history of parasomnias (in contrast to sleepwalking and sleep terrors, where a positive family history is often prominent). Moreover, dissociative disorders occur out of wakefulness (for example, in the immediate transition into sleep), rather than from established slow-wave sleep, and often span a duration that would be atypically long for an arousal parasomnia. Sleep-related dissociative disorders often lack the intense autonomic activation seen with sleep terrors, and can match prior descriptions given by others of diurnal events that were clearly unassociated with sleep.

REM behavior disorder is another parasomnia with complex and even violent movement. Patients with REM behavior disorder report dreams that have more action, intensity and violence than typical dreams [7,28]. Because of the loss of normal REM sleep atonia, these intense dreams are in turn acted out. REM behavior disorder tends to have a male predominance, with onset in middle age; this parasomnia often heralds a neurodegenerative condition, such as Parkinson's disease. REM behavior disorder is highly uncommon in children but can occur; as in adult cases, low-dose clonazepam given at bedtime is most effective in eliminating the parasomnia [29].

Epileptic seizures can begin at any age and have protean manifestations. Furthermore, seizures may occur during both wakefulness and sleep, or even exclusively during sleep. Of particular interest is nocturnal frontal lobe epilepsy (NFLE), whose features overlap with arousal parasomnias. NFLE can manifest in three patterns: (1) paroxysmal arousals, which involve abrupt, frequently recurring arousals from sleep with stereotyped movements (elevating the head, sitting, screaming, or looking about as if frightened), and dystonic posture of the limbs often occurs; (2) nocturnal paroxysmal dystonia, where sudden arousals occur with complex, stereotyped, and sometimes bizarre sequences of movements (dystonic or asymmetric tonic postures, cycling movements, kicking, twisting, or rocking of the pelvis); and (3) episodic nocturnal wanderings, where sudden awakenings with abnormal motor features are followed by agitated somnambulism (jumping, twisting, moving aimlessly). All three events will each last from 20 s to 3 min, respectively [30,31]. The mean age of onset for NFLE is 10–12 years, and affected patients usually have a history of normal psychomotor development. Establishing the diagnosis may be difficult, as neuroimaging is usually normal, and ictal or interictal EEG changes may not be present. Anti-convulsants are often effective, especially carbamazepine [7].

There is broad range of sleep-related disorders associated with abnormal sexual experiences and behaviors. Beyond sleep-related dissociative disorders, other considerations include parasomnias with abnormal sexual behaviors – particularly in the setting of confusional arousals and sleep terrors: masturbation, sexual vocalizations or shouting, fondling another person, sexual intercourse, or frank sexual assault. Sexual seizures in sleep may have many of the same manifestations (including vocalizations, masturbation), but also sexual automatisms and ictal orgasm. Moreover, a number of sleep disorders may include abnormal sexual behavior during wakefulness and sleep–wake transitions, such as Klein–Levin syndrome, severe chronic insomnia (with increased libido and compulsive sexual behaviors) and restless legs syndrome (with rhythmic pelvic movements and masturbation) [22].

Investigations

Establishing the diagnosis of sleep-related dissociative disorder can be challenging, as there is no objective test available to prove or disprove a case. Unlike arousal parasomnias such as sleepwalking, confusional arousals, and sleep terrors, there is no association with slow-wave sleep; moreover, patients remain in an EEG state of full wakefulness throughout the episode, rather than displaying an admixture of EEG frequencies denoting combined sleep–wake features as typically seen in arousal parasomnias [7]. Also, the lag time between EEG arousal and the behavior can be important in distinguishing a dissociative episode from an arousal parasomnia, since arousal parasomnias begin almost immediately after an arousal, whereas a sleep-related dissociative episode may lag by 15 s to 1 min. Patients may certainly fall asleep after either type of event. Therefore, if a typical dissociative event occurs during overnight polysomnography, then a diagnosis of a sleep-related dissociative disorder can be supported. On the other hand, a normal polysomnogram does not exclude the diagnosis, and polysomnography is not required. The diagnosis may alternatively be established based on the report of observers, especially when behavior associated with the major sleep period is similar to daytime dissociative behaviors [5].

Several questionnaires have been developed that explore the presence/tendency toward dissociative symptoms. As such, these may be useful in clinical and research evaluations of sleep-related dissociative disorders:

1. The Adolescent Dissociative Experiences Scale is a 30-item self-report measure that was developed as a screening tool for serious post-traumatic and dissociative disorders. Based on the adolescent's self-report of symptoms, each item is rated on a 1–10 scale. Excellent reliability (Cronbach's

alpha = 0.93) has been reported, with a mean score ≥4 indicating significant pathological dissociation [15,32].
2. The Child Dissociative Checklist is a 20-item, observer-completed checklist with a 3-point scale that is used as a clinical screening instrument to assess dissociation based on ratings given by caretakers/adults in close contact with the child. Studies have indicated good internal consistency (alpha = 0.86) and test–retest stability ($r = 0.65$), as well as convergent/discriminate validity [15].
3. The Dissociative Experiences Scale is a widely used 28-item self-report measure; in a meta-analysis, it was found to have an internal reliability (alpha) of 0.93 (16 studies), a test–retest reliability of 0.78–0.93 (6 studies), and a convergent validity (r) of 0.67 (26 studies) [14]. This questionnaire was designed to measure dissociative tendencies in both non-clinical and clinical samples. A variety of experiences are presented to respondents, who are then asked to estimate "what percentage of time this happens to you." Responses are graded on an 11-point scale. Factor analysis has resulted in subscales for amnesia, depersonalization, and absorption [33].
4. The Dissociative Processes Scale assesses normal-range individual differences in dissociative tendencies, with 33 items on a 5-point Likert scale. The three subscales explore detachment (feelings of depersonalization and derealization), obliviousness (mindless and automatic behavior), and imagination (absorption, imaginativeness, and fantasizing) [33,34].

Genetics

There are reports of apparent familial clustering of dissociative disorders, which in turn raises the issue of the relative roles of environmental factors versus genetic contributions. Twin studies have been used in attempts to sort out phenotypic variance due to shared environment (i.e. environmental influences that produce sibling similarity in dissociation), non-shared environment (resulting in sibling differentiation), or genetics (in monozygotic and dizygotic twins). In a study of adolescent twins, Waller and Ross reported that variance in dissociation was due to combinations of environmental factors but not to genetics [17]. Jang *et al.* in their study of adult twins describe very different results, with 48% of the variance in their twin sample being due to additive genetic influences [35]. More recently, Becker-Blease and colleagues examined child and adolescent twins, and also found that hereditability was significant at 59%, with the balance of variance attributed to the non-shared environmental component [36].

Also of interest are two studies that implicate specific genetic polymorphisms in the clinical expression of dissociation. Koenen *et al.* explored polymorphisms in *FKBP5*, which encodes a glucocorticoid receptor-regulating co-chaperone of stress proteins [37]. Two single nucleotide polymorphisms were significantly associated with peri-traumatic dissociation in medically injured children (e.g. from motor vehicle accidents, physical assaults, and falls). This significance persisted after controlling for sex, age, race, and injury severity; the proportion of the variance in dissociation explained by the polymorphisms ranged from 14 to 27% [37]. Savitz *et al.* evaluated the interaction of a catechol-*O*-methyltransferase polymorphism (Val158Met) on perceived dissociation, and found that the Val/Val genotype was associated with increasing levels of dissociation in the setting of higher childhood trauma, while the reverse was true for the Met/Met genotype (that was essentially protective from dissociation) [38].

These intriguing findings clearly need to be replicated in other sample populations before their general significance can be evaluated. Moreover, genetic studies specifically aimed at exploring sleep-related dissociative disorders should be conducted.

Pathology

The pathophysiology of dissociation is still not well established in the literature. What is clear, however, is that exposure to physical, emotional or sexual trauma, typically responsible for daytime dissociative phenomena, also applies to sleep-related dissociative disorders. A current hypothesis proposes that a functional disconnection or loss of integration among specific brain regions potentially forms the neural correlate of a psychogenic dissociation [5]. This alteration, in combination with a baseline susceptibility to physiologic and experiential dissociative phenomena across sleep stages, converges to produce and repeatedly perpetuate sleep dissociative disorders [5]. To date, no neuroimaging or post-mortem findings have been reported in sleep-related dissociative disorders.

Management

Patients with dissociative disorders are challenging to treat and require a comprehensive approach that may include cognitive-behavioral therapy, supportive psychotherapy, or post-traumatic disorder treatment. Because of the potentially sensitive nature of the causes associated with dissociative disorders, a thoughtful and rational approach is required for patients with these diagnoses. As most treatment experience has been based on adults, this is even more important for children and adolescents suffering from dissociative disorders. Since these patients have typically suffered severe physical/sexual trauma, the patients must be encouraged to develop effective coping skills before trying to explore and work through their experiences (stage-oriented therapy). Not until patients are able to tolerate intense affect, control dysfunctional behavior, maintain functioning, and sustain good collaborative relationships can they work through traumatic events. Otherwise, premature abreaction (exposure) would be largely retraumatizing. Because many patients with dissociative disorders have intense interpersonal vulnerability, therapists should use good clinical judgment to guide the therapeutic process. Late stages of treatment involve stabilization of gains and enhanced personal growth, especially in relation to the external world [39].

Early identification paired with therapeutic interventions for dissociative symptoms (such as expressive artwork) appears to be successful for children [7]. Unfortunately, systematic studies of treatment and long-term outcomes for pediatric patients who present with this symptomatology are presently lacking. Despite general population studies citing a 5% prevalence rate of diurnal dissociative symptoms in adults, little is known regarding management of sleep-related dissociative behaviors in children or adults. It is likely best for children to obtain intensive treatment as early as possible, as early identification and therapeutic intervention for dissociative symptoms in children appears to be particularly efficacious. An intensive psychiatric treatment plan, after identification of the diagnosis, appears to be helpful for supporting cognitive/emotional processing of trauma-related material in order to develop greater affect regulation capacities [11].

Psychotropic medications are usually considered adjunctive treatments for dissociative disorders, although objective studies in the literature are sparse. Virtually all classes of psychotropic medications have been used to treat dissociative disorders. Depression and anxiety symptoms have been treated with antidepressants (including fluoxetine, paroxetine, and sertraline). Anxiolytics can also be helpful. For example, 0.25–2 mg clonazepam nightly was prescribed for 33 adult patients with vigorous or dangerous nocturnal behaviors, resulting in rapid and sustained control of sleep injury for almost 6 years [6]. There is a possibility, however, that patients may develop habituation and psychological/physiological addiction, especially among those vulnerable to substance abuse. Atypical anti-psychotics (risperidone, quetiapine) have been used to treat the irritability, insomnia, and chronic anxiety in many dissociative disorder patients [39].

Conclusions

Sleep-related dissociative disorders are a group of fascinating and important parasomnias that can occur from childhood through adult life. The associated behaviors can be elaborate, bizarre, and prolonged; thematic content typically reflects or re-enacts devastatingly traumatic experiences that may be ongoing or that occurred months or years before. These disorders arise as primitive attempts at containing or compartmentalizing the trauma ultimately fail. Accordingly, sleep-related dissociative disorders should be regarded as red flags of psychiatric distress: affected patients require intensive psychiatric management and social services assistance.

In the future, prospective studies of children and adults are needed after trauma/abuse to determine the presence and frequency of dissociative disorders in general and sleep-related dissociative disorders in particular. Advances in portable monitoring, including at-home polysomnography and video recordings, may help to better define the scope of these disorders. These monitoring techniques, in turn, could help document the efficacy of psychiatric treatment modalities such as intensive psychotherapy and medications. There is a clear need for more systematic research of pharmacotherapy in patients with dissociative disorders. Finally, genetic contributions should be explored further, with regard to both individual risk for developing dissociative disorders and to individual differences in treatment response.

References

1. American Psychiatric Association. *Diagnostic and Statistical Manual of Mental Disorders*. Washington, DC: American Psychiatric Association, 2000.
2. Bernstein EM, Putnam FW. Development, reliability and validity of a dissociation scale. *J Nerv Ment Dis* 1986; **174**: 727–35.
3. Chu JA, Dill DI. Dissociative symptoms in relation to childhood physical and sexual abuse. *Am J Psychiatry* 1990; **147**: 882–92.
4. Putnam FW. *Dissociation of Children and Adolescents: A Developmental Perspective*. New York: Guilford Press, 1997.
5. American Academy of Sleep Medicine. *The International Classification of Sleep Disorders – 2*. Westbrook, IL: American Academy of Sleep Medicine, 2005.
6. Schenck C, Milner D, Hurwitz T, Bundlie S, Mahowald M. A polysomnographic and clinical report on sleep-related injury in 100 patients. *Am J Psychiatry* 1989; **146**: 1166–73.
7. Mason TBA, Pack AI. Pediatric parasomnias. *Sleep* 2007; **28**: 140–50.
8. Bremner JD, Southwick S, Brett E, Fontana A, Rosenheck R, Charney DS. Dissociation and posttraumatic stress disorder in Vietnam combat veterans. *Am J Psychiatry* 1992; **149**: 328–32.
9. Feeny N, Zoellner L, Fitzgibbons L, Foa E. Exploring the roles of emotional numbing, depression, and dissociation in PTSD. *J Trauma Stress* 2000; **13**: 489–98.
10. Cardena E, Speigel D. Dissociative reactions to the San Francisco Bay Area Earthquake of 1989. *Am J Psychiatry* 1993; **150**: 474–8.
11. Briere J. Dissociative symptoms and trauma exposure: Specificity, affect dysregulation, and posttraumatic stress. *J Nerv Ment Dis* 2006; **194**: 78–82.
12. Hartman D, Crisp AH, Sedgwick P, Borrow S. Is there a dissociative process in sleepwalking and night terrors? *Postgrad Med J* 2001; **77**: 244–9.
13. Gershuny B, Thayer J. Relations among psychological trauma, dissociative phenomena, and trauma-related distress: A review and integration. *Clin Psychol Rev* 1999; **19**: 631–57.
14. Foote B, Smolin Y, Kaplan M, Legatt M, Lipschitz D. Prevalence of dissociative disorders in psychiatric outpatients. *Am J Psychiatry* 2006; **163**: 623–9.
15. Kisiel CL, Lyons JS. Dissociation as a mediator of psychopathology among sexually abused children and adolescents. *Am J Psychiatry* 2001; **158**: 1034–9.
16. American Psychiatric Association. *Diagnostic and Statistical Manual of Mental Disorders-IV-TR*. Washington, DC: American Psychiatric Association, 2000.
17. Waller NG, Ross C. The prevalence and biometric structure of pathological dissociation in the general population: Taxometric and behavior genetic findings. *J Abnorm Psychiatry* 1997; **106**: 499–510.
18. Sar V, Kundakçi T, Kiziltan E, Bakim B, Bozkurt O. Differentiating dissociative disorders from other diagnostic groups through somatoform dissociation in Turkey. *J Trauma Dissoc* 2000; **1**: 67–80.
19. Broughton RS. Sleep disorders: Disorders of arousal? *Science* 1968; **159**: 1070–80.
20. Calamaro CJ, Mason T. Sleep-related dissociative disorder in a 6-year-old female. *Behav Sleep Med* 2008; **6**: 147–57.
21. Nakatani Y. Dissociative disorders: From Janet to DSM-IV. *Seishin Shinkeigaku Zasshi* 2000; **102**: 1–12.
22. Schenck C, Arnulf I, Mahowald M. Sleep and sex: What can go wrong? A review of the literature on sleep related disorders and abnormal sexual behaviors and experiences. *Sleep* 2007; **30**: 683–702.
23. Guilleminault C, Moscovitch A, Yuen K, Poyares DA. Atypical sexual behavior during sleep. *Psychosom Med* 2002; **64**: 328–36.
24. Agargun M, Kara H, Ozer O, Selvi Y, Kiran U, Kiran S. Nightmares and dissociative experiences: The key role of childhood traumatic events. *Psychiatr Clin Neurosci* 2003; **57**: 139–45.
25. Moldofsky H, Gilbert R, Lue F, MacLean A. Sleep related violence. *Sleep* 1995; **18**: 731–9.
26. Ohayom M, Caulet M, Priest R. Violent behavior and sleep. *J Clin Psychiatry* 1997; **58**: 369–78.
27. Broughton R. NREM arousal parasomnias. In Kryger MR and Decment W (Eds), *Principles and Practice of Sleep Medicine*. 3rd edn. Philadelphia: W.B. Saunders Co., 2000; 693–706.
28. Schenck C, Mahowald M. REM sleep behavior: Clinical, developmental and neuroscience perspectives 16 years after its formal identification in SLEEP. *Sleep* 2002; **25**: 120–38.
29. Sheldon S, Jacobsen J. REM-sleep motor disorder in children. *J Child Neurol* 1998; **13**: 257–60.
30. Provini F, Plazzi G, Tinuper P, Vandi S, Lugaresi E, Montagna P. Nocturnal frontal lobe epilepsy: A clinical and polygraphic overview of 100 consecutive cases. *Brain* 1999; **122**: 1017–31.
31. Provini F, Plazzi G, Lugaresi E. From nocturnal paroxysmal dystonia to nocturnal frontal lobe epilepsy. *Clin Neurophysiol* 2000; **111**: S2–8.

32. Armstrong J, Putnam F, Carlson E, Libero D, Smith S. Development and validation of a measure of adolescent dissociation: The Adolescent Dissociative Experiences Scale. *J Nerv Ment Dis* 1997; **185**: 491–7.

33. Watson D. Dissociations in the night: Individual differences in sleep-related experiences and their relation to dissociation and schizotypy. *J Abnorm Psych* 2001; **110**: 526–35.

34. Farrington A, Waller G, Smerden J, Faupel A. The Adolescent Dissociative Experiences Scale: Psychometric properties and difference in scores across age groups. *J Nerv Ment Dis* 2001; **189**: 722–7.

35. Jang KL, Paris J, Zweig-Frank H, Lively WJ. Twin study of dissociative experience. *J Nerv Ment Dis* 1998; **186**: 345–51.

36. Becker-Blease K, Deater-Deckard K, Eley Freyd J, Stevenson J, Plomin R. A genetic analysis of individual differences in dissociative behaviors in childhood and adolescence. *J Child Psychol Psychiatry* 2004; **45**: 522–32.

37. Koenen KC, Saxe G, Purcell S, *et al*. Polymorphisms in FKBP5 are associated with peritraumatic dissociation in medically injured children. *Mol Psychiatry* 2005; **10**: 1058–9.

38. Savitz J, Van Der Merwe L, Newman T, Solms M, Stein D, Ramesar R. The relationship between child abuse and dissociation: Is it influenced by catechol-*O*-methyltransferase (COMT) activity? *Int J Neuropsychopharmacol* 2008; **11**: 149–61.

39. Chu JA. Treatment of traumatic dissociation. In Vermetten E, Dorahy MJ, Spiegel D (Eds), *Traumatic Dissociation: Neurobiology and Treatment*. Washington, DC: American Psychiatric Publishing, 2007; 333–52.

Section 4 Chapter 18

Other parasomnias

Sleep enuresis

Oliviero Bruni, Luana Novelli, Elena Finotti and Raffaele Ferri

Clinical findings

Sleep enuresis (SE) is characterized by recurrent involuntary voiding of urine during sleep that occurs at least twice a week, for at least 3 consecutive months, in a child who is at least 5 years of age [1]. The International Children's Continence Society (ICCS) has established a clinical terminology about SE and other forms of voiding dysfunction [2]. Incontinence is an uncontrollable leakage of urine after the age of 5 years or after the age of attending bladder control, and enuresis (or night-time incontinence) is defined as an intermittent incontinence only while sleeping.

This condition is considered primary (PNE) if the involuntary discharge of urine during sleep has been present since birth and has not been interrupted by consistently dry periods, while it is considered as secondary (SNE) if the child or adult had previously been dry during sleep for six consecutive months.

In a prospective study [3], the presentation of the patient with PNE or SNE was found to be similar, suggesting that, in the majority of cases, the pathogenesis of SNE is not different from that of PNE.

The clinical severity of the disorder can be defined on the basis of the number of events that occur during a week and, specifically, is defined as: infrequent (1 or 2 events per week), moderate (3–5 events per week) and severe (6 or 7 events per week) [4,5].

When the subject has no associated daytime voiding symptoms (such as frequency, urgency or daytime incontinence), SE is defined as monosymptomatic. But, usually, when a meticulous history is obtained, the majority of children have at least some light daytime void symptoms and their SE is classifiable as non-monosymptomatic.

The exact cause of primary SE is unknown, but a variety of factors contribute to its persistence after the age at which nocturnal continence occurs: (1) disorders of arousal from sleep (children do not wake up to the sensation of a full or contracting bladder), (2) nocturnal polyuria, and (3) reduced nocturnal bladder capacity [6]. Studies attempting to establish bladder problems as the cause of PNE have been contradictory because extensive urodynamic testing has shown that bladder function falls within the normal range in children with nocturnal enuresis [7]; however, one investigation found that while real bladder capacity is identical in children with and without nocturnal enuresis, functional bladder capacity (the volume at which the bladder empties itself) may be lower in those with enuresis [8]. The bladder's capacity increases throughout the first 8 years of life [9,10] and can be influenced by toilet training methods [11]. Analyzing the prevalence of SE according to age of acquisition of daytime urinary continence, Chiozza et al. [12] observed that starting toilet training at later ages may favor the occurrence of SE.

It has been supposed that children with nocturnal enuresis have a delay in achieving the circadian (nocturnal) rise in arginine vasopressin and develop nocturnal polyuria that overwhelms the bladder's ability to retain urine until morning [13].

Congenital, structural, or anatomic abnormalities rarely present solely as enuresis. Secondary sleep enuresis is more commonly associated with organic factors such as: (1) urinary tract infections; (2) malformations of the genitourinary tract; (3) extrinsic pressure on the bladder, such as chronic constipation or encopresis; (4) medical conditions that result in polyuria (diabetes mellitus or insipidus); (5) increased urine production secondary to excessive evening fluid intake, caffeine ingestion, diuretics, or other agents; (6) neurologic diseases, like spinal cord abnormalities with neurogenic bladder; (7) sleep-disordered breathing; and (8) seizure disorders [8]. Also psychosocial stressors, such as parental divorce, neglect, physical or sexual abuse, and institutionalization have been found in children with SNE [14,15].

Natural history

Primary nocturnal enuresis has been considered to be normal and it is present in about 30% of 4-year-olds. The prevalence of SE in 5-year-old children is about 15–20% [16], and at 6 years is approximately 10%, while, in adolescence and adulthood, only 1–3% of subjects still suffer from sleep enuresis [17].

A recent study [18] reported SE prevalence data based on the Avon Longitudinal Study of Parents and Children (ALSPAC), using questionnaires completed by parents: bedwetting at least twice a week fell from 8.4% at 4.5 years to 1.5% at 9.5 years of age. Infrequent bedwetting (less than twice a week) decreased from 21.6% to 8.2% in the same age period.

Approximately 75–90% of patients with SE have PNE, whereas 10-25% have SNE [14]. SE occurs three times more often in boys than in girls under 11 years of age. After 11 years there is no difference between sexes [19]. This sex-related difference is likely to be based on more generalized differential sex-related brain or bladder development [20,21].

The spontaneous remission rate of SE during childhood is 14–19% [22], and this natural history should be kept in mind when counseling parents and children about the prognosis of their child and for the consideration of the effectiveness of various treatments.

Laboratory investigations

In SE, a correct diagnosis is essential for the success of treatment. The assessment of SE is based on history (familial predisposition and emotional standpoint), sleep habits, and also on physical examination.

The use of a sleep diary for 2–4 weeks may be useful for a correct assessment of the habits and the application of sleep hygiene rules. Evening and daytime fluid intake which might contribute to nocturnal polyuria [23] should be assessed carefully. Many parents try fluid restriction and when the wetting does not resolve, they presume this is not an influencing factor, and thus they permit large fluid intake. Many children have a bedtime snack or have dinner a few hours before bedtime; overnight, the kidneys are obliged to process the evening fluid intake and the excess fluid will result in urine production.

Physical examination includes the observation of enlarged adenoids or tonsils, bladder distension, fecal impaction, genital abnormalities, spinal cord anomaly and routine laboratory tests (urinalysis and possibly urine culture). A low specific gravity in the morning sample of urine might indicate decreased nocturnal vasopressin secretion, and urine culture is recommended if the urinalysis is abnormal [24]. Ultrasonography, bladder sphincter electromyography, and cystoscopy might be considered in some children who continue to be enuretic after 3 months of treatment or if organic causes are suspected. Nocturnal polysomnography is rarely required for the diagnosis of SE and should only be performed when other underlying sleep-related disorders (seizures and/or sleep-disordered breathing) need to be ruled out. It is essential to exclude other diseases and, in particular, medical conditions (e.g. diabetes), nocturnal seizures, neurogenic bladder (e.g. spina bifida), urinary infection and sleep-disordered breathing.

Genetics

There is a strong genetic influence in SE; when both parents suffered from SE, almost 75% of their children are expected to be also enuretic, while the prevalence of SE in the offspring of two parents who were not enuretic during childhood is only 15% [25].

Studies of twins with enuresis showed a higher concordance between monozygotic twins than between dizygotic twins. Abe *et al.* [26] showed that the concordance rate for SE in monozygotic twins was 0.9 while in dizygotic twins it was 0.5. Similar results were found by Bakwin [27] who, in a selected twin sample of 338 pairs, reported a pairwise concordance of 0.92 in monozygotic pairs and of 0.53 in dizygotic pairs. Badalian *et al.* [28] included in their study 34 pairs of twins with at least one enuretic co-twin, resulting in a pairwise concordance of 0.67 in monozygotic pairs and of 0.14 in dizygotic pairs. All these studies showed a strikingly higher rate in monozygotic than in dizygotic pairs, indicating important genetic factors for SE.

Segregation analyses of families with SE showed several multiple modes of inheritance, such as autosomal dominant with high penetrance, autosomal dominant with low penetrance, and autosomal recessive [29]. Linkage studies have shown an association of

SE with chromosome 4 (in autosomal-dominant families), and also with chromosomes 8q, 12q, 13q, and 22q [29].

Pathophysiology

Although enuresis is one of the most common and distressing sleep problems of childhood, only a few studies have evaluated sleep structure modifications. Parents often report that their children have a "very deep sleep" and, accordingly, Wolfish et al. [30] showed that enuretic patients are more difficult to awake from sleep than normal controls. This finding was supported by Hunsballe [31], who reported that enuretic children show a significant increase in sleep EEG delta power, as compared to normal controls, suggesting that they have an increased depth of sleep.

Several polysomnographic studies reported that children with SE have normal sleep architecture, in terms of proportion and distribution of sleep stages during the night [32,33]. A more recent study confirmed that sleep architecture of enuretic children does not diverge from that of controls, and the only significant differences are represented by a longer time in bed and an increased number of sleep cycles. The same authors also observed the presence of a short EEG arousal preceding micturition [34].

Nocturnal enuresis has been related also to sleep-disordered breathing and, in particular, to obstructive apnea, in both adults and children [35,36]. This association is supported by the improvement or full resolution of SE after treatment of sleep-disordered breathing (adenotonsillectomy or intranasal corticosteroids) [36,37]. Recently Alexopoulos et al. [38] revealed also that in a community sample of children, those with habitual snoring had primary nocturnal enuresis more often than those without snoring. SE also seems to be more common in children with attention deficit hyperactivity disorder and other learning and behavioral problems [39–41].

Overall, these studies confirm the idea that sleep architecture in children with SE does not differ significantly from that of non-enuretic and polysomnographically normal children and night enuresis episodes can occur in all sleep stages [42].

Management

No treatment is needed for SE before the age of 5 or 6 years, but after this age treatment may be indicated, based on the frequency and severity of the disturbance. Successful enuresis management programs use combined methods of intervention, but begin with an assessment of primary or secondary enuresis. In Figure 18.1 we propose a flow chart for the diagnosis and treatment of enuresis.

It is obvious that in secondary enuresis it is imperative to treat the underlying cause (infection of the urinary tract, sleep breathing disorders, stress and emotional factors, etc.) before starting any other specific treatment. As an example, children with recurrent cystitis benefit from hygiene efforts and might benefit from short courses of preventive antibiotic therapy. Sleep breathing disorders represent another common cause/precipitating factor. It has been reported that habitual snorers have a history of PNE more often than non-habitual snorers (7.4% vs. 2%) [38]; in another study in 1976 children with habitual snoring, 26.9% (531) had enuresis while its prevalence in non-snoring children was 11.6% [43]. Moreover, brain natriuretic peptide levels are elevated in children with enuresis. Therefore, sleep-disordered breathing should always be considered in the differential diagnosis of SE.

Following these observations, several studies showed that different treatments of sleep-disordered breathing, such as adenotonsillectomy [44] or rapid maxillary expansion [45], are able to improve enuresis.

The management of primary enuresis starts from the education of the patient and family including: supportive approach (e.g. do not punish the child for enuresis episodes), evening fluid restriction, and sleep hygiene rules.

The most widely used treatments for primary SE are: motivational therapy, conditioning therapy with enuresis alarm, bladder control training and pharmacological therapy. Psychotherapy, hypnosis or biofeedback may be tried also [46].

Motivational therapy

Motivational therapy for the management of SE involves encouraging the parents and the child, removing the guilt associated with bed-wetting and providing emotional support. The child with SE should be helped to understand the condition and to become conscious that he/she did not cause the problem but do have a role in its resolution. Positive reinforcement for desired behaviors should be established.

Section 4: Other parasomnias

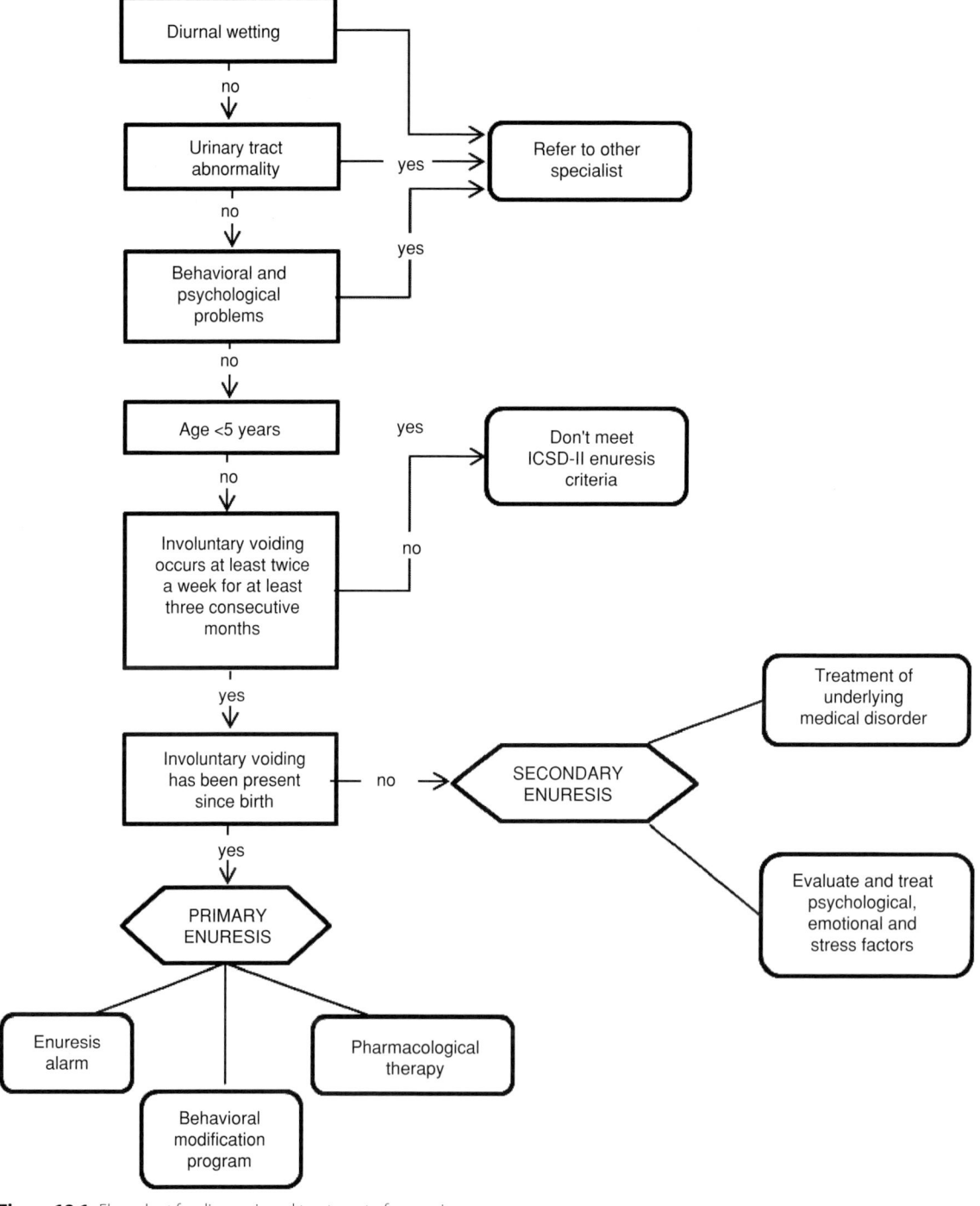

Figure 18.1 Flow chart for diagnosis and treatment of enuresis.

Conditioning therapy

Conditioning therapy in the treatment of primary SE is based on the use of an alarm device. A small electrode is placed near the genitals and when the child voids in bed, the alarm is activated and triggers a considerable noisy sound, inducing a response of waking and, hopefully, inhibiting urination. The precise mechanism of action is unclear [21]. However, approximately one-third of children successfully treated with the alarm therapy develop a pattern of nocturia, probably because the control of sleep arousal is improved, although the children still have a reduced nocturnal bladder capacity [18]. On the other hand, about two-thirds of children that become sleep dry do not have nocturia. One theoretical explanation is that these children might respond to the alarm with an arousal that is too brief to be recalled but sufficient to inhibit a detrusor contraction and prevent the wetting. Another explanation is that the improvement is related to an increase in bladder capacity and does not affect arousal [47].

Sophisticated technology is now available: one system includes a device with an ultrasonic pelvic-skin probe that creates its stimulus (transmitted to the patient) before bladder capacity is reached rather than after, thus before the child voids. All alarm systems work using the same principle of operant conditioning, with the physiologic function of bladder distension, detrusor muscle contraction, and voiding coupled to an external stimulus. The sound is intended to awaken the child, who will then stop voiding and will finish the void in the toilet. At first, the child may have difficulty waking to the sound of the buzzer or bell. A parent should help the child to wake and guide the child to the bathroom to try voiding in the toilet. If the parents are constant and continual, soon the youngster will begin to wake up with the alarm autonomously.

Considering this, it is obvious that alarm therapy requires a cooperative and motivated child and family. Parental involvement is very important when using alarm devices, including recording the child's responses to the device and monitoring his or her progress. Again, the use of a diary and a reward system may help to reinforce the desired behavior.

A Cochrane review of 56 trials [48] concluded that alarm therapy results in dryness in about two-thirds of children, demonstrating that it is the most successful treatment and the only one that resolves enuresis. On the other hand, it should be considered that the effectiveness is higher in children who are motivated and cooperative [49]. It can be used for a minimum of 3 months and can be discontinued after 3–6 months, if successful. Eventually, recurrent enuresis can be retreated. The resolution rate for enuresis with conditioning devices varies from 65 to 80%, with reversion in 10–15% of cases [14].

Alarm systems should not be used when constipation is a comorbid problem.

Bladder control training/behavioral therapy

Bladder training exercises, such as voluntarily suspending voiding midstream during micturition, may help to increase the tone of the bladder neck sphincter. This exercise increases functional bladder capacity, but has been used without consistent evidence; a recent study found that bladder-holding exercises do not increase the overall cure rate in children with monosymptomatic SE and, therefore, the authors did not recommend them [50].

At the beginning of a program of behavioral management, sufficient time must be spent to reassure the child and the parents that nobody should be blamed for SE. Interventions such as randomly waking up the child from sleep to void should be discouraged because they generally cause the persistence of the problem [15].

Children benefit from counseling on good bladder health [51,52], such as to void regularly (at least once every 1.5–2 h) and to avoid urgency and urgency incontinence. Children who prefer to sit while voiding should be counseled on the optimal posture to relax the pelvic floor muscles, to facilitate a good emptying. Boys who stand to void should be counseled to pull their zipper or their pants down such that the penis is not bent during voiding.

The aims of this therapy include achievement of good bladder health, improved arousal, and an optimal circadian rhythm of urine production. A program of about 6 months with personalized calendars of bladder and bowel parameters, a series of realistic goals between appointments, and monthly follow-up to sustain motivation improves the outcome [52]. Behavioral therapy usually increases the success rate of bedwetting alarm systems or pharmacological therapy.

Pharmacological therapy

Pharmacological therapy for the treatment of primary nocturnal enuresis is usually not indicated for children

Section 4: Other parasomnias

Table 18.1 Pharmacological treatment for enuresis.

Drug	Dose	Action	Adverse effects	Success
Desmopressin	0.2-0.6 mg oral or 10-40 µg intranasally at bedtime	Synthetic analog of the anti-diuretic hormone arginine (vasopressin), decreases nocturnal urine production and increases urinary osmolality	Water intoxication	48%
Imipramine	10 mg for 6- to 8-year-old children, and 25 mg for children older than 8 years	Increases urinary osmolality and decreases detrusor tone while increasing sphincter tone	REM sleep suppression (that can lead to daytime sleepiness), constipation	25%
Oxybutynin	5–10 mg at bedtime	Reduces or decreases the bladder's ability to contract	Dry mouth, facial flushing, drowsiness, constipation, dizziness, occasional tremulousness	Poor effect

under 7 years of age. Two approaches to drug therapy can be used: one to increase bladder capacity and the other to reduce the nocturnal polyuria.

Anti-muscarinic medications such as oxybutynin and tolteridine improve bladder capacity [53]. They must be prescribed with close and regular follow-up to screen for constipation and increased post-void residual volume, and adverse events that will worsen SE.

Desmopressin acetate, a synthetic analog of the anti-diuretic hormone arginine (vasopressin), can decrease nocturnal urine production and increase urinary osmolality [13]. The only serious adverse event reported is water intoxication [54,55]. This rare adverse effect can be avoided by reducing the fluid intake when desmopressin is taken; the children should not drink for 2 h prior to going to bed. The risk of water intoxication is greater in patients treated with the nasal spray than with the oral preparation [3], and the indication for SE has recently been removed for the nasal spray formulation.

The desmopressin initial dose is 0.2 mg at bedtime. If not successful within 2 weeks, the dose can be increased to 0.4 mg and, for older children, up to 0.6 mg. It is important to remember that the risk of hyponatremia increases with increasing dose, especially if the child fluid loads in the evening.

Desmopressin is successful in up to 48% of children with SE treated, but it is only a control therapy. A recent randomized, double-blind, placebo-controlled study [56,57] has shown that the new oral lyophilisate formulation of desmopressin in children aged 6–12 years at a small dose range (120–240 µg) is likely to control diuresis for a period corresponding to a night's sleep (7–11 h).

Tricyclic agents (such as imipramine, approved by the US Food and Drug Administration for children of 6 years of age and older) increase urinary osmolality and decrease detrusor tone while increasing sphincter tone [21]. The response rate is quite variable, and the long-term cure rate is only approximately 25%; relapses are common. Tricyclic anti-depressants significantly affect sleep cycle and result in REM sleep suppression, which can lead to daytime sleepiness. Another adverse effect of these drugs is constipation [21,58].

Imipramine treatment can affect cardiac conduction, so an ECG before starting the treatment should be performed [21,58]; if normal, treatment can be started with a dose of 10 mg for children aged 6–8 years, and 25 mg for children older than 8 years. The dose can be increased by 10–25 mg every 5 days, until dryness.

Probably, each intervention may have effects on a combination of factors; therefore, they can be used in combination, especially in children resistant to the treatment (Table 18.1).

A recent randomized, double-blind, placebo-controlled trial has evaluated a combination therapy with desmopressin and an anti-cholinergic medication for non-responders to desmopressin with monosymptomatic SE [59]. The authors observed a significant reduction in the number of wet nights per week and a 66% reduction in the propensity for wet nights after combination therapy, compared to desmopressin plus placebo.

In another trial, carbamazepine was found to be effective in the treatment of primary SE [60], but complete polysomnography or EEG was not performed prior to randomization, making the results of the study questionable.

Other forms of intervention using alternative techniques have been reported, such as hypnosis and acupuncture [61,62]. Hypnotherapy has been successfully used to treat children and adolescents with SE, but results are usually only evident after several sessions [63]. A comparative study of imipramine versus hypnosis demonstrated that patients in the hypnosis group (who continued practising self-hypnosis daily) maintained a longer positive response after termination of the active treatment. However, hypnosis and self-hypnosis strategies were found to be less effective in younger children (5–7 years old) compared to imipramine treatment [64]. In comparison with pharmacological therapy using desmopressin, Radmayr et al. [65] found that laser acupuncture should be taken into account as an alternative therapy for children with primary SE because no statistically significant differences were found between the two treatments.

Constipation may accompany enuresis, causing or aggravating the problem. In these cases it is necessary to apply an education program including: regular toileting, high water intake during the day, reduce constipating foods (e.g. milk products), specific bowel protocol to reduce constipation [66].

Conclusions

Enuresis may be considered as an unusual parasomnia; in our old study of validation of a sleep disorders questionnaire in children, we found that enuresis was the only item with a low factor loading and inter-item correlation and was therefore eliminated from the final questionnaire [67]. This finding is in agreement with other questionnaire-based studies that stated that enuresis should be considered independent from a wide range of sleep-related behaviors.

A sleep disorder is defined by some abnormal sleep pattern; strictly speaking, enuresis is not a sleep disorder. Three decades of research indicate that bedwetting children do not have abnormal sleep patterns and, although depth of sleep may be an important factor in some children, enuretic episodes are not associated with deep sleep, transition between sleep stages, or arousal. However, it seems that subjects with SE have a higher arousal threshold and are therefore considered deep sleepers [30], but their sleep is not deeper than normal from a polysomnography point of view. A neurophysiological correlate of the low arousability of subjects with SE is likely to exist and should probably be sought in the brainstem and in the activity of the autonomic nervous system [68]. This neurophysiological correlate might be evaluated by analyzing the subcortical activations and, perhaps, the sleep cyclic alternating pattern [69,70].

Although it is not yet entirely clear how and why the sleep of children with SE is disturbed, they report a bad sleep quality linked to the sleep interruptions for the wetting episodes and to the related anxiety [71].

Finally, a careful assessment is required to identify specific sleep-related subjective or objective disturbances because sleep disruption in enuretic children may lead to disturbances of daytime psychosocial functioning [68].

References

1. American Academy of Sleep Medicine. *International Classification of Sleep Disorders: Diagnostic and Coding Manual.* 2nd ed. Westchester, IL: AASM, 2005.
2. Neveus T, von Gontard A, Hoebeke P, et al. The standardization of terminology of lower urinary tract function in children and adolescents: Report from the standardization committee of the International Children's Continence Society. *J Urol* 2006; **176**: 314–24.
3. Robson WLM, Leung AKC, van Howe R. Primary and secondary nocturnal enuresis: Similarities in presentation. *Pediatrics* 2005; **115**: 956–9.
4. Yeung CK. Nocturnal enuresis in Hong Kong: Different Chinese phenotypes? *Scand J Urol Nephrol* 1997; Suppl **183**: 17–21.
5. Yeung CK, Sreedhar B, Sihoe JD, et al. Differences in characteristics of nocturnal enuresis between children and adolescents: A critical appraisal from a large epidemiological study. *BJU Int* 2006; **97**: 1069–73.
6. Robson WLM, Leung AKC. Nocturnal enuresis. *Adv Pediatr* 2001; **48**: 409–38.
7. Djurhuus JC. Definitions of subtypes of enuresis. *Scan J Urol Nephrol Suppl* 1999; **202**: 5–7.
8. Thiedke CC. Nocturnal enuresis. *Am Fam Physician* 2003; **67**: 1499–506.
9. Caldwell PH, Edgar D, Hodson E, Craig JC. Bedwetting and toileting problems in children. *Med J Aust* 2005; **182**: 190–5.
10. Jansson UB, Hanson M, Hanson E, et al. Voiding pattern in healthy children 0 to 3 years old: A longitudinal study. *J Urol* 2000; **164**: 2050–4.
11. Hjalmas K, Arnold T, Bower W, et al. Nocturnal enuresis: An international evidence based

management strategy. *J Urol* 2004; **171**: 2545–61.

12. Chiozza ML, Bernardinelli L, Caione, *et al.* An Italian epidemiological multicentre study of nocturnal enuresis. *Br J Urol* 1998; **81**(Suppl 3): 86–9.

13. Devitt H, Holland P, Butler R, *et al.* Plasma vasopressin and response to treatment in primary nocturnal enuresis. *Arch Dis Child* 1999; **80**: 448–51.

14. Sheldon SH. Sleep related enuresis. In Sheldon SH, Ferber R, Kryger MH (Eds), *Principles and Practice of Pediatric Sleep Medicine*. Philadelphia: Elsevier Saunders, 2005; 317–25.

15. Sheldon SH. Sleep-related enuresis. *Child Adolesc Psychiatr Clin North Am* 1996; **5**: 661–72.

16. Mark SD, Frank JD. Nocturnal enuresis. *Br J Urol* 1995; **75**: 427–34.

17. Laberge L, Tremblay RE, Vitaro F, Montplaisir J. Development of parasomnias from childhood to early adolescence. *Pediatrics* 2000; **106**: 67–74.

18. Butler RJ, Heron J. The prevalence of infrequent bedwetting and nocturnal enuresis in childhood: A large British cohort. *Scan J Urol Nephrol* 2007; **42**: 1–8.

19. Meadow SR. Enuresis. In Edelmann CM (Ed), *Pediatric Kidney Disease*. Boston: Little, Brown and Company, 1992; 2015.

20. Largo RH, Molinari L, von Siebenthal K, Wolfensberger U. Development of bladder and bowel control: Significance of prematurity, perinatal risk factors, psychomotor development and gender. *Eur J Pediatr* 1999; **158**: 115–22.

21. Norgaard JP, Djurhuus JC, Watanabe H, Stenberg A, Lettgen B. Experience and current status of research into the pathophysiology of nocturnal enuresis. *Br J Urol* 1997; **79**: 825–35.

22. Forsythe WI, Redmond A. Enuresis and spontaneous cure rate: Study of 1129 enuretics. *Arch Dis Child* 1974; **49**: 259.

23. Hjalmas K, Arnold T, Bower W, *et al.* Nocturnal enuresis: An international evidence based management strategy. *J Urol* 2004; **171**: 2545–61.

24. Kotagal S. Parasomnias in childhood. *Sleep Med Rev* 2008; doi:10.1016/j.smrv.2008.09.005.

25. Moffatt M. Nocturnal enuresis: A review of the efficacy of treatments and practical advice for clinicians. *J Dev Behavior Pediatr* 1997; **18**: 49–56.

26. Abe K, Oda N, Hatta H. Behavioural genetics of early childhood: Fears, restlessness, motion sickness and enuresis. *Acta Genet Med Gemellol* 1984; **33**: 303–06.

27. Bakwin H. Enuresis in twins. *Am J Dis Child* 1971; **121**: 222–5.

28. Badalian LO, Oradovskaia IV, Lipovetskaia NG. Nocturnal enuresis in twins (clinico-genetic analysis). *Urol Nefrol* 1971; **36**: 44–8.

29. Hublin C, Kaprio J. Genetic aspects and genetic epidemiology of parasomnias. *Sleep Med Rev* 2003; **7**: 413–21.

30. Wolfish NM, Pivik RT, Busby KA. Elevated sleep arousal thresholds in enuretic boys: Clinical implications. *Acta Paediatr* 1997; **86**: 381–4.

31. Hunsballe JM. Increased delta component in computerized sleep electroencephalographic analysis suggests abnormally deep sleep in primary monosymptomatic nocturnal enuresis. *Scand J Urol Nephrol* 2000; **34**: 294–302.

32. Mikkelsen EJ, Rapoport JL, Nee L, *et al.* Childhood enuresis: Sleep patterns and psychopathology. *Arch Gen Psychiatry* 1980; **37**: 1139–44.

33. Nevéus T, Stenberg A, Läckgren G, *et al.* Sleep of children with enuresis: A polysomnographic study. *Pediatrics* 1999; **106**: 1193–7.

34. Bader G, Nevéus T, Kruse S, Sillén U. Sleep of primary enuretic children and controls. *Sleep* 2002; **25**: 579–83.

35. Brooks LJ, Topol HI: Enuresis in children with sleep apnea. *J Pediatr* 2003; **142**: 515–8.

36. Weider DJ, Sateia MJ, West RP. Nocturnal enuresis in children with upper airway obstruction. *Otolaryngol Head Neck Surg* 1991; **105**: 427–32.

37. Alexopoulos EI, Kaditis AG, Kostadima E, *et al.* Resolution of nocturnal enuresis in snoring children after treatment with nasal budesonide. *Urology* 2005; **66**: 194.

38. Alexopoulos EI, Kostadima E, Pagonari I, *et al.* Association between primary nocturnal enuresis and habitual snoring in children. *Urology* 2006; **68**: 406–09.

39. Crimmins CR, Rathbun SR, Husmann DA. Management of urinary incontinence and nocturnal enuresis in attention-deficit hyperactivity disorder. *J Urol* 2003; **170**: 1347–50.

40. Robson WLM, Jackson HP, Blackhurst D, *et al.* Enuresis in children with attention-deficit hyperactivity disorder. *South Med J* 1997; **90**: 503–05.

41. Robson WLM, Leung AKC. A survey of voiding dysfunction in children with attention deficit-hyperactivity disorder. *J Urol* 2004; **172**: 388–9.

42. Sans Capdevila O, Crabtree VM, Kheirandish-Gozal L, Gozal D. Increased morning brain natriuretic peptide levels in children with nocturnal enuresis and sleep-disordered breathing: A community-based study. *Pediatrics* 2008; **121**: 1208–14.

43. Bruni O, Finotti E, Novelli L, Ferri R. Parasomnias in children. *Somnology* 2008; **12**: 14–22.
44. Weissbach A, Leiberman A, Tarasiuk A, *et al.* Adenotonsilectomy improves enuresis in children with obstructive sleep apnea syndrome. *Int J Pediatr Otorhinolaryngol* 2006; **70**: 1351–56.
45. Schütz-Fransson U, Kurol J. Rapid maxillary expansion effects on nocturnal enuresis in children: A follow-up study. *Angle Orthod* 2008; **78**: 201–08.
46. Mattelaer P, Mersdorf A, Rohrmann D, *et al.* Biofeedback in the treatment of voiding disorders in childhood. *Acta Urol Belg* 1995; **63**: 5–7.
47. Robson WLM. Current management of nocturnal enuresis. *Curr Opin Urol* 2008; **18**: 425–30.
48. Glazener CM, Evans JH, Peto RE. Alarm interventions for nocturnal enuresis in children. *Cochrane Review* 2005; **18**: CD002911.
49. Hoebeke PB, Vande Walle J. The pharmacology of paediatric incontinence. *BJU Int* 2000; **86**: 581–9.
50. Van Hoeck KJ, Bael A, Lax H, *et al.* Improving the cure rate of alarm treatment for monosymptomatic nocturnal enuresis by increasing bladder capacity: A randomized controlled trial in children. *J Urol* 2008; **179**: 1122–6.
51. Mota DM, Barros AJD. Toilet training: Methods, parental expectations and associated dysfunctions. *J Pediatr* 2008; **84**: 9–17.
52. Robson WLM, Leung AK. Urotherapy recommendations for bedwetting. *J Natl Med Assoc* 2002; **94**: 577–80.
53. Nijman RJ. Role of antimuscarinics in the treatment of nonneurogenic daytime urinary incontinence in children. *Urology* 2004; **63**: 45–50.
54. Robson WLM, Norgaard JP, Leung AKC. Hyponatremia in patients with nocturnal enuresis treated with DDAVP. *Eur J Pediatr* 1996; **155**: 959–61.
55. Robson WLM, Leung AKC, Norgaard JP. The comparative safety of oral versus intranasal desmopressin in the treatment of children with nocturnal enuresis. *J Urol* 2007; **178**: 24–30.
56. Vande Walle J, Vande Walle C, van Sintjan P, *et al.* Nocturnal polyuria is related to 24-h diuresis and osmotic excretion in an enuresis population. *J Urol* 2007; **178**: 2630–4.
57. Vande Walle JG, Bogaert GA, Mattsson S, *et al.* Desmopressin oral lyophilisate PD/PK study group. A new fast-melting oral formulation of desmopressin: A pharmacodynamic study in children with primary nocturnal enuresis. *BJU Int* 2006; **97**: 603–09.
58. Sukhai RN, Mol J, Harris AS. Combined therapy of enuresis alarm and desmopressin in the treatment of nocturnal enuresis. *Eur J Pediatr* 1989; **148**: 465–7.
59. Austin PF, Ferguson G, Yan Y, *et al.* Combination therapy with desmopressin and an anticholinergic medication for nonresponders to desmopressin for monosymptomatic nocturnal enuresis: A randomized, double-blind, placebo-controlled trial. *Pediatrics* 2008; **122**: 1027–32.
60. Al-Waili NS. Carbamazepine to treat primary nocturnal enuresis: Double-blind study. *Eur J Med Res* 2000; **5**: 40–4.
61. Glazener CM, Evans JH, Cheuk DK. Complementary and miscellaneous interventions for nocturnal enuresis in children. *Cochrane Database Syst Rev* 2005; **18**: CD005230.
62. Olness K, Kohen DP. *Hypnosis and Hypnotherapy with Children.* 3rd ed. New York: The Guilford Press, 1996.
63. Dowd ET. Hypnotherapy in the treatment of adolescent enuresis. In Lynn SJ, Kirsch I, Rhue JW (Eds), *Casebook of Clinical Hypnosis.* Washington, DC: American Psychological Association, 1996; 293–307.
64. Banerjee S, Srivastav A, Palan BM. Hypnosis and self-hypnosis in the management of nocturnal enuresis: A comparative study with imipramine therapy. *Am J Clin Hypn* 1993; **36**: 113–9.
65. Radmayr C, Schlager A, Studen M, Bartsch G. Prospective randomized trial using laser acupuncture versus desmopressin in the treatment of nocturnal enuresis. *Eur Urol* 2001; **40**: 201–05.
66. Reiner WG. Pharmacotherapy in the management of voiding and storage disorders, including enuresis and encopresis. *J Am Acad Child Adolesc Psychiatry* 2008; **47**: 491–8.
67. Bruni O, Ottaviano S, Guidetti, *et al.* The Sleep Disturbance Scale for Children (SDSC). Construction and validation of an instrument to evaluate sleep disturbances in childhood and adolescence. *J Sleep Res* 1996; **5**: 251–61.
68. Neveus T. Enuretic sleep: Deep, disturbed or just wet? *Pediatr Nephrol* 2008; **23**: 1201–02.
69. Bruni O, Ferri R, Miano S, *et al.* Sleep cyclic alternating pattern in normal school-age children. *Clin Neurophysiol* 2002; **113**: 1806–14.
70. Bruni O, Ferri R, Miano S, *et al.* Sleep cyclic alternating pattern in normal preschool-age children. *Sleep* 2005; **28**: 220–30.
71. Gozmen S, Keskin S, Akil I. Enuresis nocturna and sleep quality. *Pediatr Nephrol* 2008; **23**: 1293–6.

Section 4 Chapter 19

Other parasomnias

Catathrenia (sleep-related groaning)

Roberto Vetrugno, Giuseppe Plazzi and Pasquale Montagna

History and terminology

Sleep-related groaning was first reported in the medical literature in 1983 when De Roeck and Van Hoof described, in abstract form, the case of a young male with groaning during REM sleep as the result of forced and prolonged expiration [1]. In 2001, Vetrugno et al. described four additional patients (three males, one female) between 15 and 25 years of age and introduced the term catathrenia (from the Greek κατά = like, and θρῆνος = groan) to discriminate this unusual sleep-related behavior from other respiratory and non-respiratory disturbances during sleep [2]. In the same year, Pevernagie et al. reported 10 patients (7 males, 3 females), aged between 20 and 49 years, who had sleep-related respiratory dysrhythmia characterized by clusters of bradypneic events associated with prolonged expiration and expiratory sound production consistent with monotonous vocalization and occurring predominantly during REM sleep [3]. In 2004, Brunner and Gonzalez reported, in abstract form, eight other patients (six males, two females) who had prolonged groaning-like vocalization during sleep [4] and, in 2005, Oldani et al. described 21 patients (13 males and 8 females) between 18 and 43 years of age, highlighting that no effective treatment was available to solve nocturnal groaning [5].

In 2005, catathrenia was included by the American Academy of Sleep Medicine into *The International Classifications of Sleep Disorders Diagnostic and Coding Manual* (ICSD-2) as a parasomnia [6]. In 2006, Iriarte et al. applied nasal continuous positive airway pressure (nCPAP) therapy in a patient (a woman) described as having catathrenia plus obstructive sleep apnea syndrome (OSAS) and reported effects on both groaning and OSAS [7]. In 2007, Vetrugno et al. added six new cases (two males and four females) aged between 26 and 41 years and emphasized catathrenia as a distinctive, possibly vestigial, breathing pattern during sleep and different from other sleep-related breathing disorders [8].

As of 2008, more than 50 cases have been reported in the literature, varying from case reports to series. Variable responses to nCPAP treatment have been reported in some patients described as having catathrenia [9–14].

Clinical findings

Catathrenia is a rare disorder with exclusively expiratory groaning during sleep. Patients are usually unaware of the nocturnal noise and seek medical consultation because they feel socially embarrassed whenever they have to sleep with other people, or because of parents and/or bed partners' concerns. In a series of 10 patients (5 males) the mean age at the observation was 27 ± 7.4 years (range 15–41) and the mean age at onset of nocturnal groaning was 13.3 ± 4.6 years (range 5–19), with a mean duration of 13.7 ± 6.6 years (range 7–26) [2,8]. Groaning was reported by relatives and/or partners to occur, in clusters, almost every night and not associated with any movement or respiratory distress, the patients remained unaware of the nocturnal noise and continued to sleep unaffected. Coaxing the patient to change posture would stop the groaning, but groaning would start again later on during the same night and was unrelated to body position. The patients never reported any dream content associated with the nocturnal noise. Of the ten patients, none had physical illness including alcohol and drug abuse, diabetes mellitus, thyroid dysfunction and other metabolic/endocrine disorders. Daytime fibroscopy of the upper airway with static and dynamic vocal cord evaluation, CT/MRI of brain and

Figure 19.1 Two patients' night polysomnographic histograms showing catathrenia recurring only during REM sleep (A) and during both NREM and REM sleep (B).

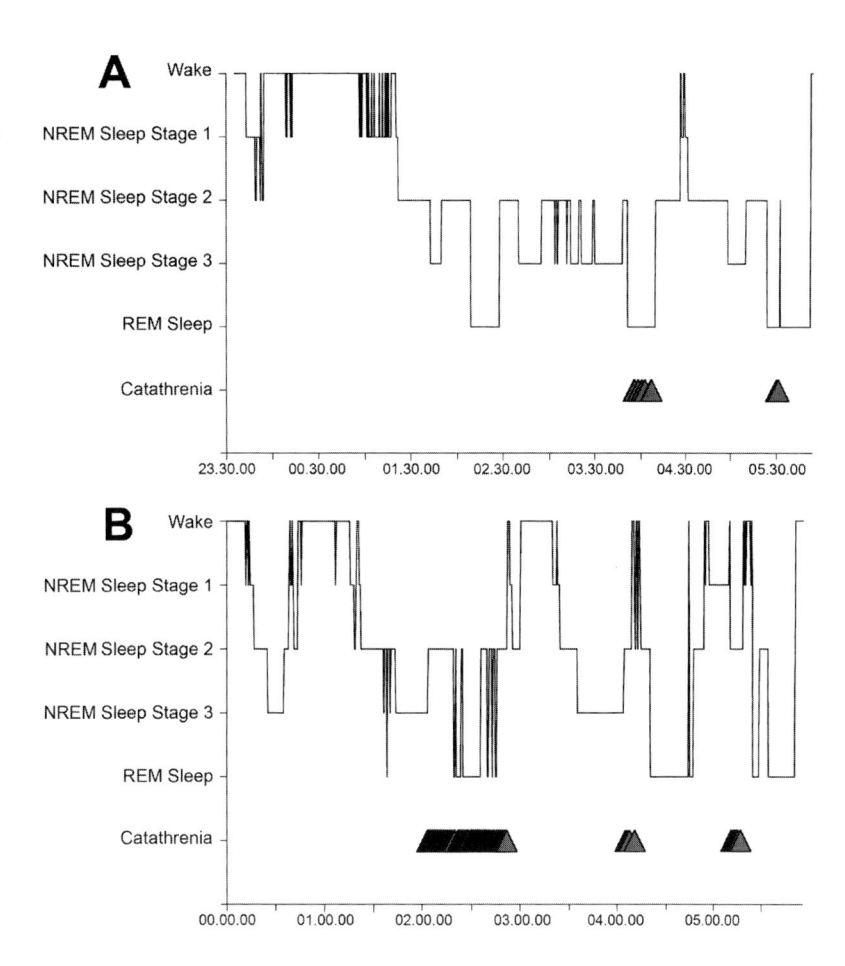

neck and physical and neurological examinations were all normal. Mean body mass index was 22.2 ± 1.7 (range: 18.8–24.5). Clinical interview disclosed normal sleep habits without mood-psychiatric disturbances, hypertension, cardiovascular disease or sexual dysfunction in any patient. Past and present daytime episodes of breath-holding spells were absent [15–17]. No patient complained of daytime sleepiness or unrefreshing sleep, fatigue or insomnia, sudden awakening with breath-holding, gasping or choking. Bed partners and/or parents denied patients' loud snoring or breathing interruptions during sleep. Four patients had a positive personal history for parasomnias (sleep-related enuresis until 7 years; sleep terrors from 6 to 10 years; sleep talking from 6 to 12 years; and sleepwalking from 5 to 11 years) and two a positive family history (sleep-related bruxism and sleep talking; sleep terrors and sleeptalking).

At video-polysomnographic investigation, all patients had a normal sleep structure: they entered sleep through NREM sleep stages, had recognizable NREM–REM sleep alternations and physiological atonia during REM sleep and did not show significant changes in total sleep time, percentages of light, deep and REM sleep phases, and arousal index (numbers of arousal per hour of sleep) versus a control group of ten age- and sex-matched normal subjects. Patients started to groan between 90 and 360 min after sleep onset. Catathrenia occurred during both NREM and REM sleep in six patients and exclusively during REM sleep in four patients. The groaning sounds lasted from 2–3 s to 20 s and recurred in clusters, 10–76 min in duration but spanning from 20 to 210 min, with the patients lying in any body position (Figure 19.1). The groaning sounds prevailed in the last third of the night and, noteworthy, during REM sleep they did not appear immediately as soon as REM sleep began but rather after several tens of seconds, waxing and waning thereafter. Patients groaned during expiration only, with continuous or fragmented sounds. An EEG arousal associated or not with a change in posture often marked the onset and the end of groaning

Section 4: Other parasomnias

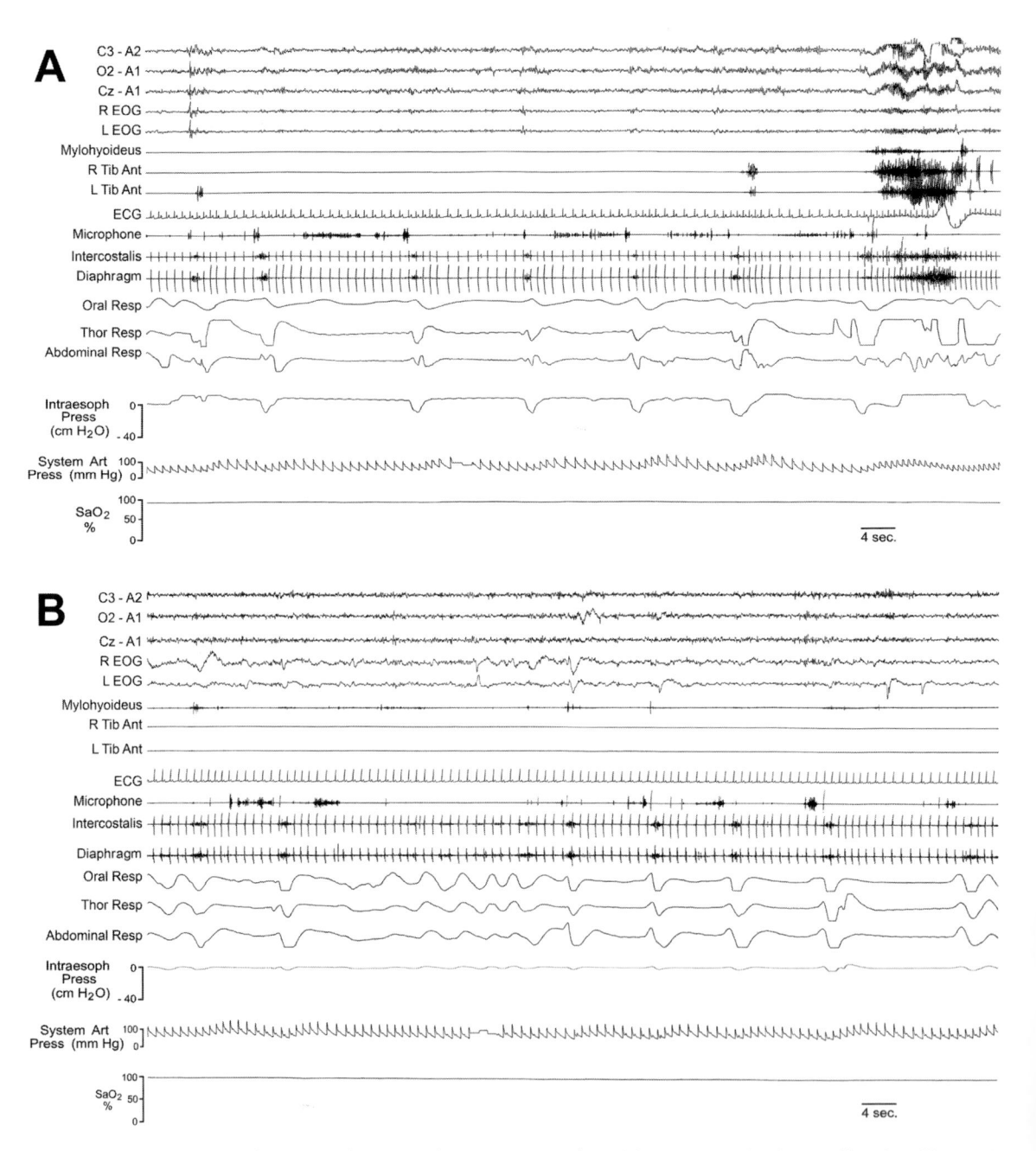

Figure 19.2 Catathrenia (microphone trace) during REM sleep recurring as a cluster (A) or interspersed with normal breathing (B). An EEG arousal signals the beginning and the end of the catathrenic cluster in A (microphone), whereas a catathrenic breathing pattern (deep inspiration followed by prolonged expiration) alternates with normal breathing in B. EOG: electro-oculogram; Tib Ant: tibialis anterior; Oral Resp: oral respirogram; Thor Tesp: thoracic respirogram; Abdominal Resp: abdominal respirogram; Intraesoph Press: intraesophageal pressure; System Art Press: systemic arterial pressure; SaO₂: oxygen saturation.

episode (Figure 19.2). No patient performed any other kind of respiratory noises or disturbances, such as snoring, stridor, wheezing, and obstructive or central apneas. In particular, cessation-reduction of airflow with ongoing respiratory effort, paradoxical movements of the ribcage and abdomen, significant endoesophageal swings between inspiratory and expiratory efforts with declining oxygen saturation and

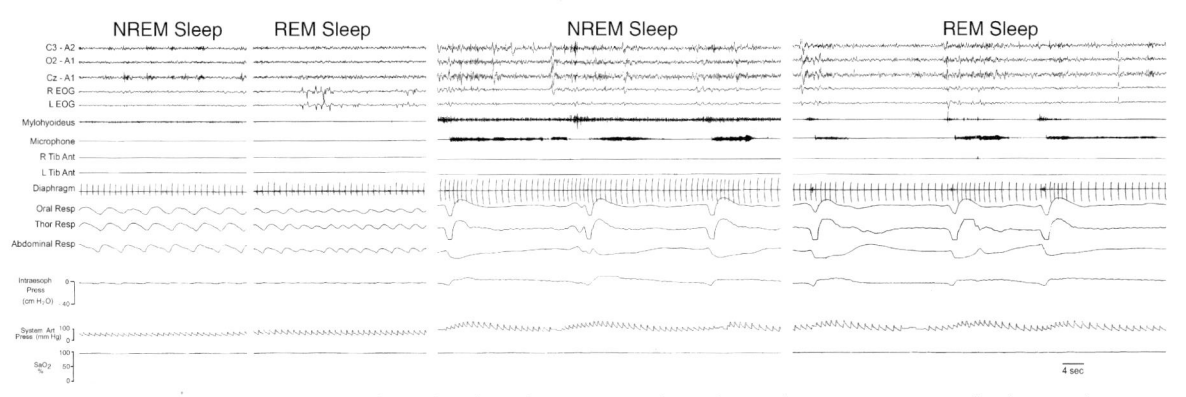

Figure 19.3 Normal breathing versus catathrenic breathing during NREM and REM sleep in the same patient. Note the dramatic slowing down of breathing rate during catathrenic breathing with the cycle length mainly occupied by the expiratory phase. Groaning sounds are shown on the microphone trace. Inspiration is associated with increased submental (Mylohyoideus) and diaphragm EMG activity, speeding up of EEG frequency, waxing in heart rate and arterial blood pressure, and negative endoesophageal pressure. After inspiration and during groaning, endoesophageal pressure shows initially slightly positive values, thereafter returning to 0 cm H$_2$O. Diaphragm EMG activity is absent, and heart rate and arterial blood pressure wane during the expiratory phase. EOG: electro-oculogram; Tib Ant: tibialis anterior; Oral Resp: oral respirogram; Thor Resp: thoracic respirogram; Abdominal Resp: abdominal respirogram; Intraesoph Press: intraesophageal pressure; System Art Press: systemic arterial pressure; SaO$_2$: oxygen saturation.

audible noises, all typical of OSAS, were not detected. No cessation in ventilatory effort and ventilation, or awakening with short-breath sensation typical of central sleep apnea syndrome, were observed. Mixed apneas were also absent.

During the respiratory groaning the respiratory pattern was distinctly abnormal, with a drastic slowing of the respiratory rate and a disproportionate increase in the length of expiration up to 85% of the respiratory cycle. Groaning was not associated with a discernible decrease in oxygen saturation. During catathrenia, each inspiratory effort was accompanied by inspiratory air flow, increased EMG activity of intercostal and diaphragmatic muscles, transient acceleration of heart rate and raising of arterial blood pressure and by normal negative swings of endoesophageal pressure. Groaning-associated prolonged expirations were accompanied by a slight decrease in heart rate and arterial blood pressure, were not associated with intercostal or diaphragmatic muscles EMG activity, and showed an initial positive swing in endoesophageal pressure, the latter falling to a plateau around 0 cm H$_2$O and remaining around zero throughout the groaning prior to the next inspiratory negative swing. This post-inspiratory positive rise in endoesophageal pressure during catathrenic breathing was not maintained throughout the groaning; it was discernibly higher than that observed during expiration in eupnoic breathing of the same patients and during eupnoic breathing in the control group subjects (Figure 19.3).

These ten patients declined any treatment, but were clinically followed for a mean period of 4.9 ± 3.5 years, still reporting the occurrence of nocturnal groaning in the absence of excessive daytime sleepiness, impairment of mood or cardiovascular, pulmonary or sexual function [2,8].

Pevernagie et al. reported ten patients (seven males) with a mean age of 32.3 ± 8.8 years (range: 20–49) whose principal clinical complaint was the making of unusual sounds during sleep. The symptom was first noticed at the mean age of 23.4 ± 9 years (range: 12–36). The vocal noises produced by the patients were indeed reported to be present from adolescence or early adulthood, to be loud, to occur on a regular basis and to be of serious annoyance to room-mates or bed partners. There was no evidence suggestive of an inherited pattern. Personal history was positive for parasomnias (bruxism) in two patients. Family history was positive for parasomnias (violent behavior during sleep; bruxism) in two patients, for nocturnal groaning in one patient, and for sudden infant death syndrome in one patient. Although patients were usually unaware of their breathing sounds during sleep, they could complain of restless sleep and mild daytime fatigue or somnolence. However, excessive daytime sleepiness was not the prime complaint in any of them. All patients denied the presence of sleep paralysis, sleep-onset hallucinations and cataplexy. None had a history of prior psychiatric illness or use of psychotropic medication. Medical and neurological examinations disclosed no particular abnormalities, except in one patient, in whom a frontal meningioma was detected (probably incidentally).

Video-polysomnography (VPSG) demonstrated the presence of clustered bradypneic events associated with prolonged expiration and expiratory sound production consistent with groaning. These episodes occurred predominantly during REM sleep (93% of the total number of groaning episodes), in the latter part of the nocturnal sleep, and showed a night-to-night consistency. In particular, normal respiration was interrupted by episodes of abnormal breathing consisting of deep inspiration followed by a prolonged expiratory phase during which a sound was produced. Endoesophageal pressure (recorded only in two patients) showed that the sustained expiratory phase was associated with a slight, gently declining elevation of the intrathoracic pressure. The bradypneic events with expiratory sound production occurred from 2 to 25 per hour during total sleep time, between 0 and 4 per hour during NREM sleep, and between 3 and 102 per hour during REM sleep, with a minimum duration of 3 s and a maximum of 49 s (mean: 10.5 s), and without evidence of motion of any part of the body. The authors stated that different empirical treatments, including pharmacotherapy (clonazepam, antidepressant drugs) and nCPAP, provided insufficient symptomatic control [3].

Oldani et al. described the clinical data of 21 patients (13 males) complaining of an expiratory groaning sound during sleep, some of them feeling socially embarrassed whenever they had to sleep with other persons. However, all patients were unaware of the disorder and were referred by family members. The mean age at observation was 31 ± 8.1 years (range: 18–48) and the mean age at onset 21.7 ± 7 years (range: 8–36). None presented neurological or pulmonary diseases and none had a history of psychiatric illness or the use of psychotropic medications. Eight patients reported a family history positive for parasomnias (bruxism, sleepwalking, sleep talking, sleep terrors) and three for nocturnal groaning. Sixteen patients underwent VPSG (none with endoesophageal pressure monitoring) and 12 of these presented episodes of nocturnal groaning, all performed during prolonged expiration. There was no specific modification of the sleep structure and architecture. The episodes of groaning were both isolated, with a duration of about 10 s, or in short sequences, lasting up to 4 min, and were not influenced by body position. Groaning occurred almost exclusively during REM sleep (89% of the total number of groaning episodes). In two cases, polysomnography showed the co-existence of bruxism. None of the patients had OSAS, and the oxygen saturation remained constantly over 90% all night long. Limb movements per hour of sleep were lower than five in all patients. In five patients, the results obtained from empirical treatments (clonazepam, gabapentin, pramipexole, trazodone) were unsatisfactory. At the follow-up visits (mean duration of follow-up: 18 months) nocturnal groaning still persisted in all patients. The authors stated that there was no association evident of nocturnal groaning with any predisposing factor or underlying disease [5].

An association between bruxism and nocturnal groaning was clinically and polysomnographically reported in a 32-year-old man with a 2-year history of strange nocturnal vocal sounds; in this patient nCPAP treatment was ineffective [18].

Iriarte et al. reported a 62-year-old woman with tremendous noises during sleep whose video-polysomnographic recording (not including endoesophageal pressure) showed a respiratory dysrhythmia during all sleep stages with obstructive sleep apnoeas (number of obstructive apnea–hypopnea per hour of sleep: 16) and intermittent hypoxia (number of oxygen desaturations per hour of sleep: 50; nadir of oxygen saturation: 79%), irregular abdominal wall movements and respiratory noise present during inspiration and expiration. A trial with nCPAP improved this condition, which the authors diagnosed as catathrenia [7]. It must be noted, however, that all of the above features (age of the patient, presence of severe OSAS with oxygen desaturation, noise present during both inspiration and expiration) were rather atypical by comparison with the previously described case series of catathrenia [2,3,5,8], thus casting doubts on the diagnosis. Indeed, since Iriarte et al. [7], other atypical cases have been reported as catathrenia.

Guilleminault et al. reported a series of seven non-obese women with a mean age of 26.7 years (range: 20–34). In these patients, sleep-related nocturnal noise was reported to be expiratory and to occur mainly during light NREM sleep and to diminish during REM sleep. Moreover, the produced sound was short-lasting (1–2 s), expiration was not prolonged, the sound was not produced during REM sleep and there was no bradypnea during "groaning". In view of the co-existence of a significant and mainly inspiratory flow limitation with anatomic evidence of a small upper airway and small jaws, the patients underwent nCPAP treatment, plus surgical intervention or oral device appliance in four of them. The treatments abolished or reduced the sleep-related hypopneas and inspiratory flow limitation and solved the respiratory noise [9].

Songu et al. described a 40-year-old woman with a body mass index of 36, daytime dyspnea, severe obstructive sleep apnea with intermittent hypoxia (apnea–hypopnea index: 38; nadir of oxygen saturation: 75%), moderate pulmonary hypertension and sleep-related nocturnal noise diagnosed as predominantly NREM sleep nocturnal groaning (only two out of the nine clusters of noise occurred during REM sleep) that was effectively treated with nCPAP [10].

According to Vetrugno [2,8], Pevernagie [3] and Oldani [5] alike, the hallmark of catathrenia can be said to consist of the fact that inspiration is followed by protracted expiration during which a prolonged or fragmented sound is produced, and this recurs predominantly during REM sleep. The features of catathrenia are quite stereotyped: a deep inspiration without sound production is followed by a prolonged expiration with groaning, usually lasting from at least 2 s up to 50 s and without any evidence for respiratory muscular effort or associated oxygen desaturation. Remarkably, nocturnal groaning alternates with normal breathing in the same night, sometimes in the same sleep state (Figure 19.2).

Natural history

Catathrenia typically appears insidiously during adolescence or early adulthood, but once established the night-to-night consistency is remarkable. No predisposing or precipitating factors have been identified and, indeed, catathrenia may go unnoticed until VPSG is carried out. Therefore, its actual incidence and prevalence are unknown. The course of catathrenia is chronic. Because of the normality of neurological, psychiatric, otorhynolaryngological and pulmonary investigations in the majority of the cases, the long-term prognosis of catathrenia remains unknown. The available follow-up data are still incomplete, but they seem to exclude a clinical progression or complication of catathrenia [5,8]. However, further studies are needed before concluding that catathrenia is harmless.

Laboratory investigations and differential diagnosis

VPSG is the investigation of choice to diagnose catathrenia and to differentiate it from other sleep-related breathing phenomena. All-night VPSG ought to include EEG, right and left electro-oculography, surface EMG of mentalis, masseter, tibialis anterior, intercostal (electrodes positioned in the third and fourth right intercostal space in the midaxillary line, 10–300 Hz band-passed) and diaphragm (electrodes positioned in the sixth and seventh right intercostal space in the anterior axillary line, 10–300 Hz band-passed), ECG, oro-nasal (thermistor), thoracic and abdominal (by means of strain-gauges placed, respectively, at the level of axilla and just superior to the iliac crest) respirograms, microphone (taped on the anterolateral part of the neck), oxygen saturation (pulse oximeter), systemic arterial pressure, and endoesophageal pressure (by means of an inflatable pressure probe transducer transnasally inserted into the lower third of the esophagus, i.e. endoesophageal balloon).

From a polysomnographic point of view, the episodes of catathrenia are characterized by a sudden switch from a eupnoic breathing to a bradypneic breathing with a recalibration of the respiratory cycle, now with prolongation of the expiratory phase, but without net gas exchange variability (i.e. normal and unchanged oxygen saturation). During this protracted expiration, continuous or fragmented sounds are produced. In particular, irregular sound production during the expiratory phase consists of high-pitched monotonous vocal noise with a crescendo pattern in some cases and an intermittent/jerky pattern in other cases, with a quite constant sound peak/sigh just prior to the next inspiration. This sound resembles a lament or groaning. The pitch and timbre of the sound may vary among patients, but are fairly constant for each individual. An EEG arousal, associated or not with a change of posture, often marks the onset and the end of a groaning episode. During the expiratory groaning sounds, neither the diaphragm nor the intercostal EMG is active and endoesophageal pressure shows an initial positive rise (3–4 cm H_2O) subsequently returning to values around 0 cm H_2O. Hemoglobin desaturation does not occur, even with prolonged groaning episodes. Groaning episodes with prolonged expiration usually occur with slightly decreased heart rate and blood pressure, and end with an inspiratory effort and an EEG arousal (Figures 19.2 and 19.3).

Section 4: Other parasomnias

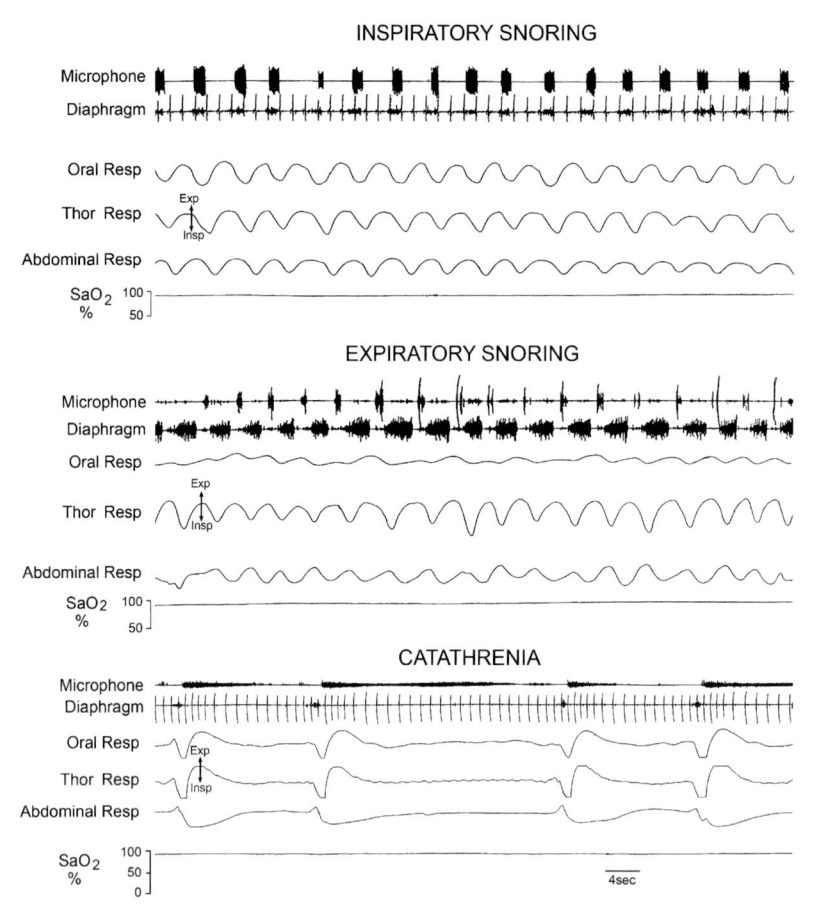

Figure 19.4 Catathrenia compared to inspiratory and expiratory snoring. The recordings are shown at the same time scale. Note: (1) the prolonged duration of the groaning sounds (microphone), (2) the prolonged expiration phase (oral, thoracic and abdominal respirograms), and (3) the bradypnoic pattern in catathrenia. Oral Resp: oral respirogram; Thor Resp: thoracic respirogram; Abdominal Resp: abdominal respirogram; SaO$_2$: oxygen saturation.

The respiratory tracings of catathrenia may be confused with a central apnea due to the apparent long cessation of flow and breathing effort, but careful inspection will show that in contrast to a central apnea, where the apneic pause is preceded by an exhalation, in catathrenia the breath preceding the apnea is a large inhalation. Due to the presence of cardiac oscillations on the airflow trace, the graphic may be interpreted as "respiratory pause"; however, during catathrenia, prominent heart rate deceleration is seen during the first part of the "respiratory pause", similar to that which occurs during the Valsalva maneuver. This, together with the sound production, is consistent with a prolonged expiration against a partially occluded upper airway.

Catathrenia is also different from the physiologic post-sigh apnea where pulse artifact persists on the graphic airflow, but the gradual cardiac deceleration has its nadir during the last third of the pause.

Stridor may also be expiratory and confused with catathrenia because of its possible recurrence in clusters during the night, but stridor does not occur as a prolonged expiration following an initial deep inspiration.

Catathrenia should be differentiated also from the vocalizations and moaning observed during epileptic seizures, from sleep-related laryngospasm and particularly from snoring [6].

Snoring, in effect, may be also expiratory with distinctive VPSG findings [19]. Narrowing of the upper airway and flow limitation are, indeed, not solely inspiratory phenomena, but they may occur with expiration in healthy subjects, and also in snorers, in patients with upper airway resistance syndrome (UARS) and in patients with OSAS [20,21]. Expiratory obstruction with expiratory snoring has been observed during sleep [20,22,23]. The effect of gravity (mainly during supine body position) on airway structures together with the relaxation of the pharyngeal dilator muscles, such as the tensor palatini and genioglossus, may promote local upper airway narrowing during expiration more frequently at the supraglottic/retroglossal level [24]. Flow limitation is associated with high-frequency oscillations of the airway wall which are propagated like a noise, i.e. expiratory snoring if during expiration. Isolated expiratory flow limitation thus recurs in breaths and coupled with inspiratory flow limitation in sleep [20] (Figure 19.4).

Genetics

Catathrenia represents less than 1% of the population referred to a sleep disorder center [3,5]. The condition may be familial. Oldani *et al.* noted a positive family history in 14.8% of their cases, with an apparent autosomal dominant pattern of inheritance in two of their families [5]. Remarkably, catathrenia may be associated with a positive personal or familial history for other parasomnias, like bruxism, sleep-related enuresis, sleep terrors, sleeptalking, sleepwalking, and violent behavior during sleep [2,3,5,8,18]. However, given the young age of the patients affected with catathrenia and considering the high prevalence of parasomnias in the young, the possibility of a casual association cannot be ruled out.

Pathology

There is no pathological report on catathrenia, and the pathophysiology of catathrenia is unknown. However, normal waking laryngoscopic examinations exclude conditions characterized by local airway disease, such as laryngomalacia, and rather suggest that catathrenia is a sleep state-specific stereotyped breathing pattern presumably influenced by neural "central pattern generator(s)" in the brainstem [8]. In cases with typical clinical and VPSG findings of catathrenia, daytime respiratory function tests performed through static and dynamic spirometry yielded normal results, and fibroscopy of the upper airways, with static and dynamic vocal cord evaluations, was normal [2,8].

The VPSG findings in catathrenia (e.g. the slightly increased endoesophageal pressure) are consistent with the abnormal sounds being generated during prolonged expiration against a partially closed glottis, and the salient features of catathrenia are, in our view, represented by its occurrence prevalently during REM sleep and its alternating with the normal breathing pattern even during the same sleep stage (Figures 19.2 and 19.3).

Catathrenia is, at least in part, reminiscent of some breathing pattern(s) of the infant. Regular breathing during sleep in infants may be interrupted at intervals by sighs usually followed by brief (less than 10 s) periods of "hypoventilation/apnea" repetitively recurring for some time with a calculated cycle length of approximately 18 s, but with stable maintenance of minute ventilation [25]. These cyclical fluctuations of breathing are more evident during REM sleep [25]. According to Adamson *et al.*, 3—13-s "pauses" in breathing occur frequently in the newborn, especially in REM sleep, and may reflect "instability" of the central rhythm generator and "plasticity" of the entire breathing system [26]. Glottal restriction has been observed endoscopically during such respiratory pauses [27], and correlated to maintenance of thyroarytenoid muscle EMG activity in the lamb [28]. Phylogenetically, the basic respiratory pattern alternates pulmonary ventilation and inspiratory breath-holding, with the glottis closed to maintain the gas exchanger full of air, thus favoring continuation of gas exchange in the absence of ventilatory movements [29]. This is relevant particularly in the preterm newborn, in which lung volume tends to decrease dramatically as soon as inspiratory muscle contractions cease, because of the presence of a highly compliant chest wall with low lung compliance [30]. In the lamb fetus in utero, periods with diaphragmatic "inspiratory" contraction (fetal breathing movements) are separated by prolonged periods with the glottis closed and absence of diaphragmatic contraction [31]. Prenatal lung growth is also dependent on the increase in tracheal pressure brought about by active glottal closure during periods without fetal breathing movements, the same mechanism enhancing postnatal lung growth in the immature newborn [32]. In these circumstances, active expiratory laryngeal closure represents an important defense mechanism in the preterm infant [33], this phenomenon being well known by the neonatologists as the expiratory grunting of the newborn. In both term and preterm infants, this peculiar breathing pattern virtually disappears by 6 months [34–36].

The similarities in breathing patterns during catathrenia, with a substantial slowing of the respiratory rate, a disproportionate increase in the length of expiration, and the alternation with normal breathing, suggest that it occurs because of an "instability" of the neural structures controlling ventilation during sleep [8,19].

Patients with catathrenia are usually young and their respiratory "instability" during sleep (eupnoic breathing interspersed with prolonged expiration with sound production) is reminiscent of the fetal pattern of respiration in which active expiratory laryngeal closure has been observed during "respiratory pauses" sufficient to maintain a high lung volume and to favor continuation of gas exchange in the absence of ventilatory movements (i.e. absence of diaphragmatic contraction) [27,29–31,33].

The proposed "two-oscillator model" of breathing posits that the "dominant" oscillator generates inspiration (via the pre-Bötzinger complex) with the other one generating expiratory activity (via the retrotrapezoid/parafacial nucleus) [37]. In "normal" conditions when there is minimal active expiratory activity the respiratory rhythm is driven by the pre-Bötzinger complex, but the retrotrapezoid/parafacial nucleus expiratory activity may also merge and drive breathing in particular conditions [37,38]. In this regard, simultaneous and erratic activations of neuron groups of the internal respiratory drive system have been observed particularly during REM sleep [39]. This hypothesis of catathrenia as a kind of vestigial breathing pattern helps to explain its prevalence in the young, its occurrence mainly during REM sleep, its alternation with eupnoic patterns, and the apparent absence of long-term clinical consequences [8]. However, it needs confirmation in follow-up studies and additional investigations on upper airway patency performed during sleep.

Management

There is no drug medication available for catathrenia. Empirical pharmacological treatments with dosulepine, trazodone, clonazepam, paroxetine, carbamazepine, gabapentin, and pramipexole have been unsuccessful or refused [3,5]. The efficacy of the nCPAP ventilation is still debated [7,40]. In particular, nCPAP treatment seems effective only when noisy breathing during sleep, diagnosed as catathrenia, is instead related to the co-existence of expiratory and inspiratory flow limitation with obstructive apneas or hypopneas and consequent intermittent hypoxia [7,9,10].

Conclusions (including future directions)

The episodic occurrence during sleep of bradypneas with prolonged expiration and sound generation constitutes an, until today, unsolved puzzle. It is important not to confuse catathrenia with other respiratory, especially obstructive, and non-respiratory disturbances during sleep, for the clear and important consequences on prognosis and treatment. Although VPSG remains the investigation of choice to diagnose this disorder, fiberoptic examination of the upper airways and vocal cords during sleep are needed to shed light on the mechanisms and physiopathology of catathrenia and on its, if any, relationship with the central, mixed or obstructive sleep apnea syndromes. Prospective and long-term follow-up is also needed in order to exclude possibly long-term health consequences of catathrenia.

References

1. De Roek J, Van Hoof E, Cluydts R. Sleep related expiratory groaning. A case report. *Sleep Res* 1983; **12**: 237.
2. Vetrugno R, Provini F, Plazzi G, et al. Catathrenia (nocturnal groaning): A new type of parasomnia. *Neurology* 2001; **56**: 681–3.
3. Pervernagie DA, Boon PA, Mariman AN, et al. Vocalization during episodes of prolonged expiration: A parasomnia related to REM sleep. *Sleep Med* 2001; **2**: 19–30.
4. Brunner DP, Gonzalez HL. Catathrenia: A rare parasomnia with prolonged groaning during clusters of central or mixed apneas. *J Sleep Res* 2004; **13**: 107.
5. Oldani A, Manconi M, Zucconi M, et al. Nocturnal groaning: Just a sound or a parasomnia? *J Sleep Res* 2005; **14**: 305–10.
6. American Academy of Sleep Medicine. *International Classification of Sleep Disorders, Diagnostic and Coding Manual*. 2nd ed. Westchester, IL: American Academy of Sleep Medicine, 2005; 165–7.
7. Iriarte J, Alegre M, Urrestarazu E, et al. Continuous positive airway pressure as treatment for catathrenia (nocturnal groaning). *Neurology* 2006; **66**: 609–10.
8. Vetrugno R, Lugaresi E, Plazzi G, et al. Catathrenia (nocturnal groaning): An abnormal respiratory pattern during sleep. *Eur J Neurol* 2007; **14**: 1236–43.
9. Guilleminault C, Hagen CC, Khaja AM. Catathrenia: Parasomnias or uncommon feature of sleep disordered breathing? *Sleep* 2008; **31**: 132–9.

10. Songu M, Ylmaz H, Yuceturk AV, et al. Effect of CPAP therapy on catathrenia and OSA: A case report and review of the literature. *Sleep Breath* 2008; **12**: 401–05.

11. Ramar K, Gay P. Catathrenia: Getting the 'cat' out of the bag. *Sleep Breath* 2008; **12**: 291–4.

12. Ramar K, Olson EJ, Morgenthaler TI. Catathrenia. *Sleep Med* 2008; **9**: 457–9.

13. Steinig J, Lanz M, Krügel R, et al. Breath holding. A rapid eye movement (REM) sleep parasomnia (catathrenia or expiratory groaning). *Sleep Med* 2008; **9**: 455–6.

14. Siddiqui F, Walters AS, Chokroverty S. Catathrenia: A rare parasomnia which may mimic central sleep apnea on polysomnogram. *Sleep Med* 2008; **9**: 460–1.

15. Lombroso CT, Lerman P. Breathholding spells (cyanotic and pallid syncope). *Pediatrics* 1967; **39**: 563–81.

16. Laxdal T, Gomez MR, Reiher J. Cyanotic and pallid syncopal attacks in children (breath-holding spells). *Dev Med Child Neurol* 1969; **11**: 755–63.

17. Livingston S. Breathholding spells in children. *J Am Med Assoc* 1970; **212**: 2231–5.

18. Manconi M, Zucconi M, Carrot B, et al. Association between bruxism and nocturnal groaning. *Mov Disord* 2008; **23**: 737–9.

19. Vetrugno R, Lugaresi E, Ferini-Strambi L, et al. Catathrenia (nocturnal groaning): what is it? *Sleep* 2008; **31**: 308–10.

20. Stanescu D, Kostianev S, Sanna A, et al. Expiratory flow limitation during sleep in heavy snorers. *Eur Respir J* 1996; **9**: 2116–21.

21. Lofaso F, Lorino AM, Fodil R, et al. Heavy snoring with upper airway resistance syndrome may induce intrinsic positive end-expiratory pressure. *J Appl Physiol* 1998; **85**: 860–6.

22. Weitzman ED, Pollak CP, Borowiecki BB, et al. The hypersomnia–sleep apnea syndrome: Site and mechanism of upper airway obstruction. In Guilleminault C, Dement WC (Eds), *Sleep Apnea Syndromes*. New York: Alan R. Liss Inc, 1978; 22–6.

23. Lugaresi E, Coccagna G, Cirignotta F. Snoring and its clinical implications. In Guilleminault C, Dement WC (Eds), *Sleep Apnea Syndromes*. New York: Alan R. Liss Inc, 1978; 13–21.

24. Woodson BT. Expiratory pharyngeal airway obstruction during sleep: A multiple element model. *Laryngoscope* 2003; **113**: 1450–9.

25. Hathorn MKS. Analysis of periodic changes in ventilation in newborn infants. *J Physiol* 1978; **285**: 85–99.

26. Adamson TM, Cranage SM, Maloney JE, Wilkinson M, Wilson FE. Periodic breathing: Its occurrence and relation to birth in preterm and term infants. *Aust Pediatr* 1984; **20**: 340.

27. Ruggins NR, Milner AD. Site of upper airway obstruction in infants following an acute life-threatening event. *Pediatrics* 1993; **91**: 595–601.

28. Renolleau S, Létourneau P, Niyonsenga T, et al. Thyroarytenoid muscle electrical activity during spontaneous apneas in preterm lambs. *Am J Respir Crit Care Med* 1999; **159**: 1396–404.

29. Shelton G, Boutilier RG. Apnea in amphibians and reptiles. *J Exp Biol* 1982; **100**: 245–73.

30. Bryan AC, Wohl ME. Respiratory mechanics in children. In Fishman AP (Ed), *Handbook of Physiology*. Section 3, Vol **III**, Part 1. Bethesda, MD: American Physiological Society, 1986; 179–91.

31. Kianicka I, Diaz V, Dorion D, et al. Coordination between glottic adductor muscle and diaphragm EMG activity in the fetal lamb in utero. *J Appl Physiol* 1998; **84**: 1560–5.

32. Harding R, Hooper SB. Regulation of lung expansion and lung growth before birth. *J Appl Physiol* 1996; **81**: 209–24.

33. Diaz V, Dorion D, Renolleau S, et al. Laryngeal dynamics during pulmonary edema in capsaicin-desensitized lambs. *J App Physiol* 1999; **86**; 1570–7.

34. Carse E, Wilkinson AR, Whyte PL, et al. Oxygen and carbon dioxide tensions, breathing and heart rate in normal infants during the first six months of life. *J Dev Physiol* 1981; **3**: 229–33.

35. Hoppenbrouwers T, Hodgemen JE, Harper RM, et al. Polygraphic studies of normal infants during the first six months of life. III. Incidence of apnea and periodic breathing. *Pediatrics* 1977; **60**: 418–25.

36. Richards JM, Alexander JR, Shinebourne EA, et al. Sequential 22-hour profiles of breathing patterns and heart rate in 110 full term infants during their first 6 months of life. *Pediatrics* 1984; **74**: 763–77.

37. Feldman JL, Del Negro CA. Looking for inspiration: New perspectives on respiratory rhythm. *Nature Rev Neurosci* 2006; **7**: 232–42.

38. Janczewski WA, Feldman JL. Distinct rhythm generators for inspiration and expiration in the juvenile rat. *J Physiol* 2006; **570**: 407–20.

39. Orem JM, Lovering AT, Vidruk EH. Excitation of medullary respiratory neurons in REM sleep. *Sleep* 2005; **28**: 801–07.

40. Ortega-Albas JJ, Diaz JR, Serrano AL, et al. Continuous positive airway pressure as treatment for catathrenia (nocturnal groaning). *Neurology* 2006; **67**: 1103.

Section 4 Chapter 20

Other parasomnias

Sleep-related hallucinations and exploding head syndrome

Satish C. Rao and Michael H. Silber

Definitions and historical perspective

Accurately processed external sensory input is a fundamental component of consciousness and normal cognition. Hallucinations occur when sensations are perceived in the absence of environmental stimuli. They are generated by the brain under a variety of relatively normal or abnormal situations, including drowsiness, sensory deprivation, use of or withdrawal from drugs or toxins, structural or metabolic brain disease, seizures or migraine, and psychiatric disorders such as schizophrenia. Hallucinations can occur with or without insight into their unreality. Consciousness may remain full or may be disturbed, especially with toxic or metabolic causes. Phenomenologically, dreaming could be considered hallucinatory, but is excluded by its occurrence as a normal physiologic experience. Hallucinations should be distinguished from illusions, which are distorted perceptions of real external stimuli. Many types of hallucinations are associated with drowsiness, sleep or the sleep–wake transition (Table 20.1).

Hallucinations that occur during sleep onset are commonly referred to as hypnagogic hallucinations, while those occurring around the time of waking are named hypnopompic hallucinations. Maury invented the phrase "hypnagogic hallucinations" over 150 years ago, characterizing his own sleep onset hallucinatory experiences [1]. Since that time, population studies have shown that these experiences are common in the normal population with a prevalence of 25–37% for hypnagogic hallucinations and 7–13% for hypnopompic hallucinations [2,3]. The most common pathologic association is with narcolepsy; approximately 59% of narcoleptics with cataplexy and 32% without cataplexy experience hypnagogic hallucinations [4].

The other major sleep-related hallucination is that of complex nocturnal visual hallucinations (CNVH). While many features suggest that this entity is different from hypnogogic or hypnopompic hallucinations, their exact relationship is at present unclear. CNVH occur after sudden awakening during the night and likely have different mechanisms from hypnagogic and hypnopompic hallucinations. These hallucinations are typically associated with underlying pathology, usually neurologic, visual, or toxic in nature [5,6]. There is a rich history of descriptions of complex visual hallucinations with variable etiologies. In 1760, the Swiss philosopher Charles Bonnet published a description of complex visual hallucinations in his grandfather who was rendered sightless from cataracts [7,8]. This condition, often referred to as Charles Bonnet Syndrome (CBS), is thought to emerge from deafferentation of visual association cortex from the central visual pathways [9]. Hallucinations and psychosis were noted as adverse effects of treatment in Parkinson's diseases in the 1950s with anti-cholinergic agents [10], and in the 1970s with dopaminergic therapy [11,12]. Spontaneous hallucinations in Lewy body dementia were recognized later [13]. These disorders are also associated with hallucinations that occur during waking hours [5]. Idiopathic complex hallucinations occurring only at night were first described in 1993 [14].

The exploding head syndrome was first described by Pearce in 1988 and is thought to likely represent a sensory variant of the hypnic jerk or sleep start [15]. Since the initial clinical description, there have been a few subsequent publications describing clinical and polygraphic characteristics. It is characterized by brief, largely auditory hallucinations at the wake–sleep transition. Although the clinical manifestations suggest that it falls within the spectrum of sleep-related hallucinations, the *International Classification of Sleep Disorders* (2nd edition) classifies it as a separate disorder [16].

Table 20.1 Hallucinations associated with sleep.

Hypnagogic and hypnopompic hallucinations
  Idiopathic parasomnia
  Associated with narcolepsy

Complex nocturnal visual hallucinations
  Idiopathic parasomnia
  Associated with medication use
  Associated with visual loss (Charles Bonnet syndrome)
  Associated with Lewy body disorders
  Associated with diencephalic/mesencephalic pathology
    (peduncular hallucinosis)
  Associated with anxiety disorder
  Associated with idiopathic hypersomnia/narcolepsy

Hallucinations due to epilepsy or migraine

Exploding head syndrome

Sleep-related hallucinations

Clinical findings and natural history

Hypnagogic and hypnopompic hallucinations

Hypnagogic and hypnopompic hallucinations (HH) are typically visual, but can be auditory, tactile or kinetic. The visual hallucinations can take elementary forms, such as points of light and geometric patterns, as well as more complex forms with human or animal figures [5]. The images are often vague, such as an indistinct figure standing in the corner of the room, but may be more realistic and detailed, such as a man dressed in guerrilla warfare attire with an automatic weapon sitting silently by the bed. Such hallucinations can be described as "dream-like" in their degree of vividness. However, HH are distinctly different from dreams in that the patients perceive themselves as either being awake or in a twilight state between wake and sleep. They usually observe the hallucinations rather than being engaged in a dream plot or reporting any significant communication with the figures [2,5]. One large study performed in a European population showed that the most common type of hypnagogic hallucination was the feeling of falling down an abyss, followed by a feeling that something or someone is present in the room [2]. The likelihood of reporting hypnagogic hallucinations was higher in women and younger subjects. There were epidemiologic associations with anxiety, mood disorders, sleep onset insomnia, perceived insufficient sleep, past alcohol use and current drug use. However, in over half of the participants (58% with hypnagogic hallucinations and 55% with hypnopompic hallucinations), there was no history of use of psychoactive substances, systemic pathology, sleep disorders or psychiatric disease. Thus hypnagogic and hypnopompic hallucinations can be a normal variant in many people. On the other hand, they can be associated with narcolepsy, but their presence is neither sensitive nor specific due to their high prevalence in the normal population and far from universal occurrence among narcoleptic patients [4].

Complex nocturnal visual hallucinations

Complex nocturnal visual hallucinations (CNVH) have somewhat different phenomenology and putative pathophysiology from HHs and can be seen in a variety of pathologic conditions. Rather than occurring during sleep onset or offset, CNVH appear when the individual wakes in the middle of the night. These hallucinations, as the name implies, are always visual and take the form of vivid, detailed images of people or animals. In a study of 12 patients with CNVH [6], examples included a "witch-like, short, baggy woman, clowns, rats and a brightly colored butterfly." The hallucinatory figures were often distorted; for example, a patient reported seeing a woman with hair on only one half of her head. The figures were relatively immobile and silent, and the hallucinations usually lasted less than 5 min. The hallucinations vanished if the lights were switched on in 11 of the 12 patients. Insight regarding the hallucinations was initially reduced in these patients, such that some patients had left their bed to investigate the phantasms, sometimes resulting in injuries. The frequency of events ranged from two to seven per week (mean 4.4). None of the 12 patients had daytime hallucinations. Eleven of the 12 patients were women. Long-term follow-up was not reported.

While CNVH may be an idiopathic parasomnia, it is often associated with a variety of underlying disorders. In patients with some of these conditions, similar hallucinations can also occur during the day. A variety of associated etiologic factors were noted in a study of 12 patients [6], including dementia with Lewy bodies (1), idiopathic hypersomnia (2), macular degeneration (1), beta adrenergic antagonist medication (3), and anxiety disorder (4). In one patient, CNVH was a life-long idiopathic parasomnia with age of onset at 5 years. The associations with visual loss (Charles Bonnet Syndrome), Lewy body disorders, and pathology of the mesencephalon and diencephalon (peduncular hallucinosis) will be discussed in more detail.

Charles Bonnet Syndrome (CBS) is a disorder characterized by complex visual hallucinations that arise in the setting of severe vision loss of any cause, most commonly macular degeneration [8]. In one large study of 505 visually handicapped patients, 60 patients met criteria for CBS [8]. Based on this and another study [17], it is widely accepted that approximately 10% of elderly subjects with significant visual impairment develop CBS. The hallucinations of CBS are strikingly variable. They range from the mundane, a motionless bottle, to the bizarre, "two miniature policemen guiding a midget villain to a tiny prison van" [8]. The hallucinations can last from seconds to hours, and in one study the frequency varied from several daily to twice per year [8]. The influence of time of day on CBS hallucinations and their relation to ambient lighting has been studied [8]. Hallucinations occurred most commonly in the evening (35%) or at night (23%), while daytime hallucinations are less common. In regards to ambient light, 65% of patients reported poor lighting and only 15% bright daylight to be favorable circumstances for hallucinations. These results confirm that a significant proportion of CBS hallucinations may occur at night and can present clinically as a sleep-related hallucination. It is important to educate the patient regarding the inter-relationship between the hallucinations, their visual impairment, and low ambient illumination in the evening and night. These patients often do well with education and reassurance about their condition [8].

Parkinson's disease (PD) and dementia with Lewy bodies (DLB) are neurodegenerative diseases associated with abnormal depositions of the protein alpha-synuclein [18]. Patients with these disorders can have hallucinations both spontaneously and as a side effect of commonly used medications in these disorders, such as levodopa. The hallucinations are usually visual and composed of animated human beings or animals [19]. Dim light can predispose to the occurrence of these hallucinations. They can occur in the day or in the form of complex nocturnal visual hallucinations. The etiology is debated with two major mechanisms hypothesized. Lewy body deposition in the brainstem may cause dysfunction of key nuclei responsible for state transitions between wakefulness, NREM and REM sleep. This, in turn, may lead to intrusion of REM phenomena (dream imagery) into wakefulness causing hallucinations. The other possible mechanism is direct deposition of Lewy bodies in neocortical neurons of the visual cortices causing loss of function and giving rise to hallucinations as a secondary release phenomenon. It is possible that both mechanisms are needed for these hallucinations to occur [19]. Diagnosing these disorders relies almost entirely on the clinical history and physical examination. Signs of Parkinsonism or dementia with fluctuating levels of awareness and often the presence of REM sleep behavior disorder help establish the diagnosis.

Peduncular hallucinosis (PH) refers to hallucinations caused by structural lesions in the pons, midbrain or thalamus. The etiology of this disorder is commonly vascular [5]. Similar to CBS, these hallucinations tend to have a diurnal pattern, occurring in the evening and remitting in the day. The visions can last from minutes to hours and be accompanied by disturbances in consciousness. Examples include a detailed trellis-work with beautiful birds flying back and forth, or more story-like hallucinations, with the patient participating [5]. A recent history of brainstem or thalamic infarction usually precedes PH by a few days and the hallucinations typically remit a few weeks later. However, other etiologies should be considered when a history of stroke is lacking. For example, there are several reports of tumors, both primary and metastatic, causing PH, and it has also been reported as a postoperative complication of brainstem surgery and angiography [20–22]. A careful history, neurological examination and a neuroimaging study will reveal the cause of PH in most cases.

Nocturnal hallucinations related to epilepsy and migraine

Epileptic hallucinations may occur at the time of sleep, as sleep is a known provocation for some seizure types [23]. In a prospective study of 613 partial seizures [24], 264 (43%) occurred out of sleep. Of these, 23% began during stage 1 non-rapid eye movement (NREM) sleep and 68% during stage 2, while seizures rarely began in slow-wave sleep, and no seizures commenced in REM sleep. Frontal lobe seizures were more common in sleep than seizures with onset from other brain regions. Key features of hallucinations caused by epileptic seizures which can aid the clinician in distinguishing them from hallucinations caused by other etiologies include the duration, stereotyped content, other semiologic features consistent with seizures (for example, progression to clonic jerking or altered awareness), and a history of secondarily generalized seizures. The vast majority of seizures are less than 2 min in duration, the mean being approximately 1 min for both complex partial and secondarily generalized tonic–clonic seizures [25,26]. A reported longer duration of hallucinations can be very helpful in ruling out epilepsy, with the rare exception of partial status epilepticus. The stereotyped nature of seizures is thought to arise from the ictal discharge activating the same neural network with each attack [27].

The pathophysiology of epileptic hallucinations is complex, but can be viewed in two simplistic categories. Seizures which activate primary sensory areas usually give rise to primitive hallucinations. For example, visual cortex hyperexcitation may cause flashing lights, and auditory cortex activation may cause a rushing sound. In contrast, seizures that arise from visual or auditory association cortex and activate a memory trace usually cause more well-formed hallucinations, such as scenery, figures or music [28]. These well-formed hallucinations include autoscopy, memory flashbacks, voices, music, and dreams of past objects, faces, and scenes. Seizure-induced hallucinations should be distinguished from epileptic illusions including déjà vu, jamais vu, macropsia, micropsia, depersonalization, derealization, time stopping or slowing, or increased awareness. These complex hallucinations and illusions most commonly localize to the temporal neocortex, mesial temporal lobe structures, and sometimes the temporo-occipital or temporo-parietal junctions [29,30]. Patients typically have insight that the hallucinations are not real [28].

Migraine must be kept in the differential diagnosis for sleep-related hallucinations, especially the variant of migraine equivalents or acephalgic migraines. These are migraine auras without the headache, which typically occur in people over the age of 50 years. In many cases, these patients have a previous history of migraine with or without aura [31]. Migraine auras are most commonly visual, and can be positive or negative phenomena. The classic example of a positive visual aura is the scintillating fortification scotoma, which consists of polychromatic, pulsating jagged lines that start in an arc near the center of the visual field and move outward. This outward movement usually evolves over 15–30 min towards the temporal visual field and is followed by a negative scotoma. A negative visual aura consists of black, gray or white spots obscuring vision, sometimes in the distribution of a hemianopia. These simple visual hallucinations in migraine are common and may occur at the time of sleep. Complex visual hallucinations associated with migraine are rare and may be associated with more complex forms of the disorder. A case in which a patient with hemiplegic migraine visualized "small, silent, white dogs running around her room" during recovery from the attack has been described [5]. It is now widely believed that cortical spreading depression is vital in the generation of migraine aura and a functional magnetic resonance imaging study (fMRI) study showed blood oxygenation level-dependent (BOLD) signal changes during migraine visual aura in humans with characteristics of cortical spreading depression [32]. Previous histories of migraine, a classic description of scintillating fortification scotoma, or the temporal association of the hallucination with migraine headache are keys to this diagnosis.

Laboratory investigations

The clinical history is critical in making the correct diagnosis of sleep-related hallucinations and in helping to select which laboratory investigations are most appropriate. For example, if the history is classic for hypnagogic hallucinations without other symptoms to suggest narcolepsy (such as daytime hypersomnolence), then no further testing is needed. Similarly, a clear history of CNVH is sufficient for a diagnosis to be made, although neurologic testing is sometimes necessary to determine the etiology. Sometimes the history may be unclear, and other parasomnias such as REM sleep behavior disorder or sleep terrors may be considered. In these cases, EEG-video polysomnography should be performed. In the few reported cases studied by polysomnography, CNVH arose from stage 2 NREM sleep and occurred while the EEG showed occipital alpha rhythm [6,14]. If there is any suspicion that the hallucinations may represent seizures, then wake and sleep EEGs and either EEG-video polysomnography or admission to an epilepsy monitoring unit may be necessary. To establish the etiology of the hallucinations, tests should be tailored to the specific clinical circumstances. If narcolepsy is suspected, then polysomnography followed by a multiple sleep latency test is needed. Magnetic resonance imaging of the head should be considered for unexplained CNVH or CNVH thought to be due to PH or cortical blindness. Neuropsychometric testing may be indicated in suspected Lewy body disease.

Genetics and pathophysiology

Familial patterns of sleep-related hallucinations have not been reported, and there are no known associations with specific genes or chromosomes. The pathophysiology of hypnagogic and hypnopompic hallucinations is believed to be REM intrusion (dream content or mentation) into wakefulness, although there is no direct evidence for this mechanism, especially in subjects who do not have narcolepsy [5,16].

CNVH have a similar phenomenology and represent a final common pathway for a variety of etiologies. Speculation regarding their pathophysiology must take into account their origin out of sleep and their occurrence in darkness or reduced ambient illumination. An attractive unifying hypothesis is that of release hallucinations, generated by the visual cortex under conditions of reduced sensory input, as a result of pathology, reduced environmental light or thalamic gating during sleep. Charles Bonnet Syndrome is the clearest model of this proposed mechanism, with deafferentation of the visual cortex causing a release phenomenon, with disinhibited cortical cells generating false images. Peduncular hallucinosis may similarly result from thalamic pathology causing reduced afferent input into the visual cortex. The pathogenesis in Lewy Body disease is unclear but, as discussed earlier, may be due to occipital cortical dysfunction causing release hallucinations [5].

An alternative hypothesis is that of sleep-state dissociation with fragmentation of the boundaries between sleep states and waking and intrusion of dream-like phenomena of REM sleep into wakefulness. Such a mechanism is thought to underlie a number of other parasomnias, including REM sleep behavior disorder and disorders of arousal. Lewy body pathology in the brainstem might produce such dissociation and similar states can be found in narcolepsy. Midbrain disease causing PH could conceivably induce similar changes in state [5,6].

The pathogenesis of hallucinations due to beta adrenergic antagonists is presumably related to blockade of central noradrenergic receptors, but the site and mechanism is unknown. The hallucinations seen in disorders mimicking CNVH, such as epilepsy and migraine, are believed to be due to direct cortical irritation. In the case of epilepsy, these arise through abnormal neuronal discharge, while in migraine they are thought to be due to cortical spreading depression.

Management

Little objective information is available regarding management of sleep-related hallucinations. Most often reassurance is sufficient for HH and CNVH. Tricyclic anti-depressants have been suggested for HH, but there are no published data on their efficacy either in isolated HH or in patients with narcolepsy. Two studies have examined the use of sodium oxybate for HH in narcolepsy. In the one uncontrolled study [33], 76% of 21 patients reported a decrease in the frequency of HH on 9 g sodium oxybate, while the second controlled study of 136 patients revealed no improvement on doses up to 9 g in comparison to placebo [34]. In one study, benzodiazepines (clonazepam and temazepam) and tricyclic anti-depressants (nortriptyline and amitriptyline) did not reduce the frequency of CNVH in two patients, while hypnosis was unhelpful in two others [6]. Further management depends on the underlying cause of the hallucinations. The treatment of specific sleep and neurological disorders such as narcolepsy, epilepsy, migraine, Parkinson's disease, dementia with Lewy bodies, and disorders causing peduncular hallucinosis are beyond the scope of this chapter. Beta adrenergic antagonists should be discontinued if hallucinations develop; three patients have been reported with complete resolution of CNVH after discontinuation of the drugs [6]. Lastly, cholinesterase inhibitors and atypical anti-psychotics can be considered for symptomatic treatment of hallucinations in the setting of PD and DLB [35], but potential benefits should be balanced with the risks of these drugs, especially the anti-psychotic agents [36].

Conclusions

Sleep-related hallucinations are a diverse collection of mostly visual experiences that can occur as both benign parasomnias and in the setting of various diseases. Diagnosing the etiologies of these disorders requires a careful clinical history and physical examination. Additional testing, such as neuroimaging, video-EEG polysomnography and electroencephalography, may be very useful in certain patients. The etiopathogenesis of sleep-related hallucinations probably represents distinct neural mechanisms with a final common product of false perceptual data. The exact pathophysiology needs further investigation, but current hypotheses focus on the concepts of release hallucinations and sleep state dissociation. Adequate trials of medications have not been conducted, but many patients obtain relief with simple reassurance. Underlying conditions should be identified and treated.

Exploding head syndrome

Clinical findings and natural history

The exploding head syndrome (EHS) is thought to be a benign condition characterized by an imagined very loud sound or explosion in the head at sleep onset or on waking during the night. Ten patients were described in the initial 1988 report [15]. One of the patients, an 80-year-old woman, described it as "strange and frightening attacks of something exploding, creating a loud bang in my head. There is no real pain, it does not hurt, but you feel there has been a massive hemorrhage and it takes a quarter of an hour before the fear passes, though the noise itself lasts only a split second." The spectrum of EHS is now recognized to include a "painless loud bang, an explosion, a clash of symbols, or a bomb exploding but occasionally may be a less alarming sound" [16]. There have been reports of associated perceptions of a flash of light, a myoclonic jerk, or brief stab of head pain [16]. These attacks may be precipitated by emotional stress in some patients [37]. This condition can start during almost any decade in life, with most patients having symptoms commence after 50 years of age [38]. There has been no neurologic morbidity reported with these symptoms and it is thus thought to be a benign condition [15,38]. However, if an individual has multiple events on a given night, insomnia can occur. EHS appears to abate in many patients over time [37,38].

Laboratory investigations

No investigations or laboratory testing is needed in typical cases. While the differential diagnosis includes headache syndromes such as idiopathic stabbing headache, hypnic headache and thunderclap headache, EHS is typically painless and easily differentiated on the patient's history alone. In rare cases with a prominent pain component suggesting the possibility of thunderclap headache, then emergent neuroimaging may be indicated to assess for subarachnoid hemorrhage.

Genetics and pathophysiology

It is not known if there is a genetic basis for this condition, nor is there a definite familial pattern [16]. Perhaps the best insights into the pathophysiology of these symptoms come from polysomnographic (PSG) recordings during the ictus. PSG recordings during attacks of EHS [37] have shown that the symptoms arise during early drowsiness or relaxed wakefulness with alpha rhythm and interspersed theta activity. During some events, arousal patterns occur immediately following the symptoms. No epileptiform activity has been reported. These findings are consistent with hypnagogic phenomenon. The phenomenology and electrophysiology have led to the currently accepted hypothesis that EHS represents a sensory variant of the more common hypnic jerk or sleep start [16,38].

Management

The cornerstone of management in EHS is reassurance and education, as this is a benign condition that remits over time in most patients. This information alone can significantly reduce the stress and anxieties regarding EHS, especially considering some patients misinterpret the symptoms as a stroke or brain hemorrhage [38]. There have been case reports describing success with tricyclic anti-depressants and calcium channel blockers in EHS; however, pharmacologic treatment is typically not needed [37,39]. If a patient experiences multiple attacks on a single night leading to insomnia, a benzodiazepine agonist hypnotic may be the most appropriate therapeutic option.

Conclusions

The EHS is a benign, usually self-limited, condition that is likely a sensory variant of the hypnic jerk. No testing or medications are necessary when the history is typical. Education and reassurance are the cornerstones of therapy. If the symptoms occur multiple times a night and cause insomnia, a hypnotic maybe useful.

References

1. Maury A. Des hallucinations hypnagogiques, ou des erreurs des sens dans l'etat intermediaire entre la veille et le sommeil. *Ann Medico-Psychol* 1848; **7**: 26–40.
2. Ohayon MM. Prevalence of hallucinations and their pathological associations in the general population. *Psychiatry Res* 2000; **97**: 153–64.
3. Ohayon MM, Priest RG, Caulet M, Guilleminault C. Hypnagogic and hypnopompic hallucinations: Pathological phenomena? *Br J Psychiatry* 1996; **169**: 459–67.

4. Silber MH, Krahn LE, Slocumb N. Clinical and polysomnographic findings of narcolepsy with and without cataplexy: A population-based study (abstract). *Sleep* 2003; **26**: A282–A3.

5. Manford M, Andermann F. Complex visual hallucinations. Clinical and neurobiological insights. *Brain Res* 1998; **121**: 1819–40.

6. Silber MH, Hansen MR, Girish M. Complex nocturnal visual hallucinations. *Sleep Med* 2005; **6**: 363–6.

7. Bonnet C. *Essai analytique sur les facultes d l'ame*. Copenhagen: Philibert; 1760.

8. Teunisse RJ, Cruysberg JR, Hoefnagels WH, *et al.* Visual hallucinations in psychologically normal people: Charles Bonnet syndrome. *Lancet* 1996; **23**: 794–7.

9. Plummer C, Kleinitz A, Vroomen P, *et al.* Of Roman chariots and goats in overcoats: The syndrome of Charles Bonnet. *J Clin Neurosci* 2007; **14**: 709–14.

10. Porteous HB, Ross DN. Mental symptoms in parkinsonism following benzhexol hydrochloride therapy. *Br Med J* 1956; **2**: 138–40.

11. Celesia GG, Barr AN. Psychosis and other psychiatric manifestations of levodopa therapy. *Arch Neurol* 1970; **23**: 193–200.

12. Damasio AR, Lobo-Antunes J, Macedo C. Psychiatric aspects in parkinsonism treated with L-dopa. *J Neurol Neurosurg Psychiatry* 1971; **34**: 502–07.

13. Perry RH, Irving D, Blessed G, *et al.* Senile dementia of Lewy body type. A clinically and neuropathologically distinct form of Lewy body dementia in the elderly. *J Neurol Sci* 1990; **95**: 119–39.

14. Kavey NB, Whyte J. Somnambulism associated with hallucinations. *Psychosomatics* 1993; **34**: 86–90.

15. Pierce JMS. Exploding head syndrome. *Lancet* 1988; **2**: 270–1.

16. American Academy of Sleep Medicine. *International Classification of Sleep Disorders, Diagnostic and Coding Manual*. 2nd ed. Westchester, IL: American Academy of Sleep Medicine, 2005.

17. Teunisse RJ, Cruysberg JR, Verbeek A, *et al.* The Charles Bonnet syndrome: A large prospective study in the Netherlands. A study of the prevalence of the Charles Bonnet syndrome and associated factors in 500 patients attending the University Department of Ophthalmology at Nijmegen. *Br J Psychiatry* 1995; **166**: 254–7.

18. Marti MJ, Tolosa E, Campdelacreu J. Clinical overview of the synucleinopathies. *Mov Disord* 2003; **18**(suppl 6): S21–7.

19. Diederich NJ, Goetz CG, Stebbins GT. Repeated visual hallucinations in Parkinson's disease as disturbed external/internal perceptions: Focused review and a new integrative model. *Mov Disord* 2005; **20**: 130–40.

20. Kumar R, Behari S, Wahi J, *et al.* Peduncular hallucinosis: An unusual sequel to surgical intervention in the suprasellar region. *Br J Neurosurg* 1999; **13**: 500–03.

21. Parisis D, Poulios I, Karkavelas G, Drevelengas A, Artemis N, Karacostas D. Peduncular hallucinosis secondary to brainstem compression by cerebellar metastases. *Eur Neurol* 2003; **50**: 107–09.

22. Rozanski J. Peduncular hallucinosis following vertebral angiography. *Neurology* 1952; **2**: 341–9.

23. Eisenman L, Attarian H. Sleep epilepsy. *Can J Neurol Sci* 1985; **12**: 317–20.

24. Herman ST, Walczak TS, Bazil CW. Distribution of partial seizures during the sleep–wake cycle: Differences by seizure onset site. *Neurology* 2001; **56**: 1453–9.

25. Theodore WH, Porter RJ, Albert P, *et al.* The secondarily generalized tonic–clonic seizure: A videotape analysis. *Neurology* 1994; **44**: 1403–07.

26. Theodore WH, Porter RJ, Penry JK. Complex partial seizures: Clinical characteristics and differential diagnosis. *Neurology* 1983; **33**: 1115–21.

27. Williamson PD, Spencer DD, Spencer SS, *et al.* Complex partial seizures of frontal lobe origin. *Ann Neurol* 1985; **18**: 497–504.

28. Kellinghaus C, Luders HO, Wyllie E. Classification of seizures. In Wyllie E, Gupta A, Lachhwani DK (Eds), *The Treatment of Epilepsy: Principles and Practice*. Philadelphia: Lippincott Williams & Wilkins, 2006; 226.

29. Mauguière F. Scope and presumed mechanisms of hallucinations in partial epileptic seizures. *Epileptic Disord* 1999; **1**: 81–91.

30. Penfield W, Jasper H. *Epilepsy and the Functional Anatomy of the Human Brain*. Boston: Little, Brown, 1954.

31. Hupp SL, Kline LB, Corbett JJ. Visual disturbances of migraine. *Surv Ophthalmol* 1989; **33**: 221–36.

32. Hadjikhani N, Sanchez Del Rio M, Wu O, *et al.* Mechanisms of migraine aura revealed by functional MRI in human visual cortex. *Proc Natl Acad Sci USA* 2001; **10**: 4687–92.

33. Mamelak M, Black J, Montplaisir J, Ristanovic R. A pilot study on the effects of sodium oxybate on sleep architecture and daytime alertness in narcolepsy. *Sleep* 2004; **27**: 1327–34.

34. The US Xyrem Multicenter Study Group. A randomized, double blind, placebo-controlled

multicenter trial comparing the effects of three doses of orally administered sodium oxybate with placebo for the treatment of narcolepsy. *Sleep* 2002; **25**; 42–9.
35. Rongve A, Aarsland D. Management of Parkinson's disease dementia: Practical considerations. *Drugs Aging* 2006; **23**: 807–22.
36. Ray WA, Chung CP, Murray KT, Kall K, Stein CM. Atypical antipsychotic drugs and the risk of sudden cardiac death. *N Eng J Med* 2009; **360**: 225–35.
37. Sachs C, Svanborg E. The exploding head syndrome: Polysomnographic recordings and therapeutic suggestions. *Sleep* 1991; **14**: 263–6.
38. Pierce JMS. Clinical features of the exploding head syndrome. *J Neurol Neurosurg Psychiatr* 1989; **52**: 907–10.
39. Jacome DE. Exploding head syndrome and idiopathic stabbing headache relieved by nifedipine. *Cephalalgia* 2001; **21**: 617–8.

Section 4 Chapter 21

Other parasomnias

Sleep-related eating disorder

John W. Winkelman

Eating and sleep are both under the control of circadian influences, such that sleep usually occurs at night and food intake predominates during the day. The recent explosion of interest in the relationship of food intake, metabolism, sleep, and circadian rhythms is based on advances in sleep and circadian physiology as well as societal increases in obesity and sleep deprivation. We will review clinical disorders in which the daily pattern of food intake is dysregulated such that eating occurs at night during the sleep period.

Historical perspective on pathological night-time eating

In 1955, Stunkard, Grace and Wolff described a pattern of eating they called "Night-Eating Syndrome" (NES) to characterize 16 obese patients whose inability to lose weight in a monitored diet program confounded them [1]. After further analysis, they discovered that the patients were consuming a substantial fraction of their daily calories at night. In the first 30 years after this initial publication, only a handful of case reports [2–4] were added to the existing literature on the topic [5]. However, in the last 20 years, there has been a renewed interest in the topic, both in the medical literature and lay media. Problematic night-time eating has been featured on multiple popular television programs and magazines, exposing the general public to the recognition of nocturnal eating as a medical disorder, in the same way that daytime eating disorders such as anorexia nervosa, bulimia nervosa, and binge-eating disorder gained both popular and scientific interest.

The three original criteria for NES were evening hyperphagia, defined as consuming a quarter or more of daily calories after the evening meal, difficulty falling asleep, and morning anorexia [1]. Although the term has remained the same, the criteria for NES have been, and continue to be, modified in areas such as the amount of calories eaten during evening hyperphagia, the timing of the eating, the state of awareness during the eating, the effect on mood, and its distinctions from bulimia nervosa and binge-eating disorder. As evidence of this, de Zwaan *et al.* found that subjects varied in the degree to which they met sets of historical and recent diagnostic criteria for nocturnal eating disorders. Some individuals in the sample met multiple sets of diagnostic criteria, and others none at all [6]. This may indicate an inadequacy in the current standards to identify and diagnose individuals suffering from night-time eating. Unfortunately, this also leads to complexities in interpreting the results of various descriptive and interventional reports, as heterogeneity in patient sample compositions can certainly influence results.

Much of the early investigation into NES was performed from the perspective that night eating was a variant of a daytime eating disorder. More recently, this work has been supplemented by investigations of patients who initially presented to sleep disorders medicine clinics. In that context, such patients are generally diagnosed with sleep-related eating disorder (SRED). Unfortunately, although they often see overlapping groups of patients, treatment of, and investigation into, nocturnal eating disorders continues to be split into these two groups of clinicians and researchers, using two sets of definitions, with two sets of diagnostic work-ups. As a result, investigators from the eating disorders community continue to describe patients with NES, who are generally characterized as having an atypical eating disorder. On the other hand, patients who predominantly have eating after nocturnal awakenings, particularly if they have alterations in the level of consciousness during eating, are seen by those in the sleep disorders community, evaluated by polysomnography (PSG), and diagnosed with SRED, according to the *International Classification of Sleep Disorders* (ICSD-2).

For the purposes of this review within a book on parasomnias, we will focus on the latter group of patients, although we will make reference to differential diagnosis with NES. However, clinicians seeing such patients will be at a great disadvantage without a perspective that includes both eating and sleep disorders, as pathological night-time eating combines features of a daytime eating disorder with those of a parasomnia. There is compulsive, driven eating, with next-day anorexia and undesirable weight gain, characteristic of eating disorders. However, additionally, patients with SRED often exhibit features of parasomnias, especially arousal disorders, such as partial arousals early in the sleep period, characterized by confusion, automatic behavior, and relative unresponsiveness to external stimuli, followed by impaired recollection of the behavior. It is this combination of behavioral features of disparate disorders which makes SRED a challenge from both pathophysiologic and therapeutic perspectives.

Definition and characteristics of SRED

The 1990 edition of the *International Classification of Sleep Disorders* (ICSD) included the diagnosis of nocturnal eating/drinking syndrome (NEDS), which at the time was "characterized by recurrent awakenings, with the inability to return to sleep without eating or drinking" [7]. More recently, the revised edition of the ICSD has removed NEDS and has added the term sleep-related eating disorder (SRED) (see Table 21.1). According to the ICSD-2, the diagnostic features of SRED include "out of control" or involuntary eating during arousals from sleep, which can occur at any point along a spectrum of level of consciousness, from partial and/or confusional awakenings from sleep, with subsequent partial recollection of the event, to full awareness during nocturnal eating, with subsequent unimpaired memory for the event. As with most behaviors classified as a disorder, negative consequences are a requirement and include ingestion of abnormal combinations of food, or toxic substances, complaints of non-restorative sleep or daytime sleepiness/fatigue, sleep-related injury, morning anorexia, or weight gain [8]. Finally, the nocturnal eating cannot be better explained by another disorder such as hypoglycemia, peptic ulcer disease, or other sleep disorders.

Table 21.1 Current ICDS-2 definition and diagnostic criteria for SRED.

A. Recurrent episodes of involuntary eating and drinking occur during the main sleep period.

B. One or more of the following must be present with the recurrent episodes of involuntary eating and drinking:
  1. Consumption of peculiar forms or combinations of food or inedible or toxic substances.
  2. Insomnia related to sleep disruption from repeated episodes of eating, with a complaint of non-restorative sleep, daytime fatigue, or somnolence
  3. Sleep-related injury
  4. Dangerous behaviors performed while in pursuit of food or while cooking food
  5. Morning anorexia
  6. Adverse health consequences from recurrent binge eating of high-caloric food

C. The disturbance is not better explained by another sleep disorder, medical or neurological disorder, mental disorder, medication use or substance use disorder (hypoglycemic states, peptic ulcer disease, reflux esophagitis, Kleine–Levin syndrome, Kluver–Bucy syndrome, and night-time extension of daytime anorexia nervosa (binge/purge subtype), bulimia nervosa, and binge eating disorder).

*(American Academy of Sleep Medicine, 2005 [8]).

Patients with SRED generally arouse from sleep and eat within the first 1–4 h after sleep onset. Eating episodes are initiated after patients "make a beeline" to the kitchen, and are characterized by rapid ingestion of food, which the patient usually reports as "out of control". A preference for high caloric foods (sweets, peanut butter, chips) is common, with ingestion of non-edible or toxic items also occasionally reported. Patients will often deny hunger associated with episodes, but rather report a drive to eat. Some will report the belief that they will be unable to return to sleep unless they eat. The level of consciousness during nocturnal eating ranges from full awareness to dense unawareness typical of a somnambulistic episode. Many patients report that episodes occur somewhere in the middle of this spectrum, describing themselves as "half-awake, half-asleep". Obviously, however, a precise description of the level of consciousness is very difficult, as it is impossible to describe oneself (at the time, or later) as unconscious. Therefore, the latter judgment is usually made by the patient based on the level of recollection for the episode in the morning. For this reason, the extent of next-day amnesia for the episode usually correlates with the self-reported level of consciousness during the episode. Further complicating this issue is that the level of awareness can vary within an episode, across episodes within one night and over the longitudinal course (often of years) of the disorder. For instance, some individuals will describe "coming to" full alertness during an episode, find themselves eating, and will then return to bed.

The most common daytime consequences of SRED are daytime fatigue from the repetitive nocturnal awakenings and weight gain due to the large number of calories consumed during these night-time eating episodes. The frequency of episodes can range from once a week to 10 times in the same night. While patients may make behavioral changes to try to control their night-time eating, such as locking cabinets or doors, compensatory behaviors, such as excessive exercise or self-induced vomiting, which are often seen in daytime eating disorders, are rarely present [9]. However, morning anorexia, or reduction in daytime caloric intake, in response to overeating throughout the night is common with SRED, at times simulating a daytime eating disorder, in this case as a secondary disorder.

Differential diagnosis of SRED and NES

As described above, it is unclear whether SRED and NES constitute independent disorders, exist along a continuum, or in fact should be lumped under the same diagnosis. Nevertheless, a better understanding of what is known about these two sets of patients may assist clinicians in defining an appropriate clinical assessment, prognosis, and treatment for pathological nocturnal eating. According to the nosologies identified by researchers in these areas, the major distinctions between NES and SRED include (1) the level of consciousness during nocturnal eating, (2) the timing of nocturnal eating, and (3) the rate of comorbid sleep disorders present in those with nocturnal eating. However, it should be recognized that these distinctions may be spurious, and based on the extent of the diagnostic workup (e.g. evaluation for primary sleep disorders).

Whereas the majority of patients with SRED in the published literature report being either "asleep" or "half-asleep" during night-time eating episodes [9,10], those with NES report being fully awake and aware during them [11]. Similarly, subsequent recall of the event is often impaired in those with SRED, whereas it is always maintained in patients with NES [11]. This lowered state of consciousness may also account for why some patients with SRED ingest inedible or toxic substances and patients with NES do not. The value of this distinguishing feature has been called into question by the variable level of consciousness seen in patients with SRED, both within a single night and across the longitudinal course of the disorder. Similarly, most investigations of patients with NES by those in the eating disorders community have not specifically addressed the level of consciousness during night-time eating, making conclusions regarding this feature of NES unreliable. Recently, an item assessing the level of awareness during nocturnal eating was added to the Night Eating Questionnaire, a psychometric scale developed to assess the severity of NES [12]. Although the item was included specifically for the purpose of distinguishing NES from SRED, the level at which ("not at all [aware]", "a little", "somewhat", "very much so", and "completely") the authors distinguished NES from SRED is not made clear. In keeping with the uncertain value of this feature of nocturnal eating as a diagnostic criterion, the revised ICSD-2 has not made a reduced level of awareness, or amnesia, diagnostic features for SRED.

The timing of nocturnal eating is another potential feature distinguishing SRED from NES. Whereas individuals with SRED, by definition, report awakenings from sleep to eat, those with NES may eat either before bed (as in the original cases of Stunkard) or at night-time awakenings, the important criterion being that greater than one-third of all calories be consumed after the evening meal [13]. Thus, whereas sleep-related awakenings are the focus of SRED, a shift in caloric consumption to night-time is the focus of NES.

Another potential characteristic distinguishing SRED from NES is the common comorbidity between SRED and sleep disorders such as sleepwalking, restless legs syndrome (RLS)/periodic limb movements of sleep (PLMS) or obstructive sleep apnea (OSA) (see below). This association is not common in patients with NES, although very few studies of NES patients have included a thorough evaluation for sleep disorders (including polysomnography), and furthermore, many of the studies of patients with NES specifically excluded those with clinical suggestion of a primary sleep disorder (e.g. sleepwalking, OSA). For instance, one polysomnographic study found that subjects with NES had complete EEG arousal during episodes of night-time eating [14]. However, this is not surprising, as, in keeping with a diagnosis of NES (which excludes SRED), subjects in this study were specifically excluded if they "lacked awareness of their night eating" or had amnesia for the episodes.

While SRED and NES may be described as independent disorders with distinct clinical presentations, in fact many of the features often overlap. This has prompted a proposed continuum of night-time eating behavior rather than a categorical differentiation of NES and SRED [15]. The current ICSD-2 nosology, by including night-time eating that occurs along the full spectrum of consciousness, is potentially a move toward viewing NES and SRED along a single continuum. In fact, many patients with NES do meet SRED criteria. On the other hand, nocturnal eating which occurs in an altered state of awareness is commonly considered exclusionary for NES.

Demographics of SRED

The prevalence of SRED in the general population is unknown. Winkelman et al. reported that 16.7% of individuals who were part of an in-patient eating disorders program, 8.7% of those in an out-patient eating disorders program, 4.6% of college students, 1.0% of obese individuals in a weight loss program, and 3.4% of those in an out-patient depression clinic reported behavior consistent with SRED [16]. Schenck et al. reviewed a sample of patients referred to a sleep disorders clinic over a 7-year period and found that 0.5% of these patients fulfilled criteria for SRED [10,17]. It should be noted, however, that these studies predated the current ICSD-2 criteria, and used clinical, and varying, definitions of SRED. On the other hand, the prevalence of NES has been investigated more frequently, both in specialized groups and in the general population. However, the prevalence has varied from 0.4 to 13.7% in community samples, and from 6 to 64% in surgical and weight loss samples [18]. When NES was specifically defined as excessive evening eating, tension and/or feeling upset during the evening hours, insomnia, and morning anorexia, the prevalence was estimated at 1.5% in the general population [19].

SRED appears to be more prevalent in women than in men, comprising two-thirds to over three-quarters of patient cases. The female predominance of SRED mimics the higher prevalence rates of daytime eating disorders (anorexia nervosa and bulimia nervosa) in women than in men. The onset of SRED generally occurs during the late teenage years or twenties, and its course is often chronic in nature. However, naturalistic longitudinal studies are lacking in SRED, and it is unclear whether the apparent chronicity is an artifact of the self-selection commonly observed in clinical settings or is truly a feature of the disorder. A number of case series, starting with Winkelman in 1993, have demonstrated a familial aspect to SRED [9,17,20,21]. One such series found that 26% of the SRED probands reported having family members who also experienced night-time eating episodes [9]. Three other series reported familial connections in 21, 19 and 27% of their SRED patients, respectively [17,21,22]. Although such data are certainly far from definitive, it is not surprising that SRED has a familial component as both daytime eating disorders and somnambulism have genetic influences [23,24].

Consequences of SRED

Weight gain is the most common, and often most troublesome, adverse effect associated with SRED, and is one of the diagnostic features of SRED in ICSD-2. This is not surprising, as consumption of high calorie foods during night-time eating episodes can certainly cause unwanted weight gain. In one case series [9], 39% of patients presenting with SRED were overweight (BMI $\geq$ 25), while in another series [21], 15% were overweight (30 > BMI $\geq$ 25) and 30% were obese (BMI $\geq$ 30). Another important consequence, psychological distress, has been noted in patients with SRED due to feelings of "lack of control", shame, guilt, and helplessness over night-time eating [5].

In terms of overall diet, medically necessary dietary restrictions (e.g. for patients with diabetes, renal/liver failure, or those on MAOI inhibitors) can be broken during uncontrolled night-time eating, either leading to, or exacerbating, pre-existing health problems [5,10].

Multiple night-time awakening and eating episodes also disrupt sleep, which can lead to daytime fatigue or frank excessive daytime sleepiness. Accidents involving falls, burns, and cuts while in search of food, during food preparation or consumption are also a concern, especially with patients who report reduced alertness during episodes. Although not the norm, some patients will also ingest non-edible and/or toxic substances such as buttered cigarettes and cleaning supplies [18,25,26].

Associations of SRED with other disorders

Sleep disorders

Polysomnographic (PSG) studies of patients with SRED demonstrate a high prevalence of concurrent sleep disorders such as somnambulism (sleepwalking), periodic limb movement disorder (PLMD), restless legs syndrome (RLS), obstructive sleep apnea (OSA) and circadian-rhythm disorders [19,27]. Schenck et al. found that 84% of SRED patients in their sample had a history of somnambulism, 13% had RLS and 10% had OSA [10,17]. Nearly half (48%) of another sample of SRED patients met criteria for somnambulism, 26% had periodic leg movements of sleep, and 13% had OSA [9]. Conversely, a recent study from Italy demonstrated that one-third of patients with RLS had a lifetime history of SRED (according to ICSD criteria), compared to only 1% of matched controls [28]. Two-thirds of the RLS patients with SRED currently met criteria for SRED, whereas one-third no longer had such symptoms. In a video-polysomnographic study of 35 patients with SRED, Vetrugno et al. demonstrated PLMS in 63% of patients, and periodic movements of facial muscles in 83% of the patients. The bruxing movements included recurrent chewing and swallowing motions that were present in all sleep stages and linked to arousal approximately 50% of the time [29].

Eating disorders

There is a high rate of comorbidity between SRED and daytime eating disorders, which include anorexia and bulimia. Two case series found that a high percentage of those with SRED also showed signs of daytime disordered eating. In the first [9], originating from a psychiatrically based sleep disorders clinic, 40% of those with SRED were also diagnosed with an eating disorder, while the second [21], composed of individuals responding to a national television program, found elevated scores on the Eating Attitudes Test (EAT) in 40% of the SRED sample. Conversely, one prevalence study [16] demonstrated that patients diagnosed with an eating disorder are more likely to have SRED than other subgroups (obese, depressed, or unselected college students), which was confirmed by Gupta, who found a 30% prevalence of SRED in patients with bulimia nervosa (BN) [30].

Mood disorders

Reports of depression and anxiety in patients with SRED have been frequent. In prevalence studies, higher rates of depression have been found in individuals with SRED than in their non-SRED counterparts [16]. In one case series, 70% of respondents had a history of depression [21]. In most such cases it is unclear if the mood disturbances preceded onset of SRED or if SRED may have caused or exacerbated the problem. Certainly, both sleep disruption and comorbid sleep disorders (e.g. RLS, OSA) are associated with an elevated rate of mood disorders.

Physiology of SRED

Very little work on the underlying physiology of SRED has been performed, which unfortunately reflects the paucity of knowledge regarding the pathophysiology of parasomnias in general. However, some avenues of investigation appear promising, including the association of SRED with primary sleep disorders, neuroendocrine studies of NES, and recent animal genetic knockouts which reflect some of the symptoms observed in SRED.

Comorbid sleep disorders and medications

Underlying sleep disorders may precipitate an episode of nocturnal eating in the same way that endogenous or exogenous stimuli may initiate an episode of somnambulism. Partial arousals caused by OSA, RLS, and PeLMS have been reported to sometimes result in a night-time eating episode [9]. Even though this connection has been noted, it is unknown why, in some patients, night-time eating results from this arousal. Vetrugno et al. noted that the prevalence of RLS, PLMS, which may be mediated dopaminergically, as well as the findings supporting some therapeutic benefit of dopaminergic agents in the treatment of SRED (discussed in the next section), may implicate dopaminergic pathways in the pathophysiology of the disorder [29].

Prescribed medications may also produce episodes of SRED. In particular, multiple case series report the onset of SRED with zolpidem use [31]. Morgenthaler and Silber described zolpidem-induced SRED in three patients with no previous history of night-time eating, and two who had previous night-time eating which worsened in frequency and in the degree of amnesia for the event. All five patients had resolution of

SRED after discontinuation of zolpidem and treatment of other current sleep disorders (all five had RLS). The fact that there were multiple simultaneous interventions in these patients make it impossible to determine causality, yet the use of zolpidem may have been the factor which induced or aggravated the presenting SRED [32]. Chiang and Krystal reported two cases in which SRED occurred while the patients were on extended-release zolpidem but not immediate-release zolpidem, indicating that it is possible for small variations in formulation to produce a differential effect on the potential precipitation of SRED for some patients [33]. Additional medications which may precipitate SRED include triazolam, first- and second-generation anti-psychotics and lithium carbonate [8].

Neuroendocrine studies in NES

The primary hypothesis regarding the origin of pathological nocturnal eating in NES is that the circadian rhythm of eating is delayed with respect to the underlying rhythms controlling sleep, which remain normal. Both out-patient (using actigraphy) and in-patient (using polysomnongraphy) studies demonstrate that sleep onset and offset in NES are similar to that of control subjects [13,14]. However, as would be expected in patients with NES, there is a temporal redistribution of daily energy intake, with consumption of food both before bedtime as well as during nocturnal awakenings. Phase delays in the circadian rhythms of the hormones leptin, insulin and melatonin have been demonstrated in patients with NES compared to normal controls [34,35]. Leptin, which usually rises nocturnally, is involved in regulation of metabolism and appetite; melatonin, which also rises nocturnally, supports and maintains sleep [36]. Elevated plasma cortisol levels were also observed in NES patients and may indicate a rise in corticotropin releasing hormone (CRH) [35]. CRH acts to suppress melatonin secretion and this rise may be the origin of the observed attenuation in the melatonin levels. However, as nocturnal awakenings and eating can both influence the underlying neuroendocrine patterns, it is difficult to tell if these physiological alterations are causes or effects of problematic night-time eating.

Genetic studies

A promising approach to understanding the pathophysiology of SRED involves the use of mutant mouse models. In two intriguing models in which clock genes are knocked out, *Clock* [37] and *mPer2* [38], mice consume substantially more food during their normally inactive (light) period. When kept on a high-fat diet, they gain substantial amounts of weight. Injections of alpha melanocyte stimulating hormone at the beginning of the light period suppress the abnormal eating. Such models should allow an increased understanding of the interrelated roles of the circadian and metabolic systems and may, in the future, play a role in testing hypotheses and even treatments for SRED.

Treatment

In the absence of adequate medical guidance related to treatment of SRED, most individuals with nighttime eating have attempted multiple "home remedies", often with little success. These may include benign approaches such as eating a meal prior to bedtime, limiting the amount and types of food in the house, locking the refrigerator and cabinets, and self-hypnosis. More exaggerated and sometimes dangerous countermeasures include tying themselves to the bed or barricading themselves in the bedroom. The recent success of some pharmacologic approaches gives sufferers with SRED more hope. Furthermore, non-pharmacological treatments which have proven valuable in daytime eating disorders (cognitive behavioral therapy) and somnambulism (hypnosis) may also have value in the future for treatment of SRED.

Pharmacologic treatments for SRED (and NES) are either derived from effective therapeutics in related disorders (e.g. bulimia nervosa or somnambulism) or those useful in disorders which are commonly comorbid with nocturnal eating disorders (e.g. RLS).

Treatment of sleep disorders that cause fragmentation of sleep, such as RLS, PLMD or OSA, may be of value in the treatment of SRED, possibly by reducing the number of arousals from sleep which may drive nocturnal eating episodes. In particular, RLS may predispose to nocturnal eating, as it produces fragmented sleep as well as the inability to stay in bed at awakenings. It is thus not surprising that Schenck *et al.* found that dopaminergic agents (carbidopa/L-dopa; bromocriptine) were effective in 52% (14/27) of his cases with SRED, five of whom had RLS or PLMD [17]. On the other hand, a randomized, double-blind, placebo-controlled crossover pilot study of pramipexole (up to .36 mg, 3 weeks each of active drug and placebo) in 11 overweight subjects with SRED demonstrated improvements in actigraphically monitored nocturnal activity and "the number of good nights of sleep per week", although eating outcomes related to SRED showed no improvement, and no weight loss was observed [22].

Benzodiazepines were of value in 37% (10/27) of all SRED cases reported by Schenck, nearly 60% of whom had a diagnosis of sleepwalking [17]. These findings must be balanced against the previous data reporting an increase in nocturnal eating with the benzodiazepine receptor agonist zolpidem. One potential explanation for this apparent inconsistency is that individuals with somnambulism may be responsive to these agents, whereas those with other underlying causes of SRED (or whose level of consciousness is less impaired than the sleepwalkers) may have their nocturnal eating worsened.

Treatments that are employed to manage daytime eating disorders may also be beneficial in controlling night-time eating episodes. Both an open-label and a double-blind, flexible dose study of sertraline (up to 200 mg) demonstrated substantial benefit for patients with NES who did not have impaired recollection for nocturnal eating and did not meet criteria for a DSM-IV eating or mood disorder [13,39]. Sertraline, at a mean dose of 127 mg, led to treatment response (much or very much improved) in 71% of subjects, whereas only 18% of those given placebo met this standard. Those given sertraline reduced nocturnal eating episodes by over 80% (from 8.3 to 1.6 episodes per week) and had mild weight loss.

Topiramate, an FDA approved anticonvulsant, was originally found to produce weight loss in treatment trials for epilepsy, bipolar disorder, and migraine headaches, and reduce binge episodes in patients with binge-eating disorder (BED) [40,41]. It was originally used in a case series of four patients with SRED, with substantial reduction in night-time eating [27]. In a larger and more recent retrospective case series, 68% of 25 patients with SRED were topiramate responders (mean dose of 135 mg) as measured by the Clinical Global Impression of Improvement (CGI-I) [42]. Although substantial weight loss was observed in over one-quarter of responders, nearly half of the responders discontinued topiramate after a mean of 12 months due to side effects, predominantly cognitive dulling, paresthesias, and daytime sleepiness. It is unclear how topiramate works to manage night-time eating behaviors; however, it was hypothesized that topiramate may work to suppress arousals produced by underlying sleep disorders (e.g. RLS) or act as an anorexigenic agent, either though glutamatergic antagonism or serotonin agonism [27]. In addition, topiramate stimulates insulin release and increases insulin sensitivity, both of which may contribute to appetite regulation and weight loss [43,44].

Additional pharmacologic interventions for SRED have included agents such as melatonin, D-fenfluramine (now off the market), gamma-hydroxybutyric acid, oxazepam, and sibutramine [8]. Further controlled clinical trials of pharmacological agents for the treatment of SRED are warranted.

Summary

Sleep-related eating disorder combines features of a sleep disorder and an eating disorder, such that individuals eat during partial or complete arousal from sleep. Those who present for clinical attention often have a chronic course, with near-nightly eating episodes, and have a variety of daytime consequences of this behavior, including weight gain, daytime fatigue, and mood disorders. Currently, treatment is directed towards underlying sleep disorders, when present, or otherwise involve the empiric use of serotonergic anti-depressants or topiramate.

References

1. Stunkard AJ, Grace WJ, Wolff HG. The night-eating syndrome; a pattern of food intake among certain obese patients. *Am J Med* 1955; **19**: 78–86.
2. Coates TJ. Successful self-management strategies toward coping with night eating. *J Behav Ther Exp Psychiatry* 1978; **9**: 181–3.
3. Guirguis WR. Sleepwalking as a symptom of bulimia. *Br Med J* 1986; **293**: 587–8.
4. Oswald IO, Adam K. Rhythmic raiding of the refrigerator related to rapid eye movement sleep. *Br Med J* 1986; **292**: 589.
5. Montgomery L, Haynes L. What every nurse needs to know about nocturnal sleep-related eating disorder. *J Psychosoc Nurs Ment Health Serv* 2001; **39**(8): 14–20.
6. de Zwaan M, Roerig DB, Crosby RD, *et al*. Night time eating: A descriptive study. *Int J Eat Disord* 2006; **39**: 224–32.
7. American Academy of Sleep Medicine. *The International Classification of Sleep Disorders (Revised): Diagnostic and Coding Manual*. Rochester, MN: American Academy of Sleep Medicine, 1990.

8. American Academy of Sleep Medicine. *The International Classification of Sleep Disorders (Revised-2): Diagnostic and Coding Manual*. Rochester, MN: American Academy of Sleep Medicine, 2005.
9. Winkelman JW. Clinical and polysomnography features of sleep-related eating disorder. *J Clin Psychiatry* 1998; **59**: 14–19.
10. Schenck CH, Hurwitz TD, Bundlie SR, *et al*. Sleep-related eating disorders: Polysomnographic correlates of a heterogeneous syndrome distinct from daytime eating disorders. *Sleep* 1991; **5**: 419–31.
11. O'Reardon JP, Peshek A, Allison KC. Night eating syndrome: Diagnosis, epidemiology and management. *CNS Drugs* 2005; **12**: 997–1008.
12. Allison KC, Lundgren JD, O'Reardon JP, *et al*. The Night Eating Questionnaire (NEQ): Psychometric properties of a measure of severity of the Night Eating Syndrome. *Eat Behav* 2008; **9**: 62–72.
13. O'Reardon JP, Ringel BL, Dinges DF, *et al*. Circadian eating and sleeping patterns in the night eating syndrome. *Obes Res* 2004; **12**: 1789–96.
14. Rogers NL, Dinges DF, Allison KC, *et al*. Assessment of sleep in women with night eating syndrome. *Sleep* 2006; **29**: 814–9.
15. Winkelman JW. Sleep-related eating disorder and night eating syndrome: Sleep disorders, eating disorders, or both? *Sleep* 2006; **29**: 876–7.
16. Winkelman JW, Herzog DB, Fava M. The prevalence of sleep-related eating disorder in psychiatric and non-psychiatric populations. *Psychol Med* 1999; **29**: 1461–6.
17. Schenck CH, Hurwitz TD, O'Connor KA, *et al*. Additional categories of sleep-related eating disorders and the current status of treatment. *Sleep* 1993; **5**: 457–66.
18. de Zwaan M, Burgard MA, Schenck CH, *et al*. Night time eating: A review of the literature. *Eur Eat Disorders Rev* 2003; **11**: 7–24.
19. Rand CS, MacGregor AM, Stunkard AJ. The night eating syndrome in the general population and among postoperative obesity surgery patients. *Int J Eat Disord* 1997; **22**: 65–9.
20. Winkelman JW. Nocturnal binge eating is a familial disorder (abstract). *Sleep Res* 1993; **22**: 68.
21. Winkelman JW. Sleep-related eating disorder: The dateline dataset (abstract). *Sleep Research* 1997; **26**: 31.
22. Provini F, Albani F, Vetrugno R, *et al*. A pilot double-blind placebo-controlled trial of low-dose pramipexole in sleep-related eating disorder. *Eur J Neurol* 2005; **6**: 432–6.
23. Hudson JI, Lalonde JK, Berry JM, *et al*. Binge-eating disorder as a distinct familial phenotype in obese individuals. *Arch Gen Psychiatry* 2006; **63**: 313–9.
24. Kales A, Soldatos CR, Bixler EO, *et al*. Hereditary factors in sleepwalking and night terrors. *Br J Psychiatry* 1980; **137**: 111–8.
25. Schenck CH, Mahowald MW. Review of nocturnal sleep-related eating disorders. *Int J Eat Disord* 1994; **4**: 343–56.
26. Schenck CH, Mahowald MW. Parasomnias: Managing bizarre sleep-related behavior among certain obese patients. *Am J Med* 2000; **19**: 78–86.
27. Winkelman JW. Treatment of nocturnal eating syndrome and sleep-related eating disorder with topiramate. *Sleep Med* 2003; **4**: 243–6.
28. Provini F, Anetlmi E, Vignatelli L, *et al*. Association of restless legs syndrome with nocturnal eating: A case-control study. *Mov Disord* 2009 **24**: 871–7.
29. Vetrugno R, Manconi M, Ferini-Strambi L, *et al*. Nocturnal eating: Sleep-related eating disorder or night eating syndrome? A videopolysomnographic study. *Sleep* 2006; **29**: 949–54.
30. Gupta MA. Sleep-related eating in bulimia nervosa: And an underreported parasomnia disorder. *Sleep Res* 1991; **20**: 182.
31. Dolder CR, Nelson MH. Hypnosedative-induced complex behaviors: Incidence, mechanisms, and management. *CNS Drugs* 2008; **22**: 1021–36.
32. Morgenthaler TI, Silber MH. Amnestic sleep-related eating disorder associated with zolpidem. *Sleep Med* 2002; **3**: 323–7.
33. Chiang A, Krystal A. Report of two cases where sleep related eating behavior occurred with the extended-release formulation but not the immediate-release formulation of a sedative-hypnotic agent. *J Clin Sleep Med* 2008; **4**: 155–6.
34. Goel N, Stunkard A, Rogers N. Circadian rhythm profiles in women with night eating syndrome. *J Bio Rhythms* 2009; **24**: 85–94.
35. Birketvedt GS, Florholmen J, Sundsfjord J, *et al*. Behavioral and neuroendocrine characteristics of the night-eating syndrome. *J Am Med Assoc* 1999; **282**: 657–63.
36. Zhdanova IV, Wurtman RJ, Marabito C, *et al*. Effects of low oral dose of melatonin, given 2–4 hours before habitual bedtime, on sleep in normal young humans. *Sleep* 1996; **19**: 423–31.
37. Turek FW, Joshu C, Kohsaka A, *et al*. Obesity and metabolic syndrome in circadian clock mutant mice. *Science* 2005; **13**: 1043–5.
38. Yang S, Liu A, Weidenhammer A, *et al*. The role of mPer2 clock gene in glucocorticoid and

feeding rhythms. *Endocrinology* 2009; **150**: 2153–60.

39. O'Reardon JP, Allison KC, Martino NS, *et al*. A randomized, placebo-controlled trial of sertraline in the treatment of night eating syndrome. *Am J Psychiatry* 2006; **163**: 893–8.

40. Shapira NA, Goldsmith TD, McElroy SL. Treatment of binge-eating disorder with topiramate: A clinical case series. *J Clin Psychiatry* 2000; **5**: 368–72.

41. McElroy SL, Guerdjikova AI, Martens B, *et al*. Role of antiepileptic drugs in the management of eating disorders. *CNS Drugs* 2009; **23**: 139–56.

42. Winkelman JW. Efficacy and tolerability of open-label topiramate in the treatment of Sleep-Related Eating Disorder: A retrospective case series. *J Clin Psychiatry* 2006; **67**: 1729–34.

43. Liang Y, Chen X, Osborne M, *et al*. Topiramate ameliorates hyperglycaemia and improves glucose-stimulated insulin release in ZDF rats and db/db mice. *Diabetes Obes Metab* 2005; **7**: 360–9.

44. Wilkes JJ, Nelson E, Osborne M, *et al*. Topiramate is an insulin-sensitizing compound in vivo with direct effects on adipocytes in female ZDF rats. *Am J Physiol Endocrinol Metab* 2005; **288**: E617–24.

Figure 3.1 SPACET findings during sleepwalking after integration into the appropriate anatomical magnetic resonance image.

The highest increases of regional cerebral blood flow (>25%) during sleepwalking compared with quel stage 3 to 4 NREM sleep are found in the anterior cerebellum – i.e. vermis (A) and in the posterior cingulate cortex (Brodmann area 23 [Tallarch coordinate $x = -4$, $y = -40$, $z = 31$]. (B). However, in relation to data from normal volunteers during wakefulness ($n = 24$), large areas of frontal and parietal association cortices remain deactivated during sleepwalking, as shown in the corresponding parametrice maps (2-threshold = −3). Note the inclusion of the dorsolateral prefrontal cortex (C), mesial frontal cortex (D), and left angular gyrus (C) within these areas.

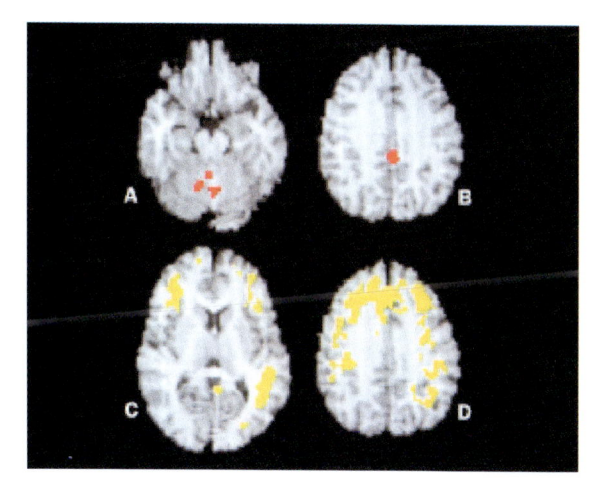

Figure 9.1 Posterior cingulate gyrus (red), active during sleepwalking, in relation to portion of the limbic system (yellow) controlling large segment of sexual behavior.

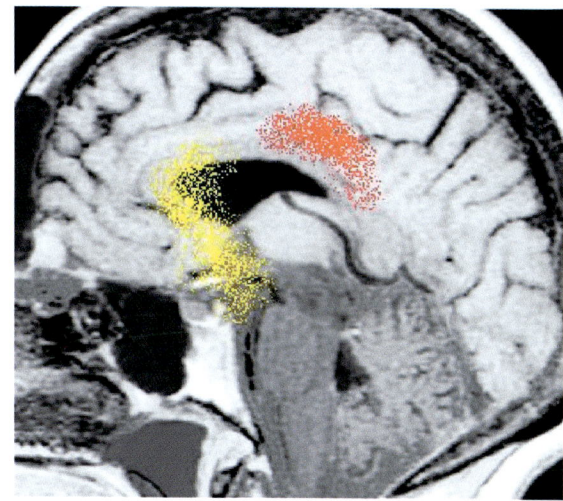

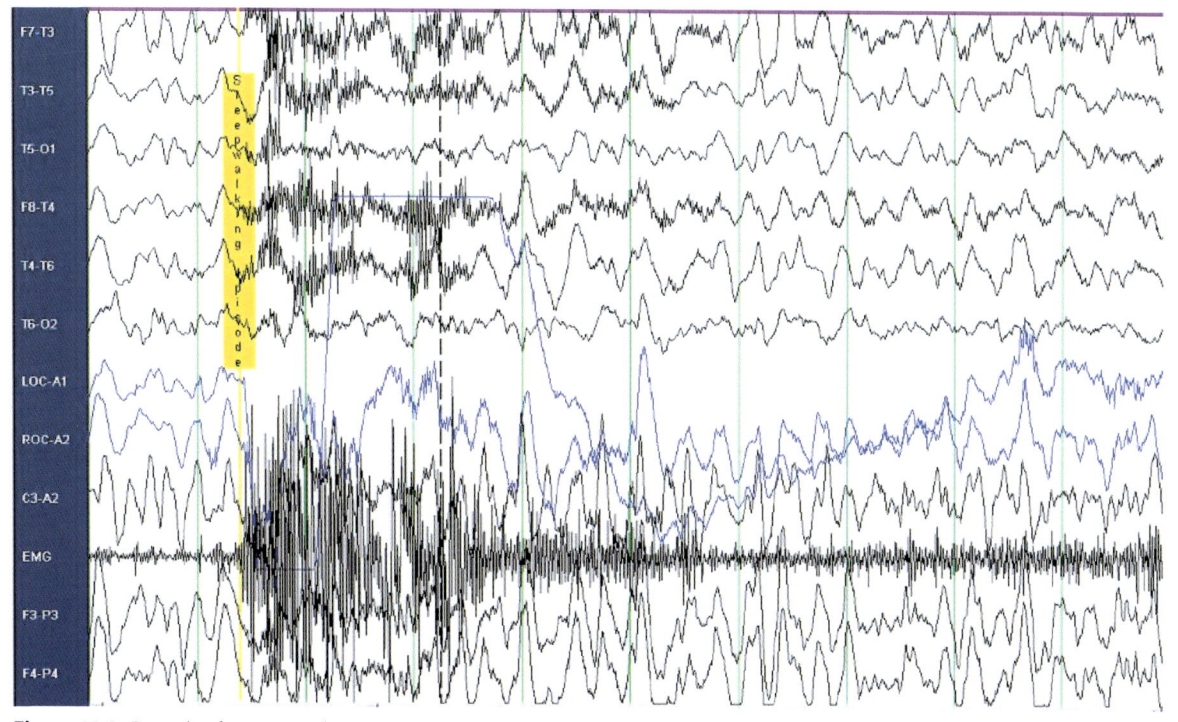

Figure 12.2 Example of post-arousal EEG pattern I during a behavioral episode from stage 4 sleep in a 19-year-old man. The EEG shows diffuse and rhythmic delta activity and is most predominant in the anterior regions.

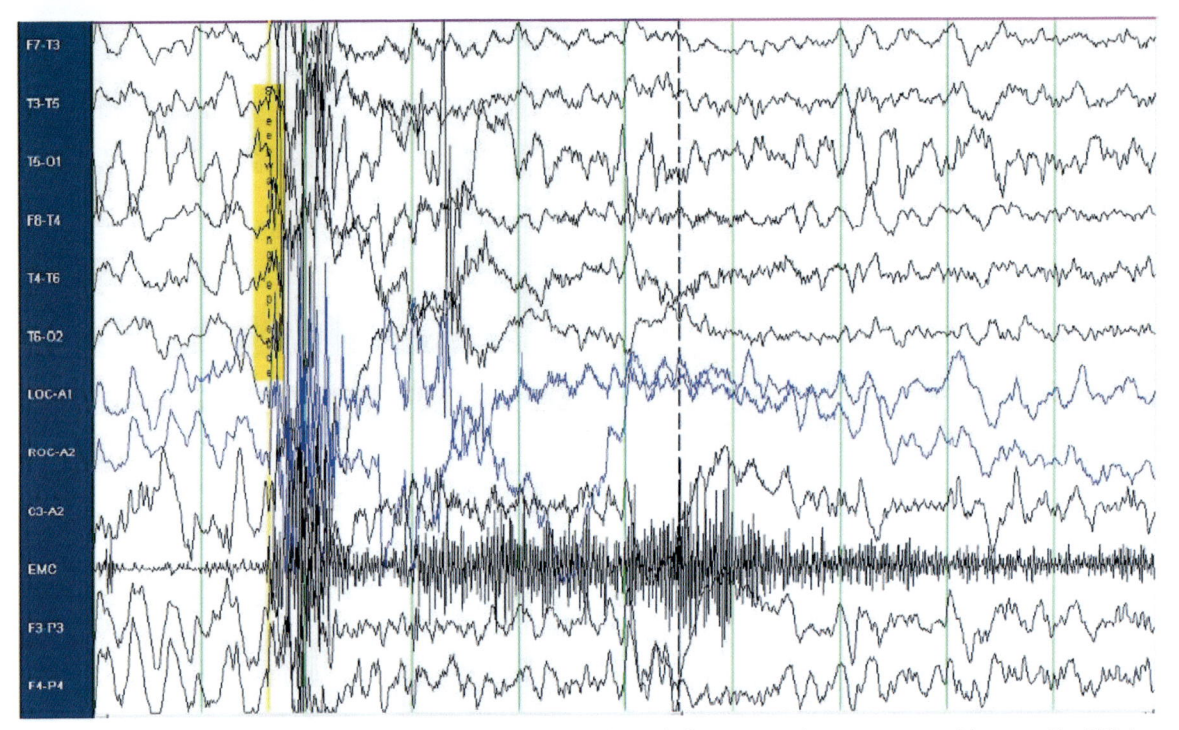

Figure 12.3 Example of post-arousal EEG pattern II during a behavioral episode from stage 4 sleep in a 23-year-old woman. The EEG shows irregular delta and theta activity intermixed with faster activity.

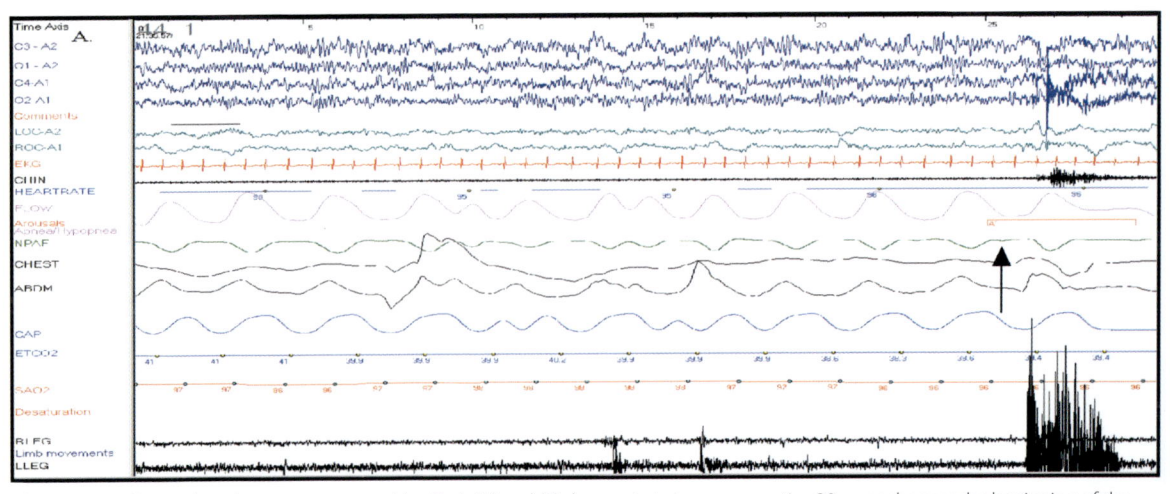

Figure 17.1 Overnight polysomnogram graphics. Both (A) and (B) demonstrate two consecutive 30-s epochs near the beginning of the study (22 min after lights out). (A) The patient is in wake–sleep transition (stage 1 NREM sleep), with fragmented alpha rhythm in the EEG and slow rolling eye movements (horizontal line). In the final 4 s of this epoch, there is an arousal (A1) marked by an increase in EEG frequencies and increased muscle activity (in the chin and leg leads). (B) The patient is awake with prominent leg movement, eye blinking, and increased baseline EEG activity. From this epoch forward, for nearly 2 h the patient remains awake and engaged in the episode described in the text.

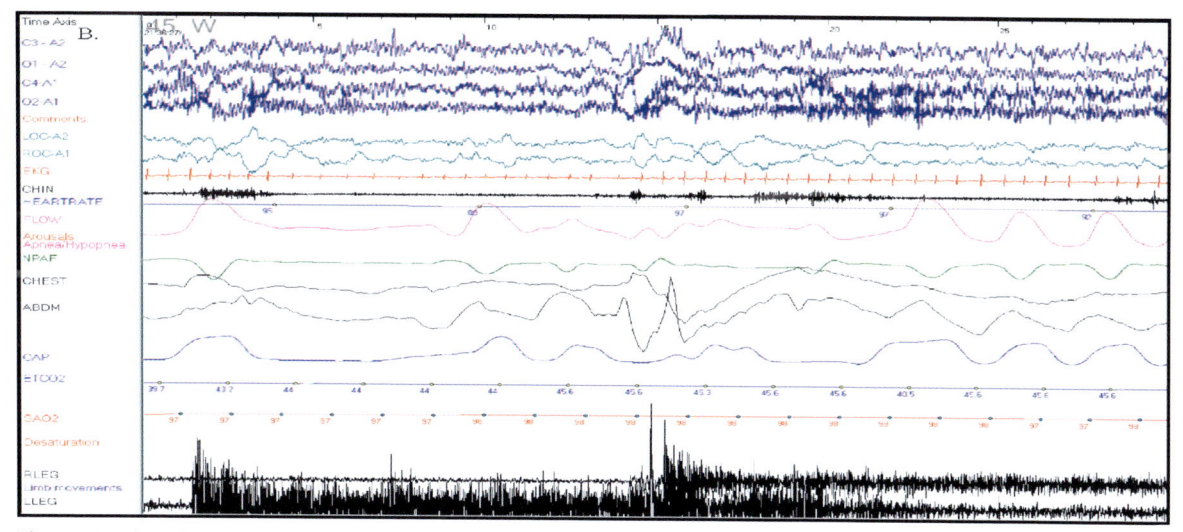

Figure 17.1 (cont.)

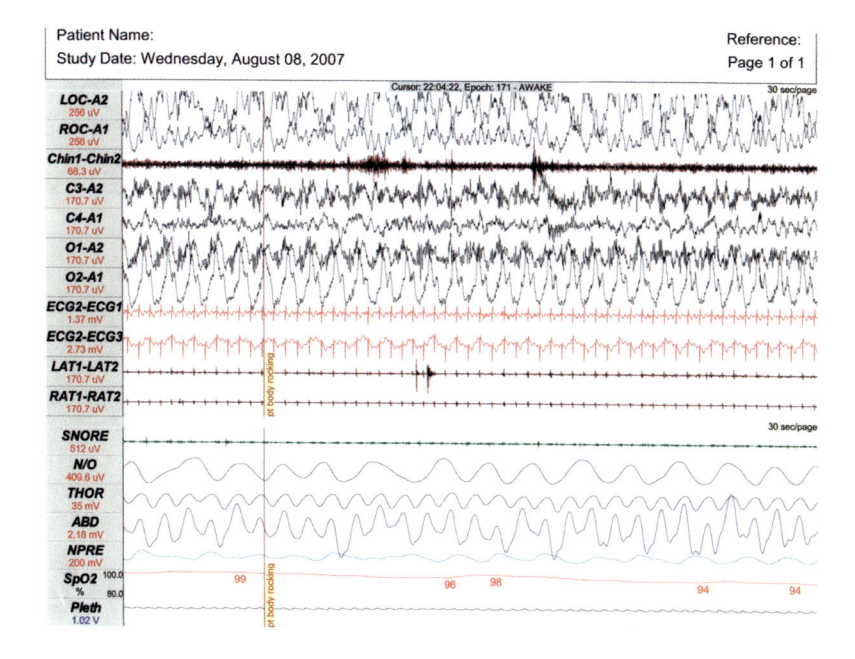

Figure 28.1 30-s PSG epoch illustrating body rocking during wakefulness in a 10-year-old girl. High amplitude 1 Hz movement artifact on EEG leads reflects rhythmic body movements.

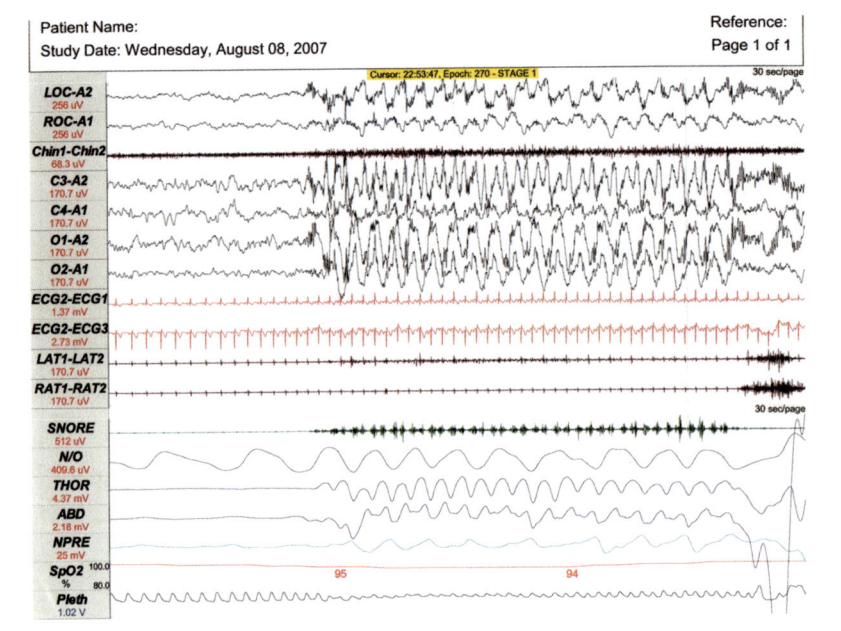

Figure 28.2 30-s PSG epoch illustrating body rocking arising from sleep in a 10-year-old girl. High amplitude 1 Hz movement artifact on EEG and EOG leads reflects rhythmic body movements. Activity on snore channel reflects vocalizations accompanying the episode.

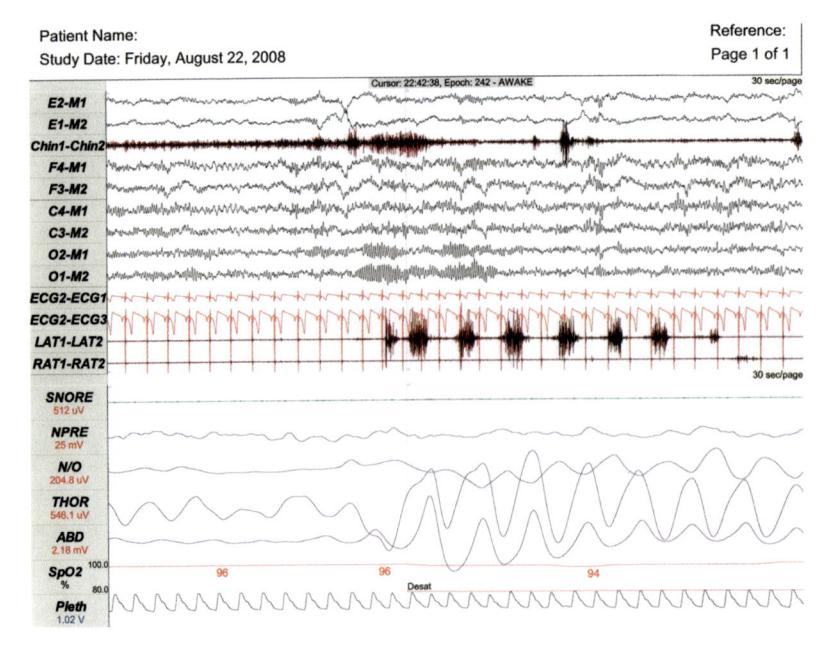

Figure 28.3 30-s PSG epoch for a 17-year-old male demonstrating leg rolling arising from wakefulness, characterized by rhythmic EMG activity seen exclusively in the left anterior tibialis lead (labeled LAT1-LAT2).

Section 5

Sleep-related movement disorders and other variants

Section 5 Chapter 22

Sleep-related movement disorders and other variants

Restless legs syndrome (RLS) and periodic leg movements (PLM)

Richard P. Allen

History

In many ways, restless legs syndrome (RLS) is a bit of an oddity in this book on parasomnias. Its inclusion here reflects the somewhat tortured history of our understanding of this major sleep–wake disorder. RLS occurs as a sensorimotor neurological disorder primarily affecting what the great neurologist Critchley referred to as the pre-dormitum, i.e. that state before sleep enabling the entry to sleep. Thus RLS presents mostly as a sensory disorder disturbing the resting wake state, although it also appears to cause awakenings during sleep. Although a sensory disorder, it has a non-specific motor sign of periodic leg movements (PLM). These leg movements occur both as periodic events while resting awake (PLMW) and during sleep (PLMS). PLMS occurring during sleep meet the classic definition of a parasomnia. Table 22.1 presents the sometimes confusing terminology used in this chapter.

The Oxford Don most famous for his description of the blood vessels at the base of the brain, the circle of Willis, in 1672 also provided the first medical description of RLS [1]. His fine description of an RLS patient still aptly describes the night-time distress with moderately severe RLS (see Table 22.2).

RLS after Willis remains largely ignored for the next 200 years. It is eventually described again in the nineteenth century in various forms often attributed to psychiatric problems, particularly anxiety [2]. The Swedish Neurologist Karl Ekbom provided the first careful description of the disorder. His monograph provided both the currently used name of restless legs syndrome and a better clinical description of the disorder [3,4]. He emphasized the sensory and even painful nature of the disorder and also its relation to iron deficiency.

The remarkable development of sleep medicine during the last half of the twentieth century was based largely on advances allowing all-night physiological recordings during sleep. These uncovered a remarkable and previously unknown abnormal movement pattern in sleep characterized as periodic leg movements. These events occurred for many but not most subjects recorded. They were first inappropriately labeled as sleep myoclonus [5]. However, they involve relatively smooth, predominately physiological flexor movements of the toes, foot and leg lasting 0.5–10 s. They do not fit the usual 'myoclonic' pattern. These were identified as a particularly common occurrence for most RLS patients [6].

Initially, there was considerable excitement about the discovery of these leg movements in sleep. It was felt they constituted in themselves a major sleep disturbance. This led to the development of the concept of a periodic limb movement disorder (PLMD) characterized by these PLMS disrupting sleep, thereby causing either insomnia at night and/or sleepiness in the daytime. Unfortunately it was soon discovered that aside from the relation to RLS there was little evidence for PLMS themselves causing a significant sleep–wake problem. The PLMS occur in other sleep disorders and with older age [7]. There may be some with PLMD, but the significance of this disorder remains to be determined. In contrast, RLS as documented below is a major common sleep-related disorder that when severe becomes very disabling.

Clinical findings

Diagnosis

RLS as a clinical syndrome relies upon identifying symptoms defining the disorder. The international restless legs syndrome study group (IRLSSG) has established the currently accepted diagnostic criteria

---

The Parasomnias and Other Sleep-Related Movement Disorders, ed. M. J. Thorpy and G. Plazzi. Published by Cambridge University Press. © Cambridge University Press 2010.

Table 22.1 Common abbreviations and terms related to RLS.

Term	Definition
PLM	Periodic leg movement: Defined as a leg movement lasting 0.5–10 s with at least 4 sequential movements occurring with the interval between onsets of 5–90 s
PLMS	Periodic leg movement occurring during sleep
PLMW	Periodic leg movement occurring during wake
PLMD	Periodic leg movement disorder: PLMS/hr usually greater than 15 associated with significant sleep or wake disturbance and not accounted for by another sleep disorder
PSG	Polysomnogram: multiple physiological recordings during sleep usually including at least recording of EEG, chin EMG and eye movements

Table 22.2 Description of probable RLS patient by Willis (*The London Practice of Physick*, 1685).

"Wherefore to some, on being a bed, they **betake themselves to sleep,** presently in the **arms and legs,** leaping and contractions of the tendons and so great a restlessness and tossings of their members ensue that the diseased are **no more able to sleep than if they were in the place of greatest torture.**"

for both adult and pediatric RLS [8] (see Table 22.3 for adult criteria). Basically, RLS presents as a focal akathisia of the legs often occurring with very peculiar sensory symptoms which patients find hard to describe. The sensory symptoms generally are deep in the leg, dynamic and unlike arthritic conditions rarely involve only or mainly the joints. Phrases patients use to describe these symptoms often refer to things like electric feelings, worms crawling or a Cola drink in the legs. The symptoms tend to occur more in the lower leg and rarely in the foot. They are usually bilateral, but sometimes in only one leg at a time, changing between the legs, and may be more pronounced in one leg. The strange feelings do not generally follow a distal pattern characteristic of peripheral neuropathy. In more severe RLS or unusual cases, the urge to move may occur in the arms or even in some rare cases in the torso and face, but there must be at least a history of an urge to move the legs.

The diagnosis requires that the urge to move the legs and any associated leg sensations are: engendered by rest (sitting or lying down), relieved by moving the legs, and worse in the evening or night. There is a "protected period" in the morning when symptoms rarely occur. When RLS gets worse the symptoms occur earlier in the evening or afternoon, but still are not generally present in the morning, i.e. between 7 and 11 a.m.

Table 22.3 RLS: diagnostic criteria (adults), with features supporting the diagnosis (from [8]).

Essential diagnostic criteria for RLS

1. An urge to move the legs, usually accompanied or caused by uncomfortable and unpleasant sensations in the legs (sometimes the urge to move is present without the uncomfortable sensations and sometimes the arms or other body parts are involved in addition to the legs)
2. The urge to move or unpleasant sensations begin or worsen during periods of rest or inactivity such as lying or sitting
3. The urge to move or unpleasant sensations are partially or totally relieved by movement, such as walking or stretching, at least as long as the activity continues
4. The urge to move or unpleasant sensations are worse in the evening or night than during the day or only occur in the evening or night (when symptoms are very severe, the worsening at night may not be noticeable but must have been previously present)

Features supporting the diagnosis

When the following is present it increases the confidence in the diagnosis of RLS

1. Family history of RLS: first- or second-degree relative with RLS

When the following are not present it decreases confidence in the diagnosis of RLS

1. Good therapeutic response at least to initial treatment with dopaminergic agents
2. Periodic leg movements in sleep

A family history of RLS supports a diagnosis of RLS. The failure to respond, at least initially, to dopaminergic treatment, and no indications for leg movements in sleep and in particular no PLM on a sleep study, cast some doubt on any diagnosis of RLS.

Differential diagnosis

The differential diagnosis for RLS requires excluding other leg pains and discomforts that can be misinterpreted as producing an urge to move. The most common are positional discomfort, leg cramps, arthritic leg pains, myalgias, and neuropathies. Anxiety responses including habitual foot tapping when sitting can often be confused with RLS symptoms. Most of these other conditions producing leg discomfort do not come with the compelling urge to move. They also, unlike RLS, usually fail to get better rapidly if not immediately with standing and walking.

Neuroleptic-induced akathisia produces many of the same symptoms as RLS, except symptoms usually involve the whole body and not predominately the legs. The differential here, however, can be easily made based on the medication history.

Other parasomnias can sometimes be confused with RLS. Sleep starts involve sudden, whole-body jerks at the onset of sleep that some perceive as leg movements disturbing sleep, but they are involuntary movements that do not include any urge to move the legs. Hypnagogic foot tremor occurring in light sleep or in a drowsy wake state also does not include any sense of an urge to move the feet or legs. These movements also usually fail the criteria for PLM. Propriospinal myoclonus like sleep starts occurs at sleep onset, but again involves involuntary movements. Myoclonic seizures occurring mostly with morning awakening usually involve involuntary whole-body jerks. None of these other parasomnias include the sensory abnormality of an urge to move the legs characteristic of RLS. These are sometimes confused with PLM, but a careful measurement of the movements generally suffices to differentiate them from PLM.

The differential diagnosis for RLS can be made with a careful medical history and exam in the clinic setting and should not pose a major problem for making the clinical diagnosis of RLS. The same is not the case for RLS evaluations done in large population-based surveys. These have mostly used questionnaires that include three to four questions covering only the basic diagnostic criteria. They ascertain samples reporting RLS symptoms that include as many or more who do not have RLS as those who do [9].

Secondary vs. primary RLS

RLS occurs not only as a primary disorder but also secondary to other medical conditions. When RLS occurs secondary to these other conditions, it develops after the other condition has started, gets better or worse in relation to the severity of the other condition, and resolves if the other condition is adequately treated. There are three major secondary causes of RLS.

1. *Pregnancy*: RLS occurs in about 11–27% of pregnancies, mostly during the last trimester, and resolves for most shortly after delivery [10].
2. *End-stage renal disease*: RLS occurs in about 20–60% of those on dialysis with rapid and complete improvement for almost all of the patients following successful transplant surgery [11]. RLS during dialysis is significantly associated with increased risk of mortality [12].
3. *Iron-deficiency anemia*: 32% or more of patients with iron-deficiency anemia have RLS which in most cases resolves with effective iron treatment [13].

RLS can be very severe in each of these conditions, particularly for end-stage renal disease and severe iron-deficiency anemia. RLS during pregnancy is often very mild, but in some cases can be severe. Patients with RLS who become pregnant or iron-deficient often report a significant worsening of their RLS symptoms that improves when the pregnancy or iron-deficiency resolves.

Clinical presentation

RLS has a wide range of severity from a mild infrequent annoying disturbance in the evening to a severely disabling inability to rest or sleep well. Figure 22.1 presents the RLS sleep log for a week in the life of one of our moderately severe RLS patients. Note the profoundly short sleep times, the presence of symptoms starting in the afternoon on bad days and in the evening on better days, but always at night and ending in the morning. The best sleep occurs in the later part of the sleep cycle. Note also that this patient who has no work or morning social responsibilities none the less gets up early every morning despite short sleep times. He does not return to bed even though in the morning he is free of RLS symptoms that would disturb rest or sleep. There appears to be a hyperarousal with this disorder compensating for the short sleep time. This may reflect more about the underlying pathology than do the diagnostic symptoms.

Moderate to severe RLS patients seen in primary care have two primary complaints: (1) insomnia in the early part of the night, contrasting with the usual pattern of early morning awakening for insomnia associated with depression; and (2) pain and discomfort in the legs when sitting and lying down for any length of time [14]. They may also complain of not being able to tolerate long car rides or evening sitting activities, e.g. movies or theatricals.

Natural history and epidemiology

Age of onset

RLS may start at any age from earliest childhood to over 100 years of age. The natural history depends on

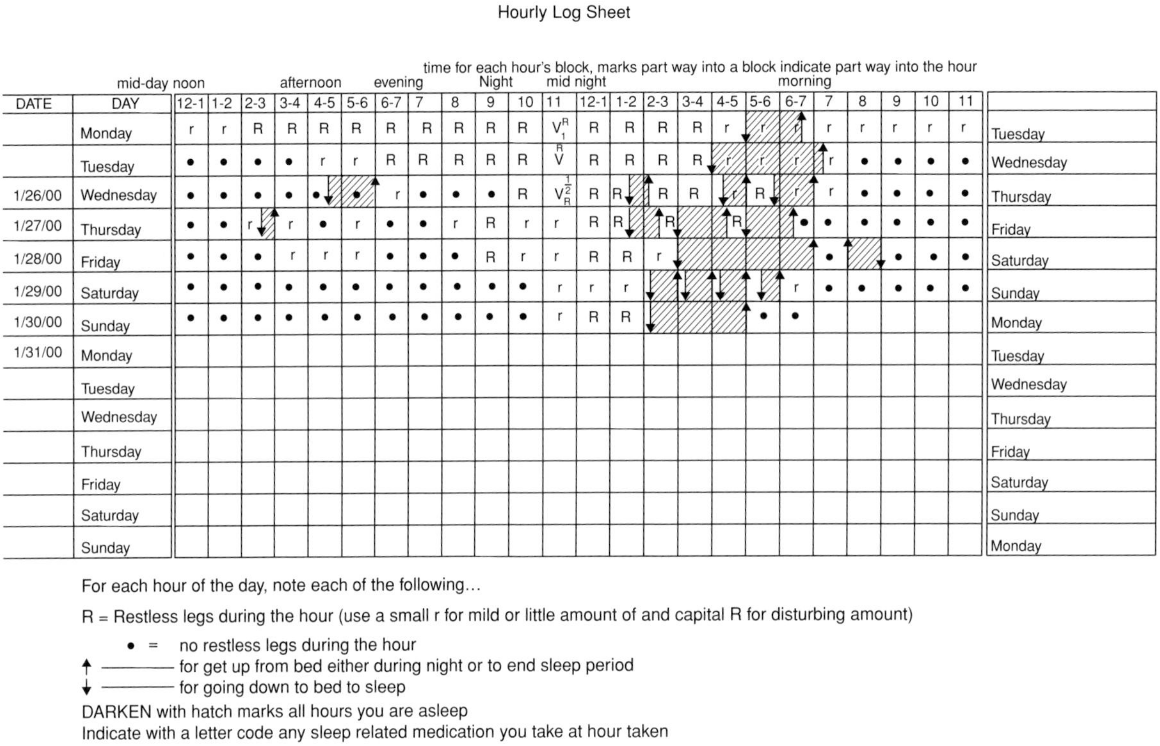

Section 5: Sleep-related disorders and others

Figure 22.1 RLS-sleep log from a patient with moderately severe RLS before starting treatment. Note the lack of symptoms in the morning, the very short sleep times and the failure to sleep late in the morning despite not having RLS symptoms.

two factors: age-of-onset of the disorder, and whether it is a primary disorder or one caused by or exacerbated by another medical condition. Primary RLS starting before age 35–45 is likely to start insidiously as an intermittent disorder gradually progressing over several years to regular events occurring most days with increasing intensity. This characteristic slow progressive pattern does not occur for all RLS patients: some appear to stabilize or even go into periods of remission. Most who report RLS symptoms starting at an early age, however, report that once RLS started it persisted throughout most of their life. The degree of progression and severity in later life varies considerably. RLS starting later in life (over age 45) is generally more rapidly progressive and often has some other medical condition exacerbating or possibly causing the expression of the RLS symptoms.

Studies of families of RLS have found that the risk of RLS for relatives of an RLS patient was about seven times greater than expected for the population if the patient had early-onset RLS and about three times greater if late-onset RLS [15]. Thus age of onset defines two different phenotypes of RLS with different natural histories, different degrees of occurrence in the same family and possibly differing pathologies [16].

Epidemiology

The better population-based surveys have found that RLS at any frequency occurs in about 7–10% of the general population in North America and Europe [17]. RLS that appears severe enough to warrant treatment (symptoms at least twice per week that are moderately to severely distressing) occurs in about 3% and the very severe RLS profoundly affecting health occurs in about 1% of the adult population [18]. The prevalence increases with age until after age 60–70, when it appears to decrease somewhat (see Figure 22.2). The prevalence is about 1.5–2.0 times greater for women than men, but this occurs only for adults over age 30 and is not present in childhood. Two studies have found that nulliparous women have the same RLS prevalence as men [19,20].

Thus epidemiology has identified three major risk factors for RLS: familial occurrence, increasing age,

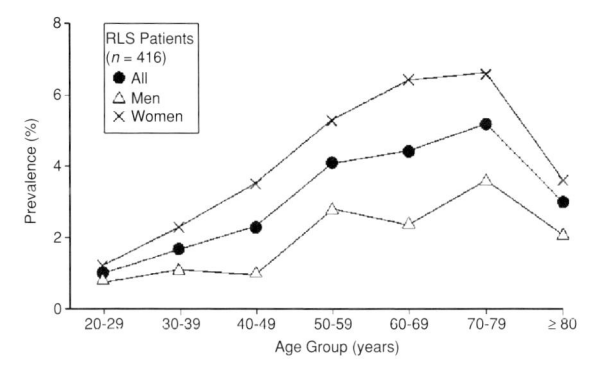

Figure 22.2 Prevalence of clinically significant RLS (RLS symptoms ≥2/week and moderately to severely distressing).

and pregnancy. How pregnancy alters the risk of developing RLS years after the pregnancy remains one of the great mysteries of RLS.

Morbidity

The face of RLS hides in the daytime. RLS expresses itself mostly in the evening and at night. The clinician sees a patient in the daytime with no apparent problems, but one who has had distressing evenings and nights. RLS affects the quality of life as much or more than other chronic disorders such as diabetes, cardiovascular disease, osteoarthritis and depression [21]. The significant sleep loss produces fatigue and increases the risks of medical problems associated with sleep loss. The PLMS of an RLS patient are associated with significant transient blood pressure increases [22]. These factors may explain in part the association between more severe RLS and cardiovascular disease. In one well-controlled study, the increased odds ratio of cardiovascular disease for RLS compared to not-RLS was 2.5 (95% confidence range 1.4–4.5) [23]. Recent studies have indicated that moderate to severe RLS patients effectively lose one working day a week because of the problems caused by their RLS. This degree of suffering and medical risk can be treated and significantly ameliorated.

Laboratory investigations

Blood tests

Serum iron measures are recommended for all RLS patients. Serum ferritin below 50 μg/l or percent transferrin saturation below 17 indicate a need for iron treatment.

Polysomnograms

The standard all-night sleep tests reveal pronounced PLM for most RLS patients with rates increasing with severity of the disorder. The PLMS are associated with arousals from sleep, and once awake while laying in bed these PLM may continue, disturbing the return to sleep. Thus the sleep studies for RLS compared to matched controls show decreased sleep times, decreased sleep efficiency, increased awakenings, increased movements in sleep and waking, and increased stage 1 and decreased stage 2 both as minutes and percentage of total sleep time. Slow-wave and REM sleep percentages are generally not significantly altered [24], but the minutes in these stages will be reduced when the sleep times become very short.

Genetics

The very common occurrence of RLS in multiple members of the same family has long been seen as an indication of a strong genetic factor producing the disorder. A monozygotic vs. dizygotic twin study found a heritability factor of about 69% for RLS [25]. It should be noted, however, that these were not twins raised separately, thus this is an upper limit of the heritability factor. The early excitement about the large number of families with multiple members having RLS led to a large series of genetic linkage studies that reported several significant results. Most of these had limited LOD scores rarely above 3 and not above 5. These now appear likely to represent type 1 errors that commonly occur with this type of genetic analysis.

Two separate large genome-wide association studies produced similar results and were published on the same day. One used mostly a sample from Iceland [26] and the other used a European and Canadian RLS sample [27]. They both reported a significant association of increased risk with one intron allelle on the BTBD9 gene encoding a BTB (POZ) domain of chromosome 6p. The Icelandic study further showed that this allele related both to increased PLMS and also decreased serum ferritin, both of which are associated with increasing severity of RLS. Thus this genetic finding related to significant characteristics of the RLS phenotype.

The European study also identified two other associations also on introns– one on the homeobox gene MEIS1 of chromosome 2p and the other on an area overlapping the mitogen-activated protein

Section 5: Sleep-related disorders and others

Table 22.4 Rates of occurrence of RLS risk allele for RLS and general populations.

Gene	Group	No. case/control	% in RLS cases	% in controls	P value	OR
MEIS1	Canadian	281/803	37.3	26.1	8.9×10^{-7}	1.7 (1.4–2.1)
	German	393/1602	36.8	25.3	4.9×10^{-10}	1.8 (1.5–2.1)
BTBD9	German	393/1602	85.0	76.1	2.2×10^{-6}	
	Canadian	281/803	84.6	70.7	0.029	1.3 (1.04–1.7)
MAP2k5/LBXCOR1	German	393/1602	75.6	66.6	3.6×10^{-6}	
	Canadian	281/803	77.8	68.7	3.9×10^{-4}	1.5 (1.2–1.9)

(Extracted from a table graciously provided by Dr. Lan Xiong, Montreal, Canada.)

kinase MAP2K5 and the transcription factor LBX-COR1 genes on chromosome 15q. A more recent association study identified a fourth locus on the PTPRD gene of chromosome 9p23–24 [28]. These studies identify ten possible risk alleles for RLS on five different genes. It is, however, important to appreciate that while these allelic variations provide an increased risk for RLS, they also commonly occur without RLS in the general population. Table 22.4 below provides for the more significant allelic variations an example of the rates of occurrence in general populations compared to the RLS populations. Clearly these will not be useful for the diagnosis of RLS. It is anticipated that these genetic findings will lead to some understanding of the pathology. Findings from association studies have to date generally contributed little to understanding disease pathology. Hopefully this will change in the future.

Pathology

Several features of RLS reveal possible underlying pathology, i.e. pharmacological treatments, PLMS, sensory disturbances, hyperarousal, secondary RLS and the response to iron treatments. Each of these provides a somewhat different perspective on the neurobiology producing RLS, but the most important have been the pharmacological treatments with dopamine and the issues of iron and secondary RLS as described below.

Pharmacological response

There are three major classes of drugs that each provide excellent reduction in RLS symptoms: dopaminergics (mainly dopamine agonists and levo-dopa), opioids, and some anti-convulsants, particularly the alpha-2-delta calcium channel drugs. Evaluating the response to dopamine has provided some insight into RLS pathology. The mechanisms by which opiates and the select anti-convulsants produce benefit for RLS remain to be determined, but have generally been viewed related to their effects on the dopaminergic system. Thus most research has focused on finding a dopamine pathology in RLS.

Dopamine pathology in RLS

The serendipitous discovery that low doses of levodopa produce dramatic relief from RLS symptoms has led to the view that dopamine pathology produces the RLS symptoms [29]. All CNS-active dopamine agonists improve RLS symptoms and centrally acting dopamine antagonists exacerbate the symptoms. Domperidone, an anti-dopaminergic drug that mostly does not cross the blood–brain barrier, has little effect on RLS symptoms. Thus the dopaminergic abnormality is seen as one of the CNS. Despite the appeal of the dopamine hypothesis, determining the pathology has been difficult. The following findings, however, now give us a better picture.

Hormones and RLS

One study reported an abnormal response to a levodopa challenge for both growth hormone and prolactin when given in the evening but not in the morning to RLS patients. The growth hormone effect, however, may reflect differences in sleep after levodopa. The prolactin response showed a significant difference at only one of the time points evaluated, and the area under the curves did not differ significantly. None the less, the changes and the circadian effects were those expected for RLS [30]. This study suggests some abnormal functioning of the tuberoinfundibular system in RLS.

CSF studies

The first two cerebrospinal fluid (CSF) studies reported no abnormalities in dopamine metabolites or dopamine-related proteins [31,32]. However, morning CSF samples showed high levels of tetrahydrobiopterin (BH4), which when compared to night samples showed a significantly greater circadian increase in BH4 for RLS than for controls [33]. Morning CSF BH4 increase would suggest increased dopamine production over the prior night. Another study reported significantly greater CSF 3-O-methyldopa (3OMD) for RLS than controls for samples obtained both at night and in the morning. Moreover, the CSF values for HVA correlated significantly with those for 3OMD [34]. Since these patients had not been taking dopamine medication and in particular not levodopa, the 3OMD increase indicates either an unlikely disruption of the normal decarboxylation of levodopa to dopamine or an overload production of levodopa. Thus we have two CSF results, both suggesting increased levodopa production in RLS.

Autopsy evaluations

Two autopsy studies of brains from RLS patients reported no indication for neurodegeneration or cell loss [35,36]. A recent report found a D2 receptor decrease in the putamen that correlated with the degree of RLS severity measured about 2–3 years before death. This study also found remarkably large increases in phosphorylated (activated) tyrosine hydroxylase (pTH) in both the putamen and the substantia nigra, and also for the nigra a substantial increase in tyrosine hydroxylase (TH) [37]. These results, like those from the CSF, indicate an overly active pre-synaptic dopamine system with increased extracellular dopamine likely.

Brain imaging

There have been several SPECT and PET studies of the striatum, producing somewhat conflicting results. SPECT striatal studies reported that D2R binding was either not different [38,39] or decreased for RLS patients [40]. PET studies using raclopride reported both reduced [41], and increased [42] D2R binding. None of the three SPECT studies found any abnormalities in binding for the pre-synaptic dopamine transporter (DAT). A recent Johns Hopkins study, however, found possible decreased striatal DAT binding using PET and a methylphenidate ligand. The PET more than SPECT studies are both more sensitive and more specific to detecting functional DAT on the cell surface at a given time point. The binding site on the DAT also differs for the PET methylphenidate ligand compared to the tropane ligands used in the SPECT studies.

In contrast to the conflicting PET and SPECT imaging data noted above, the two flurodopa studies showed the same result of decreased striatal uptake for RLS compared to controls. There is no known cell loss in RLS, and the flurodopa uptake occurs with an amino-acid transport that is unlikely to be altered. The decreased flurodopa uptake can be best explained as indicating rapid turnover and increased activity of the pre-synaptic dopamine system. The DAT decrease reported in the Hopkins study would also be consistent with a pre-synaptic dopamine pathology.

A11 system

The A11 system has cell bodies in the hypothalamus with processes descending the entire spinal column and ascending to the thalamus. It would seem likely to be a dopamine system involved in producing the RLS symptoms. A11 lesions in rats produced increased motor activity potentiated by dietary iron deficiency [43]. However, a recent autopsy study found no dopaminergic cell loss in the A11 region [44]. The A11 system, none the less, seems likely to be involved in producing many of the RLS symptoms, but it is unlikely to be the only system, and its abnormal functioning would presumably be somewhat similar to that reported above for the striatum.

Summary

RLS does not appear to be a neurodegenerative disorder. Rather, it appears to be a metabolic disorder with increased pre-synaptic dopamine activity in the nigra-striatal system and possibly increased extracellular dopamine and decreased post-synaptic dopamine responses. This may serve to exaggerate the natural circadian cycle producing relatively greater deficiency during the circadian low point of the dopamine system.

Iron and secondary RLS

Secondary RLS

The three clearly defined secondary causes of RLS (pregnancy, end-stage renal disease, and iron deficiency) share one important abnormality. They all involve impaired iron status. This has led to the general

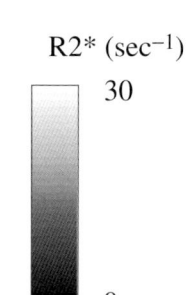

Figure 22.3 R2* images in (A) a 70-year-old RLS patient and (B) a 71-year-old control subject. Higher values of R2* (more white) indicate more iron. The substantia nigra and red nucleus both show substantially lower R2* relaxation rates, indicating less iron.

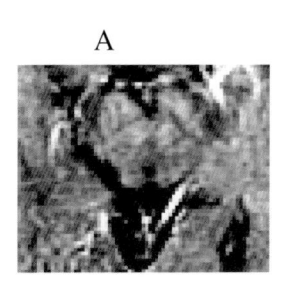

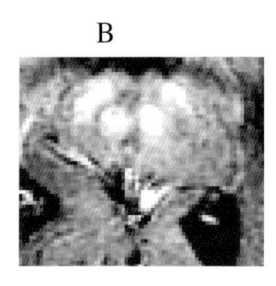

hypothesis that anything disrupting brain iron access will exacerbate or produce RLS symptoms. To date that has proven to be the case for conditions as divergent as gastric surgery and lipoprotein apheresis [45].

Iron and RLS

Iron has a central role in secondary RLS. Dramatic improvements in RLS occur with IV iron treatment using longer-acting iron formulations (e.g. iron dextran or iron ferric carboxymaltose) [46,47]. These clinical data support a fundamental hypothesis that brain iron deficiency is a primary pathology in RLS.

An MRI study demonstrated decreased brain iron for RLS compared to controls particularly for the substantia nigra as shown in Figure 22.3 [48]. The nigral iron deficiency for RLS patients has been confirmed in several studies using MRI [49] and ultrasound [50–53]. This is the best-documented neuropathology of RLS.

Autopsy studies have similarly confirmed the nigral iron deficiency and also reported several abnormalities of iron management proteins: increased H-ferritin, transferrin and iron regulatory protein 2 (IPR2), decreased divalent metal transporter 1(DMT1) and ferroportin [35,54]. One striking anomaly was an increase in transferrin receptor and an associated decrease in iron regulatory protein 1 (IRP-1). These changes are in the opposite direction usually observed for iron deficiency reflecting a cellular abnormality in iron metabolism.

CSF studies have revealed both decreased brain iron status and an interesting relation between peripheral and central iron as shown in Figure 22.4. The RLS patients in this study did not differ from controls for any peripheral measure of iron status and yet their CSF ferritin was abnormally low. Moreover, the relation between CSF and serum ferritin had not only overall much lower CSF values, but also had a much lower increase in CSF ferritin with higher serum ferritin. This difference in the slope of the lines in Figure 22.3 indicates that the brain either is not getting access to the peripheral iron or is unable to retain the iron it gets, or both.

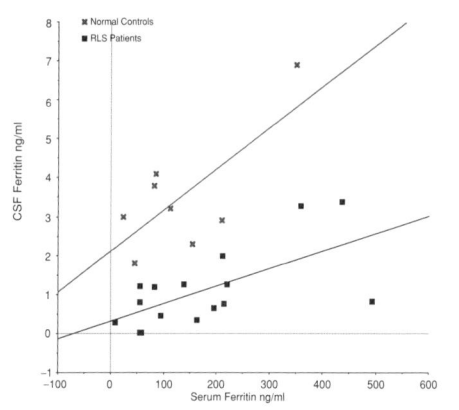

Figure 22.4 Relation between peripheral and central iron as shown by that of serum to CSF ferritin (Earley et al., Neurology, 2000).

Effects of iron deficiency on the dopamine system

If iron insufficiency is a basic pathology for RLS, then presumably the dopaminergic changes in RLS should be found in (1) animal models with dietary iron, and (2) iron chelation of cells. Both of these have now been demonstrated.

Rats placed on an iron-deficient diet show reduced brain iron and also decreased striatal D2R and functioning DAT, increased nigral TH and increased extracellular striatal dopamine [55,56]. These are changes similar to those documented above for RLS patients.

Thus the data above indicate: RLS patients have a brain iron deficiency; iron deficiency produces the dopamine pathologies observed in RLS; and treating with large doses of some formulations of IV iron provides essentially complete remission of RLS lasting several weeks.

Management

The following should be considered when evaluating and treating the RLS patient.

Laboratory tests

The medical evaluation of an RLS patient requires at least a serum ferritin, but preferably an iron panel from a fasting morning blood sample. This should include iron, ferritin, percent transferrin saturation and total iron binding capacity. C-reactive protein should also be considered as a guide to evaluate the serum ferritin value. A CBC including Hgb, Hct, and RDW is also desirable.

No other lab tests are standard for RLS but should certainly be considered as appropriate if secondary medical factors are thought to contribute to the disorder, e.g. diabetes, renal insufficiency, neuropathy, and rheumatoid arthritis.

Secondary RLS

Secondary RLS appears to respond to the same treatments as primary RLS. The only difference in management involves focusing on the underlying condition that causes the RLS and the modifications these require for the RLS treatment. Iron deficiency can be treated with IV iron for immediate relief and oral iron for delayed relief, sometimes requiring several weeks of treatment. Behavioral and nutritional (e.g. iron and folate) treatments are preferred for RLS during pregnancy. RLS during end-stage renal disease can be reduced by reasonably aggressive use of erythropoietin (EPO) and IV iron. Medications that do not rely upon renal clearance may be preferred for RLS treatments of end-stage renal disease.

Iron treatments

Oral iron should be considered for any RLS patient with a serum ferritin <50 μg/l provided there is no indication for hemochromotosis (e.g. transferrin saturation $>50\%$) or intolerance to the medication. One small controlled study has documented the benefits of oral iron treatment for reducing RLS symptoms [57]. Oral iron can be given in tablets containing 25–65 mg of elemental iron (e.g. ferrous sulfate) taken with 200 mg of vitamin C to enhance iron absorption. The tablets are most effective when taken on an empty stomach two or three times a day. It may take several weeks or even months to produce a clinically significant increase in the serum ferritin. During this time, standard pharmacological treatment could be used to reduce symptoms rather than waiting for the uncertain benefit of the oral iron treatment.

Since serum ferritin is phase-reactive it may be falsely elevated during an infection. Obtaining c-reactive protein is recommended particularly when serum ferritin values are above 50 μg/l.

It is important during initial iron treatment to monitor the patient for indications of complications, particularly the expression of hemochromotosis usually indicated by increased transferrin saturation above 50%.

Medical and medication history

It is important that development or changes in RLS symptoms are reviewed in relation to changes in medical status or medication use. Medications that can make RLS worse include most anti-depressants except for buproprion, all anti-dopaminergics that are centrally active, and all H1 anti-histamines.

Behavioral changes to a more sedentary lifestyle may also exacerbate RLS. This is often confused with lack of exercise.

Increased anxiety or depression and any significant sleep loss could exacerbate the symptoms.

When some of these factors are present, adjusting them may reduce the need for other treatments.

Frequency, time and intensity of RLS symptoms

The type of treatment depends largely upon the frequency of the symptoms and their intensity when present. Generally these three features of RLS vary together: greater frequency occurs with earlier onset in the day and greater intensity of the symptoms. The major divisions in treatment consideration involve behavioral treatment for RLS symptoms that are not intense, intermittent medications for more intense symptoms that do not occur most days and regular daily treatment for bothersome symptoms that occur most days. (See treatment algorithms in Figures 22.5 and 22.6.) The time of medication is usually determined by the time of onset of symptoms that cannot be managed with behavioral intervention.

Section 5: Sleep-related disorders and others

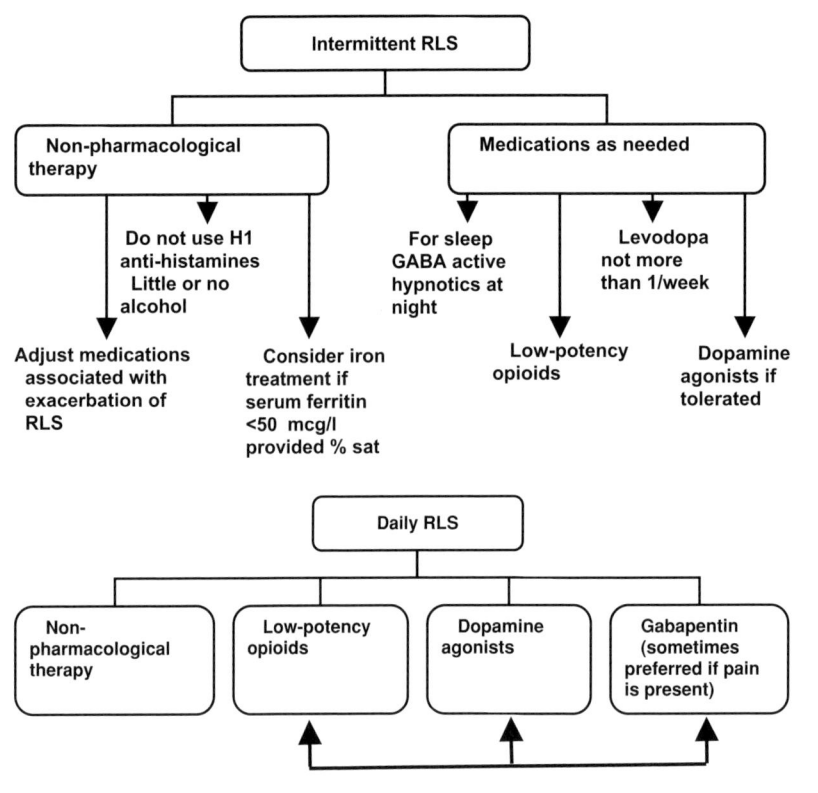

Figure 22.5 Treatment for intermittent RLS (occurring less than twice a week).

Figure 22.6 Treatment for daily or nearly daily RLS (occurring at least twice a week) (note: although dopamine agonists are the only FDA-approved drugs at this time and are considered the treatment of first choice, some clinicians prefer to start with one of the other types of drugs and then switch or add to another type).

Pharmacological treatments

The dopaminergic medications commonly used for treatment of RLS are listed with usual daily dose ranges in Table 22.5. It should be emphasized that evidence for efficacy is only adequately established for the three dopamine agonists listed in this table. The following medication treatments can be considered for RLS.

Hypnotics and benzodiazepines. These are used mostly to promote sleep, thereby treating the sleep problems of RLS. Any of these may be appropriate in the hypnotic dose range. Clonazepam has received some attention in the treatment of RLS, but there are no large clinical trials supporting its efficacy. The three major problems with hypnotic treatment of RLS are: (1) the increased risk of falls, particularly if the patient has to get up to walk around to reduce his RLS symptoms; (2) daytime sleepiness and increased risk of accidents, particularly for longer-acting hypnotics; and (3) the medications may provide little relief from the RLS symptoms themselves when the patient is awake at night not sleeping.

Levodopa. This given in combination with a peripheral dopamine-acting medication (e.g. carbidopa or benserazide) was the first dopaminergic drug to be used with RLS [29]. It also was the first to get regulatory approval for treatment of RLS, but that approval has been limited to Germany and Austria. It is dramatically effective at doses much lower than that used for treatment of Parkinson's Disease. Unfortunately it also produces significant augmentation of the RLS symptoms that occurs in 50–70% of the treated patients. It is therefore recommended only for intermittent treatment not to exceed 1–2 tablets a week at doses of no more than 200 mg.

Dopamine agonists

The older ergotamine dopamine agonists (DA) were found to have a rare adverse effect of significant cardiac

Table 22.5 Dopaminergic medications commonly used for treatment of RLS.

Rx	Start dose (mg)	Titration dose increase: amount and rate	Maximum approved or recommended dose (mg)	Minutes to peak plasma levels	Half-life hrs	Receptor activation	Percent with augmentation	Elimination
L-dopa*,**	100	100, 3–7 days	200***	30	1.5–3	All dopamine receptors	50–70	Hepatic
Pramipexole	0.125	0.125, 3–7 days	0.50 (0.75 mg in some countries)	120	8–12	D2, D3	30	Renal
Ropinirole	0.25	0.25, 3–7 days	4.0	60–120	6–7	D2, D3	Unknown	Hepatic
Rotigotine (24-h patch)	1 mg/24 h	1.0/24, 7 days	3.0/24 h	N/A	N/A	D1, D2, D3,	Unknown	Renal (some fecal)

*Not recommended for daily use. **With peripheral decarboxylation inhibitor (e.g. carbidopa, benserazide). ***Maximum doses have been used over 200 mg with RLS but the risk of augmentation increases with increasing doses. Oral medications are generally given at least 30 min before bothersome symptoms occur.

valve damage producing regurgitation. Since these medications have no advantage over the newer non-ergotamine DA, they are not recommended for use with RLS.

Two non-ergotamine DA (pramipexole and ropinirole) are the only medications currently approved by the US FDA for treatment of RLS. A third, rotigotine, is provided as a transdermal patch. It has regulatory approval for RLS treatment in Europe but not yet in the USA. The two FDA-approved dopamine agonists pramipexole and ropinirole have demonstrated efficacy and safety in large clinical trials [58,59]. They have fairly similar characteristics. Both are approved for use to be taken only once daily before bed. Clinically they are usually taken 1–3 h before bothersome symptoms start. If bothersome symptoms start before night time, then these medications are often taken twice a day, once in the afternoon or early evening and again before bed. Because of adverse effects, particularly nausea, pramipexole and ropinirole need to be titrated to the effective dose using dose increases every 3–7 days. When effective, they reduce and sometimes eliminate all of the RLS symptoms including the sensory disturbances, the urge to move and the PLMS. Pramipexole has a longer half-life than ropinirole and thus may support longer sleep. Since pramipexole relies upon renal clearance, its half-life becomes longer with decreased renal function occurring with older age as well as disease. The number of titration steps is somewhat less for pramipexole than ropinirole, but the range of possible dose adjustments to optimize treatment is greater for ropinirole.

The efficacy and safety of the rotigotine patch has now been demonstrated in two large clinical trials [60,61]. The patch is worn for 24 h and replaced every day. Mild adverse skin reactions to the patch are seen in about 20–40% of the patients, but this led to discontinuing treatment in only about 2–5% of the cases. The usual effective doses are 1 or 2 mg over 24 h with upward titration as needed after 1 week on the 1 mg dose.

The common side effects for all of the DA are nausea, headache and stuffy nose. Tolerance usually develops rapidly to these effects, but not always. In about 3–5% of patients in clinical trials nausea and headache became severe enough to lead to discontinuing treatment [58].

More significant adverse effects include peripheral edema, daytime sleepiness, compulsive behaviors (gambling, shopping, nocturnal eating, etc.) and RLS augmentation. The mild vascular effects of DA can produce significant peripheral edema in vulnerable patients that may limit use of the medication. Profound daytime sleepiness with sudden onset of sleepiness has been reported for Parkinson's patients treated with DA [62], but not for RLS patients, except for one case where this occurred when reducing the dose of pergolide (and ergotamine DA) [63]. Mild to moderate increase in daytime sleepiness has been clinically noted as an adverse effect for 12–15% of patients in clinical trials [58]. Compulsive behaviors occur for some patients as a result of DA treatment for RLS, and in some cases these involve considerable social problems and sometimes loss of money [64,65]. It is important

Section 5: Sleep-related disorders and others

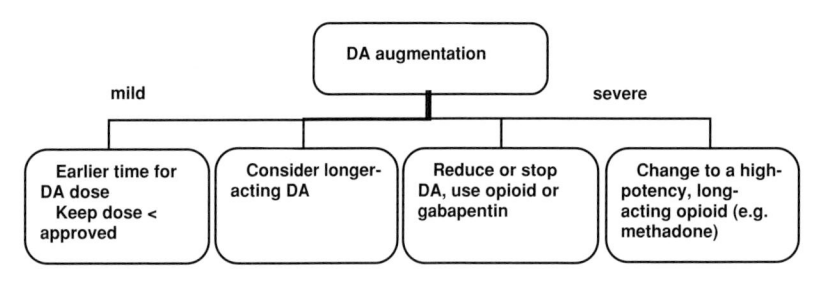

Figure 22.7 Treatment for dopamine (DA) augmentation.

to advise patients about the risk of these more significant effects. Patients need to be followed with repeated clinical visits during the first year of treatment and regularly thereafter in order to carefully evaluate them for development of these adverse effects as well as to ensure their RLS is adequately treated. It deserves note that patients may not be aware of the development of either compulsive behaviors or RLS augmentation. Thus the treatment evaluation should include specific attention to these problems rather than waiting for the patient to report them.

Some of the more severe adverse effects of DA treatment in Parkinson's Disease fortunately do not appear to occur for RLS patients, i.e. orthostatic hypotension, dyskinesias, and hallucinations.

RLS augmentation on medication

The problem of increasing severity of RLS symptoms produced by the medication treating these symptoms occurs for all of the dopaminergic medications and also for tramadol [66,67]. This has not been observed with the other medications used to treat RLS. Augmentation occurs with a worsening of all RLS symptoms that includes an earlier onset in the daytime. Since most of these medications are only taken later in the day, this symptom exacerbation is most commonly noticed by the earlier symptom onset before the usual time for taking the DA. Augmentation may also be observed from increased sleep disturbance, increased intensity of RLS symptoms when they occur, decreased ability to sit still for any length of time, and by any indication of decreased efficacy of the RLS treatment. Many things other than augmentation can produce worsening of RLS symptoms. If there are no medical or lifestyle changes that caused the worsening of RLS symptoms, then augmentation should be considered likely. In such cases it is generally recommended not to increase the DA treatment above the approved dose, but rather to add an alternate type of medication and decrease the dose or stop the DA medication.

This should lead to reduced RLS symptoms. Cases of severe augmentation with very severe RLS have been reported to respond well to gradually discontinuing the DA and starting treatment with low to moderate doses of methadone (see Figure 22.7) [68].

RLS augmentation appears to develop with both increasing dose and duration of treatment. Since we are only now developing information on the effects of very long-term treatment (over 10 years) of RLS, it remains unclear how many patients will develop augmentation or how much this will be a problem in the future.

Anti-convulsants (the alpha-2 delta medications)

One of the earliest clinical trials for treatment of RLS showed efficacy for carbamazepine in a small sample [69], but this medication has never gained any general clinical acceptance for RLS treatment. The alpha-2 delta medications are sometimes used in RLS treatment. Gabapentin, in particular, has been evaluated in several small trials and found to be effective in doses of 600–2400 mg a day (usually in divided doses when exceeding 600–800 mg/day) [70].

Two new alpha-2 delta drugs are now being considered for RLS. A pro-drug for gabapentin has been developed and now tested in large clinical double-blinded, placebo-controlled trials for efficacy and safety in treatment of RLS. It has been found to be effective in doses of 600–1200 mg taken in the early evening [71]. It has the advantage over gabapentin of longer half-life and less variability between people in the gabapentin blood levels. Pregabalin has been used in some clinical settings and has been reported to be effective in doses of 100–500 mg/day [72]. It has not been evaluated in clinical trails. It has a somewhat shorter half-life than the gabapentin pro-drug. The adverse effects of these types of drugs are mostly daytime sleepiness, although some patients report significant dysphoric reactions. Patients should be cautioned about the possible daytime sleepiness when taking these medications.

Opioids

Many of the opioids have been reported to provide effective treatment for RLS. RLS can be considered to be a pain syndrome. Patients describe the sensory symptoms as uncomfortable and painful [14]. The more severe the RLS, the more likely it will be described as painful. One [11C]diprenorphine PET study found reduced opioid receptor binding indicating greater opioid release in the medial affective pain system correlated with greater values for both RLS severity and McGill pain scores [73]. Thus treatment of RLS as a chronic pain with opioids seems reasonable.

Small open-label studies have documented the efficacy of some opioids for RLS, and there has been one small double-blinded, randomized cross-over trial showing significant treatment benefits for oxycodone compared to placebo [74]. Recently methadone, a long-acting high-potency opioid, has been reported to be effective when other treatments have failed [68]. Unlike the other opioids, the methadone dose reported to be effective was somewhat lower than that used for chronic pain. The doses reported range from 2.5 to 40 mg/day, average 15 mg/day [68].

Unfortunately, there are no large clinical trials evaluating the efficacy and safety of these medications in treatment of RLS. Long-term benefits versus dependency problems cannot at this time be determined for use of these drugs with RLS patients. The major adverse effects of these medications include daytime sedation, possible dependency, and respiratory suppression with central apneas during sleep.

Management summary

Suggested treatment algorithms are presented in Figures 22.5 and 22.6. These rely upon the assessments for frequency and severity and using the treatments described above.

The current approved treatments for RLS are the dopamine agonists, and they are usually considered the first treatment of choice when medications are needed. This situation is likely to change soon with the introduction of the alpha-2 delta medications, gabapentin pro-drug and pregabalin, both of which may prove to be effective enough to be possible first treatments for RLS.

The major problems of DA treatment that deserve special warning to the patient and special attention during follow-up are: daytime sleepiness, compulsive behaviors and RLS augmentation. Opioids have the usual problems of dependence, sleepiness and some respiratory suppression. The alpha-2 delta drugs are known to cause problems with sleepiness and may affect body weight.

Conclusions (including future direction)

RLS is a common disorder with a wide range of severity. Moderate to severe RLS is associated with significant morbidity from both profound sleep loss and major discomfort and pain in the daytime. RLS treatments largely reduce the RLS symptoms and significantly improve the life of an RLS patient, but generally they remain only partially effective. Better treatments are needed, and these may be developed based on our growing understanding of the neurobiology of the disorder.

RLS neurobiology occurs as an interesting complex, mostly metabolic, disorder. Like most complex disorders it is unlikely to have a single cause for all cases, but rather several factors interacting to produce the symptoms. There is, however, reasonable coherence of symptoms allowing diagnosis of RLS. Thus there are likely to be some neurological system abnormalities common to most if not all RLS. The dopamine abnormalities may be that commonality. We now have a better understanding of the complex nature of the dopamine pathology in RLS. There appears to be abnormally high dopamine production and release in the moderate to severe RLS. It is somewhat troubling that mild RLS may have the opposite effect, with decreased dopamine release. Future studies will be needed to sort out the relative final pathways for expression of the disorder, but these may indicate possible treatment alternatives.

For many cases, the underlying metabolic disorders disrupting the final pathways causing RLS appear to involve conditions that produce brain iron deficiency. In this view RLS patients have some disruption of the brain's access to iron or its ability to retain iron. Future studies of the basis for the iron metabolic problems in RLS may lead to better treatments and in particular better methods for delivering and maintaining iron in the RLS brain.

We now also have well-documented genetic factors contributing to RLS. The challenge will be relating these genetic factors to pathology. In particular, the relation between these genetic findings and the iron metabolic problem deserves to be carefully explored.

Other new treatments for RLS are now being developed, and we can expect to see them available in the very near future. The alpha-2 delta drugs mentioned above will likely become an option as an initial treatment that avoids the augmentation problems of the dopaminergics. Opioids combined with naloxone to reduce abuse risks and peripheral side effects are likely to be considered. Evidence for the hyperarousal in RLS may lead to better understanding of the histamine and hypocretin abnormalities in RLS. These could lead to treatments related to these neurotransmitter systems.

The most promising new development for the immediate future, however, involves treatments for RLS that will correct or reduce the brain iron deficiency. The multi-center controlled trial of IV ferric carboxymaltose for treatment of RLS showed that a large dose of IV iron produced essentially complete symptom relief lasting several weeks for about 30% of the patients [47]. Open-label studies have found similar results with dextran [46]. Repeated IV iron doses in some patients produced very long possibly indefinite RLS symptom remissions [75]. It may be that we will learn how to better correct the brain iron deficiency in RLS, and in doing so may learn how to better treat other conditions that have decreased brain iron. We may also learn about the environmental factors that contribute to the brain iron deficiency. This might permit finding interventions to prevent the development of brain iron deficiency and the development of RLS.

References

1. Willis T. *De Animae Brutorum*. London: Wells and Scott, 1672.
2. Wittmaack T. *Pathologie und therapie der sensibilitat neurosen*. Liepzig: Schafer, 1861.
3. Ekbom KA. *Restless Legs*. Stockholm: Ivar Haeggströms, 1945.
4. Ekbom KA. Restless legs syndrome. *Neurology* 1960; **10**: 868–73.
5. Symonds CP. Nocturnal myoclonus. *J Neurol Neurosurg Psychiatr* 1953; **16**: 166–71.
6. Lugaresi E, Coccagna G, Berti Ceroni G, Ambrosetto C. Restless legs syndrome and nocturnal myoclonus. In Gastaut H, Lugaresi E, Berti Ceroni G (Eds), *The Abnormalites of Sleep in Man*. Bologna: Aulo Gaggi Editore, 1968; 285–94.
7. Pennestri MH, Whittom S, Adam B, Petit D, Carrier J, Montplaisir J. PLMS and PLMW in healthy subjects as a function of age: Prevalence and interval distribution. *Sleep* 2006; **29**: 1183–7.
8. Allen RP, Picchietti D, Hening WA, Trenkwalder C, Walters AS, Montplaisir J. Restless legs syndrome: Diagnostic criteria, special considerations, and epidemiology. A report from the restless legs syndrome diagnosis and epidemiology workshop at the National Institutes of Health. *Sleep Med* 2003; **4**: 101–19.
9. Hening WA, Allen RP, Washburn M, Lesage S, Earley C. The four diagnostic criteria for the Restless Legs Syndrome are unable to exclude confounding conditions ("mimics"). *Sleep Med* 2009; **10**: 976–81.
10. Manconi M, Govoni V, De Vito A, et al. Pregnancy as a risk factor for restless legs syndrome. *Sleep Med* 2004; **5**: 305–08.
11. Kavanagh D, Siddiqui S, Geddes CC. Restless legs syndrome in patients on dialysis. *Am J Kidney Dis* 2004; **43**: 763–71.
12. Winkelman J, Chertow G, Lagos L, et al. Restless legs syndrome is associated with reduced long term survival in patients with end-stage renal dialysis. *APSS annual meeting*; 1996; Washington, DC: APSS, 1996.
13. Akyol A, Kiyilioglu N, Kadikoylu G, Bolaman AZ, Ozgel N. Iron deficiency anemia and restless legs syndrome: Is there an electrophysiological abnormality? *Clin Neurol Neurosurg* 2003; **106**: 23–7.
14. Hening W, Walters AS, Allen RP, Montplaisir J, Myers A, Ferini-Strambi L. Impact, diagnosis and treatment of restless legs syndrome (RLS) in a primary care population: The REST (RLS epidemiology, symptoms, and treatment) primary care study. *Sleep Med* 2004; **5**: 237–46.
15. Allen RP, La Buda MC, Becker P, Earley CJ. Family history study of the restless legs syndrome. *Sleep Med* 2002; **3**: S3–7.
16. Allen RP, Earley CJ. Defining the phenotype of the restless legs syndrome (RLS) using age-of-symptom-onset. *Sleep Med* 2000; **1**: 11–19.
17. Allen RP, Walters AS, Montplaisir J, et al. Restless legs syndrome prevalence and impact: REST general population study. *Arch Intern Med* 2005; **165**: 1286–92.
18. Allen RP, Stillman P, Myers AJ. Physician-diagnosed restless legs syndrome in a large sample of primary medical care patients in Western Europe: Prevalence and characteristics. *Sleep Med*. in press.
19. Berger K, Luedemann J, Trenkwalder C, John U, Kessler C. Sex and the risk of restless legs syndrome in the general population. *Arch Intern Med* 2004; **164**: 196–202.

20. Pantaleo NP, Hening WA, Allen RP, Earley CJ. Pregnancy accounts for most of the gender differences in prevalence of familial RLS. *Sleep Med* in press.

21. Abetz L, Allen R, Follet A, et al. Evaluating the quality of life of patients with restless legs syndrome. *Clin Ther* 2004; **26**: 925–35.

22. Siddiqui F, Strus J, Ming X, Lee IA, Chokroverty S, Walters AS. Rise of blood pressure with periodic limb movements in sleep and wakefulness. *Clin Neurophysiol* 2007; **118**: 1923–30.

23. Winkelman JW, Shahar E, Sharief I, Gottlieb DJ. Association of restless legs syndrome and cardiovascular disease in the Sleep Heart Health Study. *Neurology* 2008; **70**: 35–42.

24. Saletu B, Gruber G, Saletu M, et al. Sleep laboratory studies in restless legs syndrome patients as compared with normals and acute effects of ropinirole. 1. Findings on objective and subjective sleep and awakening quality. *Neuropsychobiology* 2000; **41**: 181–9.

25. Xiong L, Jang K, Montplaisir J, et al. Canadian restless legs syndrome twin study. *Neurology* 2007; **68**: 1631–3.

26. Stefansson H, Rye DB, Hicks A, et al. A genetic risk factor for periodic limb movements in sleep. *N Engl J Med* 2007; **357**: 639–47.

27. Winkelmann J, Schormair B, Lichtner P, et al. Genome-wide association study of restless legs syndrome identifies common variants in three genomic regions. *Nat Genet* 2007; **39**: 1000–06.

28. Schormair B, Kemlink D, Roeske D, et al. PTPRD (protein tyrosine phosphatase receptor type delta) is associated with restless legs syndrome. *Nat Genet* 2008; **40**: 946–8.

29. Akpinar S. Treatment of restless legs syndrome with levodopa plus benserazide. *Arch Neurol* 1982; **39**: 739.

30. Garcia-Borreguero D, Larrosa O, Granizo JJ, de la Llave Y, Hening WA. Circadian variation in neuroendocrine response to L-dopa in patients with restless legs syndrome. *Sleep* 2004; **27**: 669–73.

31. Earley CJ, Hyland K, Allen RP. CSF dopamine, serotonin, and biopterin metabolites in patients with restless legs syndrome. *Mov Disord* 2001; **16**: 144–9.

32. Stiasny-Kolster K, Moller JC, Zschocke J, et al. Normal dopaminergic and serotonergic metabolites in cerebrospinal fluid and blood of restless legs syndrome patients. *Mov Disord* 2004; **19**: 192–6.

33. Earley CJ, Hyland K, Allen RP. Circadian changes in CSF dopaminergic measures in restless legs syndrome. *Sleep Med* 2006; **7**: 263–8.

34. Allen RP, Connor JR, Hyland K, Earley CJ. Abnormally increased CSF 3-Ortho-methyldopa (3-OMD) in untreated restless legs syndrome (RLS) patients indicates more severe disease and possibly abnormally increased dopamine synthesis. *Sleep Med* 2009; **10**: 123–8.

35. Connor JR, Boyer PJ, Menzies SL, Dellinger B, Allen RP, Earley CJ. Neuropathological examination suggests impaired brain iron acquisition in restless legs syndrome. *Neurology* 2003; **61**: 304–09.

36. Pittock SJ, Parrett T, Adler CH, Parisi JE, Dickson DW, Ahlskog JE. Neuropathology of primary restless leg syndrome: Absence of specific tau-and alpha-synuclein pathology. *Mov Disord* 2004; **19**: 695–9.

37. Connor JR, Wang X, Allen RP, et al. Altered dopaminergic profile in the putamen and substantia nigra in restless leg syndrome. *Brain* in press.

38. Eisensehr I, Wetter TC, Linke R, et al. Normal IPT and IBZM SPECT in drug-naive and levodopa-treated idiopathic restless legs syndrome. *Neurology* 2001; **57**: 1307–09.

39. Tribl GG, Asenbaum S, Happe S, Bonelli RM, Zeitlhofer J, Auff E. Normal striatal D2 receptor binding in idiopathic restless legs syndrome with periodic leg movements in sleep. *Nucl Med Commun* 2004; **25**: 55–60.

40. Michaud M, Soucy JP, Chabli A, Lavigne G, Montplaisir J. SPECT imaging of striatal pre-and postsynaptic dopaminergic status in restless legs syndrome with periodic leg movements in sleep. *J Neurol* 2002; **249**: 164–70.

41. Turjanski N, Lees AJ, Brooks DJ. Striatal dopaminergic function in restless legs syndrome: 18F-dopa and 11C-raclopride PET studies. *Neurology* 1999; **52**: 932–7.

42. Cervenka S, Palhagen SE, Comley RA, et al. Support for dopaminergic hypoactivity in restless legs syndrome: A PET study on D2-receptor binding. *Brain* 2006; **129**: 2017–28.

43. Ondo WG, He Y, Rajasekaran S, Le WD. Clinical correlates of 6-hydroxydopamine injections into A11 dopaminergic neurons in rats: A possible model for restless legs syndrome. *Mov Disord* 2000; **15**: 154–8.

44. Earley C, Allen RP, Connor JR, Ferrucci L, Troncoso J. The dopaminergic neurons of the A11 system in RLS autopsy brains appear normal. *Sleep Med* in press.

45. Happe S, Tings T, Schettler V, Canelo M, Paulus W, Trenkwalder C. Low-density lipoprotein apheresis and restless legs syndrome. *Sleep* 2003; **26**: A335–6.

46. Earley CJ, Heckler D, Horská A, Barker PB, Allen RP. The treatment of restless legs syndrome with intravenous iron dextran. *Sleep Med* 2004; **5**: 231–5.

47. Allen RP, Butcher A, Du W. Double-blind, placebo-controlled multi-center evaluation of restless legs syndrome (RLS) treatment with 1,000 mg of IV iron (ferric carboxymaltose –FCM). *Sleep* 2009; in press.

48. Allen RP, Barker PB, Wehrl F, Song HK, Earley CJ. MRI measurement of brain iron in patients with restless legs syndrome. *Neurology* 2001; **56**: 263–5.

49. Earley CJ, Barker PB, Horska A, Allen RP. MRI-determined regional brain iron concentrations in early-and late-onset restless legs syndrome. *Sleep Med* 2006; **7**: 459–61.

50. Schmidauer C, Sojer M, Seppi K, *et al.* Transcranial ultrasound shows nigral hypoechogenicity in restless legs syndrome. *Ann Neurol* 2005; **58**: 630–4.

51. Godau J, Schweitzer KJ, Liepelt I, Gerloff C, Berg D. Substantia nigra hypoechogenicity: Definition and findings in restless legs syndrome. *Mov Disord* 2007; **22**: 187–92.

52. Godau J, Wevers AK, Gaenslen A, *et al.* Sonographic abnormalities of brainstem structures in restless legs syndrome. *Sleep Med* 2008; **9**: 782–9.

53. Godau J, Klose U, Di Santo A, Schweitzer K, Berg D. Multiregional brain iron deficiency in restless legs syndrome. *Mov Disord* 2008; **23**: 1184–7.

54. Connor JR, Wang XS, Patton SM, *et al.* Decreased transferrin receptor expression by neuromelanin cells in restless legs syndrome. *Neurology* 2004; **62**: 1563–7.

55. Chen Q, Beard JL, Jones BC. Abnormal rat brain monoamine metabolism in iron deficiency anemia. *J Nutritional Biochem* 1995; **6**: 486–93.

56. Erikson KM, Jones BC, Hess EJ, Zhang Q, Beard JL. Iron deficiency decreases dopamine D1 and D2 receptors in rat brain. *Pharmacol Biochem Behav* 2001; **69**: 409–18.

57. Wang J, O'Reilly B, Venkataraman R, Mysliwiec V, Mysliwiec A. Efficacy of oral iron in patients with restless legs syndrome and a low-normal ferritin: A randomized, double-blind, placebo-controlled study. *Sleep Med* 2009; **10**: 973–5.

58. Trenkwalder C, Garcia-Borreguero D, Montagna P, *et al.* Ropinirole in the treatment of restless legs syndrome: Results from the TREAT RLS 1 study, a 12 week, randomised, placebo controlled study in 10 European countries. *J Neurol Neurosurg Psychiatry* 2004; **75**: 92–7.

59. Oertel WH, Stiasny-Kolster K, Bergtholdt B, *et al.* Efficacy of pramipexole in restless legs syndrome: A six-week, multicenter, randomized, double-blind study (effect-RLS study). *Mov Disord* 2007; **22**: 213–9.

60. Oertel WH, Benes H, Garcia-Borreguero D, *et al.* Efficacy of rotigotine transdermal system in severe restless legs syndrome: A randomized, double-blind, placebo-controlled, six-week dose-finding trial in Europe. *Sleep Med* 2008; **9**: 228–39.

61. Trenkwalder C, Benes H, Poewe W, *et al.* Efficacy of rotigotine for treatment of moderate-to-severe restless legs syndrome: A randomised, double-blind, placebo-controlled trial. *Lancet Neurol* 2008 Jul; **7**: 595–604.

62. Lang AE, Hobson DE, Martin W, Rivest J. Excessive daytime sleepiness and sudden onset sleep in Parkinson's disease: A survey from 18 Canadian movement disorders clinics. *Neurology* 2001; a: S40.001.

63. Bassetti C, Clavadetscher S, Gugger M, Hess CW. Pergolide-associated 'sleep attacks' in a patient with restless legs syndrome. *Sleep Med* 2002; **3**: 275–7.

64. Quickfall J, Suchowersky O. Pathological gambling associated with dopamine agonist use in restless legs syndrome. *Parkinsonism Relat Disord* 2007; **13**: 535–6.

65. Ondo WG, Lai D. Predictors of impulsivity and reward seeking behavior with dopamine agonists. *Parkinsonism Relat Disord* 2008; **14**: 28–32.

66. Vetrugno R, La Morgia C, D'Angelo R, *et al.* Augmentation of restless legs syndrome with long-term tramadol treatment. *Mov Disord* 2007; **22**: 424–7.

67. Earley CJ, Allen RP. Restless legs syndrome augmentation associated with tramadol. *Sleep Med* 2006; **7**: 592–3.

68. Ondo WG. Methadone for refractory restless legs syndrome. *Mov Disord* 2005; **20**: 345–8.

69. Lundvall O, Abom PE, Holm R. Carbamazepine in restless legs. A controlled pilot study. *Eur J Clin Pharmacol* 1983; **25**: 323–4.

70. Garcia-Borreguero D, Larrosa O, de la Llave Y, Verger K, Masramon X, Hernandez G. Treatment of restless legs syndrome with gabapentin: A double-blind, cross-over study. *Neurology* 2002; **59**: 1573–9.

71. Kushida CA, Becker PM, Ellenbogen AL, Canafax DM, Barrett RW. Randomized, double-blind, placebo-controlled study of XP13512/GSK1838262 in patients with RLS. *Neurology* 2009; **72**: 439–46.

72. Sommer M, Bachmann CG, Liebetanz KM, Schindehutte J, Tings T, Paulus W. Pregabalin in restless legs syndrome with and without neuropathic pain. *Acta Neurol Scand* 2007; **115**: 347–50.

73. von Spiczak S, Whone AL, Hammers A, *et al.* The role of opioids in restless legs syndrome: An [11C]diprenorphine PET study. *Brain* 2005; **128**: 906–17.

74. Walters AS, Winkelmann J, Trenkwalder C, *et al.* Long-term follow-up on restless legs syndrome patients treated with opioids. *Mov Disord* 2001; **16**: 1105–09.

75. Earley CJ, Heckler D, Allen RP. Repeated IV doses of iron provides effective supplemental treatment of restless legs syndrome. *Sleep Med* 2005; **6**: 301–05.

Section 5 Sleep-related movement disorders and other variants

Chapter 23: Sleep starts

Sudhansu Chokroverty and Divya Gupta

Introduction

Sleep starts, also known as somnolescent starts, hypnic starts, hypnagogic jerk or hypnic jerks, cause a sudden "start" or excitation of the motor centers at the moment of sleep onset. Weir Mitchell is credited with the earliest description of sleep starts in 1890, and also mentioned the possibility of sleep-onset insomnia as a result of these starts [1]. Gallavardin, cited by the early French neurologist Roger, gave a clinical description of hypnic jerks [2], and Oswald in 1959 described the electroencephalographic (EEG) correlates of these hypnic jerks [3]. In 1965, Gastaut and Broughton described these episodic sensory-motor phenomena of sleep onset with simultaneous polygraphic recordings [4]. Broughton later used the term "intensified hypnic jerks" in 1988 causing sleep-onset insomnia in some of the subjects, as was also mentioned by Weir Mitchell in 1890 [5,6]. Purely sensory sleep starts at sleep onset were clearly documented by Sander et al. in 1998 [7]. The exploding head syndrome is probably a variant of sensory sleep starts and was first mentioned by Armstrong-Jones in 1920 as a "snapping of the brain" [8], and was later brought to the attention of the medical community by Pearce in 1989 [9]. Another variant of sensory sleep starts is probably what Lance called the "blip" syndrome of transient sensation of impending loss of consciousness at sleep onset [10].

Clinical subtypes and descriptions

Sleep starts may be divided into the following six subtypes (Table 23.1):

1. Motor sleep starts ("hypnic jerks")
2. Sensory-motor types
3. Pure sensory sleep starts
4. Intensified hypnic jerks
5. Exploding head syndrome
6. "Blip" syndrome

The most common type is the motor sleep starts and sensory-motor sleep starts. Sleep starts are classified under the category of Section VII (isolated symptoms, apparently normal variants, and unresolved issues) in the *International Classification of Sleep Disorders*, second edition [11].

Motor sleep starts ("hypnic jerks")

Hypnic jerks or motor sleep starts are seen in many normal adults and are physiological phenomena without any pathologic significance [11]. At the moment of falling asleep, there is a sudden transient jerk usually involving the limbs or the trunk, sometimes also the head, and could be symmetrical but more often seen asymmetrically. The jerks last a few seconds. Sometimes the jerks can repeat after sleep onset. Some patients also describe these jerks after waking up in the middle of the night and on falling asleep again. On some rare occasions patients have described these transient myoclonic jerks at the moment of sleep onset during daytime naps. These myoclonic jerks are non-stereotyped, abrupt, and characterized by brief flexion or extension movements. These jerks are often triggered by fatigue, stress, sleep deprivation, vigorous exercise and stimulants like caffeine and nicotine. Probably most adults at some time or other have experienced these jerks and the literature quotes up to 70% of the adult population have experienced these transient jerks at sleep onset. There is no family history and there is no sex preference. This is a benign condition and it generally disappears without any abnormal neurological findings, except occasionally this could be intensified causing sleep-onset insomnia

Table 23.1 Subtypes of sleep starts.

- Motor sleep starts ("hypnic jerks")
- Sensory-motor type
- Pure sensory sleep starts
- Intensified hypnic jerks
- Exploding head syndrome
- "Blip" syndrome

and anxiety (see later). Sometimes these are accompanied by sensory phenomena such as the sensation of falling and occasionally accompanied by inner electric shock, unexplained fear or alarm. Rarely, these jerks may cause mild injury, such as bruising of the feet. These transient hypnic jerks may resemble a physiological startle response, although these occur without any apparent triggering stimulus. Physiologically, these jerks may utilize the same startle reflex pathway (see below under pathophysiology). These hypnic jerks are transiently accompanied by autonomic activation as manifested by tachycardia and tachypnea and are immediately followed by transient arousal with reappearance of the alpha activities in adult EEG.

Sensory-motor types

The sensory-motor type is characterized by a combination of muscle jerks accompanied by various types of sensations (e.g. sensation of falling through space, fear of falling, a light flash, an electric shock-like feeling, or a dream-like sensation of falling) at the moment of sleep onset [11].

Pure sensory sleep starts

Purely sensory sleep starts without a muscle jerk have been described occurring exclusively at sleep onset [7]. Prior to this report by Sander et al., the only literature reference to sensory phenomena without a body jerk is an anecdotal comment within a review article [12]. Sander et al. described two patients with purely sensory complaints restricted to onset of sleep. The first patient is a 42-year-old college professor with a 12-year history of 5–30-s spells occurring weekly to monthly. These episodes always occurred upon falling asleep. She described the episodes as non-radiating electric shock-like sensation in the chest, sometimes accompanied by a sense of suffocation and occasionally with a feeling of numbness on the medial side of the right arm, ring and little finger. She would be immediately alerted after the initial sensation. She has had extensive investigations at an outside hospital including electrocardiogram, prolonged video-EEG monitoring and magnetic resonance imaging of the brain, all with normal findings. She was diagnosed with sensory seizures and prescribed anti-convulsants, but she refused. After the consultation she was given reassurance and an extensive explanation of the benign physiological phenomenon, and eventually she overcame the fear of the sensory sleep starts. The second patient was a woman with focal itchy, sharp, pin prick-like sensation occurring anywhere in the body at the moment of falling asleep. The initial sensation awakened the patient. In both these patients, the spells occasionally occurred during periods of daytime sleep or drowsiness. Stress, fatigue and sleep deprivation were often provoking factors. These two patients never had any associated tongue biting, urinary incontinence or body movements during these spells. The occurrence of the sensory phenomena exclusively at sleep onset should prompt the consideration of sensory sleep starts. The recognition of this unusual syndrome may eliminate unnecessary diagnostic testing and avoid unnecessary anti-convulsant therapy. There is also a report of acoustic sleep starts (see below) with sleep-onset insomnia related to a brain stem lesion [13].

Intensified hypnic jerks

Occasionally, patients may have an unusual presentation of hypnic jerks with intensification or excessive hypnic jerks which may be misdiagnosed as myoclonic seizures [14]. Weir Mitchell described patients suffering from apparent intensification of the physiological hypnic jerks or sleep starts at sleep onset and one of these patients also had sleep-onset insomnia [1]. In 1988, Broughton confirmed this observation and described two such patients. The first patient was a 55-year-old man with a 3-year history of excessive hypnic jerks at sleep onset which would recur several times. His second patient was a 40-year-old woman with a similar history for 18 months. She had similar jerks on awakening in the middle of the night and falling asleep. Both had sleep-onset insomnia. Conigliari et al. also briefly described two such patients in 1999 misdiagnosed as myoclonic seizure [14]. The first patient was a 29-year-old man; the second a 38-year-old man. The jerks sometimes started on one side and then spread to the opposite side with occasional occurrence during daytime naps. An overnight polysomnographic (PSG) study including ten channels of EEG showed a mixture of myoclonic and dystonic EMG bursts in patient 1, mostly in the arms at sleep onset and transition from awakening to NREM stage 1 sleep. The patients improved following reassurance. The intensified hypnic jerks may interfere with sleep onset causing sleep-onset insomnia, fear of falling asleep and chronic anxiety.

Exploding head syndrome

This most likely represents a variant of purely sensory sleep starts although it is classified among other parasomnias in the ICSD-2 [11]. As mentioned previously, this condition was probably first described by Armstrong-Jones in 1920 as a "snapping of the brain" and is characterized by sensations of explosions occurring in the head, awakening the patient from sleep, and these sensations last for several seconds [8]. In 1989, Pearce gave a comprehensive description of exploding head syndrome which most commonly occurs in persons over 50 years of age. Several other authors have also described this condition since then [15–17]. The sensations are variously described by patients as a terrifying loud bang or bomb-like explosions inside the head at the moment of sleep onset. This loud banging noise awakens the patient with intense anxiety. These can occur more than once per night, lasting for several weeks to months, with prolonged or total remissions. Sachs and Svanborg documented polysomnographically the occurrence of these attacks during normal sleep stages including REM sleep and during the transition from wakefulness to sleep [16]. Our patient with exploding head syndrome was seen in consultation at the age of 54 years [17]. She began to have terrifying sensations inside the head after sleep onset at the age 28 years. She described the sensations as "rapid fire explosions," "feeling of an explosion or a sensation of bursting," "thunder-like or loud banging inside the head with sensations of flashing light in the field of vision," and sometimes "electric shock-like sensations" throughout the body. These nocturnal episodes always occurred at sleep onset or at sleep–wake transition states, and sometimes similar episodes occurred during the daytime at sleep onset. The frequency of occurrence of these episodes was irregular with one to two times per week or every one to two months, and sometimes there were intervals of infrequent occurrence and even remission. These spells would last for seconds but often several times in a row; she would have these spells lasting for a total of 10–15 min. All these symptoms caused her intense anxiety and sleep disturbance and she complained of daytime fatigue and tiredness. Neurological examination and family history were unremarkable. She denied any jerky movements, urinary incontinence, tongue biting or confusion immediately after the thunder-like sensations. The only triggering factor identified was stress. She had numerous EEGs including prolonged video-EEG monitoring in an epilepsy unit during symptomatic periods, which were all normal without any epileptiform discharges. Her MRI of the brain was normal. Overnight PSG study including ten channels of EEG showed non-specific sleep architectural changes with occurrence of these sensations at the onset of stage 1 NREM sleep during the recording. Several neurologists at multiple centers diagnosed the condition as nocturnal seizure, and over the years she was treated with a variety of anti-convulsants without any benefit. She finally received firm assurance and understanding about the condition and felt better, but still had some intermittent episodes. The main distinction between exploding head syndrome and nocturnal seizures is the occurrence of the spells at the moment of sleep onset and they always occur at the transition between wake and sleep, whereas nocturnal seizures can occur at any sleep stage and sometimes during the daytime.

Some unusual manifestations

The "blip" syndrome

This is also probably a variant of sensory sleep starts described by Lance in 1996 [10]. The syndrome is characterized by a momentary sensation of impending loss of consciousness, particularly when the subjects were relaxed, without any obvious cardiorespiratory or cerebrovascular cause, or without any indication of an epileptic seizure.

Repetitive sleep starts in neurologically impaired children

Fusco *et al.* described sleep starts occurring repetitively in three epileptic children with spastic–dystonic diplegia and mental retardation [18]. Repetitive sleep starts began at age 18 months in two children and at 9 months in the third. All three children had seizures which were controlled by anti-epileptic medication. The authors documented clusters of sleep starts during the transition between wakefulness and

Table 23.2 Conditions mimicking sleep starts.

- Propriospinal myoclonus at sleep onset
- Physiologic fragmentary or partial hypnic myoclonus (PFHM)
- Excessive fragmentary hypnic myoclonus (EFHM)
- Myoclonic seizures
- Benign sleep myoclonus of infancy
- Hypnagogic foot tremor
- Alternating leg muscle activation (ALMA)
- Rhythmic movement disorder (RMD)
- Restless legs syndrome (RLS)
- Periodic limb movement in sleep (PLMS)
- Hereditary hyperexplexia syndrome
- Essential startle disease of Gastaut and Villeneuve

sleep by video-EEG recordings in all three children during the afternoon nap. Clusters lasted 4–15 min and comprised from 20 to 29 contractions. The EEG showed an arousal response but no epileptiform discharges during these spells. The authors suggested that repetitive sleep starts should be recognized and clearly differentiated from epileptic seizures, particularly if these episodes are seen in epileptic subjects. The authors speculated that in neurologically compromised patients, these repetitive spells may represent an intensification of an otherwise normal event in patients with corticospinal tract lesion in the absence of strong inhibitory influence.

Acoustic sleep starts

Salih et al. [13] described an acoustic sleep start with sleep-onset insomnia in a 64-year-old woman related to a brain stem lesion. The patient presented with sleep-onset insomnia related to the sensation of a startling, cracking sound and fear of sleep onset for the past 12 years. Her MRI of the brain revealed an unchanging, non-enhancing symmetric T2-hyperintense pontomesencephalic lesion around the periaqueductal gray which was etiologically thought to be related to her residual sarcoidosis diagnosed 12 years ago. She responded to clonazepam 0.5 mg at bedtime.

Differential diagnosis of sleep starts

Sleep starts should be differentiated from a variety of conditions mimicking sleep starts based on the history and physical examination and appropriate laboratory tests. Table 23.2 lists conditions mimicking sleep starts.

Propriospinal myoclonus at sleep onset

Propriospinal myoclonus at sleep onset (PSM) closely resembles sleep starts or hypnic jerks and may be difficult to differentiate without an electrophysiological investigation. In 1997, Montagna et al. described three patients, aged 71, 50 and 41 years, presenting with myoclonic activity arising in the relaxation period preceding sleep onset and causing severe insomnia [19]. Subsequently the same group of investigators led by Vetrugno gave a detailed description of the condition, including the electrophysiological findings, labeling it as a new parasomnia [20]. This is now classified in the category of sleep-related movement disorders [11]. This is a condition which occurs during the period which McDonald Critchley called "predormitum" [21], and is characterized by transient sudden muscle jerks involving predominantly the axial muscles. Patients complain of sleep-onset insomnia. PSM may be a special type of spinal myoclonus originating from a myoclonic generator in the midthoracic region with propagation up and down the spinal cord at a very slow speed (3–16 m/s). As soon as the patient falls asleep (moment of sleep onset) PSM disappears, differentiating it from hypnic jerks. Furthermore, physiologically, PSM is propagated by the propriospinal pathways, but the hypnic jerks are probably propagated by reticulospinal fibers (see below). However, PSM may sometimes reappear during intra-sleep wakefulness and upon awakening in the morning.

Physiologic fragmentary or partial hypnic myoclonus (PFHM)

PFHM was first described by De Lisi in 1932 [22], who described this as sudden sporadic spontaneous, asynchronous and asymmetrical brief myoclonic twitchings involving different body parts, especially distal limb and facial muscles. The muscle discharges of PFHM appear as bursts of motor unit action potentials with or without visible movements during NREM sleep stage 1 [23], and during REM sleep [24]. It is easy to differentiate PFHM from hypnic jerks, as PFHM represents a simple motor phenomenon during sleep, mostly during stage 1 NREM and REM sleep, causing very little or no visible movements. PFHM represents physiological escape from the state-dependent motor inhibition causing the descending volleys within the brain stem reticulospinal system into the spinal alpha motor neurons.

Excessive fragmentary hypnic myoclonus (EFHM)

EFHM is simply a pathological enhancement of PFHM characterized by myoclonic muscle twitches throughout all sleep stages which may cause small movements of the fingers, toes or corners of the mouth without gross displacement across the joint space [25–27]. EFHM resembles PFHM but is seen in all sleep stages and states (NREM and REM). The clinical significance of EFHM remains uncertain and is seen in a variety of sleep disorders. EFHM is predominantly a polysomnographic (PSG) finding consisting of brief myoclonic jerks (75–150 ms) of more than five potentials per minute sustained for at least 20 min during NREM sleep [28].

Myoclonic seizures

Sleep starts may sometimes be misdiagnosed as myoclonic or other nocturnal seizures. An important condition to differentiate sleep starts is juvenile myoclonic epilepsy of Janz [29]. The characteristic manifestation is generalized massive myoclonic jerks, which are most commonly seen in the morning shortly after awakening. Sometimes jerks occur in the middle of the night. The condition is usually seen in young adults between 13 and 19 years of age and responds very well to valproic acid. EEG shows characteristic multiple spike and wave discharges seen synchronously and symmetrically which differentiate this from sleep starts or hypnic jerks. Also, the myoclonic seizure is not restricted to the sleep onset only.

Benign sleep myoclonus of infancy

Benign neonatal sleep myoclonus occurs during the first few weeks of life and is generally seen in NREM sleep but also during REM sleep [30]. Episodes often occur in clusters involving arms, legs and sometimes the trunk. The movements consist of jerky flexion, extension, abduction and adduction. The EEG is normal. The condition is benign and it resolves by the third or fourth month of life, and definitely before the end of the first year.

Hypnagogic foot tremor

This condition is characterized by rhythmic movement of feet or toes, but occurs at the transition between wake and sleep or during NREM stages 1 and 2 [5,11].

This is a relatively common finding and the clinical significance remains unknown. This may be a variant of rhythmic movement disorder. PSG findings consist typically of EMG bursts of 1–2 Hz (0.3–4.0 Hz) in one or both feet with a minimum of four consecutive bursts and a duration of 250–1000 ms lasting for 10 or more seconds in trains [28]. The clinical and PSG findings clearly differentiate this from sleep starts.

Alternating leg muscle activation (ALMA)

ALMA consists of brief activation of the tibialis anterior muscle in one leg alternating with similar activation in the other leg during sleep or arousals from sleep [31]. This is a PSG finding with a frequency of 0.5–3.0 Hz with an individual activation duration between 100 and 500 ms. A minimum of four alternating activations with less than 2 s between the activations is recorded for diagnosis, and each sequence may last up to 30 s [28]. The clinical significance of this entity is not known.

Rhythmic movement disorder (RMD)

RMD is characterized by stereotyped repetitive movements involving large axial muscles typically occurring immediately before sleep onset and persisting into light sleep. The most common types are head banging, head rolling and body rocking. Other movements which may occur include leg rolling and leg banging. RMD may occur at any sleep stage including REM sleep and is most often seen during drowsiness persisting into a lighter stage of sleep [11]. The movements occur with a frequency of 0.5–2.0 Hz and persist for a few minutes to many hours during sleep. A minimum of four consecutive activations with an amplitude twice the background EMG activity is needed for scoring. RMD most commonly occurs in children and generally resolves by the age of 4, but sometimes persists into adulthood. The characteristic clinical and PSG features differentiate RMD from sleep starts.

Restless legs syndrome (RLS)

RLS is characterized by an urge to move with or without accompanying uncomfortable feeling in the legs and occurring most commonly during inactivity and in the evening, and relieved at least temporarily by movements. The RLS is a disease of quiescence and relaxed wakefulness and is not present during sleep, in contrast to hypnic jerks. RLS patients may sometimes also have myoclonic movements of the legs during rest.

Periodic limb movements in sleep (PLMS)

PLMS should not be mistaken for sleep starts, as these movements are not present during pre-dormitum or sleep onset, but are present mostly during NREM sleep and occurring in a periodic manner at 5–90 s apart with a movement duration of 0.5–10 seconds consisting typically of dorsiflexion of the foot, but also sometimes accompanied by flexion of the knees or hip joints, and must be present consecutively for four limb movements in the PSG [11]. PLMS is a PSG phenomenon and may be associated with EEG arousals. PLMS is present in 80% of the RLS patients.

Hereditary hyperekplexia syndrome

Hereditary hyperekplexia may be associated with excessive startling response to stimuli spontaneously at night or during wakefulness and may be accompanied by hypnic jerks. The minor form of hereditary hyperekplexia may be mistaken for sleep starts [32]. The minor form is characterized by excessive startle response without any signs of body stiffness. The occasional occurrence of the minor form in other families has been confirmed, but whether the minor form represents a variation in expression of the same gene defect in the major form remains conjectural [33]. The startle response in hyperekplexia has not been restricted to the moment of sleep onset only, unlike that noted in sleep starts. Clinical and physiological observations support a brainstem origin for the hyperekplectic startle response [33]. The only difference from the normal response is that in hyperekplexia there is impairment of the habituation and exaggerated startle response in these patients.

Non-familial hyperekplexia or essential startle disease of Gastaut and Villeneuve [34]

Sporadic cases of hyperekplexia without a genetic basis have been described by Gastaut and Villeneuve. The case described by Chokroverty *et al.* in a 67-year-old patient with a 4–6-year history of incapacitating startle conforms to the category of essential startle disease [35]. The startle reflex showed impaired habituation and exaggerated response.

Polysomnographic findings

Electrophysiological correlates of sleep starts were first recorded by Oswald [3], and later polygraphic recordings were made by Gastaut and Broughton [4] and by Broughton [6]. Hypnic jerks occur during transition from wakefulness to sleep as well as on falling asleep. Surface EMG recordings including multiple muscle recordings show bursts of muscle potentials with a duration of 75–250 ms both in the agonist and antagonist muscles as a single burst or in succession. The EEG channels show movement artifacts as a result of these body jerks. EEG during these spells typically show the stage 1 sleep pattern and may show a vertex wave. Following the jerks, the patient briefly awakens with return of the alpha activity (figure 1). There is also autonomic activation of tachycardia and tachypnea. PSG recording is not needed most of the time, but occasionally intensified hypnic jerks or sleep starts may be mistaken for myoclonic seizures and then PSG recording with a seizure montage is needed to exclude any evidence of electrographic epileptiform discharges.

Pathophysiology of sleep starts

At sleep onset, a variety of physiological changes occur in the body caused by activation of sleep-promoting neurons and inhibition of neurons responsible for wakefulness with blockage of the afferent stimuli at the thalamic level creating a momentary unstable state in the body physiologically with steady but progressive motor inhibition. In sleep starts there is a sudden inhibition of such normal motor atonia coupled with a sudden "whirlwind" of excitation of the cortical and subcortical motor structures producing a myoclonic jerk. This may happen spontaneously or in response to a stimulus (exogenous or endogenous), causing vertex sharp waves in the EEG. These jerks accompany sleep starts followed by autonomic activation (e.g. tachycardia and tachypnea) and cortical arousal (reappearance of alpha waves). Sleep starts may be similar to a normal physiological startle response, utilizing the same startle reflex pathways in the brainstem, causing patterned symmetrical muscle responses bilaterally in the body. The classical audiogenic startle reflex pathway as defined in animal studies, mostly in rats, involves the structures in the brainstem [36,37]. The reflex pathway begins in the auditory nerve and involves the following structures: ventral cochlear nucleus (first synapse), ventral nucleus of the lateral lemniscus (second synapse), nucleus reticularis pontis caudalis (third synapse) and divergent pathways which include bulbar reticular tracts and motor neurons of the facial and other lower cranial nuclei as well as reticulospinal tracts, spinal interneurons, ventral motor neurons, spinal motor nerves and ultimately, the neuromuscular junctions (last synapse) before the inputs finally reach the muscles. The point against this hypothesis is the presence of asymmetrical and sometimes unilateral muscle jerks. On falling asleep, certain sensory centers within the cortex or subcortex may be facilitated or disinhibited; thus the sensory phenomena and the motor manifestations of sleep starts at sleep onset may correspond to excitation or disinhibition of sensory-motor pathways.

Treatment

Sleep starts are common physiological phenomenon affecting up to 70% of the adult population and the course is benign, resolving without any neurological sequela. Therefore reassurance and counseling are all that is needed to calm the patient down. The patient should also be advised to follow a strict sleep–wake schedule, avoid sleep deprivation and follow common-sense sleep hygiene measures, avoiding stimulants and heavy exercise in the evening. In some rare subjects, intensified hypnic jerks may give rise to anxiety and sleep-onset insomnia. Even in these cases, an adequate explanation and reassurance may help the patient but some patients may require a small dose of clonazepam (0.5–1 mg at bedtime) to ameliorate the symptoms on a short-term basis.

References

1. Mitchell SW. Some disorders of sleep. *Int J Med Sci* 1890; **100**: 109.
2. Roger H. *Les Troubles du Sommeil*. Paris: Masson et Cie, 1932; 201.
3. Oswald I. Sudden bodily jerks on falling asleep. *Brain* 1959; **82**: 92.
4. Gastaut H, Broughton R. A clinical and polygraphic study of episodic phenomena during sleep. In Wortis J (Ed), *Recent Advances in Biology and Psychiatry*, Volume 7, New York: Plenum Press, 1965; 197–222.
5. Broughton R. Pathological fragmentary myoclonus, intensified hypnic jerks and hypnagogic foot tremor: three unusual sleep-related movement disorders. In Koella WP, Obal M, Shulz H, Visser P (Eds), *Sleep '86*. Stuttgart: G Fischer Verlag, 1988; 240–2.
6. Broughton RJ. Behavioral parasomnias. In Chokroverty S (Ed), *Sleep Disorders Medicine; Basic Science, Technical Considerations and Clinical Aspects*. Boston: Butterworth/Hinemann, 2000; 636.
7. Sander HW, Geisse H, Quinto C, Sachdeo R, Chokroverty S. Sensory sleep starts. *J Neurol Neurosurg Psychiatry* 1998; **64**: 690.
8. Armstrong-Jones R. Snapping of the brain. *Lancet* 1920; **196**: 720.
9. Pearce JM. Clinical features of the exploding head syndrome. *J Neurol Neurosurg Psychiatry* 1989; **52**: 907–10.
10. Lance JW. Transient sensations of impending loss of consciousness: the "blip" syndrome. *J Neurol Neurosurg Psychiatry* 1996; **60**: 437–8.
11. American Academy of Sleep Medicine. *The International Classification of Sleep Disorders*, second edition. Westchester, IL: AASM, 2005.
12. Mahowald MW, Schenck CH. NREM sleep parasomnias. *Neuro Clin* 1996; **14**: 675–96.
13. Salih F, Klingebiel RD, Zschenderlein RD, Grosse P. Acoustic sleep starts with sleep onset insomnia related to a brain stem lesion. *Neurology* 2008; **70**: 1935–7.
14. Conigliari M, Quinto C, Masdeu J, Chokroverty S. An unusual presentation of hypnic jerks misdiagnosed as myoclonic seizure. *Neurology* 1999; **52**(Suppl 2): A80.
15. Montagna P. Physiologic body jerks and movements at sleep onset and during sleep. In Chokroverty S, Hening W, Walters A (Eds), *Sleep and Movement Disorders*. Boston: Butterworth/Heinemann, 2003.
16. Sachs C, Svanborg E. The exploding head syndrome: polysomnographic recordings and therapeutic suggestions. *Sleep* 1991; **14**: 263–6.
17. Bhatt M, Quinto C, Sachdeo R, Chokroverty S. Exploding head syndrome misdiagnosed as nocturnal seizures. *Neurology* 2000; **54**(Suppl 3): A403.
18. Fusco L, Pachatz C, Cusmai R, Vigevano F. Repetitive sleep starts in neurologically-impaired children: an unusual non-epileptic manifestation in otherwise epileptic subjects. *Epileptic Disord* 1999; **1**: 63–7.
19. Montagna P, Provini F, Plazzi G, et al. Propriospinal myoclonus upon relaxation and drowsiness: a cause of severe insomnia. *Mov Dis Ord* 1997; **12**: 66–72.
20. Vetrugno R, Provini F, Meletti S, et al. Propriospinal myoclonus at the sleep–wake transition: a new type of parasomnia. *Sleep* 2001; **24**: 835–43.
21. Critchley M. The predormitum. *Rev Neurol (Paris)* 1955; **93**: 101–06.
22. DeLisi L. Su di un fenomeno motorio constante del sonno normale: le mioclonie ipniche fisiologiche. *Riv Patol Nervosa e Mentale* 1932; **39**: 481–96.

23. Dagnino N, Loeb C, Massazza G, Sacco G. Hypnic physiological myoclonus in man: an EEG-EMG study in normals and neurological patients. *Eur Neurol* 1969; **2**: 47–58.

24. Montagna P, Liguori R, Zucconi M, *et al*. Physiological hypnic myoclonus. *Electroencephalogr Clin Neurophysiol* 1988; **70**: 172–6.

25. Broughton R, Tolentino MA. Fragmentary pathological myoclonus in NREM sleep. *Electroencephalogr Clin Neurophysiol* 1984; **57**: 303–09.

26. Broughton R, Tolentino MA, Krelina M. Excessive fragmentary pathological myoclonus in NREM sleep: a report of 38 cases. *Electroencephalogr Clin Neurophysiol* 1985; **61**: 123–33.

27. Lins O, Castonguay M, Dunham W, *et al*. Excessive fragmentary myoclonus: time of night and sleep stage distributions. *Can J Neurol Sci* 1993; **20**: 142–6.

28. Iber C, Ancoli-Israel S, Chesson Al Jr, Quan SF. *The AASM Manual for the Scoring of Sleep and Associated Events: Rules, Terminology and Technical Specifications*. Westchester, IL: American Academy of Sleep Medicine, 2007.

29. Janz D. Epilepsy with impulsive petit mal (juvenile myoclonic epilepsy). *Acta Neurol Scand* 1985; **72**: 449.

30. Courter DL, Allen RG. Benign neonatal sleep myoclonus. *Arch Neurol* 1982; **13**: 191.

31. Chervin RD, Consens FB, Kutluay E. Alternating leg muscle activation during sleep and arousals: a new sleep-related motor phenomenon? *Mov Disord* 2003; **18**: 551–9.

32. Andermann F, Keene DL, Andermann E, Quesney LF. Startle disease or hyperekplexia; further delineation of the syndrome. *Brain* 1980; **103**: 984–97.

33. Brown P. Hyperekplexia. In Hallett M (Ed), *Movement Disorders: Handbook of Clinical Neurophysiology*. Amsterdam: Elsevier, 2003, vol. 1, 479–89.

34. Gastaut H, Villeneuve A. The startle disease or hyperekplexia. *J Neurol Sci* 1967; **5**: 523–42.

35. Chokroverty S, Walczak T, Henning W. Human startle reflex: technique and criteria for abnormal response. *Electroencephalogr Clin Neurophysiol* 1992; **85**: 236–42.

36. Leitner DS, Powers AS, Hoffman HS. The neural substrate of the startle response. *Physiol Behav* 1980; **25**: 291–7.

37. Davis M, Gendelman DS, Tischler MD, Gendelman DM. A primary acoustic startle circuit: vision and stimulation studies. *J Neurosci* 1982; **2**: 791–895.

Section 5 Chapter 24

Sleep-related movement disorders and other variants

Fragmentary myoclonus

Pasquale Montagna and Roberto Vetrugno

History and terminology

Excessive fragmentary myoclonus (EFM) was reported as a pathological motor activity of small myoclonic twitches and fasciculation potentials during NREM sleep, polygraphically difficult to distinguish from the physiologic FM except for greater EMG activity [1]. EFM has been incorporated in section VII, among the "isolated symptoms, apparently normal variants and unresolved issues", of the new *International Classification of Sleep Disorders* [2]. Alternate names include "fragmentary NREM myoclonus," "excessive fragmentary hypnic myoclonus," and "sleep-related twitching." EFM is characterized by small "quiver" movements of the corners of the mouth, finger, toes or limbs that usually do not cause gross movement across a joint space. Patients are typically unaware of the occurrence of these movements during sleep and may be totally asymptomatic during the daytime, apart from some rare cases with daytime sleepiness or fatigue (Figure 24.1). Nevertheless, it is difficult to establish a causative relationship between EFM and, when present, daytime impairments, as many patients have other associated disorders of sleep (Figure 24.2). The course of EFM is not well known, and longitudinal studies regarding progression and/or consequences of the disorder are lacking.

Clinical findings

At rest, during wakefulness, muscle tone, while abolished in the voluntary muscles, still persists in the antigravitary muscles. During transition from wakefulness to NREM sleep and during NREM sleep, muscle tone is diminished and spontaneous motor activity reduced [3].

De Lisi (1932) was the first to observe in humans and in domestic animals such as cats and dogs brief, fine, twitch-like movements involving various body areas in asynchronous and asymmetric fashion at sleep onset and at times during sleep [4]. He called these twitch-like movements "physiologic hypnic myoclonias" (PHM).

Using surface EMG electrodes, potentials of 50–200 μV in amplitude and less than 150 ms in duration were recorded [5,6]. The twitches resembled fasciculation potentials when they remained confined to the muscle belly and assumed a myoclonic aspect when large enough to displace the segment involved, such as lip and fingers [7]. These twitches were particularly prominent in small babies and children and in muscles of the extremities. They were especially frequent during NREM sleep stage 1, peaking during REM sleep and decreasing during deep sleep [7]. PHM closely resemble the brief jerky motor activity observed in the cat during phasic REM sleep periods, which were thought to derive from strong excitatory volleys descending from the reticular formation.

Dagnino *et al.* performed a quantitative study of FM in humans, and calculated its incidence in the different sleep stages by means of a myoclonic index in the opponens pollicis muscles in 29 normal volunteers [6]. They also examined 18 patients with various neurological diseases of neural, spinal, or pyramidal and extrapyramidal origin. The greatest myoclonic index was found in stage 1 NREM sleep, decreasing progressively in REM sleep, and in stages 2, 3 and 4 NREM sleep. There were no differences between phasic and tonic (e.g. associated or not with bursts of rapid eye movements) REM sleep periods. FM could also be recorded from patients with peripheral nerve lesions or with spinal paraplegia, whereas it was not observed in two patients with tabe dorsalis, in whom muscle proprioceptive input was probably abolished. In six patients with ischemic hemiparesis FM was absent on

The Parasomnias and Other Sleep-Related Movement Disorders, ed. M. J. Thorpy and G. Plazzi. Published by Cambridge University Press. © Cambridge University Press 2010.

237

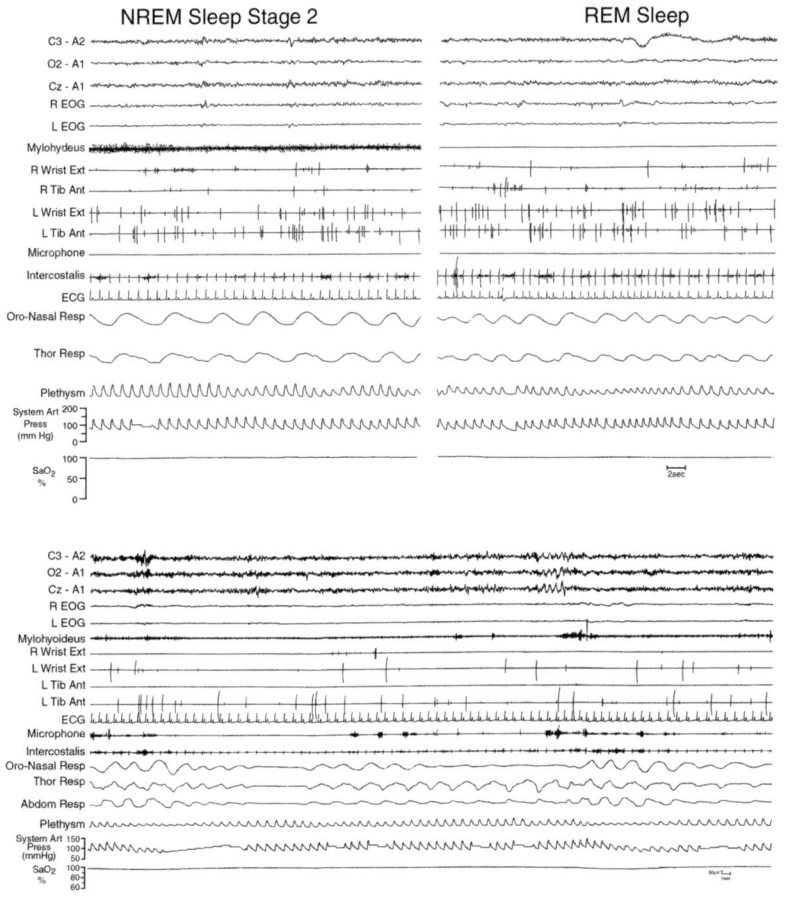

Figure 24.1 Excessive fragmentary myoclonus occurring in the right and left limbs as an isolated phenomenon during sleep, without significant EEG changes and with persistent chin atonia (Mylohyoideus) during REM sleep. EOG: electro-oculogram; Wrist Ext: wrist extensor; Tib Ant: tibialis anterior; ECG: electrocardiogram; Oro-Nasal Resp: oro-nasal respirogram; Thor Resp: thoracic respirogram; Plethysm: plethysmogram; System Art Press: systemic arterial pressure; SaO$_2$: oxygen saturation; R: right; L: left.

Figure 24.2 Excessive fragmentary myoclonus recorded as brief high amplitude EMG potentials in the right and left limbs in a patient with obstructive sleep apnea. EOG: electro-oculogram; Wrist Ext: wrist extensor; Tib Ant: tibialis anterior; ECG: electrocardiogram; Oro-Nasal Resp: oro-nasal respirogram; Thor Resp: thoracic respirogram; Plethysm: plethysmogram; System Art Press: systemic arterial pressure; SaO$_2$: oxygen saturation; R: right; L: left.

the affected side, whereas it was greatly increased in six patients with Parkinson's disease and in one patient with Wilson's disease. Five patients who underwent thalamotomy did not show any change in the amount of FM.

Therefore, FM can be considered to represent a universal phenomenon in normal subjects, where it is most apparent during stage 1 NREM sleep, in contrast to studies in cats in which the highest peak of FM is reached during REM sleep [8]. Moreover, FM originates in the muscle endplate [9], but undergoes a supraspinal modulation [6,8], because it does not occur in muscles paralyzed because of a peripheral nerve, spinal, or pyramidal lesion, it is increased in extrapyramidal diseases such as Parkinson's disease, and remains unaffected by changes in muscle spindle afferents brought about by dorsal root lesions (tabes dorsalis).

Another quantitative analysis in seven healthy subjects documented that FM was more frequent during stage 1 NREM sleep and peaked during REM sleep, in keeping with the experimental studies in animals. There was, again, no difference between phasic and tonic REM sleep periods. EMG activity identical to FM could also be recorded but to a much lesser degree during quiet wakefulness and persisted, at this level, during stages 2, 3 and 4 NREM sleep. FM was especially abundant in muscles such as the tibialis anterior and the triangularis labii, rather than in more proximal muscles such as the deltoideus [7].

Askenasy et al. (1988) compared the ocular versus the tibialis anterior muscles and found discharges in both muscles, but those in the ocular muscles were 14 times more common during REM sleep. Phasic discharges were, however, a constant feature of REM sleep in the tibialis anterior muscles [10].

In cats, the hypnic twitches observed during REM sleep are probably caused by a descending volley within the reticulospinal system that impinges on the spinal alpha motoneurons [8]. Indeed, destruction of the reticulospinal tract abolished the myoclonic activity which was left unchanged by lesioning of the dorsal root, red nucleus, or pyramidal tract. Pyramidal tract lesions had a temporary inhibiting effect. Thus, it seems that, in animals, hypnic twitches represent the motor accompaniment of the tonic electroencephalographic desynchronization transmitted from the reticular substance to the spinal cord [8]. Gastaut proposed the pontine tegmentum as the site of origin of this kind of myoclonus [11].

In the baboon during light sleep, myoclonias are almost always accompanied by electroencephalographic paroxysmal discharges of the fronto-rolandic cortex, which disappear, together with the myoclonus, during deep-sleep stages. During REM sleep, hypnic myoclonus again becomes well evident, unassociated, however, with cortical discharges. Therefore in the baboon, hypnic myoclonus seems not to be tightly linked to the cortical discharges, but rather coupled to them during light sleep by a hypothetical subcortical pacemaker [12]. It must be remarked, however, that these myoclonias described in the baboon as being like FM are phenomenologically more similar to hypnic jerks.

Dagnino *et al.* (1969) proposed a role of the corticospinal tract in the transmission of the excitatory volleys responsible for the FM, in keeping with the spatial distribution of the hypnic myoclonias that were especially evident in distal and facial muscles [6].

Physiologic FM thus consists of sudden, arrhythmic, asynchronous and asymmetric brief twitches involving various body areas, in particular distal limbs and face, occurring during sleep [4], but also during relaxed wakefulness and with an inverse relationship with the degree of EEG synchronization [5–7]. The muscle discharges of FM appear as bursts of unit action potentials of the facial and other muscles with visible movement when >150 μV in amplitude.

EFM can be recorded in 5–10% of patients suffering from excessive daytime sleepiness, in most cases adults, and is predominantly found in males. Pathological FM was reported for the first time by Broughton and Tolentino in 1984 in a 42-year-old patient exhibiting marked amounts of brief, multifocal and aperiodic myoclonus throughout NREM sleep, associated with excessive daytime sleepiness. At polysomnography, the myoclonus was very brief (less than 150 ms in duration), aperiodic and recurred in an asynchronous and asymmetrical fashion over the legs, arms and face, with equal frequency in all stages of NREM sleep and with some degree of sleep fragmentation. The EMG contractions often corresponded to visible brief leg twitches and were dissimilar from any physiologic motor activity or from the jerks of periodic limb movements during sleep (PLMS). Although the authors noted the difference from physiological FM previously described as predominant in stage 1 of NREM sleep, they stated that it could conceivably represent an abnormal intensification of that entity [1]. Subsequently, EFM was described in 38 consecutive patients, predominantly males (36/38), and was found associated with sleep-related respiratory problems (sleep apnea obstructive and/or central in 12 cases) (Figure 24.2), periodic movements in sleep (in 11 cases) (Figure 24.3), narcolepsy (in 6 cases), insomnia (in 2 cases), and excessive daytime sleepiness (in 6 cases). The phenomenon was present throughout all stages of NREM sleep, with a frequency never below five twitches per minute (over a sustained period of 20 min), and could be polymyoclonic in shape. It recurred randomly over the two sides and, when of larger magnitude, was accompanied by visible twitches, but never during pre-sleep wakefulness, and without any specific EEG changes. The twitches showed no relationship to nocturnal hypoxia, even though in some cases they intensified during periods of decreased oxygen saturation. Thus, it appeared that EFM represented a distinct polysomnographic abnormality associated with excessive daytime sleepiness or insomnia, perhaps facilitated by hypoxia. It was considered as a pathological "spillover" of the physiologic FM sometimes encountered in light stages of NREM sleep in normals [13].

A quantitative index of EFM has also been proposed to monitor its modification as a function of sleep stages and time. This FM index (FMI) was defined as the calculated mean of 3-s epochs with one or more myoclonic potentials exceeding 50 μV averaged for each 30-s scoring epoch and across sleep stages [14]. In 11 patients, the FMI was significantly higher than in a control group during all sleep stages, but with a somewhat lower frequency in slow-wave sleep. FMI reached the highest score during REM sleep and showed no relationship to age of the patients. FMI exhibited a significantly lower rate in the first hour after sleep onset compared to later hours. Interestingly, there was no evidence for greater sleep fragmentation or lighter sleep compared to a matched patient group in whom EFM had not been noted [14].

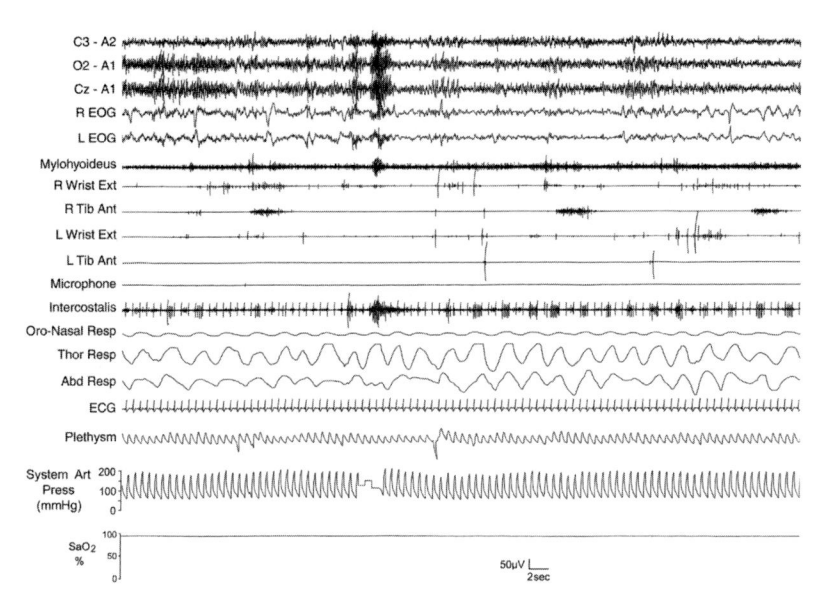

Figure 24.3 Co-existence of periodic limb movements during sleep and excessive fragmentary myoclonus in a patient with restless legs syndrome. EOG: electro-oculogram; Wrist Ext: wrist extensor; Tib Ant: tibialis anterior; ECG: electrocardiogram; Oro-Nasal Resp: oro-nasal respirogram; Thor Resp: thoracic respirogram; Abd Resp: abdominal respirogram; Plethysm: plethysmogram; System Art Press: systemic arterial pressure; SaO$_2$: oxygen saturation; R: right; L: left.

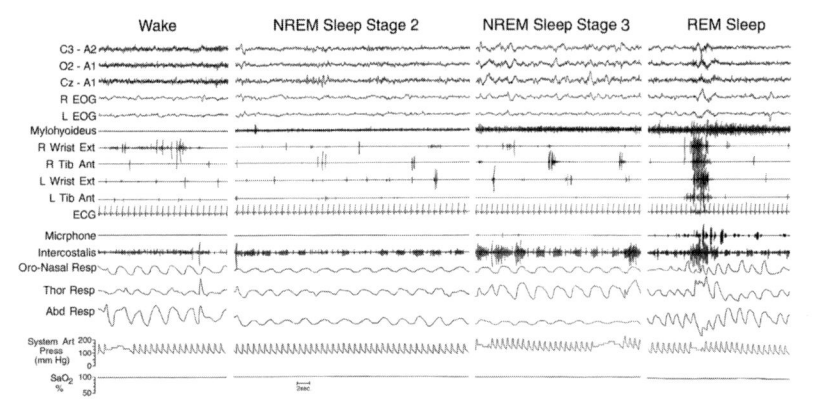

Figure 24.4 Polysomnographic samples from relaxed wakefulness (Wake), NREM sleep stage 2, NREM sleep stage 3 and REM sleep in a patient showing excessive fragmentary myoclonus throughout all the states and culminating into a REM sleep behavior disorder episode during REM Sleep. EOG: electro-oculogram; Wrist Ext: wrist extensor; Tib Ant: tibialis anterior; ECG: electrocardiogram; Oro-Nasal Resp: oro-nasal respirogram; Thor Resp: thoracic respirogram; Abd Resp: abdominal respirogram; System Art Press: systemic arterial pressure; SaO$_2$: oxygen saturation; R: right; L: left.

EFM has been reported as an isolated finding in a 71-year-old man with a 4-year history of "quiver" movements affecting primarily the hands and face, and as associated with REM sleep behavior disorder (RBD) in a 53-year-old man with a 3-year history of episodic elaborate movements during sleep and associated daytime sleepiness [15]. Both patients had no neuromuscular abnormalities at EMG-ENG investigation during wake. Polysomnographic study documented RBD in the second patient and EFM in both patients. EFM was present in all sleep stages, but prevailed in the second part of the night. Back-averaging of myoclonic activity during sleep did not disclose any EMG-related cortical activity. Carbamazepine (200 mg at bedtime) reduced the number of quiver movements during the night in the first patient, and clonazepam (2 mg at bed time) reduced all kinds of movements during the night in the second patient; in both patients therapy also improved the quality of sleep [15].

EMG patterns quite similar to EFM have also been observed in patients with restless legs syndrome (RLS) (Figure 24.3) [16], extrapyramidal syndromes [17], RBD (Figure 24.4) [18], status dissociatus [19,20], children with Niemann–Pick disease type C [21], and mitochondrial encephalomyopathy [22].

PHM must be distinguished from the sleep starts (also termed hypnic jerks) which occur at sleep onset but consist of simultaneous contractions of the whole-body or one or asymetrically more body segments [2] and that may be erroneously identified as FM [8]. PHM also differs from other pathological forms of sleep-related myoclonus such as the epileptic myoclonus that can occur during sleep and is associated with an EEG discharge, the propriospinal myoclonus that consists of sudden muscular jerks involving mainly axial muscles with flexion of the trunk occurring at the transition from wakefulness to sleep [23,24], the minipolymyoclonus seen with some degenerative disease and some neuropathic and myopathic conditions, and the tardive dyskinesia, dystonia, choreoathetosis, and various spasms that are more intense and slower movements.

Natural history

There is insufficient information about the natural history of EFM. EFM is indeed a sleep-related phenomenon that still lies at the borderline between normal and abnormal events. Its course is not well studied, and whether it is benign or progressive remains unsolved.

Laboratory investigations

For patients with suspected EFM, multiple muscle EMGs from all four limbs are essential during polysomnographic investigation. The upper and lower limb surface electrodes should be placed over wrist extensor and tibialis anterior muscles, respectively, with a distance of 2–2.5 cm between the two electrodes. The electrode impedance should be less than 5 KΩ with a high-frequency filter of 90 Hz and a low-frequency filter of 5.0 Hz, and with a sensitivity of at least 50 μV per centimeter. Simultaneous videorecording is mandatory to document and clearly differentiate any kind of sleep-related abnormal movements, EFM included. On video-polysomnography, EFM is detected as asymmetrical, asynchronous EMG potentials that when exceeding 200 μV in amplitude or when repetitive (more than 150 ms in duration) can be associated with visible local twitches of the fingers, toes, or corners of the mouth. If smaller, without overt movement, EFM may resemble fasciculation potentials (Figures 24.1 and 24.2). Even when movements are present, the patient may be totally unaware of them. Occasionally, the EMG activity is already present in drowsiness prior to sleep onset and may persist during EEG periods of wakefulness after sleep onset. The EMG findings of EFM resemble the phasic REM twitches that are a normal finding in REM sleep, except that they exist in all stages of sleep and are not clustered as in normal REM sleep, but are more evenly spaced across individual epochs. It is never associated with cortical epileptic activity and seems to be independent from infra-slow oscillations of sleep-related EEG activity like K-complexes and transient EEG arousal, without any ocular or autonomic accompaniments. More than five potentials per minute sustained for at least 20 min of NREM sleep stages 2, 3, or 4 are necessary to score the presence of EFM during polysomnography (ICSD-2).

Genetics and pathology

Whether there is a genetic or other basis predisposing individuals to develop EFM is unknown. No familial cases of "pure" EFM have been described to date. Likewise, pathology is unknown, since no cases have come to autopsy because of EFM.

Management

There is no known treatment, but the need for treatment remains unclear, and it is better to decide according to each patient's history. Clonazepam and carbamazepine seem to reduce EFM clinically and polysomnographically [15,19]. SSRIs can cause EFM-like motor activity during sleep [25], their withdrawal resulting in normalization of excessive motor activity during sleep.

Conclusions (including future direction)

The exact origin and significance of FM still remains unclear, and despite it being a common finding in polysomnography, it is often asymptomatic. Therefore, the overall significance of EFM is unknown, in particular whether it occurs as a consequence of sleep disruption or whether it is an independent cause of sleep disruption and daytime symptoms. The pathological relevance of EFM should therefore be evaluated in the frame of the clinical findings displayed by each patient. In particular, its association with RBD deserves attention in relation to a possible common pathogenetic mechanism (Figure 24.4). Many patients with RBD, indeed, display prominent aperiodic movements of all extremities in every conceivable combination during all stages of NREM sleep. These aperiodic movements are similar to, and even more intense than EFM [18]. It has also been observed that patients with RBD may develop, with time, chronic status dissociatus with persistent motor activity and quivering movements throughout the night that polygraphically resemble EFM [20]. Likewise, after surgery for tegmental pontomesencephalic cavernoma, a 36-year-old patient developed status dissociatus with sleep-related complex abnormal motor patterns and behaviors including EFM, diffuse myoclonic jerks and RBD [19]. These observations suggest that the derangement of neural structures responsible for motor control during sleep may be responsible for both EFM and RBD, for the blowing of EFM into RBD or for the "dissolving" of RBD into EFM. Indeed, functional depression or destruction of the brainstem structures responsible for atonia, and reduced activity or destruction of brainstem serotonergic or noradrenergic structures responsible for inhibiting phasic activity, may result in motor activity during sleep and determine the evolution, even in the same patient, of one kind of sleep-related motor disorder into another [20,26]. Remarkably, leg muscle twitches have been reported to increase during REM sleep as a result of emotional distress and anxiety in humans suffering from post-traumatic stress disorder (PTSD) [27–30]. These observations seem to be consistent with the view that a disregulation of REM sleep, particularly its phasic event generation, may be involved in the pathogenesis of EFM and its association with other motor disorders (especially RBD and PLMS) in the same patient. Further studies should be aimed at the definition, if any, of the cut-off between physiological FM, as seen in many normal individuals, versus EFM, and at investigating EFM as a possible marker of neurodegeneration and/or abnormal central nervous system motor excitability.

References

1. Broughton R, Tolentino MA. Fragmentary pathological myoclonus in NREM sleep. *Electroenceph Clin Neurophysiol* 1984; **57**: 303–09.
2. International Classification of Sleep Disorders. *Diagnostic and Coding Manual*. 2nd ed. Westchester, IL: American Academy of Sleep Medicine, 2005; 218–20.
3. Chase MH, Morales FR. The control of motoneurons during sleep. In Kryger MH, Roth T, Dement WC (Eds), *Principles and Practice of Sleep Medicine*. Philadelphia: Saunders, 1989; 74–85.
4. De Lisi. Su di un fenomeno motorio costante del sonno normale: le mioclonie ipniche fisiologiche. *Riv Pat Nerv* 1932; **39**: 481–96.
5. Loeb C, Massazza G, Sacco G, et al. Etude polygraphique des 'myoclonies hypniques' chez l'homme. *Rev Neurol* 1964; **10**: 258–68.
6. Dagnino N, Loeb C, Massazza G, et al. Hypnic physiological myoclonias in man: An EEG-EMG study in normals and neurological patients. *Eur Neurol* 1969; **2**: 47–58.
7. Montagna P, Liguori R, Zucconi M, et al. Physiological hypnic myoclonus. *Electroenceph Clin Neurophysiol* 1988; **70**: 172–6.
8. Gassel MM, Marchiafava PL, Pompeiano O. Phasic changes in muscular activity during desynchronized sleep in unrestrained cats. An analysis of the pattern and organization of myoclonic twitches. *Arch Ital Biol* 1964; **102**: 449–70.
9. Buchthal F, Rosenfalck P. Spontaneous electrical activity of human muscles. *Electroenceph Clin Neurophysiol* 1966; **20**: 231–2.
10. Askenasy JJ, Yahr MD, Davidovitch S. Isolated phasic discharges in anterior tibial muscle: A stable feature of paradoxical sleep. *J Clin Neurophysiol* 1988; **5**: 175–81.
11. Gastaut H. Les myoclonies – Séméiologie des myoclonies et nosologie analytique des syndromes myocloniques. *Rev Neurol* 1968; **119**: 1–30.
12. Cepeda C, Naquet R. Physiological sleep myoclonus in baboons. *Electroencephalogr Clin Neurophysiol* 1985; **60**: 158–62.
13. Broughton R, Tolentino MA, Krelina M. Excessive fragmentary myoclonus in NREM sleep: A report of 38 cases. *Electroenceph Clin Neurophysiol* 1985; **61**: 123–33.
14. Lins O, Castonguay M, Dunham W, et al. Excessive fragmentary myoclonus: Time of night and sleep stage distribution. *Can J Neurol Sci* 1993; **20**: 142–6.
15. Vetrugno R, Plazzi G, Provini F, et al. Excessive fragmentary hypnic myoclonus: Clinical and neurophysiological findings. *Sleep Med* 2002; **3**: 73–6.
16. Coccagna G, Lugaresi E, Tassinari CA, et al. La sindrome delle gambe senza riposo (restless legs). *Omnia Med Ther* 1966; **44**: 619–87.
17. Tassinari CA, Broughton R, Poiré R, et al. Sur l'évolution des mouvements anormaux au cours du summeil. In Fishgold H, et al. (Eds), *Le sommeil de nuit normal et pathologique. Electrencephalographie Neurophysiologie Clinique* Paris: Masson, 1965; 314–33.
18. Mahowald MW, Schenck CH. REM sleep parasomnias. In Kryger MH, Roth T, Dement WC (Eds), *Principles and Practice of Sleep Medicine*. 3rd ed. Philadelphia, PA: W.B. Saunders, 2000; 724–41.
19. Provini F, Vetrugno R, Pastorelli F, et al. Status dissociatus after surgery for tegmental

ponto-mesencephalic cavernoma: A state-dependent disorder of motor control during sleep. *Mov Disord* 2004; **19**: 719–23.

20. Vetrugno R, Alessandria M, D'Angelo R, et al. Status dissociatus evolving from REM sleep behavior disorder in multiple system atrophy. *Sleep Med* 2009; **10**: 247–52.

21. Vankova J, Stepanova I, Jech R, et al. Sleep disturbances and hypocretin in Niemann–Pick disease type C. *Sleep* 2003; **26**: 427–30.

22. Pincherle A, Mantoani L, Villani F. Excessive fragmentary hypnic myoclonus in a patient affected by a mitochondrial encephalomyopathy. *Sleep Med* 2006; **7**: 663.

23. Montagna P, Provini F, Plazzi G, et al. Propriospinal myoclonus upon relaxation and drowsiness: A cause of severe insomnia. *Mov Disord* 1997; **12**: 66–72.

24. Vetrugno R, Provini F, Meletti S, et al. Propriospinal myoclonus at the sleep–wake transition: A new type of parasomnia. *Sleep* 2001; **24**: 835–43.

25. Jordan LM, Liu J, Hedlund PB, Akay T, Pearson KG. Descending command systems for the initiation of locomotion in mammals. *Brain Res Rev* 2008; **57**: 183–91.

26. Hishikawa Y, Sugita Y, Iijima S, et al. Mechanisms producing "stage 1-REM" and similar dissociations of REM sleep and their relation to delirium. *Adv Neurol Sci (Tokyo)* 1981; **25**: 1129–47.

27. Ross RJ, Ball WA, Sullivan KA, Caroff SN. Sleep disturbance as the hallmark of posttraumatic stress disorder. *Am J Psychiatry* 1989; **146**: 697–707.

28. Ross RJ, Ball WA, Dinges DF, et al. Motor dysfunction during sleep in posttraumatic stress disorder. *Sleep* 1994; **17**: 723–32.

29. Ross RJ, Ball WA, Dinges DF, et al. Rapid eye movement sleep disturbance in posttraumatic stress disorder. *Biol Psychiatry* 1994; **35**: 195–202.

30. Mellman TA, Nolan B, Hebding J, Kulick-Bell R, Dominguez R. A polysomnographic comparison of veterans with combat-related PTSD, depressed men, and non-ill controls. *Sleep* 1997; **20**: 46–51.

Section 5 Chapter 25

Sleep-related movement disorders and other variants

Sleep-related leg cramps

Renee Monderer and Michael J. Thorpy

Introduction

Leg cramps are defined as involuntary painful contractions that usually occur in the calf, but may sometimes affect the thighs or feet [1]. These episodes can last anywhere from a few seconds to 10 min and then remit spontaneously. Tenderness and pain can last for several hours after the cramping. Although cramps can occur during the daytime, they are more frequent at night. Most people experience leg cramps at some time in their life, but they are usually very sporadic. While the cramps may be painful at the time, because they are infrequent, there is usually little concern about the episodes. However, occasionally patients have frequent nocturnal leg cramps causing much distress and night-time disturbance. The simplest remedy that is often discovered by the patient is forceful stretching. Painful cramps and remedies used to relieve the pain can delay sleep onset and awaken the patient from sleep. The discomfort that persists after a cramp can delay subsequent return to sleep.

Epidemiology

Nocturnal leg cramps are common, especially among the elderly. Naylor and colleagues studied 218 subjects and found the overall prevalence of cramps was 37% among patients 50 years and older [2]. The cramps increased with age, with those over age 80 having a prevalence of 54%. No significant difference in prevalence was noted between men and women.

The above study also describes the clinical features reported by these patients [2]. Those patients who reported leg cramps described symptoms in their leg, foot or thigh muscles. Seventy-three per cent of patients reported having cramps only at night, whereas 20% reported rest cramps during the day and night, and only 7% had symptoms exclusively during the day.

Nine minutes was the average duration of the cramps (95% CI 6.7–11.2). Thigh cramps tended to last longer when compared to those in the foot or leg. The majority of cramp sufferers reported symptoms occurring less than once per week, but 40% experienced cramps more than three times per week and 6% reported daily leg cramps.

Oboler and colleagues looked at the prevalence of nocturnal leg cramps in 515 veterans. Of these patients, 95% were men with a mean age of 60.4 years (range 26–91). In this survey, 56% reported nocturnal leg cramps [3]. Thus, a similar prevalence was found in this population.

Another population that often reports leg cramps is pregnant women. Young and colleagues found that up to 50% of pregnant women experience leg cramps [4]. These cramps tended to increase in frequency as the pregnancy progressed. Many women reported that the leg cramps were most distressing at night and disturbed their night-time sleep.

Leg cramps not only occur in adults and become more frequent with age, but they can occur in children too. Leung and colleagues evaluated 2527 healthy children and found that the overall incidence of leg cramps was 7.3% [5]. Children as young as 8 years reported cramps, but the incidence increased at age 12 and peaked at ages 16–18. Most children (81.6%) reported only experiencing cramps 1–4 times a year and they typically lasted for about 2 min. This study showed that nocturnal leg cramps are a problem in children, but the clinical characteristics are significantly different than those seen in adults.

Pathophysiology

The pathophysiologic mechanism underlying leg cramps remains unclear. Electromyography during

The Parasomnias and Other Sleep-Related Movement Disorders, ed. M. J. Thorpy and G. Plazzi. Published by Cambridge University Press. © Cambridge University Press 2010.

leg cramps shows bursts of high-voltage and high-frequency discharges. Spontaneous firing of groups of anterior horn cells, followed by contraction of motor units, has been implicated in the pathophysiology [6]. Other mechanisms that have been proposed involve motor unit hyperactivity possibly due to spinal disinhibition, abnormal terminal motor nerve excitability, or enhanced muscle contraction propagation through cross-activation of neurons [7]. It has been suggested that cramps occur when a maximally contracted muscle is stimulated, and is therefore shortened beyond physiologic tolerance [8]. Pain may occur from an accumulation of metabolites or from focal ischemia [7].

Inadequate stretching exercise or muscle and tendon shortening with age have been proposed as possible contributors to the development of nocturnal cramps [9]. The squatting hypothesis suggests that modern habits of failure to squat when sitting or using the bathroom lead to inadequate stretching of the muscles. This in turn may cause muscle and tendon shortening leading to nocturnal leg cramps. The basis for this theory comes from the knowledge that stretching the affected muscle helps prevent or reduce cramps.

Risk factors

Most cases of leg cramps are idiopathic. However, there are many secondary causes of leg cramps, including endocrine, metabolic, neuromuscular, vascular and congenital disorders (Table 25.1). Disorders such as thyroid disease (both hyperthyroidism and hypothyroidism), diabetes mellitus, peripheral vascular disease, iron deficiency anemia, McArdle's disease, autosomal dominant cramping disease and Parkinson's disease can be associated with leg cramps [10]. Electrolyte imbalance from low magnesium, calcium, sodium or phosphate or volume depletion secondary to sweating, diarrhea, diuretics, or hemodialysis can also precipitate leg cramps. Neuromuscular disorders such as nerve root compression, motor neuron disease, mononeuropathies, polyneuropathies and dystonia are also known secondary causes of cramps. Many medications such as nifedipine, beta-blockers, steroids, morphine, cimetidine, penicillamine, statins, oral contraceptives and lithium have been reported to cause leg cramps [7]. Leg cramps may also develop secondary to repetitive movements or after strenuous activity such as in runners [1]. The clinical features of cramps are essentially identical regardless of whether they are idiopathic or due to a secondary cause.

Table 25.1 Conditions associated with NLC.

Neurologic
Neuropathy, dystonia, Parkinson's disease, nerve root compression, motor neuron disease, multiple sclerosis

Endocrine
Hypothyroidism, hyperthyroidism, diabetes mellitus, Addison's disease

Metabolic
Hypoglycemia, hypocalcemia, hyperkalemia, hypokalemia, hyponatremia, dialysis, diarrhea

Vascular
Peripheral vascular disease, Reynaud's

Drugs
Nifedipine, diuretics, ethanol, phenothiazines, penacillamine, steroids, lithium, statins, fibrates, terbutaline, cimentadine, oral contraceptives, morphine withdrawal

Toxins
Lead toxicity, strychnine poisoning, tetanus

Congenital
Autosomal dominant cramping disease, McArdle's disease

Diagnosis

The best diagnostic approach to leg cramps includes a careful history and a thorough exam. Cramps can sometimes be confused with disorders such as restless legs syndrome (RLS), periodic limb movements, dystonia, vascular claudication, or peripheral neuropathy. The typical features usually allow differentiation from these other disorders.

Restless legs syndrome can be confused with cramps because both conditions occur during the sleep period and involve leg pain. However, RLS presents as more continuous discomfort, whereas nocturnal leg cramps cause acute sudden onset of pain. It can also be differentiated from nocturnal leg cramps in that movement of the legs mostly relieves RLS, whereas nocturnal leg cramps require vigorous stretching of the muscle to relieve the pain. Similarly, nocturnal leg cramps can be differentiated from periodic limb movements because of the muscle hardening, pain and necessity of strong stretching seen with cramps.

Certain nocturnal leg cramps, especially those in the feet, can look like dystonias. However, unlike dystonia, nocturnal leg cramps do not involve agonist and

Table 25.2 Medications for NLC.

Medication	Dose	Comments
Quinine sulfate	200–500 mg	Clinically appears effective, but FDA advisory about use
Magnesium sulfate	300–900 mg	May be beneficial for pregnancy-related leg cramps
Verapamil	120 mg	Limited data, but appears to be beneficial
Diltiazem	30 mg	Limited data, but appears to be beneficial
Vitamin E	400–800 IU	May be effective in dialysis patients
Vitamin B complex	See text	Limited data
Naftidrofuryl	30 mg	Limited data; not available in the USA
Orphenadrine citrate	100 mg	Limited data
Gabapentin	400–1600 mg	May be beneficial for cramps secondary to neurologic disease

antagonist muscle co-contraction and are relieved by muscle stretching.

Peripheral vascular disease causes intermittent claudication that also needs to be differentiated from nocturnal leg cramps. Claudication generally occurs during limb use and is relieved by rest, whereas cramps occur during rest. Occasionally claudication can cause cramps at rest or during sleep. It is important to examine the patient's legs for weak pulses or cold extremities to assist in this differentiation.

It is important to note that many of the disorders that mimic leg cramps can also be a secondary cause of leg cramps. For example, symptoms of peripheral neuropathy can be confused with cramps, but neuropathy can also cause cramps through nerve damage, muscle fiber pathology or disturbance of electrolytes responsible for nerve and muscle excitability [10].

Work-up

A detailed history should screen for the presence of secondary causes of cramping, such as diabetes mellitus, renal failure, thyroid disease, electrolyte imbalance and iron-deficiency anemia. Careful questioning about medication use, occupation, and physical routines can be helpful in making a diagnosis. The physical exam should look for signs of thyroid disease (goiter), dehydration (orthostatic hypotension, tachycardia), tetany, muscle wasting, dystonia, peripheral neuropathy, and peripheral pulses.

Blood tests can be useful if the history or physical exam points to a secondary etiology. Laboratory investigations such as iron studies, ferritin, and serum chemistry including sodium, potassium, calcium, and magnesium can be sent. Thyroid function tests as well as BUN and creatinine can also be helpful.

Additional testing such as duplex scans of the lower extremities in patients experiencing claudication and magnetic resonance imaging of the lumbar spine may help diagnose nerve root entrapment. Nerve conduction and electromyography may reveal neuropathies or motor neuron disease.

Polysomnographic studies are not routinely recommended for isolated nocturnal leg cramps. Patients with chronic nocturnal leg cramps may have non-periodic bursts of gastrocnemius EMG activity recorded on the polysomnogram.

Treatment

A vast array of treatments, both non-pharmacologic and pharmacologic, has been used in an attempt to treat nocturnal leg cramps. The first step should include treating any primary disorders that may be causing leg cramps. Withdrawal of medications suspected to be causing leg cramps may alleviate symptoms. Non-pharmacologic therapy, such as walking, stretching and massage, is recommended as first-line treatment [11,12]. Pharmacologic treatments that have been studied for nocturnal leg cramps include quinine, magnesium, calcium-channel blockers, sympathetic inhibitors, vitamin E, vitamin B complex and anti-epileptic medications. See Table 25.2.

Non-pharmacologic treatments

Cramps can be acutely managed by stretching the muscle. Forcible flexion of the foot with the knee extended can provide immediate relief. This is often the simplest treatment, which patients come to discover on their own. The use of stretching as a preventative measure has been studied in a limited number of studies reviewed below.

William Daniell first proposed stretching exercises to prevent night-time cramps [13]. He conducted a small, uncontrolled study that introduced patients to a regular program of stretching exercises to be performed three times per day. Patients were instructed to stand without their shoes, face a wall two to three feet away and then lean forward, using their hands and arms to regulate their forward tilt and keeping their heels on the floor. The stretching position was held for 10 s and then repeated after a 5-s period of relaxation. Daniell reported that all 44 patients were cured within one week and all remained almost cramp-free for as long as one year.

Based on the above study, Coppin and colleagues designed a study to evaluate the effect of calf-stretching exercises on nocturnal leg cramps [14]. The study randomized 191 patients, previously prescribed quinine for night-time cramps, into four groups, defined by whether or not they started exercise stretching programs and whether or not they stopped quinine. Follow-up at 12 weeks showed no significant difference between both advice on stretching and advice to stop quinine on the number of cramps reported. Thus, calf stretching was not shown to be effective in reducing night-time cramps. However, the authors concluded that patients on quinine might be able to stop medication without significant problems.

Other non-pharmacologic measures that have been proposed include raising the head of the bed and raising the feet on pillows. Neither of these methods has been evaluated formally. Other anecdotal treatments include lying in a prone position with the feet hanging over the end of the bed. However, this may be impractical, as most people reposition during the night [10].

Quinine sulfate

Quinine, an alkaloid agent, has been used to treat nocturnal leg cramps for many decades. The exact mechanism of action is unclear. Quinine is thought to increase the refractory period of skeletal muscle contractions resulting in a reduced response to titanic stimulation. Additionally, quinine decreases the excitability of the motor end plate to nerve stimulation [15].

Studies investigating the effectiveness of quinine for nocturnal leg cramps have yielded conflicting results. Man-Son-Hing and colleagues conducted a meta-analysis to assess the efficacy of quinine compared to placebo [11]. Data from a total of 107 general ambulatory patients from six randomized, double-blind, cross-over published studies was compiled. Treatment with 200–500 mg of quinine resulted in a significant reduction in the number of leg cramps for a 4-week period (8.83 fewer cramps; 95% confidence interval 4.3–13.5). Treatment did not result in a significant change in severity or duration of individual leg cramps. Serious side effects were reported in one patient. That person experienced nausea, myalgia, leucopenia and thrombocytopenia that resolved 3 days after stopping the medication. The authors concluded that quinine is effective for nocturnal leg cramps. However, patients should be monitored for at least 4 weeks to assess the benefits and risks for each patient individually, because these may not be apparent until the fourth week of treatment [11].

Mon-Son-Hing and colleagues published a second meta-analysis three years later that included data from three unpublished studies as well as four published studies used in the previous meta-analysis [12]. Combining data from the above studies, patients had 3.6 (95% confidence interval 2.2–5.1) fewer cramps in a 4-week period when taking quinine compared to control. Interestingly, the estimated benefit of quinine found in the published trials (8.83 fewer cramps: 95% CI 4.16–13.49) was larger than that derived from unpublished trials (2.45 fewer cramps; 95% CI 1.03–3.87). Hence, the addition of data from unpublished studies to the original published studies reduced the estimate of quinine efficacy, but the results remained significant. As seen in the original study, the longer the treatment period of a study, the larger its estimate of quinine benefit in reducing the frequency of leg cramps ($p = 0.1$). The analysis showed that tinnitus occurred at a significantly higher frequency when patients took quinine compared to controls ($p = 0.1$). After this second meta-analysis, the authors concluded that non-pharmacologic treatment, such as stretching, should be tried initially. If this fails and the patient's quality of life is significantly affected, then quinine should be tried [12].

Interestingly, both meta-analyses showed a large heterogeneity between the individual studies. One study by Connolly et al. was responsible for this heterogeneity. This study showed the largest effect of quinine on the frequency of nocturnal leg cramps. When this study was removed from the analysis, the estimated efficacy of quinine was 2.62 fewer cramps (95% CI 1.32–3.91) in a 4-week period. Notably, this study was the only one with exclusively male subjects and used the largest total dose of quinine (200 mg at supper and 300 mg at bedtime) [12].

In 2002, Diener and colleagues performed a double-blind, placebo-controlled trial to determine the effectiveness of quinine for nocturnal leg cramps [15]. Ninety-eight patients with more than six muscle cramps in 2 weeks were enrolled. A 2-week period without treatment was followed by 2 weeks with 400 mg of quinine or placebo and a washout period of 2 weeks without treatment. Eighty per cent of patients in the quinine group and 53% in the placebo group had a reduction of at least 50% in the number of muscle cramps. This points to a powerful placebo effect. The therapeutic effect continued in the washout period for the quinine group, but not for the placebo group, which possibly points to a pharmacologic action. No significant differences were found between the placebo and quinine group with respect to side effects, although the treatment period was only two weeks. It is noteworthy that this study used a high dose of quinine, which may account for the powerful effect seen in reducing the frequency of nocturnal leg cramps.

Recently, Woodfield and colleagues performed an N-of-1 trial in 13 general practice patients already prescribed quinine [16]. N-of-1 trials compare two treatments on each patient in a randomized, double-blind, multiple cross-over study. Following a 2-week washout period, quinine sulfate 200–300 mg/day and matched placebo capsules were compared in three 4-week treatment blocks (each block consisted of 2 weeks of active drug and 2 weeks of placebo in random order). Patients were randomly assigned to one of eight possible treatment sequences of active drug and placebo in a cross-over design. Ten people completed the study. Three patients showed significant benefits from quinine ($p < 0.05$), six showed non-significant benefits and one showed no benefit. Blood quinine levels were drawn and there was no correlation between steady-state plasma quinine and the number of cramps reported. The incidence of side effects was not significantly different between the quinine and placebo group. Interestingly, even after the results were presented to the patients at the conclusion of the study, no one decided to stop using quinine. This suggests that once patients are using quinine for leg cramps, they may be reluctant to stop the medication.

Significant debate surrounds the risk-to-benefit ratio of quinine, especially because the side effects are considerable. Thrombocytopenia is a rare but potentially fatal side effect. The Food and Drug Administration analysis of published and unpublished studies found evidence of thrombocytopenia in between 1:1000 and 1:3500 users [7]. Other hypersensitivity reactions include cinchonism, impaired vision, nausea, vomiting, epigastric pains, granulomatous hepatitis, cardiovascular effects and hemolytic uremic syndrome. There are no known factors that predispose patients to hypersensitivity reactions. These side effects may occur after a single dose or after months or years of use. A recent study found quinine-dependent IgG antibodies against platelets in two patients and against granulocytes in one patient who developed hypersensitivity reactions to quinine [17]. Additionally, quinine is capable of increasing serum digoxin levels by decreasing clearance of the drug [18]. Quinine can also interact with medications used in patients with renal failure or who are on dialysis, such as aluminum hydroxide, cimetidine, and heparin [18]. In 1995, after determining that the risk of quinine outweighed the possible benefits, the Food and Drug Administration ordered a stop to marketing of quinine for the prevention or treatment of nocturnal leg cramps. Quinine is still available for the treatment of malaria. Physicians can still use quinine for the treatment of nocturnal leg cramps, but the patient must understand the risks involved.

Due to the side effect profile of quinine, many researchers decided to conduct studies on alternative treatments for nocturnal leg cramps. Medications such as magnesium sulfate, calcium channel blockers, vitamin E and B and gabapentin have been studied as possible remedies. The research on these medications is reviewed below.

Magnesium sulfate

It is common practice in countries in Latin America and Europe to use magnesium sulfate for nocturnal leg cramps. Magnesium sulfate was first shown to be effective in treating nocturnal leg cramps in pregnant women. A double-blind, –placebo-controlled randomized study in pregnant women showed an improvement in leg cramps when taking magnesium [19]. The major side effect noted in this study was diarrhea.

Frusso and colleagues first studied the efficacy of using magnesium sulfate in non-pregnant patients in a cross-over randomized double-blind, placebo-controlled trial [20]. Forty-five patients were randomized to receive either 900 mg of magnesium citrate twice daily for one month followed by a matching placebo for one month, or the placebo first, followed by magnesium. No significant difference was found between placebo and magnesium in the number of cramps, nor in the duration or severity of cramps. Interestingly, there was a significant decrease in cramps between the first and second months of treatment regardless of treatment received. The authors attributed this period effect bias to a combination of natural variability of symptoms, regression to the mean, and a true placebo effect. Diarrhea was seen as a side effect of magnesium. Based on this study it appears that magnesium is not an effective treatment for nocturnal leg cramps. Presumably, the pathophysiology of leg cramps in pregnant women is different than that of the general population.

Roffe and colleagues did a second randomized double-blind placebo-controlled cross-over trial looking at the effect of magnesium [21]. Forty-seven patients received either 300 mg of magnesium for 6 weeks followed by placebo or placebo followed by magnesium. This study differed from Frusso's study in that there was a longer treatment period, and magnesium levels and compliance were monitored. As seen in the previous study, no significant decrease in number, severity or duration of cramps was found, but there was a trend towards fewer cramps on magnesium ($p = 0.07$). Additionally, significantly more patients thought that treatment had helped after magnesium (78%) than after placebo (54%) ($p = 0.03$). This study also had a significant period effect ($p = 0.008$). Diarrhea was seen as a side effect of magnesium. The authors concluded that magnesium may be an effective treatment and further studies were needed to evaluate its efficacy as a treatment for nocturnal leg cramps.

Calcium channel blockers

Baltodano and colleagues decided to study the effects of verapamil in leg cramps, based on the observation that when patients were being treated for angina with verapamil their leg cramps improved [22]. An open-label study with eight elderly patients (aged 62–87 years) experiencing frequent nocturnal leg cramps and refractory to quinine sulfate were placed on verapamil 120 mg at bedtime for 8 weeks. In 7 out of 8 patients, the nocturnal leg cramps completely resolved. There were no reported adverse events.

Voon and Sheu were pioneers in the use of calcium channel blockers and decided to study the effectiveness of diltiazem for nocturnal leg cramps [23]. The study evaluated 12 patients for 2 months in a randomized double-blind, placebo-controlled cross-over trial. Even with only 12 patients, the study showed a significant reduction in the frequency of nocturnal leg cramps with diltiazem (–5.84) as compared to placebo (–0.16) ($p = 0.040$). No side effects were reported.

It is interesting to note that nifedipine can induce leg cramps, but diltiazem and verapamil can relieve cramps. This distinction might be attributable to the fact that diltiazem and verapamil block neuromuscular transmission via inhibition of neurotransmitter release, but nifedipine does not [23]. This difference or a combination of mechanisms may account for the different effects of calcium channel blockers on nocturnal leg cramps.

Vitamin E

The idea of trying vitamin E for nocturnal leg cramps came from an incidental finding when patients taking vitamin E reported relief from cramping [24]. Ayers and Mihan described complete or almost complete resolution of leg cramps in 82% of their patients taking vitamin E [24]. Roca and colleagues had similar results when they performed a small, randomized, double-blind study using 400 IU of vitamin E taken at night in a group of dialysis patients [25]. This study found that vitamin E was just as effective as quinine in relieving leg cramps, but had fewer side effects. The authors concluded that vitamin E should be the initial treatment of choice for dialysis patients with leg cramps.

Connolly and coworkers compared the efficacy and safety of quinine sulfate, vitamin E, and placebo in a randomized, double-blind, placebo-controlled crossover trial [26]. Twenty-seven male veterans, aged 38–73 years, who reported frequent night-time leg cramps, completed this study. In a random order, patients were given quinine sulfate (200 mg at supper and 300 mg at bedtime), vitamin E (800 U at bedtime) or placebo for 4-week periods. The authors found that quinine reduced the frequency of leg cramps, but vitamin E was not effective in reducing the frequency of leg cramps.

Based on the above studies, it appears that although vitamin E at first seemed promising in an uncontrolled study, a randomized, controlled crossover trial showed vitamin E to be ineffective in reducing leg cramps in the general population. However, vitamin E may be effective for dialysis patients in relieving leg cramps.

Vitamin B complex

Only one randomized study was conducted to assess the efficacy and safety of vitamin B complex as a treatment for leg cramps. Chan and colleagues conducted a double-blind, placebo-controlled, randomized study using vitamin B complex (fursulthiamine 50 mg, hydroxocobalamin 250 μg, pyridoxal phosphate 30 mg and riboflavin) in 28 elderly patients with hypertension who had severe leg cramps [27]. Medications were taken three times daily. Eighty-six per cent of patients reported prominent remission of leg cramps compared to the placebo group, where no significant difference from baseline was found. This study appears promising, but further studies are needed to confirm the benefit of vitamin B complex for nocturnal leg cramps.

Naftidrofuryl oxalate and orphenadrine citrate

Small studies were done on naftidrofuryl oxalate, a vasodilator, and orphenadrine citrate, an anticholinergic muscle relaxant in patients with nocturnal leg cramps. Naftidrofuryl is available for treatment of cramps in England. A study out of England was conducted to examine the efficacy of naftidrofuryl oxalate in leg cramps. A double-blind, placebo-controlled study with 14 patients found that naftidrofuryl oxalate 30 mg twice daily significantly reduced cramp frequency (median naftidrofuryl = 5; median placebo = 17; $p < 0.004$) and significantly increased cramp-free days by a third ($p < 0.004$) [28]. Orphenadrine citrate decreased leg cramps frequency by 30% in 90% of 59 patients in a double-blind cross-over trial [29].

Anti-epileptic medications

Anti-epileptic medications were first studied in patients with leg cramps secondary to neurologic diseases. Chang and coworkers first reported an 18-year-old man with Issac's syndrome who had remarkable improvement with phenytoin therapy [30]. Next, Mueller and colleagues presented a study of 15 patients with multiple sclerosis who had severe leg cramps and spasticity [31]. They found that patients treated with 400 mg of gabapentin administered three times daily had significant improvement of symptoms. Gabapentin was well tolerated.

Based on the above reports, Serrao and colleagues performed an open-label trial with 30 patients who had frequent leg cramps associated with neurologic diseases such as neuropathy, radiculopathy, familial cramps, multiple sclerosis, and Parkinson's disease [32]. Patients started on gabapentin at 600 mg/day and titrated up to an average of 892 ± 180 mg/day at 3 months. After 3 months of therapy, patients reported a 100% disappearance of leg cramps. The mean frequency of cramps per week dropped from 18.6 ± 17.6 at baseline to 6.0 ± 8.5 ($p < 0.01$) at 1 month to 0.3 ± 0.5 at 3 months ($p < 0.001$). After 6 months the mean frequency was 0.2 ± 0.4 ($p < 0.001$). There was a similar response in pain ratings and sleep ratings. Gabapentin was generally well tolerated, with the exception of two patients who reported somnolence and drowsiness. These findings appear to be promising. Further studies in patients with idiopathic leg cramps are needed.

Conclusion

Nocturnal leg cramps is a common condition that become more frequent with age. The exact cause of leg cramps is unknown, but they can be associated with multiple diseases and medications. Therefore, it is important to identify any treatable causes for leg cramps. To date there are no studies proving the efficacy of non-pharmacologic methods in preventing leg cramps. Nevertheless, a therapeutic trial can be tried with patients given the benign nature of such treatments.

The safety and efficacy of quinine sulfate for leg cramps remains unclear. Some studies have shown that quinine is effective, while others have not shown a significant benefit from quinine use. There is significant debate about the risk/benefit ratio of this medication given the side effects that have been reported. Multiple other pharmacologic treatments have been studied, although no one treatment has sufficient research studies to prove its efficacy. Promising alternatives include diltiazem, verapamil, vitamin B complex, and orphenadrine citrate. Gabapentin has been shown to significantly reduce leg cramps in patients with neurologic diseases, but its usefulness in idiopathic leg cramps remains to be seen. Further research is needed to find a medication that is both safe and effective in preventing nocturnal leg cramps.

References

1. Riley JD, Anthony SJ. Leg cramps: Differential diagnosis and management. *Am Fam Physician* 1995; **52**: 1794–8.
2. Naylor JR, Young JB. A general population survey of rest cramps. *Age Ageing* 1994; **23**: 418–20.
3. Oboler SK, Prochazka AV, Meyer TJ. Leg symptoms in outpatient veterans. *West J Med* 1991: **155**; 256–9.
4. Young GL, Jewell D. Interventions for leg cramps in pregnancy. *Cochrane Database Syst Rev* 2002; **1**: CD000121.
5. Leung AK, Wong BE, Chan PY, Cho HY. Nocturnal leg cramps in children: Incidence and clinical characteristics. *J Natl Med Assoc* 1999; **91**: 329–32.
6. Criggs RC. Episodic muscle spasms, cramps, and weakness. In Fauci AS, Braunwald E, Isselbaucher KJ, et al. (Eds), *Harrison's Principles of Internal Medicine*. 14th ed. New York: McGraw Hill International, 1998; 119.
7. Bulter JV, Mulkerrin EC, O'Keeffe ST. Nocturnal leg cramps in older people. *Postgrad Med J* 2002; **78**: 596–8.
8. Weiner IH, Weiner HL. Nocturnal leg muscle cramps. *J Am Med Assoc* 1990; **150**: 511–8.
9. Sontag SJ, Wanner JN. The cause of leg cramps and knee pains: A hypothesis and effective treatment. *Med Hypoth* 1988; **25**: 35–41.
10. Kannan N, Sawaya R. Nocturnal leg cramps: Clinically mysterious and painful – but manageable. *Geriatrics* 2001; **56**: 34–42.
11. Man-Son-Hing M, Wells G. Meta-analysis of efficacy of quinine for treatment of nocturnal leg cramps in elderly people. *Br Med J* 1995; **310**: 13–17.
12. Man-Son-Hing M, Wells G, Lau A. Quinine for nocturnal leg cramps: A meta-analysis including unpublished data. *J Gen Intern Med* 1998; **13**: 600–06.
13. Daniell HW. Simple cure for nocturnal leg cramps. *N Eng J Med* 1979; **301**: 216.
14. Coppin RJ, Wicke DM, Little PS. Managing nocturnal leg cramps – calf stretching exercises and cessation of quinine treatment: A factorial randomised controlled trial. *Br J Gen Pract* 2005: **55**: 186–91.
15. Diener HC, Dethlefsen U, Dethlefsen-Gruber S, et al. Effectiveness of quinine in treating muscle cramps: A double-blind, placebo-controlled, parallel-group, multicentre trial. *Int J Clin Pract* 2002; **56**: 243–6.
16. Woodfield R, Goodyear-Smith F, Arroll B. N-of-1 trials of quinine efficacy in skeletal muscle cramps of the leg. *Br J Gen Pract* 2005; **55**: 181–5.
17. Halfdanarson TR, Sigfusson A, Haraldsdottir V, et al. Severe adverse effects of quinine: Report of seven cases. *Laeknabladid* 2002; **88**: 717–22.
18. Mandal AK, Abernathy T, Nelluri SN, et al. Is quinine effective and safe in leg cramps? *J Clin Pharmacol* 1995; **35**: 588–93.
19. Dahle LO, Berg G, Hammer M, et al. The effect of oral magnesium substitution on pregnancy-induced leg cramps. *Am J Obstet Gynecol* 1995; **173**: 175–80.
20. Frusso R, Zarate M, Augustovski F, et al. Magnesium for the treatment of nocturnal leg cramps: A crossover randomized trial. *J Fam Pract* 1999; **48**: 868–71.
21. Roffe C, Sills S, Crome P, et al. Randomised, cross-over, placebo controlled trial of magnesium citrate in the treatment of chronic persistent leg cramps. *Med Sci Monit* 2002; **8**: CR326–30.
22. Baltodano N, Gallo BV, Weidler DJ. Verapamil vs. quinine in recumbent nocturnal leg cramps in the elderly. *Arch Intern Med* 1988; **148**: 1969–70.
23. Voon WC, Sheu SH. Diltiazem for nocturnal leg cramps [letter]. *Age Ageing* 2001; **3**: 91–2.
24. Ayers S Jr, Mihan R. Leg cramps (systremma) and "restless legs" syndrome. Response to vitamin E (tocopherol). *Calif Med* 1969; **111**: 87–91.
25. Roca AO, Jarjoura D, Blend D, et al. Dialysis leg cramps. Efficacy of quinine versus vitamin E. *ASAIO J* 1992; **38**: 481–5.
26. Connolly PS, Shirley EA, Wasson JH, et al. Treatment of nocturnal leg cramps. A crossover trial of quinine vs. vitamin E. *Arch Intern Med* 1992; **152**: 1877–80.
27. Chan P, Huang TY, Chen YJ, et al. Randomized, double-blind, placebo-controlled study of the safety and efficacy of vitamin B complex in the treatment of nocturnal leg cramps in the elderly patient with hypertension. *J Clin Pharmacol* 1998; **38**: 1151–4.
28. Young JB, Connolly MJ. Naftidrofuryl treatment of rest cramps. *Postgrad Med J* 1993; **69**: 624–6.
29. Latta D, Turner E. An alternative to quinine in nocturnal leg cramps. *Curr Ther Res* 1989; **45**: 833–7.
30. Chang YJ, Wu CL, Chen RS, et al. Case of Issacs syndrome successfully treated with phenytoin. *J Formos Med Assoc* 1993; **92**: 1010–2.
31. Mueller ME, Gruenthal M, Olson WL, et al. Gabapentin for relief of upper motor neuron symptoms in multiple sclerosis. *Arch Phys Med Rehabil* 1997; **78**: 521–4.
32. Serrao M, Rossi P, Cardinali P, et al. Gabapentin treatment for muscle cramps: An open-label trial. *Clin Neuropharmacol* 2000; **23**: 45–9.

Section 5 Chapter 26

Sleep-related movement disorders and other variants

Sleep-related bruxism

Nelly Huynh

History

Sleep bruxism (SB) is categorized as a sleep-related movement disorder in the *International Classification of Sleep Disorders* [1], but it is also widely considered a parasomnia [2]. Sleep-related movement disorders are characterized by simple, stereotyped movements during sleep [3], while parasomnias are disorders of arousals or partial arousals during sleep. Some of the sleep-related movement disorders, such as bruxism, can also occur during wakefulness or sleep, although with a different presentation. SB, defined as "an oral activity characterized by grinding or clenching of the teeth during sleep, usually associated with sleep arousals," is also known as nocturnal bruxism, nocturnal tooth grinding, tooth clenching, or brycose [1]. The term "sleep bruxism" is more correctly used, as bruxism is taken from the Greek term "brychein" meaning "to gnash the teeth," and it occurs during sleep whether diurnal or nocturnal, whereas the terms "bruxomania" or "tooth grinding during wakefulness" are used to describe the neurotic bruxism habit present during wakefulness [2].

Clinical findings

Primary SB is possibly an extreme presentation of normal mastication muscle movements during sleep associated with tooth grinding noise [2], while secondary bruxism can be associated with the use of psychoactive medications (e.g. most selective serotonin reuptake inhibitors, haloperidol, flunarizine or other antiarrhythmia medications), drugs (e.g. cocaine, ecstasy) or some medical conditions (e.g. epilepsy, Parkinson's disease, oromandibular or cervicofacial myoclonus, oral tardive dyskinesia or dystonia, Huntington's disease, cerebellar hemorrhage, coma, Rett syndrome, depression, and anxiety disorders) [2,4,5].

During normal sleep, repetitive or phasic jaw muscle contractions can occur 1–2 times per hour in 60% of "healthy" subjects [6]. This is known as normal "rhythmic masticatory muscle activity" (RMMA) without tooth grinding [6]. An RMMA episode consists of phasic (at least three rhythmic contractions at 1 Hz frequency), tonic (sustained) or mixed (phasic and tonic) masticatory muscle activity and is considered an SB episode when this motor activity is associated with tooth-grinding sounds during sleep [7].

SB can be associated with the following consequences: abnormal tooth wear, dental pain, temporomandibular pain and headaches. In some instances, SB is not only a problem for the patient, but is also a source of sleep disruption for his or her bed partner, as the teeth grinding noise can be loud and unpleasant [1]. Often, patients with SB do not even realize the occurrence of this motor activity since patients with idiopathic SB are reported to have regular sleep architecture in comparison to age-matched control subjects [8–10].

Clinical features

A positive history of SB occurs with the presence of: (1) a family member or a bed partner reporting a tooth-grinding noise, (2) clinical observation of abnormal tooth wear (but could be less reliable in the absence of current bed partner or family member reports of tooth grinding noises), and (3) a patient complaint of jaw muscle tenderness or fatigue (possible association with occasional tension headaches) [2]. Over 50% of children with tension-type headaches report SB or tooth grinding [11]. The orofacial physical evaluation should include an evaluation of the teeth (abnormal wear, fracture, chipping, broken restoration), of the tongue (indentation), inside of the cheek (ridge-like bite mark), temporomandibular joint sound or limited jaw opening, and masseter muscle hypertrophy upon jaw clenching [2]. However, these are more or less reliable indicators of SB and are secondary to reports of tooth-grinding noises by a sleep partner or family member. It is necessary to distinguish between tooth clenching while awake and tooth grinding during sleep, since they have different pathophysiology.

A recent study examined tooth-grinding patterns during sleep in association with dental status [12]. The researchers found that laterotrusive grinding, specifically incisor–canine–premolar–molar, and mediotrusive grinding patterns had more deteriorative consequences on clinical gum attachment level, tooth mobility, non-carious cervical lesions and hypersensitivity.

Differential diagnosis

SB should be differentiated from facio-mandibular myoclonus (which can be seen in 10% of SB patients), respiratory disturbances, REM sleep behavior disorder, sleep-related abnormal swallowing, night terrors, confusional arousals, daytime dyskinetic movements (e.g. dystonia, tremor, chorea, dyskinesia), and sleep epilepsy [1]. Partial complex or general seizures are often associated with rhythmic jaw muscle contractions, which are different from SB [1].

Risk factors

SB has various concomitant risk factors, such as psychological factors, other sleep-related disorders, oral habits, temporomandibular pain, mental disabilities, medications, and recreational drugs. Psychological factors, such as anxiety and stress, have been noted to exacerbate SB frequency [13,14]. A survey paper reported that anxiety seemed more prevalent in adults with SB [15]. A case-controlled study showed an odds ratio of 5 (CI 2.8–8.8) for SB and stress [16]. Epinephrine and dopamine, both associated with stress response, were found in higher concentrations in the urine of patients with SB in comparison to control subjects [17,18]. However, no direct cause–effect link has been demonstrated, possibly because of the multifactorial pathophysiology of SB. A recent study evaluated chromogranin A as a salivary stress biomarker level in patients with SB, although there were no simultaneous audio-video recordings to distinguish SB from other orofacial activities [19]. The association of SB with REM sleep behavior disorder, although reported [2], is still controversial [20]. Furthermore, sleep apnea has also been associated with SB in some patients [15,21,22]. Similar to obstructive sleep apnea (OSA), nearly 74% of SB episodes occur in the supine position [23]. Some oral habits, like smoking and nail biting, have been linked to a higher prevalence of SB. Patients with SB may have a higher risk than the general population of suffering from temporomandibular pain or jaw movement limitations [24,25]. This increases with the degree of severity of SB, as more than half of patients with moderate SB report morning pain, while patients with severe SB have a higher RMMA index but less reported pain [6,25,26]. The prevalence of SB in a population with developmental disabilities seems to be similar to the prevalence in the general population [27]. Children with SB were reported to have a higher prevalence of attention deficit and somatic disorders [28].

Natural history

Primary SB can be reported as soon as upper and lower teeth appear in a child [1]. The reported subjective prevalence of primary SB is found to decline with age with a 14–20% prevalence in children under 11 years of age, 13% in young adults 18–29 years of age and finally 3% in mature adults over 60 years of age [29–31]. Thus, the overall prevalence of SB in adults is estimated to be 8% [31]. SB in adults is often a continuation of childhood SB in over 86.9% of cases [32]. In children, subjective reports also underlined the presence of SB concomitant oral activities such as 9–28% of nail biting, 21% of thumb sucking and 14% of snoring [29,30]. Although the literature seems slightly conflicted, generally there seems to be no statistical difference in SB prevalence between genders [2].

It is possible that these epidemiological data have been underestimated, since many subjects with SB are unaware that they grind their teeth (they may sleep alone; the bed partner or parents may be unaware of SB in the patient), and because of the higher prevalence of dentures in relation to aging. Moreover, the prevalence of SB in the general population may be further underevaluated since night-to-night variability of tooth-grinding noises has been estimated to be greater than 50%, and 25% for RMMA [1,33]. When compiling an SB history, reports of tooth-grinding noise from the family or bed partner are a good indicator, but the clinician should also report the presence of abnormal tooth wear in association with current motor activity, masseter muscle hypertrophy, possible temporomandibular joint disorder (e.g. pain and sensitivity, clicking noise or movement limitation) and possible orofacial pain (e.g. headaches) [1].

Ambulatory and laboratory investigations

To confirm the diagnosis of SB, the patient recording can be done with an ambulatory at-home device or in a sleep laboratory. Ideally, either of these recording options should be accompanied by a simultaneous audio-video recording (under black light conditions) focused on the patient's head, in order to distinguish orofacial movements and other sounds (e.g. snoring, throat grunting, teeth tapping, smiling, sighing) from SB episodes. The audio-video recordings help to confirm SB episodes and to distinguish them from other non-specific orofacial activities (up to 30%) [34].

Ambulatory and laboratory recordings can help to rule out, or to document the co-occurrence, of other sleep disorders such as sleep apnea, PLMS, epilepsy and REM sleep behavioral disorder. One case report described rhythmic tooth grinding induced by temporal lobe seizures, in which case SB was an epileptic-related motor event [35]. Parallel EMG recording of masseter and temporal muscles is necessary to discriminate any artifacts of temporal muscle activity that can be present during temporal lobe seizures.

For the purpose of detecting SB, recordings are more sensitive in severe cases than in mild to moderate cases because of the night-to-night variability in SB and RMMA [1,33].

Ambulatory recordings range from a single masseter muscle EMG to a multi-channel recording (EMG, ECG, respiration, EEG). The main advantages of ambulatory recording are home-based patient comfort and lower costs [36]. However, the main limitations of this method are the lack of specificity due to the absence of audio-video recording, and fewer recorded channels; up to 30% of orofacial movements are not specific to SB (e.g. swallowing, grunting, sighs, yawning, sleep talking and smiling) [34].

Polysomnographic recording is strongly indicated when the presence of SB is suspected in association with possible sleep-disordered breathing, REM sleep behavior disorder, night terrors, facio-mandibular myoclonus or epilepsy. A polysomnographic recording of SB should include: (1) at least two EMG (masseter and temporalis muscles) for SB scoring and a chin EMG for REM sleep hypotonia scoring, (2) EEG (C3A2 and O2A1), (3) EOG (left and right), (4) nasal airflow, (5) chest respiratory effort belt, (6) pulse oximetry, and (7) simultaneous audio-video recording. Calibration of the polysomnographic recording should include voluntary tooth tapping, maximum jaw contraction, swallowing and coughing before the lights are turned off [9,26].

From these recordings, SB can be scored as: (a) phasic activity – 1 Hz frequency lasting between 0.25 and 2 s; (b) tonic activity – sustained contraction lasting over 2 s; and (c) mixed activity. If an EMG burst lasts less than 0.25 s, it is scored as myoclonus. Approximately 10% of patients with SB also have myoclonia which can often be confused with epileptic spikes [2]. Each SB episode is separated by at least 3-s intervals with no SB-associated EMG activity. Simultaneous audio-video recordings help confirm EMG activity with tooth grinding noises. SB diagnosis can be made with the presence of at least four episodes of SB per hour of sleep, or at least 25 individual muscle bursts per hour of sleep; this EMG activity needs to be accompanied by at least two tooth-grinding noises during the sleep recording. Based on 20 years of laboratory investigation of SB, it has been the experience of Gilles Lavigne and colleagues that the chin EMG (suprahyoid muscle) recorded alone is not reliable enough to score SB, but should be associated with masseter EMG and/or temporal EMG [37].

Although SB episodes can occur in all sleep stages, they more often occur in light sleep stages 1 and 2, in up to 80% of the time, but less often in REM sleep (under 10%). However, SB can be more prevalent in REM sleep in some individuals [1]. Interestingly, 15–20% of SB episodes occur during the transition from light sleep stages to REM sleep [4,38].

Genetics

Strong familial associations have been reported for SB, with 20–50% of SB patients reporting at least one family member with a history of SB [1]. Studies in twins showed that monozygotic twins had a higher prevalence of SB than dizygotic twins [32,39]. However, a specific genetic marker has yet to be attributed to SB, although there is a large environmental influence [40]. Genetic pedigrees would be required in order to establish the genotype and type of inheritance of SB.

Pathophysiology and etiology

The exact pathophysiology and etiology of SB still remains unclear although it is strongly believed to be multifactorial. One of the predisposing factors seems to be personality type. A higher prevalence of SB has been reported in association with personality type A, highly motivated and vigilant individuals [1,41]. Patients with SB seem to be task-oriented due to their personality type and stress/anxiety coping style [2]. Dental malocclusion has often been reported to be either a predisposing or a precipitating factor, although no scientific study has been able to prove or disprove this [1]. Stress, anxiety, smoking and caffeine have been shown to exacerbate the occurrence of SB [1].

Normality

As mentioned above, 60% of normal sleepers present RMMA [6]. This masticatory muscle activity during sleep has also been reported in patients with somnambulism, sleep terrors and REM sleep behavior disorder [8,9]. SB has been said to be an extreme manifestation [2] of these phasic RMMAs with a higher frequency, stronger EMG contraction and accompanying tooth-grinding noises [1]. Even so, comparative studies between healthy young patients with SB matched with control subjects showed normal sleep macrostructure: sleep efficiency, sleep latency, total sleep time, sleep stages distribution and number of awakenings [22,38,42,43].

Physiologic sequence

Recent studies have shown that a sequence of physiological events precedes and succeeds SB episodes: (1) minus 4 min: increased sympathetic and decreased parasympathetic activities; (2) minus 4 s: EEG arousal; (3) minus 1 s: increased amplitude of respiration, increased heart rate; (4) onset of activity in jaw – opening and closing muscles; (5) SB episode followed by saliva swallowing [44–47].

Arousal-related

SB episodes do not trigger EEG arousals, but rather are simultaneous or secondary to them. Using polygraphic and audio-video recordings it was shown that nearly 90% of the SB episodes were associated with an EEG arousal, which occurred at a frequency within normal range [1,22,48]. The association between SB and EEG arousal was further confirmed when 86% of experimentally induced EEG arousals were linked to SB episodes [49]. The majority of SB episodes (80%) were associated with the EEG cyclic alternating pattern (CAP) [38,50]. CAPs are brief cyclic brain patterns associated with autonomic and motor activation, that tend to occur every 20–60 s [2]. They are NREM behavioral and polygraphic markers of sleep instability characterized by transient high-amplitude arousals (phase A) and low-amplitude background activity (phase B) [51]. Phase A is divided into three subtypes: A1 containing K-complexes and other slow-wave activities, A2 with slow and fast EEG, and A3 with fast EEG, the latter associated with increased heart rate.

Neurochemical link

Dopaminergic and adrenergic neurotransmitters have been associated with SB pathophysiology. The administration of levodopa, a dopamine precursor, was first reported to induce SB in a patient with Parkinson's disease [52]. However, a controlled study showed that levodopa reduced the frequency of SB episodes by 30% as well as EMG tone within each SB episode [53]. In addition to older studies with wake/sleep bruxism [17,18], a recent study found higher levels of urinary catecholamines – adrenaline, noradrenaline and dopamine – in patients with SB in comparison to controls [54]. Haloperidol, a dopaminergic receptor blocker, and some other dopaminergic anti-psychotic medications induced tooth grinding in awake subjects, but has not been reported to induce SB [55]. Yet, when administering bromocriptine, a dopamine agonist, the frequency of SB episodes did not decrease or increase [56]. Propranolol, an adrenergic beta-blocker, was reported in a case report and in secondary SB to reduce SB [57,58]. However, a controlled study showed no effect of propranolol on SB or on sleep variables [59]. Other neurotransmitters that could possibly play a role in the pathophysiology of SB are serotonin, cholecystokinin, and gamma-aminobutyric acid, while medications that increase SB are selective serotonin reuptake inhibitors (SSRIs), dopamine antagonists and calcium channel inhibitors [44,55,60].

Swallowing

Since most SB episodes conclude with saliva swallowing at the end of the episode, it is possible that this activity is responsible for lubricating tissues in the esophagus and mouth. One hypothesis is that xerostomia may trigger SB, but this needs to be demonstrated.

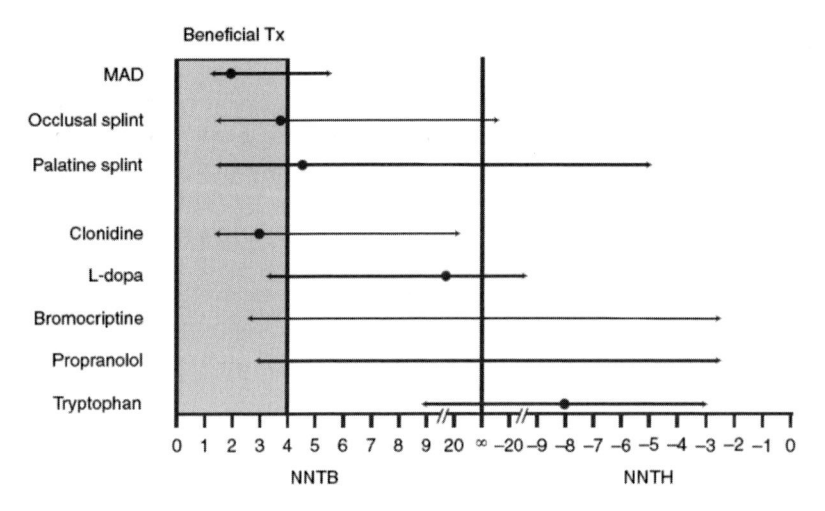

Figure 26.1 Diagram of various oral appliances and medications. Different randomized controlled trials of SB treatments were compared by the number needed to treat (NNT) which is the number of patients who need to receive the SB treatment in comparison with patients receiving a placebo/other treatment, in order to reduce SB in one patient. NNTB is NNT to benefit, and NNTH is NNT to harm. Arrows show ±95% confidence interval. Shaded box shows the range of NNT where the treatment is considered beneficial. (Modified from [81].)

Sleeping subjects swallow up to 12 times less in comparison to awake subjects [61]. Low saliva levels during tooth grinding may increase tooth wear [62].

Sleep-disordered breathing

A recent study demonstrated that SB episodes were associated with an increase in respiration amplitude [47]. As described above, SB has also been associated with OSA. In a large population survey, patients with SB reported a 2–3 times higher prevalence of sleep apnea [15]. Since OSA is caused by a reduction of upper airway patency, it has been hypothesized that the rhythmic contractions of the jaw muscles might be a way to re-establish the patency by repositioning the retruded jaw and re-establishing EMG tone in the tongue during swallowing [4].

Management

As there is no cure for SB, the clinician's role is to manage the associated symptoms of SB and exclude other neurological or sleep disorders as described above. Firstly, patients with SB should be made aware of its definition, causes, associated consequences and possible management strategies [2].

Lifestyle and sleep hygiene

Among possible SB management strategies, behavioral changes can be suggested, such as sleep hygiene or relaxation exercises [63]. Other alternative treatments have been reported to reduce SB, such as hypnotherapy [64], or auditory biofeedback [65,66], although they have not been studied in randomized controlled trials.

Prevention of damage

Occlusal appliances can be used in order to prevent further orodental deterioration. It is recommended that the soft mouth guard be used as a short-term solution, since degradation can occur rather quickly due to SB, while the hard occlusal stabilization splint offers more protection, especially in patients with severe SB or tooth clenchers [2]. While an appliance with 3 mm vertical thickness at the central incisors has been associated with reports of better tolerance and a decrease in SB, an appliance with 6 mm vertical thickness resulted in an increase of temporal EMG activity [67]. However, an occlusal appliance is not recommended for everyone, since one study showed a maxillary appliance exacerbated OSA [68]. The mandibular advancement appliance is an alternative oral appliance that has recently shown promise as an SB treatment (see Figure 26.1). By pulling the lower jaw slightly forward, this appliance may improve respiratory function and decrease secondary SB episodes [69]. Other alternatives yet to be studied in randomized controlled trials are appliances that in response to excessive tooth contact activate with electric shock, vibration or a bad taste in order to reduce the number of SB episodes [66,70–72]. In patients with removable partial dentures, night dentures (splint-like and removable) were reported to be effective in four case reports [73].

Although the efficacy of reducing occlusal interference through tooth equilibrium has yet to be proven in a randomized controlled trial, it has been previously suggested [74]. Orthodontic treatment and/or dental restoration can possibly improve comfort, respiration and oral health but there is no evidence yet of an effect on SB.

Use of medication

As previously stated, there is currently no known long-term preventive treatment for SB. Despite this, pharmacologic treatment can be considered as a possible short-term treatment for SB. Medications that act on the central nervous system taken at bedtime, like benzodiazepam (e.g. diazepam) or muscle relaxants (e.g. methocarbamol), have been reported to reduce SB [5,7], but a randomized controlled trial has yet to be performed for these medications. The main associated side effect is morning drowsiness [2]. Tricyclic anti-depressants have also been reported as a possible short-term treatment for SB [55], although two controlled studies with amitriptyline showed no effect on SB [75,76] (see Figure 26.1). Inversely, SSRIs, like sertraline, fluoxetine and citalopram, have been reported to increase wake tooth clenching [2]. Other medications acting on serotonin (fenfluramine) and L-tryptophan have been associated with exacerbated or no changes in SB, respectively [55].

Dopamine-related medications have different effects on SB. For example, L-dopa seemed to decrease SB episodes in young otherwise healthy subjects with SB, while bromocriptine did not influence SB in a similar population [53,56] (see Figure 26.1). A sustained slow-release form of L-dopa could be an alternative to prevent taking two doses of medication – at bedtime and in the middle of the night [2]. However, further studies are needed before using this medication as a long-term pharmacological treatment, since it is possible to have a SB rebound later during the night or the next day, as is the case for PLMS [2]. A case report in a patient with severe SB indicated that pergolide, a dopamine receptor agonist, reduced SB [77].

Adrenergic medications have also been associated to SB. Propranolol, a beta-adrenergic antagonist, was reported to reduce SB in two case reports [57,78], but a controlled study showed no difference in SB in young healthy subjects [59]. Clonidine, an alpha-2 agonist, decreased SB by over 60%, but clinical use was hampered by near complete REM sleep inhibition in most patients and morning hypotension in some [59]. Botulin toxin injected directly into the muscle has been suggested in the literature as a means to prevent SB episodes, although controlled studies and safety issues need to be addressed before botulin toxin becomes a widely used treatment for SB [2,5].

An interesting recent study in postmenopausal women described the positive results from hormone therapy with progesterone and estrogen versus estrogen alone; among the results, the researchers observed a decrease in the prevalence of bruxism (11% vs. 0%), periodic limb movements (8% vs. 3%), arousals from sleep, daytime somnolence and breathing irregularities [79]. However, it remains unclear whether the hormones have a direct link to SB or whether they act primarily on sleep [80].

Conclusions

Sleep-related movement disorders, such as SB, have consequences for patients' quality of life when they are associated with pain and/or headaches. SB probably remains underdiagnosed due to the limited knowledge of patients, family members and clinicians. Better management will become possible by means of inter-disciplinary communication and education. It remains for researchers to gather more information on the multifactorial pathophysiology of SB and to study new management therapies.

References

1. AASM. Sleep related bruxism. In: Medicine AAoS (Ed.) *ICSD-2 International Classification of Sleep Disorders: Diagnosis and Coding Manual*. 2nd ed. Westchester, IL: American Academy of Sleep Medicine, 2005; 189–92.
2. Lavigne GJ, Manzini C, Kato T. Sleep bruxism. In Kryger HM, Roth T, Dement WC (Eds), *Principles & Practice of Sleep Medicine*. Philadelphia: Elsevier Saunders, 2005; 946–59.
3. AASM. *International Classification of Sleep Disorders*. 2nd ed. Westchester, IL: American Academy of Sleep Medicine, 2005.
4. Lavigne GJ, Kato T, Kolta A, Sessle BJ. Neurobiological mechanisms involved in sleep bruxism. *Crit Rev Oral Biol Med* 2003; **14**: 30–46.
5. Kato T, Thie NM, Montplaisir JY, Lavigne GJ. Bruxism and orofacial movements during sleep. *Dent Clin North Am* 2001; **45**: 657–84.
6. Lavigne GJ, Rompre PH, Poirier G, Huard H, Kato T, Montplaisir JY. Rhythmic masticatory muscle activity during sleep in humans. *J Dent Res* 2001; **80**: 443–8.
7. Rugh JD, Harlan J. Nocturnal bruxism and temporomandibular disorders. In Jankovic J, Tolosa E

(Eds), *Advances in Neurology*. New York: Raven Press, 1988; 329–41.

8. Sjoholm T, Lehtinen II, Helenius H. Masseter muscle activity in diagnosed sleep bruxists compared with non-symptomatic controls. *J Sleep Res* 1995; **4**: 48–55.

9. Lavigne GJ, Rompre PH, Montplaisir JY. Sleep bruxism: Validity of clinical research diagnostic criteria in a controlled polysomnographic study. *J Dent Res* 1996; **75**: 546–52.

10. Macaluso GM, Guerra P, Di Giovanni G, Boselli M, Parrino L, Terzano MG. Sleep bruxism is a disorder related to periodic arousals during sleep. *J Dent Res* 1998; **77**: 565–73.

11. Vendrame M, Kaleyias J, Valencia I, Legido A, Kothare SV. Polysomnographic findings in children with headaches. *Pediatr Neurol* 2008; **39**: 6–11.

12. Tokiwa O, Park BK, Takezawa Y, Takahashi Y, Sasaguri K, Sato S. Relationship of tooth grinding pattern during sleep bruxism and dental status. *Cranio* 2008; **26**: 287–93.

13. Pierce CJ, Chrisman K, Bennett ME, Close JM. Stress, anticipatory stress, and psychologic measures related to sleep bruxism. *J Orofacial Pain* 1995; **9**: 51–6.

14. Major M, Rompre PH, Guitard F, *et al*. A controlled daytime challenge of motor performance and vigilance in sleep bruxers. *J Dent Res* 1999; **78**: 1754–62.

15. Ohayon MM, Li KK, Guilleminault C. Risk factors for sleep bruxism in the general population. *Chest* 2001; **119**: 53–61.

16. Ahlberg J, Savolainen A, Rantala M, Lindholm H, Kononen M. Reported bruxism and biopsychosocial symptoms: A longitudinal study. *Community Dent Oral Epidemiol* 2004; **32**: 307–11.

17. Clark GT, Rugh JD, Handelman SL. Nocturnal masseter muscle activity and urinary catecholamine levels in bruxers. *J Dent Res* 1980; **59**: 1571–6.

18. Vanderas AP, Menenakou M, Kouimtzis T, Papagiannoulis L. Urinary catecholamine levels and bruxism in children. *J Oral Rehab* 1999; **26**: 103–10.

19. Makino M, Masaki C, Tomoeda K, Kharouf E, Nakamoto T, Hosokawa R. The relationship between sleep bruxism behavior and salivary stress biomarker level. *Int J Prosthodont* 2009; **22**: 43–8.

20. Abe S, Rompre PH, Gagnon JF, Montplaisir JY, Lavigne GJ. Absence of tooth grinding in REM sleep behaviour disorder patients. Abstract presented at IADR 2009.

21. Gold AR, Dipalo F, Gold MS, O'Hearn D. The symptoms and signs of upper airway resistance syndrome: A link to the functional somatic syndromes. *Chest* 2003; **123**: 87–95.

22. Bader GG, Kampe T, Tagdae T, Karlsson S, Blomqvist M. Descriptive physiological data on a sleep bruxism population. *Sleep* 1997; **20**: 982–90.

23. Ware JC, Rugh JD. Destructive bruxism: Sleep stage relationship. *Sleep* 1988; **11**: 172–81.

24. Dao TT, Lund JP, Lavigne GJ. Comparison of pain and quality of life in bruxers and patients with myofascial pain of the masticatory muscles. *J Orofac Pain* 1994; **8**: 350–6.

25. Lavigne GJ, Rompre PH, Montplaisir JY, Lobbezoo F. Motor activity in sleep bruxism with concomitant jaw muscle pain. A retrospective pilot study. *Eur J Oral Sci* 1997; **105**: 92–5.

26. Rompré PH, Daigle-Landry D, Guitard F, Montplaisir JY, Lavigne GJ. Identification of a sleep bruxism subgroup with a higher risk of pain. *J Dent Res* 2007; **86**: 837–42.

27. Richmond G, Rugh JD, Dolfi R, Wasilewsky JW. Survey of bruxism in an institutionalized mentally retarded population. *Am J Mental Deficiency* 1984; **88**: 418–21.

28. Herrera M, Valencia I, Grant M, Metroka D, Chialastri A, Kothare SV. Bruxism in children: Effect on sleep architecture and daytime cognitive performance and behavior. *Sleep* 2006; **29**: 1143–8.

29. Abe K, Shimakawa M. Genetic and developmental aspects of sleeptalking and teeth-grinding. *Acta Paedo-psychiatry* 1966; **33**: 339–44.

30. Laberge L, Tremblay RE, Vitaro F, Montplaisir J. Development of parasomnias from childhood to early adolescence. *Pediatrics* 2000; **106**: 67–74.

31. Lavigne GJ, Montplaisir JY. Restless legs syndrome and sleep bruxism: Prevalence and association among Canadians. *Sleep* 1994; **17**: 739–43.

32. Lindqvist B. Bruxism in twins. *Acta Odontol Scand* 1974; **32**: 177–87.

33. Lavigne GJ, Guitard F, Rompre PH, Montplaisir JY. Variability in sleep bruxism activity over time. *J Sleep Res* 2001; **10**: 237–44.

34. Dutra KMC, Pereira FJ, Rompré PH, Huynh N, Fleming N, Lavigne GJ. Oro-facial activities in sleep bruxism patients and in normal subjects: A controlled polygraphic and audio-video study. *J Oral Rehab* 2009; **36**: 86–92.

35. Meletti S, Cantalupo G, Volpi L, Rubboli G, Magaudda A, Tassinari CA. Rhythmic teeth grinding induced by temporal lobe seizures. *Neurology* 2004; **62**: 2306–09.

36. Doering S, Boeckmann JA, Hugger S, Young P. Ambulatory polysomnography for the assessment of sleep bruxism. *J Oral Rehabil* 2008; **35**: 572–6.

37. AASM. *The AASM Manual for the Scoring of Sleep and Associated Events: Rules, Terminology and Technical Specifications.* Westchester, IL: American Academy of Sleep Medicine, 2007.
38. Reding GR, Zepelin H, Robinson JEJ, Smith VH, Zimmerman SO. Sleep pattern of bruxism: A revision. *APSS Meeting* 1967; **4**: 396.
39. Kuch EV, Till MJ, Messer LB. Bruxing and non-bruxing children: A comparison of their personality traits. *Pediatric Dent* 1979; **1**: 182–7.
40. Hublin C, Kaprio J, Partinen M, Koskenvuo M. Sleep bruxism based on self-report in a nationwide twin cohort. *J Sleep Res* 1998; **7**: 61–7.
41. Restrepo CC, Vasquez LM, Alvarez M, Valencia I. Personality traits and temporomandibular disorders in a group of children with bruxing behaviour. *J Oral Rehabil* 2008; **35**: 585–93.
42. Reding GR, Zepelin H, Robinson JE, Jr., Zimmerman SO. Nocturnal teeth-grinding: All-night psychophysiologic studies. *J Dent Res* 1968; **47**: 786–97.
43. Tosun T, Karabuda C, Cuhadaroglu C. Evaluation of sleep bruxism by polysomnographic analysis in patients with dental implants. *Int J Oral Maxillofac Implants* 2003; **18**: 286–92.
44. Kato T, Rompre P, Montplaisir JY, Sessle BJ, Lavigne GJ. Sleep bruxism: An oromotor activity secondary to micro-arousal. *J Dent Res* 2001; **80**: 1940–4.
45. Huynh N, Kato T, de Champlain J, *et al.* Sleep bruxism is associated with a higher sympathetic and a lower parasympathetic tone before the onset of masticatory muscle activation. *Sleep* 2003; **26**: A320-No.0804.M.
46. Miyawaki S, Lavigne GJ, Pierre M, Guitard F, Montplaisir JY, Kato T. Association between sleep bruxism, swallowing-related laryngeal movement, and sleep positions. *Sleep* 2003; **26**: 461–5.
47. Khoury S, Rouleau GA, Rompré PH, Mayer P, Montplaisir J, Lavigne GJ. A significant increase in breathing amplitude precedes sleep bruxism. *Chest* 2008; **134**: 332–7.
48. Boselli M, Parrino L, Smerieri A, Terzano MG. Effect of age on EEG arousals in normal sleep. *Sleep* 1998; **21**: 351–7.
49. Kato T, Montplaisir JY, Guitard F, Sessle BJ, Lund JP, Lavigne GJ. Evidence that experimentally induced sleep bruxism is a consequence of transient arousal. *J Dent Res* 2003; **82**: 284–8.
50. Tani K, Yoshii N, Yoshino I, Kobayashi E. Electroencephalographic study of parasomnia: Sleep-talking, enuresis and bruxism. *Physiol & Behav* 1966; **1**: 241–3.
51. Terzano MG, Parrino L, Spaggiari MC. The cyclic alternating pattern sequences in the dynamic organization of sleep. *Electroenceph Clin Neurophysiol* 1988; **69**: 437–44.
52. Magee KR. Bruxism related to levodopa therapy. *J Am Dent Ass* 1970; **214**: 147.
53. Lobbezoo F, Lavigne GJ, Tanguay R, Montplaisir JY. The effect of catecholamine precursor L-dopa on sleep bruxism: A controlled clinical trial. *Mov Disord* 1997; **12**: 73–8.
54. Seraidarian P, Seraidarian PI, das Neves Cavalcanti B, Marchini L, Claro Neves AC. Urinary levels of catecholamines among individuals with and without sleep bruxism. *Sleep Breath* 2009; **13**: 85–8.
55. Winocur E, Gavish A, Voikovitch M, Emodi-Perlman A, Eli I. Drugs and bruxism: A critical review. *J Orofac Pain* 2003; **17**: 99–111.
56. Lavigne GJ, Soucy JP, Lobbezoo F, Manzini C, Blanchet PJ, Montplaisir JY. Double-blind, crossover, placebo-controlled trial of bromocriptine in patients with sleep bruxism. *Clin Neuropharmacol* 2001; **24**: 145–9.
57. Sjoholm TT, Lehtinen I, Piha SJ. The effect of propranolol on sleep bruxism: Hypothetical considerations based on a case study. *Clin Auton Res* 1996; **6**: 37–40.
58. Amir I, Hermesh H, Gavish A. Bruxism secondary to antipsychotic drug exposure: A positive response to propranolol. *Clin Neuropharmacol* 1997; **20**: 86–9.
59. Huynh N, Lavigne GJ, Lanfranchi P, Montplaisir J, de Champlain J. The effect of two sympatholytic medications, propranolol and clonidine, on sleep bruxism: Experimental randomized controlled trials. *Sleep* 2006; **29**: 295–304.
60. Glaros AG, Rao SM. Bruxism: A critical review. *Psychol Bull* 1977; **84**: 767–81.
61. Lichter I, Muir RC. The pattern of swallowing during sleep. *Electro Clin Neurophysiol* 1975; **38**: 427–32.
62. Thie NM, Kato T, Bader G, Montplaisir JY, Lavigne GJ. The significance of saliva during sleep and the relevance of oromotor movements. *Sleep Med Rev* 2002; **6**: 213–27.
63. Pierce CJ, Gale EN. A comparison of different treatments for nocturnal bruxism. *J Dent Res* 1988; **67**: 597–601.
64. Clarke JH, Reynolds PJ. Suggestive hypnotherapy for nocturnal bruxism: A pilot study. *Am J Clin Hypnosis* 1991; **33**: 248–53.
65. Hudzinski LG, Walters PJ. Use of a portable electromyogram integrator and biofeedback unit in the treatment of chronic nocturnal bruxism. *J Prosth Dent* 1987; **58**: 698–701.
66. Jadidi F, Castrillon E, Svensson P. Effect of conditioning electrical stimuli on temporalis

electromyographic activity during sleep. *J Oral Rehabil* 2008; **35**: 171–83.

67. Abekura H, Yokomura M, Sadamori S, Hamada T. The initial effects of occlusal splint vertical thickness on the nocturnal EMG activities of masticatory muscles in subjects with a bruxism habit. *Int J Prosthodont* 2008; **21**: 116–20.

68. Gagnon Y, Mayer P, Morisson F, Rompre PH, Lavigne GJ. Aggravation of respiratory disturbances by the use of an occlusal splint in apneic patients: A pilot study. *Int J Prosthodont* 2004; **17**: 447–53.

69. Landry ML, Rompré PH, Manzini C, Guitard F, de Grandmont P, Lavigne GJ. Reduction of sleep bruxism using a mandibular advancement device: An experimental controlled study. *Int J Prosthodont* 2006; **19**: 549–56.

70. Watanabe T, Baba K, Yamagata K, Ohyama T, Clark GT. A vibratory stimulation-based inhibition system for nocturnal bruxism: A clinical report. *J Prosthet Dent* 2001; **85**: 233–5.

71. Nishigawa K, Kondo K, Takeuchi H, Clark GT. Contingent electrical lip stimulation for sleep bruxism: A pilot study. *J Prosthet Dent* 2003; **89**: 412–7.

72. Nissani M. Can taste aversion prevent bruxism? *Appl Psychophysiol Biofeedback* 2000; **25**: 43–54.

73. Baba K, Aridome K, Pallegama RW. Management of bruxism-induced complications in removable partial denture wearers using specially designed dentures: A clinical report. *Cranio* 2008; **26**: 71–6.

74. Yustin D, Neff P, Rieger MR, Hurst I. Characterization of 86 bruxing patients and long term study of their management with occlusal devices and other forms of therapy. *J Orofacial Pain* 1993; **7**: 54–60.

75. Raigrodski A, Christensen L, Mohamed S, Gardiner D. The effect of 4-week administration of amitriptyline on sleep bruxism. A double-blind crossover clinical study. *J Craniomandib Pract* 2001; **19**: 21–5.

76. Mohamed SE, Christensen LV, Penchas J. A randomized double-blind clinical trial of the effect of amitriptyline on nocturnal masseteric motor activity (sleep bruxism). *J Craniomandib Pract* 1997; **15**: 326–32.

77. Van Der Zaag J, Lobbezoo F, Van Der Avoort PG, Wicks DJ, Hamburger HL, Naeije M. Effects of pergolide on severe sleep bruxism in a patient experiencing oral implant failure. *J Oral Rehabil* 2007; **34**: 317–22.

78. Amir I, Hermesh H, Gavish A. Bruxism secondary to antipsychotic drug exposure: A positive response to propranolol. *Clin Neuropharmacol* 1997; **20**: 86–9.

79. Hachul H, Bittencourt LR, Andersen ML, Haidar MA, Baracat EC, Tufik S. Effects of hormone therapy with estrogen and/or progesterone on sleep pattern in postmenopausal women. *Int J Gynaecol Obstet* 2008; **103**: 207–12.

80. Van Cauter E. Endocrine physiology. In Kryger MH, Roth T, Dement WC (Eds), *Principles and Practice of Sleep Medicine*. 4th ed. Philadelphia, PA.: Elsevier Saunders, 2005; 266–82.

81. Huynh N, Rompré P, Montplaisir J, Lavigne GJ. Comparison of various treatments for sleep bruxism using determinants of number needed to treat and effect size. *Int J Prosthodont* 2006; **19**: 435–41.

Section 5 Sleep-related movement disorders and other variants

Chapter 27

Propriospinal myoclonus

Giuseppe Plazzi and Roberto Vetrugno

History and terminology

The term myoclonus was derived from the longer term *paramyoklonus multiplex* that was first used in a case report by professor Nikolaus Friedreich in Heidelberg in 1881 with the intent to describe symmetric (*para*) and quick (*clonus*) movements of muscles (*myo*) occurring in multiple sites (*multiplex*) over the body [1]. Lowenfeld, in 1883, was the first to use the term *myoclonus* by shortening paramyoklonus multiplex, as quoted by Seelingmüller in 1886 [2]. Myoclonus is a clinical sign encompassing a vast range of etiologies, anatomical sources, and pathophysiological features. Muscle jerks can also be produced by the spinal cord where the motor system is organized on two levels, spinal and propriospinal. The spinal segmental system may became hyperexcitable, and the result is spinal "segmental" myoclonus involving one or two contiguous spinal myotomes that is particularly resistant to supraspinal influences, such as voluntary movement, mental activity and sleep [3–5]. The propriospinal system is a slowly conducting intraspinal pathway that connects multiple segmental levels. Involvement of this system [6] leads to predominantly axial jerks [7] that, unlike spinal segmental myoclonus, is particularly influenced by mental activity and sleep [8,9].

Bussel et al., in 1988, described a patient in whom rhythmic extension movements of the trunk and lower limbs started 15 months after a traumatic section of the spinal cord, verified by MRI, at the lower cervical cord. The timing of the muscle activation in different muscles remained "fixed," but was not measured. Nevertheless, such a pattern would be consistent with spread of activation from a single source and was probably the first electrophysiological description of a long propriospinal pathway propagated spinal myoclonus [10]. Subsequently, Brown et al., in 1991, reported three patients with non-rhythmic repetitive axial jerks causing symmetric flexion of the neck, trunk, hips and knees, observed the influence of the posture (jerks were especially brought about by reclining or lying down), and described the detailed electrophysiology of this new type of spinal myoclonus that they termed propriospinal myoclonus [7]. In 1992, Davies et al. described a 59-year-old man with a 30-year history of an unusual movement disorder characterized by involuntary axial spasms that occurred only in recumbency. The authors defined this movement disorder as a tic because of the associated urge to move and its suppression by voluntary effort, but indeed it much resembled propriospinal myoclonus because movements were suppressed promptly when the patient was given mental arithmetic tasks or when he performed simple motor tasks, such as leg or hand movements, or replied to questions [11].

In 2000, Vetrugno et al. reported a case in which myoclonus was sometimes confined to abdominal muscles as in spinal segmental myoclonus, while in others the jerks from the abdominal muscles spread slowly up and down the cord to involve muscles in the neck and leg. They postulated that the same generator was involved in both types of jerk and that under conditions of heightened excitability jerks spread away from the area of the primary focus [12]. Schulze-Bonhage et al., in 1996, described a case with a purely stimulus-sensitive propriospinal myoclonus in which stimuli to the back and abdomen could provoke axial jerks at short latency with spread to rostral and caudal segments of the cords [13]. Then, in 1997, Montagna et al. outlined and highlighted the tight association that propriospinal myoclonus may have with relaxation and drowsiness with consequent sleep disruption [8]. In particular, propriospinal myoclonus was observed to occur exclusively at the transition from wakefulness to sleep and did not seem to relate to

---

The Parasomnias and Other Sleep-Related Movement Disorders, ed. M. J. Thorpy and G. Plazzi. Published by Cambridge University Press. © Cambridge University Press 2010.

posture, because the jerks could be promptly abolished by mental activation even with the patients sitting comfortably in an armchair or lying down, and immediately restarted when the patients were left alone undisturbed and lying down [8].

In 2001, Vetrugno *et al.* confirmed that propriospinal myoclonus may remain restricted to the particular neurophysiologic and mental state of transition from wakefulness to sleep (i.e. the predormitum), whereas it is absent during alert wakefulness and sleep proper. They proposed propriospinal myoclonus at sleep onset as a new parasomnia causing insomnia and altered sleep structure [9]. In 2005, propriospinal myoclonus was introduced into the American Academy of Sleep Medicine nomenclature and included into The International Classifications of Sleep Disorders Diagnostic and Coding Manual section VII – Isolated Symptoms, apparently normal variants and unresolved issues [14].

Clinical findings

Propriospinal myoclonus defines a syndrome of spontaneous or, in rare instances, stimulus-sensitive, axial myoclonic jerks that originate at a spinal segmental level and spread up and down the spinal cord via supposedly propriospinal pathways [7]. Jerks are typically slow, rhythmic, bilateral and synchronous with flexion, and rarely extension, of trunk and limbs. Brown *et al.* described three patients with non-rhythmic repetitive axial myoclonic jerks causing symmetric flexion of the neck, trunk, hips and knees [7]. They did not find any electrophysiological evidence of a cortical or brainstem reticular origin for the myoclonus. In the first patient, the axial jerks occurred only spontaneously. Paroxysmal bouts of axial flexion jerks of the trunk and hips lasted up to 3 h and repeated every minute. The inter-muscle latencies of the recruited muscles during the jerks indicated that the discharge arose in the mid thoracic cord and then slowly spread at about 5 m/s up and down the cord to involve rostral and caudal segments. No structural lesion was identified in this patient. In the second patient, spontaneous and reflex axial jerks developed following the excision of a cervical hemangioblastoma. In the stimulus-induced jerks (taps to the abdominal wall), the relative latencies of muscles innervated by rostral and caudal spinal segments suggested that the myoclonus originated between the upper cervical and mid thoracic cord. In the last patient, EMG activity during sponta-neous and stimulus-induced jerks commenced in the rectus abdominis, and was followed by later activity in muscles innervated by rostral spinal segments, suggesting that the myoclonus originated in the mid thoracic cord. No structural lesion was identified in this patient. Thus, electrophysiological evidence argued for a spinal origin for these axial jerks in all three cases, with striking features common both to this form of human myoclonus and to long propriospinal pathways identified in animals [7,15].

In a later paper, the clinical and electrophysiological characteristics of eight other patients with trunkal jerks were described [16]. Myoclonus developed within days or weeks of cervical trauma in half of the patients. Seven cases had axial flexion, and one axial extension jerks. Myoclonic EMG activity consisted of repetitive bursts with a frequency of 1–7 Hz. The jerks in three of the cases were comprised of alternating and rhythmic bursts of EMG activity in the rectus abdominis and paraspinal muscles. From these new observations, the authors speculated that, like in Bussel *et al.* [10], the cervical damage might have released a "pattern generator" in the lower thoracic cord capable of recruiting muscles through long propriospinal pathways into complex rhythmic activity.

Since then, there have been several reports of patients with propriospinal myoclonus and a slow spread of activity from a restricted section of the spinal cord [13,17–20].

Most patients with propriospinal myoclonus have no recognizable cause; however, in other cases a lesion can be detected, such as cervical hemangioblastoma, mild cervical myeloradiculopathy, spinal arteriovenous fistula, or trauma [7,16,21,22], post-traumatic tetraplegia [20], multiple sclerosis [23], thoracic herpes zoster [17], Lyme neuroborreliosis [24] and HIV infection [25]. Symptomatic propriospinal myoclonus secondary to a vertebral fracture of T11 has been reported to evolve in an acute and life-threatening "myoclonic status" with respiratory failure and loss of consciousness [26]. Propriospinal myoclonus has also been reported as a paraneoplastic symptom [27], in paraproteinemic polyneuropathy [28], after exposure to inhaled cannabis [29], ciprofloxacin [30], alpha interferon [31], and enteropathogenic toxin [32]. Moreover, a similar propriospinal pattern of propagation has been found on neurophysiologic studies of other motor activities apparently of spinal origin, such as the spasms of the stiff-man syndrome [33], some involuntary movements encountered in syringomyelia

Figure 27.1 Polysomnographic study showing propriospinal myoclonus recurring during pre-hypnic wakefulness and during infra-hypnic and post-hypnic wakefulness. Propriospinal myoclonus is transiently suppressed by mental exercise (*) and vanishes during sleep. Upper trace: wake–sleep histogram; middle trace: body position (S, supine position; R, lying on the right side; L, lying on the left side); lower trace: histogram of myoclonic jerks per minute.

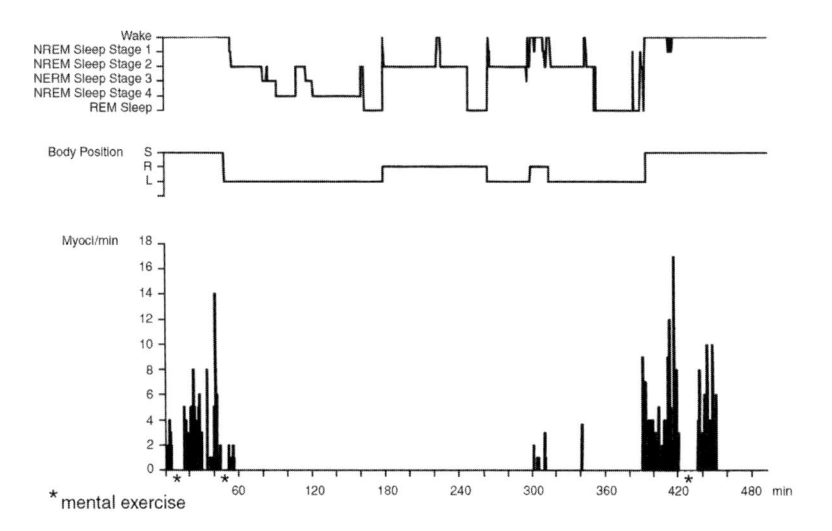

and syringobulbia [34], and even in some involuntary movements associated with restless legs syndrome (RLS) [35,36].

At the present time, therefore, propriospinal myoclonus remains a heterogeneous neurologic condition. It is not clear what distinguishes the pattern of damage that produces a prevalent myoclonic activity from that which produces a prevalent sustained muscle contraction, or what factors are involved in facilitating the spread of myoclonic activity in the propriospinal form.

A feature in some cases of propriospinal myoclonus, emphasized in the original reports, was an exacerbation when patients sat or lay flat [7,37]. In a series of eight cases, jerks disappeared or diminished upon standing in seven of them, and this was interpreted as a consequence of the effect of posture [16]. In 1997, Montagna et al. reported three patients (males) aged 71, 50 and 41 who presented propriospinal myoclonus appearing only when they were seated or lying down, but in which the triggering factor could be traced to the reduction in vigilance level at the transition from alert to relaxed wakefulness [8]. The myoclonic jerks during drowsiness were so annoying as to preclude the patients from falling asleep and caused severe insomnia. The clinical and EMG features of this myoclonic activity were typical of propriospinal myoclonus with onset of EMG activity in abdominal or cervical muscles and variable propagation at slow conduction velocity to other spinally innervated muscle in a fashion incompatible with purely descending volleys from the cerebral cortex or the reticular region.

Polygraphic studies documented that myoclonic activity appeared only during recumbency, but was not ascribed only to the effect of posture. Indeed, movements were suppressed promptly when the patients were given mental arithmetic tasks or when they performed simple motor tasks such as leg or hand movements or replied to questions. Jerks arose during relaxed wakefulness when EEG alpha activity spread from posterior occipital to anterior frontal areas, to disappear again with sleep onset, when EEG changed to theta activity, and throughout sleep proper (Figure 27.1). On magnetic resonance imaging (MRI), one patient had an arachnoid cyst at the level of the T8 posterior root. The authors emphasized the relationship between propriospinal myoclonus and the relaxed wakefulness state prior to falling sleep, the so-called "pre-dormitum", according to Critchley [38], that represents a remarkable transitional state associated with peculiar sensory and motor manifestations facilitated by removal of influences from mesopontine, posterior hypothalamic, and basal forebrain activation systems [39,40].

A similar case of propriospinal myoclonus arising in the thoracic muscles only during mental relaxation and drowsiness and causing insomnia was reported by Tison et al. in a 52-year-old woman [41]. Vetrugno et al. reported five additional patients (males) with propriospinal myoclonus, aged 24–57, in whom the peculiar relationship with relaxed wakefulness and the ensuing disturbance of sleep allowed the proposition that propriospinal myoclonus may represent a disorder of the sleep–wake transition period [9]. In all patients detailed neurophysiological examination

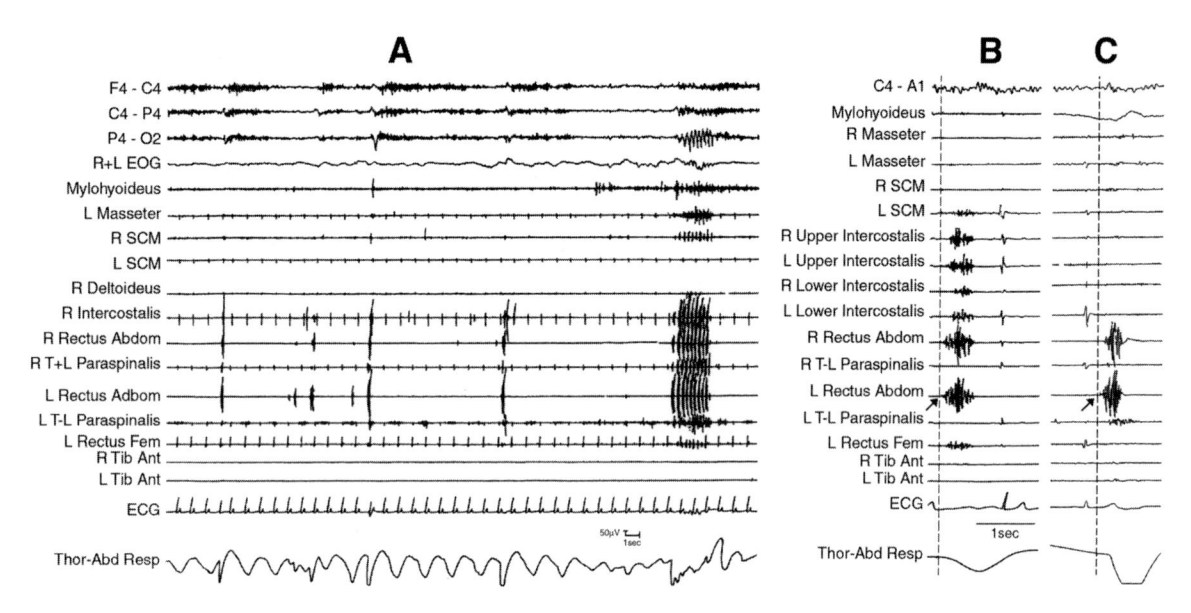

Figure 27.2 Polysomnographic recordings of propriospinal myoclonus recurring isolated or in clusters (A). At higher paper speed, it is evident that jerks always start in the left rectus abdominis muscle with (B) or without (C) spreading to more rostral and caudal muscles. Arrows show onset of activity. EOG: electro-oculogram; SCM: sternocleidomastoideus; Rectus Abdom: rectus abdominis; T-L Paraspinalis: thoraco-lumbar paraspinal; Rectus Fem: rectus femoris; Tib Ant: tibialis anterior; ECG: electrocardiogram; Thor-Abd Resp: thoraco-abdominal respirogram. L: left; R: right.

included EEG, EMG of limb and axial muscles, nerve conduction velocities, somatosensory evoked potentials (SEPs), and transcranial magnetic stimulation, which were normal. Neurophysiologically documented propriospinal myoclonus occurred solely at the transition from wake to sleep, or during intra-sleep arousals or upon awakening (Figure 27.1). There were no time-locked cortical correlates in back-averaged EEG activity preceding the spontaneous jerks which, moreover, did not involve distal hand and foot muscles, as is typical of cortical myoclonus. The diffusion of the jerks to involve multiple spinal segments, their origin in axial muscles (intercostalis, rectus abdominis, paraspinalis, sternocleidomastoideus), the long duration of the EMG bursts (100–300 ms, but sometimes longer and with polymyoclonic shape), the marked jitter in intermuscle latencies and the low spinal conduction velocities (2–16 m/s) were all characteristic of axial myoclonus of propriospinal origin. Remarkably, in some patients and in some instances, jerks could remain restricted to some muscles only (always including the originator muscle) and become propagated to more rostral and caudal levels only in the more intense jerks (Figure 27.2). In all patients, the jerks had a clear relationship with the wake–sleep transition period, arising in a semi-rhythmic fashion only during the relaxed phase prior to sleep (Figure 27.3), and disappearing with the earliest stages of sleep and throughout all sleep stages. In two cases, propriospinal myoclonus reappeared briefly during intra-sleep wakefulness and upon awakening in the morning. Mental and sensory stimulation during relaxed wakefulness stopped the jerks concomitantly with the disappearance of the EEG alpha activity and independently of any postural changes. Myoclonus thereafter reappeared as the patients were left undisturbed and the EEG alpha activity returned (Figure 27.1). An ocular myopathy and cervical myelopathy were observed in two patients, but were judged to be fortuitous associations. All patients received clonazepam, with only partial efficacy, and no particular effect was obtained by the administration of barbiturates or oral opioids (tramadol). In all patients, propriospinal myoclonus, once begun, proved to represent a chronic disorder, to be refractory to treatment, and to cause severe disability in the form of insomnia.

Propriospinal myoclonus has also been described in patients with a long history of restless legs syndrome (RLS). Vetrugno et al. reported three patients (two women), aged 36–83, with a 25-, 15-, and 5-year history of RLS and periodic limb movements during

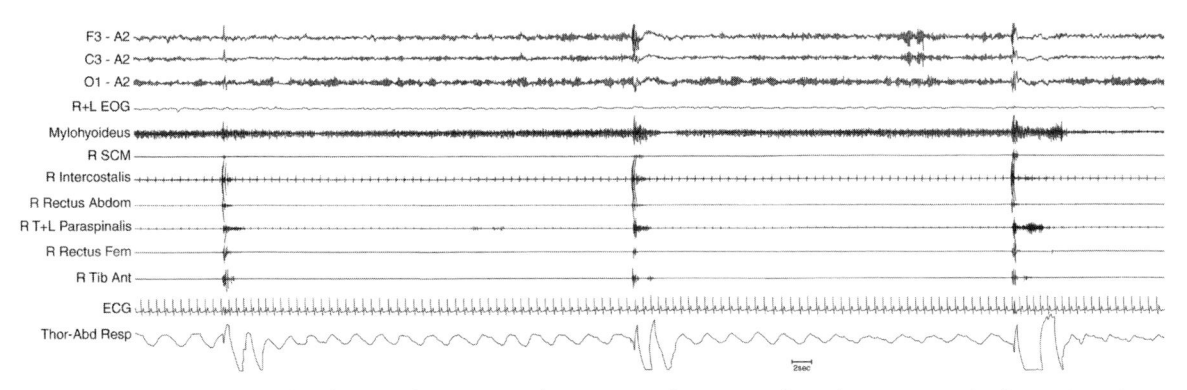

Figure 27.3 Polygraphic recording depicting the quasi-periodic recurrence of propriospinal myoclonus associated with spreading of EEG alpha activity to the anterior brain region. EOG: electro-oculogram; SCM: sternocleidomastoideus; Rectus Abdom: rectus abdominis; T-L Paraspinalis: thoraco-lumbar paraspinalis; Rectus Fem: rectus femoris; Tib Ant: tibialis anterior; ECG: electrocardiogram; Thor-Abd Resp: thoraco-abdominal respirogram.

sleep (PLMS) [36]. For 1, 4, and 5 years, the patients had complained of additional involuntary trunk and limb jerks preceding falling asleep and occasionally during intra-sleep wakefulness. Videopolysomnography revealed jerks during relaxed wakefulness arising in axial muscles with a caudal and rostral propagation at a slow conduction velocity, characteristic of propriospinal myoclonus. Jerk-related EEG-EMG back-averaging did not disclose any preceding cortical potential. During relaxed wakefulness preceding falling asleep and during intra-sleep wakefulness, propriospinal myoclonus co-existed with motor restlessness and sensory discomfort in the limbs. Propriospinal myoclonus disappeared when spindles and K-complexes appeared on the EEG. At this time, typical PLMS appeared every 20–40 s, especially during light sleep stages. PLMS EMG activity was now limited to leg, especially tibialis anterior muscles, and did not show any propriospinal propagation. Jerks with a propriospinal pattern may, thus, be associated with the RLS, in a tight relationship with relaxed wakefulness preceding sleep onset, and may co-exist though during different time windows with PLMS in the same patient [36].

Natural history

Propriospinal myoclonus at sleep onset consists of sudden axial jerks arousing during drowsiness preceding falling asleep and, rarely, during intra-sleep relaxed wakefulness and upon awakening in the morning (Figure 27.1). The jerks may be variable in frequency, recurring in clusters separated by long gaps of time or quasi-periodically every 10–20 s during the transition from wakefulness to sleep. Rhythmic or arrhythmic, flexion, rarely extension, movements of the axial muscles of the body rarely may remain segmentally located but, often, spread to the limbs excluding the cranially innervated muscles (except for the sterno-cleido-mastoideus). Movements tend to occur in the chest and abdomen and, typically, are not associated with vocalization. Neurological examination, brain and spinal MRI are usually normal. The jerks are most often spontaneous, sudden, shock-like, with variable regularity. The muscle jerks are rarely triggered by noise or external sources. The intensity of the muscle jerks may vary. The disorder can make it very hard to fall asleep with consequent insomnia. Patients may develop a fear of falling asleep, anxiety and depression. Injury to oneself or to a bed partner may occur. In all patients, propriospinal myoclonus set on in midlife and represent a chronic disorder, only in part responding to treatments. Notwithstanding, propriospinal myoclonus is a rare disorder. There are few data to determine how common it is and who is at risk for developing it. It appears to be more common in men than in women, and there are no reports of this disorder in children.

Laboratory investigations and differential diagnosis

For patients with suspected propriospinal myoclonus, multiple muscle EMGs from cranial, axial and limb muscles are essentials at polysomnographic investigation. The EMG surface bipolar silver/silver chloride electrodes should be placed 2 cm apart longitudinally over the relevant muscle bellies. The EEG electrodes should be placed at least over anterior F3 and F4, central C3 and C4, vertex Fz and Cz, and posterior O2 and O1 areas according to the International 10–20 system. Use of additional EEG electrodes, if possible, is helpful to better analyze the functional relation between the EEG activities, the consciousness state(s), and the movements studied. The polygraph should be connected to a computerized system for off-line analysis of acquired data (16-bit resolution, sampling rate 1024 Hz; EEG band pass 0.1–60 Hz; EMG band-pass 50–300 Hz). Simultaneous video-recording is mandatory to document and clearly differentiate any other kind of sleep-related abnormal movements.

Videopolysomnography demonstrates that the myoclonic activity is restricted to the wakefulness period preceding sleep or during intra-sleep wakefulness (Figure 27.1). Propriospinal myoclonus occurs as trunk flexion or, less frequent, extension with axial muscle activation. Proximal limb muscles are often involved in the jerk bilaterally, but the predominant action is in the axial muscles. Isolated or repetitive jerks may occur (Figure 27.2). The EMG discharges last typically 100–300 ms, but sometimes longer. Both reciprocal and co-contracting agonist–antagonist activity has been observed. The major characteristic of the EMG discharges is a simultaneous bilateral rostral and caudal recruitment from the area of spinal cord origin, sparing the cranial muscles. The activation speed of consecutive muscles is slower than that of the corticospinal pathway, in the range of 2–16 m/s and therefore in agreement with a propriospinal pattern of propagation. Jitter occurs from jerk to jerk with regard to the relative timing of the various EMG discharges within each episode of myoclonus. No EEG abnormalities in the routine recording or upon back-averaging have been reported. The jerks disappear with sleep onset and are not observed during sleep. During the relaxed wakefulness the myoclonic activity appears when EEG alpha rhythm spreads from the posterior to the anterior cortical areas or when it drops out. Jerks may recur at quasi-periodic intervals (every 5–40 s) and this pattern may repeat itself over a hundred times with consequent delayed sleep onset and sleep fragmentation (Figure 27.3). Mental activation with the patient comfortably lying down or sitting (asking the patient to think, speak, count, and perform simple or complex motor tasks such as waving a hand or writing) desynchronizes the EEG activity and makes the jerks disappear. Myoclonus thereafter reappears as soon as the patient is left undisturbed and relaxed and EEG alpha activity spreads or drops out.

Additional neurophysiologic investigations, including EMG of limb and axial muscles, nerve conduction velocities, SEPs and transcranial magnetic stimulation, and spinal cord and brain MRI are usually normal [8,9].

Absence of a cortical pre-movement potential, lack of involvement of cranial muscles, pattern of propagation, variable delay between different muscles, and slow propagation are all features that distinguish propriospinal myoclonus from cortical and reticular reflex myoclonus [42].

Focal abnormal involuntary movements of the abdominal wall reported under the term "diaphragmatic flutter," "moving umbilicus syndrome," and "belly dancer's dyskinesia" have different EMG patterns from those observed in patients with propriospinal myoclonus, as they consist of irregular or writhing contraction of the affected muscles at rates as high as 30–90/min [43].

Painful legs and moving toes identify a condition characterized by severe pain of the feet with a burning sensation and repetitive semicontinuous movements of the toes, with irregular EMG bursts in small muscles of the foot and leg, and not necessarily worsening at night or relieved by activity [44].

Periodic limb movements may appear during relaxed wakefulness, but in such cases they continue during light sleep stages. However, the motor pattern is different, as periodic movements in sleep consist of dorsiflexion of the big toe and foot and flexion of the knee and hip [45,46], even if they may co-exist with propriospinal myoclonus in some patients with RLS [36].

Sleep starts or hypnic jerks also deserve mention in the differential diagnosis with propriospinal myoclonus. They are non-periodic myoclonic movements, usually involving asynchronically different and isolated body segments, as a normal accompaniment of sleep and associated with a K-complex or EEG arousal. They do not primarily involve the abdominal muscles [47], even though they have been reported to cause insomnia when intensified [48]. However, the lack of detailed polygraphic data on the sleep starts makes the similarities with propriospinal myoclonus just a suggestion.

Excessive fragmentary myoclonus refers to the muscular twitches involving the fingers, toes, and the corners of the mouth, and persisting in all stages of sleep. The movements sometimes resemble muscle fasciculations with no movement across a joint space. In some cases, excessive fragmentary myoclonus is diagnosed strictly as an incidental finding on polysomnography, and no visible movement is present. Even when movements are present, the patient may be totally unaware of their presence. The EMG findings in excessive fragmentary myoclonus resemble the phasic REM twitches that are a normal finding in REM sleep, except that they exist in all stages of sleep and are not clustered as in normal REM sleep, but are more evenly spaced across individual epochs [48,49].

A psychogenic etiology also should be considered because the motor pattern of propriospinal myoclonus can be mimicked voluntarily [50,51].

Genetics and pathology

No familial cases of propriospinal myoclonus have been described to date, and the genetic or other basis predisposing individuals to develop this movement disorder at the wake–sleep transition are unknown. Also unexplained is the male prevalence in propriospinal myoclonus, as for many other NREM sleep and REM sleep parasomnias [14], and what pathological changes that supervene in life underlie the onset of the disease. MRI of the spinal cord and brain, indeed, does not disclose abnormalities in the majority of cases. According to the neurophysiological evidence available, propriospinal myoclonus at sleep onset must originate at a spinal level, but it must be set into motion by neurophysiological mechanisms specific to the transitional period between wake and sleep, the pre- and post-dormitum. Vigilance level is an important factor for the manifestation and variability of many movement disorders. The pre- and post-dormitum periods in particular are characterized by vigilance level fluctuations which modulate the state-dependent motor behavior. Propriospinal myoclonus may, indeed, be precipitated by drowsiness. Pre- and post-dormitum possess intrinsic cerebral metabolic patterns [39], and mental [38] and neurophysiological [40,52] characteristics that, with the relative changes in firing patterns of many neuronal motor-related supraspinal populations, could act to release a spinal pacemaker responsible for propriospinal myoclonus.

Management

There is no known effective treatment for propriospinal myoclonus. It responds only in part to clonazepam (up to 2 mg at night) treatment. Other treatment options includes carbamazepine (up to 400 mg/day), gabapentin (up to 800 mg/day), levetiracetam (up to 2000 mg), pramipexole (up to 0.7 mg at night) and tramadol (up to 100 mg at night) [8,9,28].

Transcutaneous electrical nerve stimulation (TENS) (80 Hz, 150-μse pulse width) with electrical current delivered over the area controlled by the low-thoracic spinal level has been reported to be effective in suppressing propriospinal myoclonus in a 50-year-old man with a 6-year history of abdominal movements which worsened when lying down and caused severe disability and insomnia [53].

Conclusions (including future directions)

Propriospinal myoclonus at wake–sleep transitions remains an idiopathic condition, often a lifelong one, in which no structural abnormality of the brain or spinal cord has been demonstrated. The long-term prognosis and natural history of the disease are still unclear and, moreover, chances for treatments are limited. Future studies are needed to better define the etiopathogenesis of propriospinal myoclonus. Conventional and functional neuroimaging studies could detect neural structures responsible for the initiation of the myoclonic jerks. Indeed, impairment to segments of the spinal cord, particularly if it involves loss of or changes in excitability of spinal interneurons, can release activity that produces spontaneous and often rhythmic bursts of muscle jerking. The impairment may either be direct, or it may involve changes in the input to spinal segments from other structures both peripheral and supraspinal. The latter could, for example, release intrinsic spinal pattern generators from external control or could provoke plastic reorganization of cord circuits to favor rhythmic and patterned discharges.

References

1. Friedreich N. Neuropathologische Beobachtung beim paramyoklonus multiplex. *Virchow's Arch Pathol Anat Physiol Klein Med* 1881; **86**: 421–34.
2. Seelingmüller A. Ein fall von paramyoklonus multiplex (Friedreich) (myoclonia congenita). *Dtsch Med Woch Enschr* 1886; **12**: 405–08.
3. Halliday AM. The neurophysiology of myoclonic jerking: A reappraisal. In Charlton HH (Ed), *Myoclonic Seizures*. Amsterdam: Excerpta Medica, 1975; 1–29.

4. Jankocic J, Pardo R. Segmental myoclonus. *Arch Neurol* 1986; **43**: 1025–31.

5. Brown P. Spinal myoclonus. In Marsden CD, Fahn S (Eds), *Movement Disorders 3*. London: Butterworth and Heineman International Medical Reviews, 1996; 459–76.

6. Meink HM, Piesiur-Strehlow B. Reflexes evoked in leg muscles from arm afferents: A propriospinal pathway in man? *Exp Brain Res* 1981; **43**: 78–86.

7. Brown P, Thompson PD, Rothwell JC, *et al*. Axial myoclonus of propriospinal origin. *Brain* 1991; **114**: 197–214.

8. Montagna P, Provini F, Plazzi G, *et al*. Propriospinal myoclonus upon relaxation and drowsiness: A cause of severe insomnia. *Mov Disord* 1997; **12**: 66–72.

9. Vetrugno R, Provini F, Meletti S, *et al*. Propriospinal myoclonus at the sleep–wake transition: A new type of parasomnia. *Sleep* 2001; **24**: 835–43.

10. Bussel B, Roby BA, Azouvi P, Biraben A, Yakovleff A, Held JP. Myoclonus in a patient with spinal cord transection. Possible involvement of the spinal stepping generator. *Brain* 1988; **111**: 1235–45.

11. Davies L, King PJL, Leicester J, *et al*. Recumbent tic. *Mov Disord* 1992; **7**: 359–63.

12. Vetrugno R, Provini F, Plazzi G, *et al*. Focal myoclonus and propriospinal propagation. *Clin Neurophysiol* 2000; **111**: 2175–9.

13. Schulze-Bonhage A, Knott H, Ferbert A. Pure stimulus sensitive truncal myoclonus of propriospinal origin. *Mov Disord* 1996; **11**: 87–90.

14. AASM. *International Classification of Sleep Disorders. Diagnostic and Coding Manual*. 2nd ed. Westchester, IL: American Academy of Sleep Medicine, 2005; 216–7.

15. Vasilenko DA. Propriospinal pathways in the ventral funicles of the cat spinal cord: Their effects on lumbosacral motoneurones. *Brain Res* 1975; **93**: 502–06.

16. Brown P, Rothwell JC, Thompson PD, *et al*. Propriospinal myoclonus: Evidence for spinal "pattern" generators in humans. *Mov Disord* 1994; **9**: 571–6.

17. Chokroverty S, Walters A, Zimmerman T, *et al*. Propriospinal myoclonus: A neurophysiologic analysis. *Neurology* 1992; **42**: 1591–5.

18. Nishiyama K, Ugawa Y, Takeda K, *et al*. Axial myoclonus mediated by the propriospinal tract: A case report. *Eur Neurol* 1994; **34**: 48–50.

19. Pisano F, Miscio G, Romorini A, *et al*. Abdominal propriospinal myoclonus of unknown etiology. *Rev Neurol* 1995; **151**: 209–11.

20. Fouillet N, Wiart L, Arné P, *et al*. Propriospinal myoclonus in tetraplegic patients: Clinical, electrophysiological and therapeutic aspects. *Paraplegia* 1995; **33**: 678–81.

21. Nogués MA. Spontaneous electromyographic activity in spinal cord lesions. *Muscle Nerve* 2002; **Suppl 11**: 77–82.

22. Capelle HH, Wöhrle JC, Weigel R, *et al*. Propriospinal myoclonus due to cervical disc herniation. Case report. *J Neurosurg Spine* 2005; **2**: 608–11.

23. Kapoor R, Brown P, Thompson PD, *et al*. Propriospinal myoclonus in multiple sclerosis. *J Neurol Neurosurg Psychiatry* 1992; **55**: 1086–8.

24. de la Sayette V, Schaeffer S, Queruel C, *et al*. Lyme neuroborreliosis presenting with propriospinal myoclonus. *J Neurol Neurosurg Psychiatry* 1996; **61**: 420.

25. Lubetzki C, Vidailhet M, Jedynak CP, *et al*. Propriospinal myoclonus in a HIV seropositive patient. *Rev Neurol* 1994; **150**: 70–2.

26. Manconi M, Sferrazza B, Iannaccone S, *et al*. Case of symptomatic propriospinal myoclonus evolving toward acute "myoclonic status". *Mov Disord* 2005; **20**: 1646–50.

27. Salsano E, Ciano C, Romano S, *et al*. Propriospinal myoclonus with life threatening tonic spasms as paraneoplastic presentation of breast cancer. *J Neurol Neurosurg Psychiatry* 2006; **77**: 422–4.

28. Vetrugno R, Liguori R, D'Alessandro R, *et al*. Axial myoclonus in paraproteinemic polyneuropathy. *Muscle Nerve* 2008; **38**: 1330–5.

29. Lozsadi DA, Forster A, Fletcher NA. Cannabis-induced propriospinal myoclonus. *Mov Disord* 2004; **19**: 708–09.

30. Post B, Koelman JH, Tijssen MA. Propriospinal myoclonus after treatment with ciprofloxacin. *Mov Disord* 2004; **19**: 595–7.

31. Benatru I, Thobois S, Andre-Obadia N, *et al*. Atypical propriospinal myoclonus with possible relationship to alpha interferon therapy. *Mov Disord* 2003; **18**: 1564–8.

32. Espay AJ, Ashby P, Hanajima R, *et al*. Unique form of propriospinal myoclonus as a possible complication of an enteropathogenic toxin. *Mov Disord* 2003; **18**: 942–8.

33. Meinck HM, Ricker K, Hülser PJ, *et al*. Stiff man syndrome: Neurophysiological findings in eight patients. *J Neurol* 1995; **242**: 134–42.

34. Nogués MA, Leiguarda RC, Rivero AD, *et al*. Involuntary movements and abnormal spontaneous EMG activity in syringomyelia and syringobulbia. *Neurology* 1999; **52**: 823–34.

35. Trenkwalder C, Bucher SF, Oertel WH. Electrophysiological pattern of involuntary limb movements in the restless legs syndrome. *Muscle Nerve* 1996; **19**: 155–62.

36. Vetrugno R, Provini F, Plazzi G, et al. Propriospinal myoclonus: A motor phenomenon found in restless legs syndrome different from periodic limb movements during sleep. *Mov Disord* 2005; **20**: 1323–9.

37. Brown P, Thompson PD, Rothwell JD, et al. Paroxysmal axial spasms of spinal origin. *Mov Disord* 1991; **6**: 43–8.

38. Critchley M. The predormitum. *Rev Neurol* 1955; **93**: 101–06.

39. Braun AR, Balkin TJ, Wesenten NJ, et al. Regional cerebral blood flow throughout the sleep–wake cycle. An H2(15)O PET study. *Brain* 1997; **120**: 1173–97.

40. Llinas RR, Steriade M. Bursting of thalamic neurons and states of vigilance. *J Neurophysiol* 2006; **95**: 3297–308.

41. Tison F, Arné P, Dousset V, et al. Propriospinal myoclonus induced by relaxation and drowsiness. *Rev Neurol* 1998; **154**: 423–5.

42. Caviness JN, Brown PB. Myoclonus: current concepts and recent advances. *Lancet Neurol* 2004; **3**: 598–607.

43. Iliceto G, Thompson PD, Day BL, et al. Diaphragmatic flutter, the moving umbilicus syndrome, and "belly dancer's" dyskinesia. *Mov Disord* 1990; **5**: 15–22.

44. Montagna P, Cirignotta F, Sacquegna T, et al. "Painful legs and moving toes" associated with polyneuropathy. *J Neurol Neurosurg Psychiatry* 1983; **46**: 399–403.

45. Lugaresi E, Cirignotta F, Coccagna G, Montagna P. Nocturnal myoclonus and restless legs syndrome. In Fahn S (Ed), *Myoclonus*. New York: Raven Press, 1986; 295–307.

46. Provini F, Vetrugno R, Meletti S, et al. Motor pattern of periodic limb movements during sleep. *Neurology* 2001; **57**: 300–04.

47. Oswald I. Sudden bodily jerks on falling asleep. *Brain* 1959; **82**: 92–103.

48. Broughton R. Pathological fragmentary myoclonus, intensified hypnic jerks and hypnagogic foot tremor: Three unusual sleep-related movement disorders. In Koella WP, Obal F, Shulz H, Visser P (Eds), *Sleep '86*. Stuttgart: G Fischer Verlag, 1988; 240–3.

49. Vetrugno R, Plazzi G, Provini F, et al. Excessive fragmentary hypnic myoclonus: Clinical and neurophysiological findings. *Sleep Med* 2002; **3**: 73–6.

50. Kang SY, Sohn YH. Electromyography patterns of propriospinal myoclonus can be mimicked voluntarily. *Mov Disord* 2006; **21**: 1241–4.

51. Williams DR, Cowey M, Tuck K, et al. Psychogenic propriospinal myoclonus. *Mov Disord* 2008; **23**: 1312–3.

52. Montagna P, Lugaresi E. Sleep benefit in Parkinson's disease. *Mov Disord* 1998; **13**: 751–2.

53. Maltête D, Verdure P, Roze E, et al. TENS for the treatment of propriospinal myoclonus. *Mov Disord* 2008; **23**: 2256–7.

Section 5 Sleep-related movement disorders and other variants
Chapter 28: Sleep-related rhythmic movement disorder

Timothy F. Hoban

Introduction

"The mother then noticed that, after the child had been asleep for a couple of hours, he would turn over on his right side, drawing the right arm above his head, and applying the left hand over the left ear. Once in this position, he would begin to oscillate his head on the pillow from right to left, in a perfectly rhythmical manner. The oscillation would be maintained for about half an hour, and then the child slept quietly again. From the time this phenomenon was first observed, no night passed without its occurrence..."

M. Putnam-Jacobi, 1880, describing "nocturnal rotary spasm" in a 3-year-old boy [1].

Sleep-related rhythmic movement disorder (RMD) represents a parasomnia characterized by slow and sustained rhythmic movements involving major muscle groups. It is unique among the parasomnias in its propensity to span both wakefulness and sleep. Episodes may occur during wakefulness, drowsiness, any stage of sleep, or in association with arousal from sleep. Although most common in younger children, RMD occasionally persists into adulthood – sometimes in dramatic form. The condition has received little scientific study, so only limited progress has been achieved towards understanding the underlying causes and consequences of the disorder. This chapter will examine the clinical manifestations, natural history, and polysomnographic findings for RMD. Possible causes and putative treatments for the condition will also be examined.

Clinical manifestations of RMD

RMD is characterized by recurrent episodes of stereotyped body movements in association with sleep. Movements may involve the head, neck, trunk, or limbs in isolation or combination, often accompanied by synchronous humming or moaning vocalizations. The cadence of movements is strikingly regular, usually at a frequency of 0.5–2 Hz [2].

The duration of rhythmic movement episodes may be as short as several seconds or as long as several hours, however most episodes abate within 15 min [2,3]. Episodes may arise during predormital wakefulness, drowsiness, or any stage of sleep and sometimes span the wake–sleep transition. Episodes arising from wakefulness have been reported to last longer than those arising during sustained sleep [4].

Published accounts of RMD date to the late nineteenth century, as excerpted above [1]. Some authors attribute the initial report of the condition to Wepfer as early as 1727 [5]. More detailed descriptions of the condition commenced in 1905 with independent reports by Zappert and Cruchet [6,7]. Zappert described sleep-related head banging as "jactatio capitis nocturna", a name still commonly used for the condition. Cruchet described sleep-related rhythmic movements as "tics dans le sommeil" and "rhythmie du sommeil" in two early case series [6,8].

Several distinct varieties of RMD have been described based on the predominant pattern of movements exhibited. *Head banging* (jactatio capitis nocturna) is characterized by forward and backward head movement which can be either gentle or vigorous in nature. Movements typically cause the head to strike the pillow or bed surface with each cycle, or less commonly the headboard or wall. Head banging usually occurs in the prone or supine positions but has been reported in the sitting and hands–knees positions as well [9].

Other varieties of RMD include *head rolling* and *body rolling*, which are characterized by rhythmic side-to-side turning, usually from the supine position.

Table 28.1 ICSD-2 diagnostic criteria for sleep-related rhythmic movement disorder [15].

1) Movements are characterized by repetitive, stereotyped, and rhythmic motor activity.
2) Movements involve large muscle groups.
3) Movements are predominantly sleep-related, occurring near sleep onset or during drowsiness or sleep.
4) The movements or behaviors result in at least one referable complaint:
    a. Interference with normal sleep;
    b. Significant impairment of daytime function;
    c. Self-inflicted bodily injury (or risk of injury without use of protective measures).
5) Rhythmic movements are not better explained by an alternative sleep or medical disorder, neurological or psychiatric disorder, or by medication or substance use.

Body rocking is a dramatic form of RMD consisting of vigorous in-line body movements from the hands–knees position. Occasionally encountered forms of RMD include *leg rolling, leg banging*, and rhythmic striking of the head with the hands [10,11]. Rhythmic sleep-related episodes of tongue biting, tongue movements, and pelvic movements have also been reported [12–14].

Diagnostic criteria for RMD were established in the International Classification of Sleep Disorders, second edition, summarized in Table 28.1 [15]. In addition to specifications regarding the nature and circumstances of sleep-related motor activity, these criteria also require that evidence of clinically significant consequences – disturbed sleep quality, impaired daytime function, or risk of injury – be present in order for a diagnosis of RMD to be established. It has been proposed that the term *rhythmic movements of sleep* (RMS) be used to describe the benign or self-limited forms of rhythmic sleep behaviors that are frequently observed in healthy infants and younger children [16].

Epidemiology and natural history of RMD

Sleep-related rhythmic movements may be observed in up to two-thirds of infants, but usually resolve before 5 years of age [17]. Clinically significant RMD is also most prevalent during early childhood, with persistence into adulthood occasionally reported [18,19]. Onset of symptoms is typically during the first year of life and only occasionally after 18 months of age [3,20,21]. Several reports suggest that head banging is more common in boys than girls at a 3:1 ratio, whereas other varieties of RMD are equally frequent in males and females [20–22]. RMD may be more common and more persistent in individuals with developmental disabilities [23,24]. A familial history of RMD is reported in up to 20% of cases [4,20,25].

Cross-sectional studies assessing the prevalence of RMD in different pediatric populations are summarized in Table 28.2. These studies suggest that 3–5% of children may exhibit sleep-related head banging and that 12–19% demonstrate body rocking. The prevalence of RMD in the adult population remains unknown.

A few longitudinal studies of children with RMD have assessed how the condition changes and often subsides with advancing age. In a prospective study of 212 randomly selected Swedish children followed from 9 through 60 months of age, the prevalence of

Table 28.2 Cross-sectional studies assessing prevalence of rhythmic movement disorder during childhood.

Study	Head banging (%)	Body rocking (%)	Head rolling (%)	Any RMD (%)	Population studied
Levy and Patrick, 1928 [65]	2.6				Pediatric screening clinic
Lourie, 1949 [46]	10				Pediatric private practice
Lourie, 1949 [46]	15–20				Unselected pediatric clinic population
Kravitz et al., 1960 [20]	3.6				Private pediatric practice
Lissovoy, 1961 [22]	2.9	12.3			Children aged 19–32 months
Sallustro and Atwell, 1978 [21]	5.1	19.1	6.3		Children aged 3 month to 6 years
Abe et al., 1984 [51]	1.5				Three-year-old children
Laberge et al., 2000 [44]		17.2			Children aged 3–13 years
Neveus et al., 2001 [66]				8.3	Children aged 6–10 years

sleep-related body rocking declined from 43% to 3%, the prevalence of head banging from 28% to 2%, and the frequency of any type of rhythmic sleep behavior from 66% to 6% [17]. Similar age-related changes were seen in a group of 1353 children assessed for body rocking. In this cohort, prevalence of body rocking was 15.3% for ages 3–10 years, declining to 3.1% at age 11 years and 3% by age 13 years.

Complications of RMD

Most children and adults with RMD who are otherwise healthy are at low risk for serious injury resulting from their sleep-related movements, although minor bruising or abrasions are occasionally reported for patients exhibiting more vigorous behaviors. Reports of serious injury from sleep-related head banging are rare, but include accounts of dermal scarring/fibrosis and suppurative wounds [10,11]. Cataracts, retinal detachment, MRI abnormalities, and bony skull injury have also been reported in association with head banging, although these accounts do not specify whether the inciting behavior was diurnal or sleep-related in nature [26–28].

Comorbidity of RMD

Sleep-related RMD usually affects children – and occasionally, adults – who are otherwise healthy and developmentally normal. Sleep-related RMD is occasionally encountered in individuals with developmental disabilities or autism spectrum disorders who also exhibit similar stereotypical movements arising during circumstances unrelated to sleep.

Acquired RMD is uncommon, but has been reported in association with head injury, herpes encephalitis, and underlying epilepsy [18,29,30]. Atypical varieties of sleep-related movements have also been reported in association with restless legs syndrome (pelvic thrusting) and Costello syndrome (tongue movements) [12,13].

Several case series have reported the association of RMD and attention deficit hyperactivity disorder (ADHD). In one group of seven children with RMD studied with video-PSG, three had a clinical history of ADHD [31]. In another group of children and adults referred for evaluation of RMD, 6 of 10 met formal diagnostic criteria for ADHD [4]. In a study of sleep problems affecting children attending several psychiatry clinics, 6 of 14 children with ADHD were reported to have a history of sleep-related head banging [32]. Although these findings provide plausible support for an association between RMD and ADHD, the data must be interpreted with due attention to the small sample sizes studied.

Polysomnography in RMD

The diagnosis of RMD is usually established on the basis of the clinical history – sometimes supplemented by home video recording – rather than polysomnography (PSG). PSG is nevertheless indicated in cases where the clinical diagnosis is uncertain, in cases where concurrent sleep disorders such as obstructive sleep apnea (OSA) may be present, and in cases where additional data are required to determine to what extent sleep-related movements impair sleep quality or daytime function.

When PSG is performed as part of the diagnostic assessment, use of concurrent video recording provides the most exact correlation between clinical and polysomnographic findings. The use of additional limb EMG leads or parasomnia montages provides valuable detail regarding limb movements which can aid the polysomnographer in distinguishing RMD from similar parasomnias, such as alternating leg muscle activation (ALMA) [33]. Use of 16-lead EEG during PSG is also advisable if there is substantial clinical suspicion that sleep-related motor activity might be the result of seizure.

Rhythmic movement events recorded during PSG exhibit several characteristic findings. Episodes may occur during wakefulness (Figure 28.1), during sleep (Figure 28.2), or following arousal from sleep. Head and body movements are typically associated with rhythmic high amplitude wave forms on EEG and EOG channels having a frequency of 0.5–2 Hz. Leg and body rolling are usually associated with rhythmic bursts of activity on limb EMG leads (Figure 28.3). RMD-associated vocalizations – when present – are sometimes reflected in the snore channel (Figure 28.2).

Published accounts of PSG findings for patients with RMD report that episodes most often arise during wakefulness, drowsiness, and light non-REM (NREM) sleep [18,19,31,34,35]. Occasional patients exhibit RMD which occurs primarily or exclusively during REM sleep [3,36–38]. Rhythmic movement episodes have also been reported in association with the cyclic alternating pattern and following apnea-associated arousals [19,39].

Figure 28.1 The color version of this figure can be found in the color plate section. 30-s PSG epoch illustrating body rocking during wakefulness in a 10-year-old girl. High amplitude 1 Hz movement artifact on EEG leads reflects rhythmic body movements.

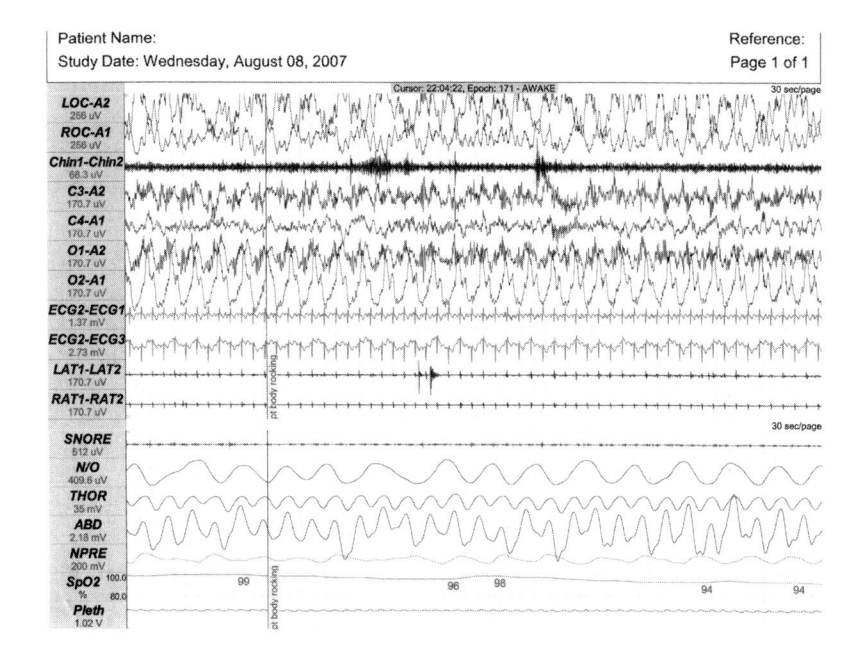

Figure 28.2 The color version of this figure can be found in the color plate section. 30-s PSG epoch illustrating body rocking arising from sleep in a 10-year-old girl. High amplitude 1 Hz movement artifact on EEG and EOG leads reflects rhythmic body movements. Activity on snore channel reflects vocalizations accompanying the episode.

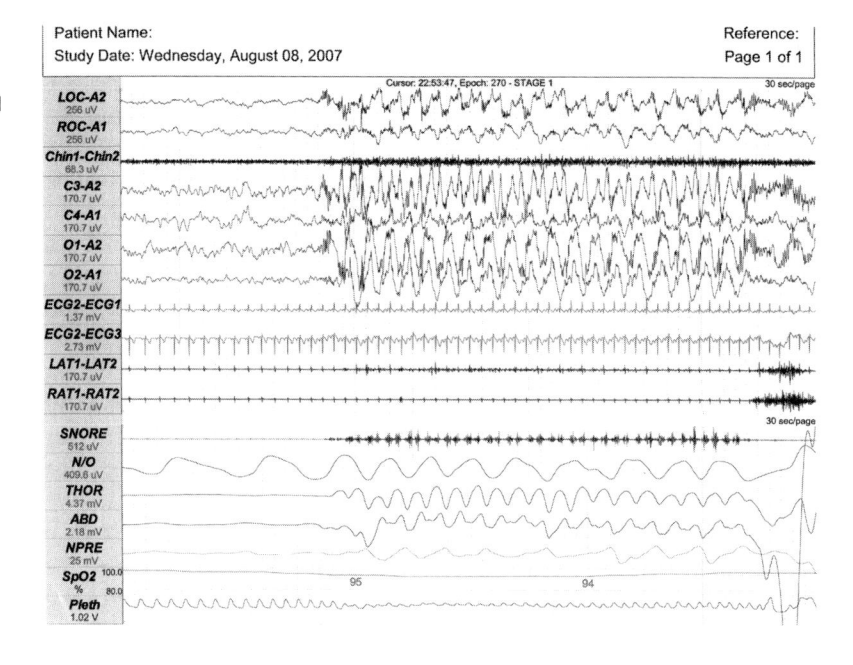

Postulated causes of RMD

The specific causes and physiologic mechanisms that underlie RMD remain uncertain. Because associated organic illness is absent in the great majority of cases, many theories have been advanced proposing behavioral or psychological causes for the condition. Older hypotheses that RMD represents autoerotic gratification, anxiety relief, self-directed aggression, or a reaction to physical restraint have not been validated [34,40–43], except for a single study that identified high anxiety scores for children with body rocking or other parasomnias compared to children without

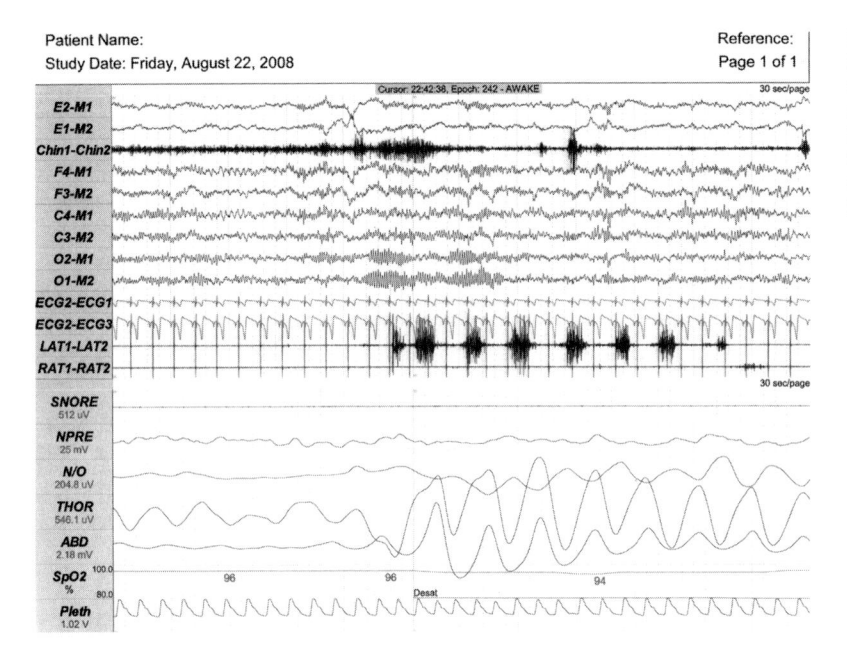

Figure 28.3 The color version of this figure can be found in the color plate section. 30-s PSG epoch for a 17-year-old male demonstrating leg rolling arising from wakefulness, characterized by rhythmic EMG activity seen exclusively in the left anterior tibialis lead (labeled LAT1-LAT2).

parasomnias [44]. Despite the absence of significant underlying psychopathology in most patients with RMD, several reports suggest that RMD may worsen during times of stress [11,45].

Alternative theories have postulated that RMD might represent a learned variety of self-soothing behavior, in which spontaneous rhythmic activity causes pleasurable sensations which positively reinforce the likelihood that the behavior will be sustained [46,47]. A recently advanced hypothesis proposes that RMD is linked to arousal fluctuations and mediated via central motor pattern generators of the brain stem [48].

Some authors have proposed that vestibular stimulation from RMD might benefit motor development during infancy via reinforcement of vestibulo-ocular reflexes [47,49,50], but clinical studies assessing young children with RMD for developmental precocity have yielded inconsistent results [21,51].

Differential diagnosis for sleep-related rhythmic movements

The diagnosis of RMD can usually be established with a high degree of certainty based on the clinical history or home video recording. In cases where sleep-related movements are atypical, violent, or particularly prolonged, a broader differential diagnosis may be appropriately considered.

Several conditions are associated with diurnal rhythmic movements which may mimic those seen in RMD prior to sleep onset. *Stereotypic movement disorder* – often exhibited by individuals with autism or other developmental disabilities – may feature prominent head banging or body rocking that is usually more clearly associated with wakefulness than sleep [52]. *Spasmus nutans*, a transient neurological syndrome which can cause head bobbing in infants, can be distinguished from RMD by the presence of concurrent head tilt or nystagmus.

When sustained or vigorous rhythmic movements are reported to arise during sleep, several elements of the history help distinguish between RMD and *sleep-related epilepsy* as possible causes. Seizure-related movements usually demonstrate tonic or tonic–clonic character and are often accompanied by gaze deviation, chewing movements, incontinence, and tongue or cheek laceration. *Nocturnal frontal lobe epilepsy* (NFLE) represents an occasional exception to this dictum. In this condition, seizures may occur multiple times per night and feature complex or atypical rhythmic behaviors – such as rocking of the body – which may resemble those seen in RMD [53].

A number of parasomnias that feature excessive motor activity during sleep may also result in relatively rhythmic behaviors which can mimic those of RMD (Table 28.3).

Table 28.3 Conditions which can mimic rhythmic movement disorder.

Stereotypic movement disorder
Motor tics
Spasmus nutans
Propriospinal myoclonus at sleep onset
Hypnagogic foot tremor
Periodic limb movement disorder
REM sleep behavior disorder
Alternating leg muscle activation during sleep
Benign sleep myoclonus of infancy
Sleep-related epilepsy

Treatment of RMD

Most children and adults with RMD do not require treatment for the condition, provided that the condition does not substantially affect sleep quality or daytime function. For patients with developmental disabilities or particularly violent forms of RMD, judicious padding around the bed or use of a protective helmet is sometimes appropriate.

Drug therapy for RMD has not been studied rigorously, although a small number of case reports have been published. Several reports have documented significant clinical improvement for adults and children with RMD with use of clonazepam 1 mg qhs [5,35,45,54], whereas others have reported either no effect [55], or the necessity of a higher dose [56]. Use of oxazepam at doses of 10–20 mg nightly was reported to produce significant but unsustained improvement of nocturnal body rocking for an 8-year-old girl [42]. Successful treatment of childhood RMD has also been reported with use of citalopram and imipramine [29,57,58].

Behavioral therapies have received limited investigation in the treatment of RMD. Case reports have documented successful treatment with use of omission training, selective reinforcement of desired behaviors, hypnosis, and forced awakening [59–62]. Attempts to suppress rhythmic movements through use of a metronome set to an identical frequency have yielded variable results [9,34,46]. Several small case series focusing on children with RMD reported dramatic improvement of symptoms with use of a water bed or following a three-week program of controlled sleep restriction [63,64].

Conclusion

This chapter has examined the limited data available regarding the clinical manifestations, pathophysiology, and treatment of sleep-related rhythmic movement disorder. Although recent research has provided valuable insights regarding RMD, few data are available regarding the impact of the condition upon daytime function apart from several case series reporting association between RMD and ADHD [4,31,32], and case reports identifying excessive daytime sleepiness in some affected patients [38,45]. Further investigation will be required to better understand the neurocognitive sequelae and causative mechanisms of the condition.

References

1. Putnam-Jacobi M. Case of nocturnal rotary spasm. *J Nerv Ment Dis*, 1880; **7**: 390–402.
2. Dyken ME, Rodnitzky RL. Periodic, aperiodic, and rhythmic motor disorders of sleep. *Neurology* 1992; **42**(7 Suppl 6): 68–74.
3. Thorpy MJ, Spielman AJ. Persistent jactatio nocturna. *Neurology* 1984; **34**(Suppl 1): 209.
4. Stepanova I, Nevsimalova S, Hanusova J. Rhythmic movement disorder in sleep persisting into childhood and adulthood. *Sleep* 2005; **28**: 851–7.
5. Alves RS, Aloe F, Silva AB, Tavares SM. Jactatio capitis nocturna with persistence in adulthood. Case report. *Arq Neuro-Psiquiatria* 1998; **56**: 655–7.
6. Cruchet R. Tics et sommeil. *Presse Med* 1905; **13**: 33–6.
7. Zappert J. Uber nactliche Kopfbewegungen bei kindern (jactatio capitis nocturna). *Jahrb Kinderheilk* 1905; **62**: 70–83.
8. Cruchet R. Six nouveaux cas de rhythmies du sommeil (les rhythmies a la caserne). *Gaz Hebd Sci Med* 1912; **33**: 303–08.
9. Lissovoy VD. Head banging in early childhood. *Child Dev* 1962; **33**: 43–56.
10. Sormann GW. The headbangers tumour. *Br J Plast Surg* 1982; **35**: 72–4.
11. Whyte J, Kavey NB, Gidro-Frank S. A self-destructive variant of jactatio capitis nocturna. *J Nerv Mental Dis* 1991; **179**: 49–50.
12. Della Marca G, Rubino M, Vollono C, et al. Rhythmic tongue movements during sleep: A peculiar parasomnia in Costello syndrome. *Mov Disord* 2006; **21**: 473–8.
13. Lombardi C, Provini F, Vetrugno R, Plazzi G, Lugaresi E, Montagna P. Pelvic movements as rhythmic motor

manifestation associated with restless legs syndrome. *Mov Disord* 2003; **18**: 110–13.

14. Tuxhorn I, Hoppe M. Parasomnia with rhythmic movements manifesting as nocturnal tongue biting. *Neuropediatrics* 1993; **24**: 167–8.

15. AASM. Sleep related rhythmic movement disorder. In *The International Classification of Sleep Disorders*. Westchester, IL: American Academy of Sleep Medicine: 2005, 193–5.

16. Picchietti DL. Personal communication, 2003.

17. Klackenberg G. Rhythmic movements in infancy and early childhood: Head banging, head turning, and rocking. *Acta Paed* 1971; **60**: 74–83.

18. Happe S, Ludemann P, Ringelstein EB. Persistence of rhythmic movement disorder beyond childhood: A videotape demonstration. *Mov Disord* 2000; **15**: 1296–8.

19. Mayer G, Wilde-Frenz J, Kurella B. Sleep related rhythmic movement disorder revisited. *J Sleep Res* 2007; **16**: 110–16.

20. Kravitz H, Rosenthal V, Teplitz Z, Murphy JB, Lesser RE. A study of head-banging in infants and children. *Dis Nerv Syst* 1960; **21**: 203–08.

21. Sallustro F, Atwell CW. Body rocking, head banging, and head rolling in normal children. *J Pediatr* 1978; **93**: 704–08.

22. Lissovoy VD. Head banging in early childhood. *J Pediatr* 1961; **58**: 803–05.

23. Matin MA, Rundle AT. Physiological and psychiatric investigations into a group of mentally handicapped subjects with self-injurious behaviour. *J Ment Defic Res* 1980; **24**: 77–85.

24. Mitchell R, Etches P. Rhythmic habit patterns (stereotypies). *Dev Med Child Neurol* 1977; **19**: 545–50.

25. Kavey NB, Jewitch DE, Bloomingdale E, Gidro-Frank S. Jactatio capitis nocturna: A longitudinal study of a boy with a familial history. *Sleep Res* 1981; **10**: 208.

26. Bemporad JR, Sours JA, Spalter HF. Cataracts following chronic headbanging: A report of two cases. *Am J Psychiatry* 1968; **125**: 245–9.

27. Carlock KS, Williams JP, Graves GC. MRI findings in headbangers. *Clin Imaging* 1997; **21**: 411–13.

28. Stuck KJ, Hernandez RJ. Large skull defect in a headbanger. *Pediatr Radiol* 1979; **8**: 257–8.

29. Drake ME, Jr. Jactatio nocturna after head injury. *Neurology* 1986; **36**: 867–8.

30. Guilleminault C, Silvestri R. Disorders of arousal and epilepsy during sleep. In Sterman MB, Shouse XN, Passouant P (Eds), *Sleep and Epilepsy*, New York: Academic Press, 1983, 513–31.

31. Dyken ME, Lin-Dyken DC, Yamada T. Diagnosing rhythmic movement disorder with video-polysomnography. *Ped Neurol* 1997; **16**: 37–41.

32. Simonds JF, Parraga H. Sleep behaviors and disorders in children and adolescents evaluated at psychiatric clinics. *J Dev Behav Pediatr* 1984; **5**: 6–10.

33. Chervin RD, Consens FB, Kutluay E. Alternating leg muscle activation during sleep and arousals: A new sleep-related motor phenomenon? *Mov Disord* 2003; **18**: 551–9.

34. Evans J. Rocking at night. *J Child Psychol Psychiatry* 1961; **2**: 71–85.

35. Manni R, Tartara A. Clonazepam treatment of rhythmic movement disorder. *Sleep* 1997; **20**: 812.

36. Anderson KN, Smith IE, Shneerson JM. Rhythmic movement disorder (head banging) in an adult during rapid eye movement sleep. *Mov Disord* 2006; **21**: 866–7.

37. Gagnon P, De Koninck J. Repetitive head movements during REM sleep. *Biol Psychiatry* 1985; **20**: 176–8.

38. Kempenaers C, Bouillon E, Mendlewicz J. A rhythmic movement disorder in REM sleep: A case report. *Sleep* 1994; **17**: 274–9.

39. Manni R, Terzaghi M, Sartori I, Veggiotti P, Parrino L. Rhythmic movement disorder and cyclic alternating pattern during sleep: A video-polysomnographic study in a 9-year-old boy. *Mov Disord* 2004; **19**: 1186–90.

40. Freud A, Burlingham DT. *Infants without Families*. New York: International Universities Press, 1973.

41. Levy DM. On the problem of movement restraint (tics, stereotyped movements, hyperactivity). *Am J Orthopsychiatry* 1944; **14**: 651–69.

42. Walsh JK, Kramer M, Skinner JE. A case report of jactatio capitis nocturna. *Am J Psychiatry* 1981; **138**: 524–6.

43. Silberstein RM, Blackman S, Mandell W. Autoerotic head banging; a reflection on the opportunism of infants. *J Am Acad Child Psychiatry* 1966; **5**: 235–42.

44. Laberge L, Tremblay RE, Vitaro F, Montplaisir J. Development of parasomnias from childhood to early adolescence. *Pediatrics* 2000; **106**: 67–74.

45. Chisholm T, Morehouse RL. Adult headbanging: Sleep studies and treatment. *Sleep* 1996; **19**: 343–6.

46. Lourie RS. The role of rhythmic patterns in childhood. *Am J Psychiatry* 1949; **105**: 653–60.

47. Thorpy MJ, Glovinsky PB. Parasomnias. *Psychiatr Clin North Am* 1987; **10**: 623–39.

48. Manni R, Terzaghi M. Rhythmic movements during sleep: A physiological and pathological profile. *Neurol Sci* 2005; **26**: s181–5.

49. Clark DL, Kreutzberg JR, Chee FK. Vestibular stimulation influence on motor development in infants. *Science* 1977; **196**: 1228–9.

50. Gregg CL, Haffner ME, Korner AF. The relative efficacy of vestibular-proprioceptive stimulation and the upright position in enhancing visual pursuit in neonates. *Child Dev* 1976; **47**: 309–14.

51. Abe K, Oda N, Amatomi M. Natural history and predictive significance of head-banging, head-rolling and breath-holding spells. *Dev Med Child Neurol* 1984; **26**: 644–8.

52. APA. *Diagnostic and Statistical Manual of Mental Disorders, fourth edition, text revision (DSM-IV-TR)*. Washington, DC: American Psychiatric Association, 2000.

53. Provini F, Plazzi G, Montagna P, Lugaresi E. The wide clinical spectrum of nocturnal frontal lobe epilepsy. *Sleep Med Rev* 2000; **4**: 375–86.

54. Merlino G, Serafini A, Dolso P, Canesin R, Valente M, Gigli GL. Association of body rolling, leg rolling, and rhythmic feet movements in a young adult: A video-polysomnographic study performed before and after one night of clonazepam. *Mov Disord* 2008; **23**: 602–07.

55. Kaneda R, Furuta H, Kazuto K, Arayama K, Sano J, Koshino Y. An unusual case of rhythmic movement disorder. *Psychiatry Clin Neurosci* 2000; **54**: 348–9.

56. Hashizume Y, Yoshijima H, Uchimura N, Maeda H. Case of head banging that continued to adolescence. *Psychiatry Clin Neurosci* 2002; **56**: 255–6.

57. Freidin MR, Jankowski JJ, Singer WD. Nocturnal head banging as a sleep disorder: A case report. *Am J Psychiatry* 1979; **136**: 1469–70.

58. Vogel W, Stein DJ. Citalopram for head-banging. *J Am Acad Child Adolesc Psychiatry* 2000; **39**: 544–5.

59. Frankel F, Moss D, Schofield S, Simmons JQ. Case study: Use of differential reinforcement to suppress self-injurious and aggressive behavior. *Psychol Rep* 1976; **39**: 843–9.

60. Jeannet PY, Kuntzer T, Deonna T, Roulet-Perez E. Hirayama disease associated with a severe rhythmic movement disorder involving neck flexions. *Neurology* 2005; **64**: 1478–9.

61. Rosenberg C. Elimination of a rhythmic movement disorder with hypnosis – a case report. *Sleep* 1995; **18**: 608–09.

62. Weiher RG, Harman RE. The use of omission training to reduce self-injurious behavior in a retarded child. *Behav Ther* 1975; **6**: 261–8.

63. Etzioni T, Katz N, Hering E, Ravid S, Pillar G. Controlled sleep restriction for rhythmic movement disorder. *J Pediatr* 2005; **147**: 393–5.

64. Garcia J. Waterbeds in treament of rhythmic movement disorders: Experience with two cases. *Sleep Res* 1996; **25**: 243.

65. Levy DM, Patrick HT. Relation of infantile convulsions, head banging and breath holding to fainting and headaches in the parents. *Arch Neurol Psychiatr* 1928; **19**: 865.

66. Neveus T, Cnattingius S, Olsson U, Hetta J. Sleep habits and sleep problems among a community sample of schoolchildren. *Acta Paediatr* 2001; **90**: 1450–5.

Section 5, Chapter 29

Sleep-related movement disorders and other variants

Sleep panic arousals

Ravi Singareddy and Thomas W. Uhde

Definition

Sleep panic arousals (SPA) are characterized by full awakening from sleep with panic anxiety, myriad somatic symptoms and secondary fear-associated cognitions.

Phenomenology and epidemiology

Panic disorder is a common anxiety disorder with recurrent spontaneous episodes of intense anxiety (panic attacks) and persistent apprehension or worry about having a future panic attack and/or the consequences of the panic attacks [1]. Lifetime prevalence ranges from 1.5 to 5% for panic disorder and 3–5.6% for panic attacks. Most patients with panic disorder experience the largest percentage of their panic attacks during wakeful states. However, approximately 60–70% of patients with panic disorder have at least one lifetime sleep panic attack and 30–45% report recurrent SPA [2–3]. A small subset of patients may present with only recurrent SPA, although the clinical characterization and course of illness in this subgroup remains to be studied. Clearly, there are individuals whose illness-onset is heralded by SPA who later develop daytime-wake panic attacks. In addition, SPA are reported in patients with post-traumatic stress disorder [4,5]. Women are 2–3 times more likely than men to suffer from sleep panic arousals.

The early descriptions of sleep panic arousals were published in the 1980s. Several of these early reports described nocturnal-sleep panic, which was initially identified while investigating the sleep of patients with panic disorder [6–9]. Panic disorder is an anxiety disorder typically characterized by recurrent, daytime "wake" panic attacks with the secondary development of anticipatory anxiety and avoidance behaviors (i.e. agoraphobia). Research groups studying panic attacks became interested in sleep panic arousals, which are similar symptomatically to daytime or wake panic attacks, and thus provide an opportunity to study panic attacks without expectancy bias or other external sources of variance. Initial studies independently confirmed that these sleep panic arousals occurred during NREM sleep, rather than in REM-stage sleep, and were not associated with dream recall or vivid imagery. Since its identification and phenomenological characterization, different terms have been used to describe these arousals such as "panic attacks during sleep," "sleep panic," "nocturnal panic," "sleep panic attacks," and "nocturnal panic attacks." In this chapter, we will use the term sleep panic arousals (SPA) to describe these sleep events.

Clinical features

Sleep panic arousals almost always occur during the first half of the sleep period, usually within 3 h of sleep onset [8,10]. These awakenings are abrupt and complete arousals from sleep with intense anxiety, fear, or panic, and typically last 2–8 min. Most patients report a feeling of anxiety or fear simultaneous with the arousal, without any foregoing dream content or cognitions. Along with intense anxiety or panic, these arousals are associated with myriad symptoms such as heart pounding, increased heart rate, chest discomfort or pain, sweating, shortness of breath or choking sensations, lightheadedness, hot or cold flashes and headaches. Psychosensory symptoms are frequently associated with panic attacks (depersonalization, strange rising feelings in stomach) and tend to be highly individualized but internally consistent across episodes. Sleep panic arousals awaken patients from sleep and then can be secondarily associated with a cascade of increasing worry and associated fearful cognitions such as "going crazy," "losing control" or "dying" from a medical condition, typically from a myocardial infarction. Early in the course of illness, patients with SPA may seek treatment in emergency medical departments.

During these arousals the individual is fully aware of his surroundings and can later accurately recall the events and nature of the fearful awakening. There is no confusion or sleepwalking associated with SPA. After SPA, patients are often restless and unable to return to the sleep environment, particularly early in the course of illness, and the majority of patients develop secondary fears of sleeping and/or the sleep environment. Not surprisingly, patients with SPA often ask their partners or friends to watch them while sleeping and some report keeping the lights/TV on while sleeping in order to "obtain rest without sleeping." Thus, a pattern of chronic, intermittent sleep deprivation is a complication of SPA [3]; moreover, sleep deprivation further exacerbates wake panic attacks and SPA [3,11].

Approximately two-thirds of patients with panic disorder report difficulty sleeping. Among panic disorder patients subjective sleep complaints are more prevalent in patients with SPA compared to patients with only wake panic attacks [2,12]. Patients with SPA report both sleep initiation and maintenance difficulty and overall poor subjective sleep quality [12,13].

Sleep panic arousals have been reported in nonclinical populations [14,15]. However, no epidemiological studies have been conducted to assess the long-term clinical course or work and social functions of such individuals.

Comorbidity

Compared to panic disorder patients without sleep panic attacks, a positive history of SPA has been associated with childhood or adult trauma or other significant life events in some but not all investigations [4,16]. While depression has generally been found to be more prevalent in patients with SPA compared to panic disorder patients without SPA, the rates are very high in both subgroups [17–21]. Using the NIMH-PQ inventory [22], we recently found in a survey of 773 individuals who met DSM-IV criteria for panic disorder that depression is more common in panic disorder patients with SPA and worsens underlying sleep disturbances. Specifically, panic disorder patients with both sleep panic arousals and a history of depression more commonly reported sleeping 5 h or less (20.6%) compared to patients with only daytime panic attacks (2.5%), daytime panic attacks plus depression (9.6%) or those patients with sleep panic attacks without a history of depression (9.2%) [2].

While clinicians tend to focus on insomnia as part of their work-up and management of panic disorder, recent evidence suggests that hypersomnia or oversleeping also may be a problem in a subgroup of panic disorder patients. Although this association appears to be most evident in patients with comorbid wake panic attacks and depression, hypersomnia was previously reported to be characteristic of patients with primary dysthymia or "atypical" depressions [23]. Within this context, features of "atypical" depression reported in the earlier literature such as somatization, interpersonal sensitivity, and anger hostility have been more recently found by Sarisoy and colleagues (2008) to be more severe in panic patients with SPA compared to patients without sleep panic arousals [24]. Conversely, patients suffering from hypersomnia also have higher rates of panic disorder [25].

Taken together, these observations highlight the need to investigate the relationship between panic disorder, with a focus on patients with SPA, and a spectrum of mood, anxiety, and sleep disorders.

Polysomnography (PSG)

Sleep panic arousals occur during the first third of the sleep period from NREM sleep, in the first or second NREM sleep cycle. These arousals occur in stage 2 sleep or within the first few minutes of stage 3 sleep, typically during transition from stage 2 to stage 3 sleep. Some electroencephalographic (EEG) slowing is observed before these arousals when they occur in stage 2 sleep [8]. Polysomnographic EEG does not show any epileptiform or other paroxysmal activity during these arousals.

Early polysomnography studies in subjects with SPA reported increased sleep latency, decreased total sleep time, decreased sleep efficiency, and both increased and decreased stage 4 sleep. Recently, however, Landry and colleagues studied sleep panic patients who were medication-free for at least a month using a two-night PSG protocol [26]. They did not find any differences in the polysomnographic measures in sleep panic subjects compared to normal controls. Largely consistent with the early investigations of Mellman and Uhde and Hauri and coworkers, all the sleep panic arousals occurred during stage 2 sleep [6,8].

Pathophysiological considerations

Patients with panic disorder have abnormalities in respiratory physiological indices including higher respiratory frequency, tidal volume, minute ventilation and sigh breaths (defined as >2.0 times the mean tidal volume) and decreased end tidal CO_2 ($P_{ET}CO_2$) levels [27–29]. These patients also have greater irregularities in respiratory rate and tidal volume in comparison to healthy volunteers [30]. Additionally, normoxic CO_2 inhalation produces more panic attacks and/or anxiety during wake state in panic disorder patients compared to normal controls [31–34]. These CO_2 inhalation-induced panic attacks resemble natural wake panic attacks [34]. Almost 50–60% of patients with panic disorder have a wake panic attack with CO_2 inhalation compared to only 10% of healthy volunteers. Even though studies evaluating respiratory physiology and CO_2 sensitivity during sleep in SPA are lacking, it is estimated that 50–65% of panic disorder subjects enrolled in CO_2 inhalation studies of panic disorder suffered from SPA.

Arterial concentration of CO_2, a major chemical regulating breathing during sleep and a known panic-inducing substance, increases during sleep, especially stage 3 and 4 sleep [35–37]. Sleep panic arousals, which are symptomatically similar to wake panic attacks, also occur during the transition from stage 2 to stage 3 sleep [6,38,39]. Based on these observations, we have hypothesized that relative increases in CO_2 during stages of increasing relaxation and during the transition from stage 2 to 3 sleep is the immediate trigger for SPA. Of interest, panic disorder patients with SPA have more respiratory symptoms, such as shortness of breath and choking or smothering sensations, during panic arousals compared to patients with only wake panic attacks [10,40,41]. These data from panic disorder and the evidence that CO_2 concentration increases from light to deeper stages of sleep suggests that SPA could be a result of increased upregulation of CO_2 chemoreceptors. However, SPA do not occur every night in these patients. Therefore, it is also likely that other neurochemical mechanisms or a certain threshold of CO_2 level may be necessary for precipitating SPA. In this regard, based on preliminary findings of decreased movement time during the nights with SPA, Brown and Uhde postulated that increased movements may prevent SPA by delaying stage 2 to 3 sleep transition and allowing more time for the CNS chemoreceptors to acclimate to the increase in CO_2 during sleep [42].

Other possible biological mechanisms of SPA include autonomic nervous system instability and disturbances in cholecystokininergic (CCK) and adenosinergic systems. Non-invasive measures to assess autonomic nervous system balance (heart period variability) indicates that parasympathetic (vagal) tone is decreased during NREM sleep in SPA patients, which in turn may lead to sympathetic overdrive [43,44]. Pharmacological challenge with caffeine [45], cholecystokinin-4 (CCK-4) [46], and pentagastrin (a synthetic analog of CCK-4) [47,48] trigger both wake panic and sleep panic arousals. Individuals with recurrent panic attacks are more prone to pharmacologically induced (e.g. pentagastrin, caffeine) panic attacks [48,49], including those with SPA [45,50]. NREM sleep is more prone than REM sleep to SPA induced by pharmacological challenges [46]. Both CCK-4 and pentagastrin induce these arousals within seconds (never more than 180 s) of infusion. Caffeine infusion triggers limited symptom SPA immediately and full symptom SPA in 4–52 min. These preliminary data indicate the possible role of CNS respiratory centers, movements during sleep, autonomic nervous system, adenosinergic and cholecystokinin systems in the pathophysiology of SPA.

Differential diagnosis

Nocturnal seizures

From a theoretical and practical perspective, perhaps the most relevant medical disorder to rule out is nocturnal seizures. From a symptomatic perspective, there are fascinating overlaps between panic attacks and partial seizures in relation to the total number and types of psychosensory symptoms such as distortions in light and sound intensity, derealization, depersonalization, gustatory and visceral feelings, sensations of floating, turning, or moving, and déjà vu or jamais vu experiences [51]. Of interest, sleep deprivation precipitates or worsens many of these same symptoms in both panic disorder and partial seizure patients [11,51]. Panic disorder patients with SPA report increased sensitivity to sleep deprivation compared to panic disorder patients without SPA, and many panic disorder patients report extreme fatigue and exhaustion after panic attacks, which bear some resemblance to the postictal somnolence in seizure patients [21,52]. Also, drowsiness and/or relaxation may be associated with the onset of both sleep panic attacks and partial seizures. Interestingly, nearly all SPA and a subgroup of patients with partial seizures have their peak occurrences during the early part of the sleep cycle [51,53] and during NREM sleep [54,55].

Despite the impressive symptomatic and sleep-cycle overlap between SPA and some nocturnal seizures, scalp and nasopharyngeal electrodes have failed to identify epileptiform discharges during inter-panic periods [11,56]. In practice, therefore, it is extremely rare to document epileptiform seizures in patients with uncomplicated daytime panic attacks, i.e. the typical panic disorder patient. To our knowledge, it is unknown whether depth electrodes or even surface electrodes in patients with primary or exclusive SPA might yield different findings, and it is this subgroup of panic disorder patients who share phenomenological similarities with patients who suffer from partial and nocturnal seizures (e.g. psychosensory and psychomotor disturbances, relaxation and sleep deprivation worsening, caffeine sensitivity) [51].

Until more definitive information is established, it is reasonable to rule out partial or nocturnal seizures in the *atypical* panic disorder patient [51,57], perhaps especially those with exclusive or primary SPA. Certainly, patients with atypical SPA or fearful sleep arousals (i.e. arousals characterized by stereotypic motor abnormalities (tonic posturing) or fearful arousals during the latter half of the sleep cycle or urinary/fecal incontinence, or an inability to recall their panic-like awakenings or failure to respond to standard anti-panic agents) should be evaluated by PSG with seizure montage [51,57–64]. If polysomnography is unable to clarify the diagnosis, 24-h video electroencephalography might be beneficial in distinguishing SPA from nocturnal seizures.

Sleep paralysis

Both sleep paralysis and sleep panic attacks are profoundly frightening; however, unlike episodes of sleep paralysis, SPA are not associated with an inability to move. Often individuals with SPA sit up or get out of bed in a "flight or fight"-type response and have the cognitive belief that moving around may somehow decrease or eliminate their anxiety. In contrast, during episodes of sleep paralysis the person is unable to move, as would be expected of a REM-related event characterized as "sleep consciousness" [65]. People with recurrent sleep paralysis often develop highly individualized strategies (e.g. concentrating on small muscle groups to jostle themselves out of their state of paralysis) [65]. Also unlike SPA, sleep paralysis may be associated with either visual or auditory hallucinatory (and, more rarely, olfactory-gustatory) experiences [66].

Beyond the profound anxiety, there are some similarities between SPA and sleep paralysis, mainly the self-perception of clarity in thinking immediately after the episodes. That is, in both types of fearful arousals there is an absence of confusion or clouding of consciousness.

Individuals with sleep paralysis and SPA, respectively, typically report "already being awake" versus "being awakened by" these events. Thus, the subjective experience of the panic patient is that these are "sleep events", whereas the individual with sleep paralysis often views these as a "wake" event. Within this context, it is interesting that a majority of patients with SPA develop context-specific fears of sleeping or the sleep environment, whereas this is much less evident, based upon our clinical experience, in patients with sleep paralysis, even in those sufferers with frequent, recurrent episodes of sleep paralysis [65].

Paroxysmal nocturnal dyspnea

Nocturnal dyspnea attacks are characterized by severe shortness of breath awakening the individual from sleep. These attacks can be frightening to the patient. Patients may report extreme anxiety and dread. These attacks are often associated with cough and wheezing. These attacks are a result of worsening of existing pulmonary congestion. A clinical history of cardiopulmonary disease and thorough physical examination is helpful in delineating these from SPA.

Nocturnal angina

Angina (cardiac chest pain) typically occurs with exertion; however, it can also occur at rest and during sleep. During nocturnal angina, patients may wake up with chest pain or discomfort associated with anxiety, sweating and difficulty breathing or dyspnea and palpitations. A comprehensive history and physical examination, specifically history of coronary artery disease and other cardiac risk factors, may help differentiate these from SPA.

Nocturnal asthma

Nocturnal worsening of asthma is common. Asthmatic episodes during sleep can lead to arousal with cough, wheezing, and difficulty breathing. Clinical examination including pulmonary examination may clarify the diagnosis. In some cases pulmonary function tests may be needed.

Nocturnal gastroesophageal reflux

Almost 80% of patients with gastroesophageal reflux have nocturnal episodes of reflux. These episodes can lead to arousal associated with cough, choking and difficulty breathing. The characteristic pain and/or "sour taste" associated with gastroesophageal reflux usually make this diagnosis easily differentiated from SPA.

Sleep-related laryngospasm

These arousals are associated with stridor, difficulty in breathing, choking, fear, agitation, cough, and other signs of respiratory distress [67]. Stridor helps differentiate these. Gastroesophageal reflux seems to be a common cause of laryngospasm during sleep.

NREM partial arousals (sleep terrors, somnambulism, confusional arousals)

These arousals are partial and individuals with these arousals typically cannot recall the episode the next morning. In contrast, nocturnal-sleep panic arousals are complete arousals and the patient vividly recalls the episode(s) the following morning. Polysomnographically, NREM partial arousals usually occur in deep sleep, mostly stage 4 sleep, and possibly during the transition from deep sleep stages to REM sleep [68], unlike SPA which occur in late stage 2, early stage 3, or during transitions from stage 2 to 3 sleep.

Nightmare disorder

Individuals with nightmare disorder have repeated awakening from sleep and recall frightening dreams preceding these awakenings. Subsequent to these awakenings, they may report anxiety/fear with autonomic symptoms similar to SPA. In contrast, patients with SPA do not recall any dream content associated with their arousal. Further, SPA occur during the first half of the sleep period in NREM sleep while nightmares predominantly occur during REM sleep, and thus are more common during the second half of sleep. Individuals who suffer from both recurrent nightmares and SPA consistently identify these fearful events when recorded in the sleep laboratory, as REM and REM-related events, respectively.

REM sleep behavior disorder

Individuals with REM sleep behavior disorder may report excessive anxiety and/or other autonomic symptoms similar to SPA. However, REM sleep behavior disorder occurs during REM and is associated with dreaming and thrashing movements of upper and/or lower extremities or other parts of the body. Often, a bed partner can recall the patient frequently verbalizing content related to their dream that they seem to be enacting. Videorecording in the sleep laboratory may be useful in addition to PSG, which may show increased muscle activity in REM sleep during such an episode.

Sleep apnea

It is possible that individuals with sleep apnea may have an arousal preceded by complete or partial cessation in breathing, leading to similar anxiety symptoms found in SPA. Therefore, sleep apnea needs to be excluded before diagnosing SPA. Information from the patient, as well as the bed partner, might be useful to differentiate SPA from sleep apnea. Specifically, a history of snoring, witnessed breath cessation during sleep, along with findings on physical examination of high BMI and neck circumference increases the likelihood of sleep apnea. An overnight PSG is the gold standard to confirm the diagnosis of sleep apnea. Unlike patients with SPA, patients with sleep apnea rarely report anxiety during arousals from apneas or hypopneas and almost never complain about the fear of sleep.

Occasionally, however, the sleep expert will be asked to evaluate a patient who suffers from both severe sleep apnea and undiagnosed SPA. It is important not to attribute the SPA to hypoxia-associated anxiety. Rather, such patients are likely to be experiencing worsening of their SPA due to the sleep deprivation caused by poorly controlled apnea. Under such circumstances, the patient will require targeted and independent treatment of both their sleep apnea and SPA.

Night sweats

Night sweats may be associated with full arousals accompanied by anxiety. The anxiety usually focuses on embarrassment and concerns about the underlying causes of the sweating. Mold and coworkers, however, found in a multivariate analysis of 2267 individuals with night sweats that panic attacks and hot flashes were factors associated with pure night sweats in women [69]. The relationship between wake panic attacks, SPA and night sweats remains unclear and deserves further investigation.

Management

Sleep panic arousals is a diagnosis of exclusion. It is important that other possible causes which may present with similar symptoms are ruled out prior to making the diagnosis of sleep panic arousals. As discussed in the differential diagnosis section of this chapter, sleep apnea (apneas/hypopneas), sleep paralysis, night sweats, nocturnal seizures, NREM parasomnias (particularly sleep terrors), and REM sleep behavior disorder may lead to an arousal with autonomic symptoms of increased heart rate, difficulty breathing, sweating, chest tightness, etc. In some cases, the patient may not be aware of such a trigger. For example, it is possible that individuals may be unaware that they have sleep apnea (apneas/hypopneas) and may actually present with complaints of arousals associated with autonomic symptoms and excessive anxiety/worry related to these awakenings. However, the cognitive symptoms of dread such as fear of losing control, fear of death or fear of going crazy are usually not present in these cases.

In most cases, the diagnosis of SPA can be made by collecting a comprehensive clinical history. The likelihood of SPA increases if the individual also provides a personal history of daytime wake panic attacks and meets criteria for panic disorder (i.e. that the panic attacks are not exclusively occurring during sleep). In some cases an overnight PSG may be required when there are indications of possible sleep apnea, nocturnal seizures, or other parasomnias (REM behavior disorder, NREM partial arousal parasomnias) and the clinical history does not provide adequate diagnostic clarification.

Although little is known about patients with exclusive SPA (i.e. patients with SPA but without co-occurring daytime, wake panic attacks), such individuals do exist and may more frequently seek treatment from primary care physicians or sleep treatment centers. Until we learn more about the natural course of the *exclusive SPA syndrome*, these people should perhaps receive a more comprehensive diagnostic and PSG evaluation, as clinically indicated, to rule out underlying medical or sleep disorders. Such an evaluation should include an assessment of the presence/absence of co-existing anxiety (e.g. PTSD) or sleep disorders (e.g. sleep apnea, nocturnal seizures). Furthermore, anxiety disorders in general and panic disorder and post-traumatic stress disorder more specifically have increased comorbidity of alcohol and other substance use disorders and mood disorders (bipolar disorder and depression). Therefore, SPA patients should be screened for these disorders to plan the most effective individualized treatment. For example, if an individual with panic disorder and SPA has comorbid bipolar disorder, starting them on an anti-depressant (selective serotonin reuptake inhibitors (SSRIs), tricyclic anti-depressants (TCA), etc.) could potentially precipitate a manic/hypomanic episode if the patient is not on a mood-stabilizing medication.

Medical disorders which may present with anxiety like symptoms during sleep such as nocturnal asthma, nocturnal gastroesophageal reflux, nocturnal angina, paroxysmal nocturnal dyspnea, thyroid disease, hypoglycemia, chronic obstructive pulmonary disease, arrhythmias and other cardiac conditions, hypoparathyroidism, and pheochromocytoma should be ruled out with a comprehensive clinical examination and/or additional laboratory tests. The overall management of SPA should be comprehensive rather than simply the SPA in isolation.

Clinicians should be particularly careful not to inadvertently "minimize" the impact of SPA when treating such patients. Well-intended but offhanded comments such as "these things are nothing to worry about" can harm an otherwise positive doctor–patient relationship. The clinician should keep in mind that patients with SPA often experience significant distress and resultant work and social dysfunctions. A successful treatment outcome often requires working with the patient over many years in a supportive "maintenance" fashion, with the ultimate goal of achieving a healthy lifestyle and sense of wellness.

Components of the treatment may require the following:

a. *Education.* Patients should be informed about the non-life-threatening nature of these arousals after ruling out other possible medical conditions (nocturnal angina, nocturnal asthma, sleep apnea) which may present with anxiety symptoms. One of the major patient concerns in SPA is the worry about a possible life-threatening physical condition (e.g. fear of a heart attack) and this needs to be addressed.

b. *Pharmacological treatment.* Few studies have investigated the pharmacological treatment of SPA. To date, no double-blind, placebo-controlled studies in SPA have been conducted. One open-label, small-sample ($n = 7$) study found imipramine, a tricyclic anti-depressant, to be beneficial [52]. Another study reported that in three patients, nortriptyline fully remitted their SPA [70]. Lastly, a case report indicated that alprazolam, a benzodiazepine, was helpful in treating SPA. As a result of lack of evidence, currently the pharmacological treatment approach for SPA is similar to wake panic attacks/panic disorder.

There are no FDA-approved drugs for treating SPA. However, if a patient with SPA is already on an anti-depressant/anti-anxiety medication such as an SSRI (fluoxetine, fluvoxamine, paroxetine, sertraline, citalopram, escitalopram) or dual reuptake inhibitor of serotonin and norepinephrine (duloxetine, venlafaxine) or a tricyclic anti-depressant (amitriptyline, doxepine, imipramine, nortriptyline, protriptyline) for underlying anxiety or a mood disorder, increasing the dose should be considered. If a patient is not on any medications, an SSRI may be considered as a first-line consideration, as substantial evidence indicates that these medications are effective in treating panic disorder. If the first SSRI tried is ineffective or if the patient is unable to tolerate the medication, another may be tried. While all the SSRIs have similar mechanisms of action and adverse events, a patient failing to achieve therapeutic benefit from one SSRI may respond to another. Dual reuptake inhibitors may be considered if SSRIs fail, or as a first-line drug. Both SSRIs and dual reuptake inhibitors are generally well tolerated and have similar adverse effects. Tricyclic anti-depressants are known to be effective in panic disorder; however, they have more adverse side effects and are less well tolerated and should be considered if SPA are not responsive to other medications. Starting on an SSRI, dual reuptake inhibitor or a tricyclic anti-depressant should be accomplished while closely monitoring for adverse reactions. Typically patients with anxiety disorders, including those with SPA, have difficulty tolerating the activating properties of medications so all medications in general should be initiated at very low dose and gradually titrated to achieve therapeutic response.

Benzodiazepines are frequently employed to treat panic disorder and other anxiety syndromes. However, benzodiazepines may induce muscle relaxation and sedation, which could potentially worsen or precipitate SPA [42,52]. However, this is merely theoretical, and thus the use of benzodiazepine in treating SPA should be assessed on a case-by-case basis. In our clinical practice, some patients with SPA have improved on benzodiazepines.

If sleep initiation or maintenance disturbances continue after the aforementioned interventions, the physician should consider other medications to improve sleep. Both the FDA-approved medications (zolpidem, zaleplon, eszopiclone, ramelteon) as well as non-FDA-approved medications (low dose trazodone (12.5–100 mg), mirtazepine (3.75–15 mg), low dose doxepine (2.5–10 mg)) may be helpful in improving sleep disturbances.

c. *Cognitive behavioral therapy (CBT).* Although cognitive influences are minimal during sleep, patients with SPA express significant catastrophic thinking in regards to the consequences of SPA (e.g. an individual with SPA may fear that they are having a heart attack based on their perception of a pounding heart beat). Maladaptive cognitive thinking plays a critical role in worsening of the SPA, secondary impairment in sleep, and overall worry. CBT of SPA involves educating the patient about increased perception of physiological sensations, addressing maladaptive patterns of thinking including catastrophic thinking, and helping the patient change thinking patterns related to SPA. Only one published randomized controlled trial has investigated CBT for SPA [71,72]. This study consisted of 43 panic disorder patients with SPA (average of at least six SPA over the past 6 months), who were assigned to either treatment with CBT or to a wait-list control group. CBT significantly reduced the frequency of SPA in the treatment group compared to the wait-list control group and these benefits continued at the 9-month follow-up visit.

A major practical problem with CBT is lack of accessibility to trained CBT therapists. There are very few well-trained CBT therapists in many regions of the US. In most medical academic centers, SPA are treated pharmacologically. It is reasonable to speculate that a combination of pharmacotherapy and CBT might be the most effective approach in terms of long-term treatment outcome, but there have been no controlled studies to affirm this notion.

d. *Sleep hygiene.* Patients with recurrent SPA develop maladaptive sleep habits such as having the TV/lights "on" while sleeping, delaying their sleep onset time, etc. In most sleep treatment manuals, a high priority is placed on the assessment of sleep habits and the resultant establishment of healthy sleep hygiene. From a chronological perspective, however, it appears that the origin of poor sleep habits in patients with SPA emerges as a consequence of, rather than being a cause for, sleep panic attacks. In terms of patient compliance (e.g. turning off lights, television, and radio), the clinician will be ineffective in maintaining good sleep hygiene until the core problem of SPA has been effectively removed with educational support and pharmaco- and/or cognitive-behavioral therapeutic interventions. *Until SPA-sufferers are confident they will not die from a medical event during their sleep, measures targeting an improvement in sleep hygiene will be ineffective.* For these reasons, we give a higher priority to educating the patient about SPA (and panic disorder) and managing the SPA with anti-panic medication and/or CBT prior to instituting sleep hygiene measures.

Conclusion and future directions

Sleep panic arousals are full arousals to complete consciousness, which occur during NREM sleep without any obvious trigger. These arousals are associated with extreme anxiety, increased physiological arousal and secondary cognitions of impending doom. Individuals with SPA often develop conditioned fears of sleeping and downstream poor sleep hygiene. Chronic-intermittent sleep deprivation is a common problem. Sleep deprivation worsens anxiety symptoms, including more severe and frequent SPA. The diagnostic assessment of SPA should include ruling out possible medical, neuropsychiatric, and sleep disorders, including other parasomnias. Treatment of SPA should be individualized and must take into account any co-occurring anxiety (e.g. PTSD), mood or substance use disorders. Anti-depressant medications and/or CBT are generally beneficial in treating SPA. If needed, hypnotics may be used to target insomnia.

A potential fruitful area for future research is the investigation of a possible relationship between panic disorder and narcolepsy, a neurological disorder associated with excessive daytime drowsiness, sleep paralysis, sleep-related hallucinations and cataplexy [73]. Many experts view a positive history of cataplexy to be sufficient to diagnose narcolepsy, particularly cataplexy triggered by laughing, hearing or telling a joke or associated with anger (i.e. "classic" cataplexy) [74]. Early in the course of illness, narcoleptics often report that anxiety, fear or stress-related events trigger muscle atonia [73,75]. Excessive drowsiness is also found in a subgroup of patients with anxiety or anxiety disorders [76–78]. Recently, Flosnik and coworkers found that 33% of patients with primary anxiety disorders, including a group of patients with panic disorder, reported a history of combined "classic" cataplexy plus excessive daytime drowsiness. None of the normal controls reported a similar history of both classic cataplexy plus excessive daytime drowsiness [79]. In a separate study of 1118 self-reported panic disorder patients, individuals with a history of freezing/immobilization panic attacks were almost twice as likely to report a history of SPA [80].

Taken together, these "pieces" of divergent information justify a systematic investigation into the possible link between panic disorder, particularly in patients with SPA, and narcolepsy. Until such research is conducted, it will be prudent for the sleep medicine expert to make an assessment of co-existing sleep paralysis and freezing/immobilization behaviors, cataplexy, excessive daytime drowsiness and hypnagogic and hypnopompic hallucinations in patients who present with sleep panic arousals.

Acknowledgments

The authors thank Dr. Bernadette Cortese for her scientific advice and ongoing collaborations.

References

1. American Psychiatric Association. *Diagnostic Statistical Manual of Mental Disorders*, 4th rev. ed. Washington, DC: American Psychiatric Association, 2000.
2. Singareddy R, Uhde TW. Nocturnal sleep panic and depression: Relationship to subjective sleep in panic disorder. *J Affect Disord* 2009; **112**: 262–6.
3. Uhde TW. The anxiety disorders. In Kryger MH, Roth T, Dement W (Eds), *Principles and Practice in Sleep Medicine*, third edition. Philadelphia, PA: W.B. Saunders, 2000; 1123–39.
4. Freed S, Craske MG, Greher MR. Nocturnal panic and trauma. *Depress Anxiety* 1999; **9**: 141–5.
5. Mellman TA, Kulick-Bell R, Ashlock LE, Nolan B. Sleep events among veterans with combat-related post-traumatic stress disorder. *Am J Psychiatry* 1995; **152**: 110–5.
6. Hauri PJ, Friedman M, Ravaris CL. Sleep in patients with spontaneous panic attacks. *Sleep* 1989; **12**: 323–37.
7. Mellman TA, Uhde TW. Sleep panic attacks: New clinical findings and theoretical implications. *Am J Psychiatry* 1989; **146**: 1204–07.
8. Mellman TA, Uhde TW. Electroencephalographic sleep in panic disorder. A focus on sleep-related panic attacks. *Arch Gen Psychiatry* 1989; **46**: 178–84.
9. Uhde TW, Roy-Byrne P, Gillin JC, *et al.* The sleep of patients with panic disorders: A preliminary report. *Psychiatr Res* 1984; **12**: 251–9.
10. Crake MG, Barlow DH. Nocturnal panic. *J Nerv Ment Dis* 1989; **177**: 160–8.
11. Roy-Byrne PP, Uhde TW, Post RM. Effects of one night's sleep deprivation on mood and behavior in panic disorder. *Arch Gen Psychiatry* 1986; **43**: 895–9.
12. Overbeek T, Diest R, Schruers K, Kruizinga F, Griez E. Sleep complaints in panic disorder. *J Nerv Ment Disord* 2005; **193**: 488–93.
13. Schredl M, Kronenberg G, Nonell P, Heuser I. Sleep quality in patient with panic disorder: Relationship to nocturnal panic attacks. *Somnologie* 2002; **6**: 149–53.
14. Craske MG, Kreuger M. Prevalence of nocturnal panic in a college population. *J Anxiety Disord* 1990; **4**: 125–39.
15. Norton GR, Dorward J, Cox BJ. Factors associated with panic attacks in nonclinical subjects. *Behav Ther* 1986; **17**: 239–52.
16. Albert U, Maina G, Bergesio C, Bogetto F. Nocturnal panic and recent life events. *Depress Anxiety* 2005; **22**: 52–8.
17. Agaragun MY, Kara H. Recurrent sleep panic, insomnia, and suicidal behavior in patients with panic disorder. *Compr Psychiatry* 1998; **39**: 149–51.
18. Labbate LA, Pollack MH, Otto MW, Lamgenauer S, Rosenbaum JF. Sleep panic attacks: An association with childhood anxiety and adult psychopathology. *Biol Psychiatry* 1994; **36**: 57–60.
19. Stein MB, Tancer ME, Uhde TW. Major depression in patients with panic disorder: Factors associated with course and recurrence. *J Anxiety Disord* 1990; **19**: 287–96.
20. Vollrath M, Angst A. Outcome of panic and depression in a 7-year follow up: Results of the Zurich Study. *Acta Psychiatr Scand* 1989; **80**: 591–9.
21. Uhde TW, Boulenger J-P, Roy-Byrne PP, Geraci MF, Vittone BJ, Post RM. Longitudinal course of panic disorder: Clinical and biological considerations. *Prog Neuro-Psychopharmacol Biol Psychiatry* 1985; **9**: 39–51.
22. Scupi BS, Maser JD, Uhde TW. The National Institute of Mental Health Panic Questionnaire (NIMH-PQ): An instrument for assessing clinical characteristics of panic disorder. *J Nerv Men Dis* 1992; **180**: 566–72.
23. Akiskal HS, Lemmi H, Dickson H, King D, Yerevanian B, Van Valkenburg, C. Chronic depressions. Part 2. Sleep EEG differentiation of primary dysthymic disorders from anxious depressions. *J Affect Disord* 1984; **6**: 287–95.
24. Sarisoy E, Boke O, Arik AC, Sahin AR. Panic disorder with nocturnal panic attacks: Symptoms and comorbidities. *Eur Psychiatry* 2008; **23**: 195–200.
25. Matza LS, Revicki DA, Davidson JR, Stewart JW. Depression with atypical features in the National Comorbidity Survey: Classification, description, and consequences. *Arch Gen Psychiatry* 2003; **60**: 817–26.
26. Landry P, Marchand L, Mainguy N, Marchand A, Montplaisir J. Electroencephalography during sleep of patients with nocturnal panic disorder. *J Nerv Ment Disord* 2002; **190**: 559–62.
27. Gorman JM, Fyer MR, Goetz R, *et al.* Ventilatory physiology of patients with panic disorder. *Arch Gen Psychiatry* 1988; **45**: 31–9.
28. Hegel MT, Ferguson RJ. Psychophysiological assessment of respiratory function in panic disorder: Evidence for a hyperventilation subtype. *Psychosom Med* 1997; **59**: 224–30.
29. Papp LA, Martinez JM, Klein DF, *et al.* Respiratory psychophysiology of panic disorder: three respiratory challenges in 98 subjects. *Am J Psychiatry* 1997; **154**: 1557–65.
30. Wilhelm FH, Trabert W, Roth WT. Physiologic instability in panic disorder and generalized anxiety disorder. *Biol Psychiatry* 2001; **49**: 596–605.

31. Gorman JM, Browne ST, Papp LA, *et al.* Effects of antipanic treatment on response to carbon dioxide. *Biol Psychiatry* 1997; **42**: 982–91.

32. Griez I, Lousberg H, Van Den Hout MA, Zandbergen J. CO_2 vulnerability in panic disorder. *Psychiatry Res* 1987; **20**: 87–95.

33. Perna G, Battaglia M, Garberi A, Arancio C, Bertani A, Bellodi L. Carbon dioxide/oxygen challenge test in panic disorder. *Psychiatry Res* 1994; **52**: 159–71.

34. Sanderson WC, Weltzer S. Five percent carbon dioxide challenge: Valid analogue and marker of panic disorder? *Biol Psychiatry* 1990; **27**: 689–701.

35. Bulow K. Respiration and wakefulness in man. *Acta Physiol Scand Suppl* 1963; **209**: 1–110.

36. Meadows GE, Dunroy HMA, Morrell MJ, Corfield DR. Hypercapnic cerebral vascular reactivity is decreased, in humans, during sleep compared to wakefulness. *J Appl Physiol* 2003; **94**: 2197–202.

37. Morrell MJ, Harty HR, Adams L, Guz A. Changes in total pulmonary resistance and PCO_2 between wakefulness and sleep in normal human subjects. *J Appl Physiol* 1995; **78**: 1339–49.

38. Roy-Byrne PP, Mellman TA, Uhde TW. Biologic findings in panic disorder. *J Anxiety Disord* 1988; **2**: 17–29.

39. Uhde TW, Mellman TA. Commentary on "Relaxation-induced panic (RIP): When resting isn't peaceful". *Integr Psychiatry* 1988; **6**: 147–9.

40. Craske MG, Barlow DH. Nocturnal panic: Response to hyperventilation and CO_2 challenges. *J Abnorm Psychol* 1990; **99**: 302–07.

41. Singareddy R, Uhde TW. Sleep deprivation in nocturnal panic attacks. *Biol Psych* 2005; **57**: S8.

42. Brown TM, Uhde TW. Sleep panic attacks: A micromovement analysis. *Depress Anxiety* 2003; **18**: 214–20.

43. Sloan EP, Natarajan M, Baker B, *et al*. Nocturnal and daytime panic attacks – comparison of sleep architecture, heart rate variability, and response to sodium lactate challenge. *Biol Psychiatry* 1999; **45**: 1313–20.

44. Aikins DE, Craske MG. Sleep-based heart period variability in panic disorder with and without nocturnal panic attacks. *J Anxiety Disord* 2008; **22**: 453–63.

45. Koenigsberg HW, Pollak CP, Ferro D. Can panic be induced in deep sleep? Examining the necessity of cognitive processing for panic. *Depress Anxiety* 1998; **8**: 126–30.

46. Kronenberg G, Schredl M, Fiedler K, Heuser I. In healthy volunteers responses to challenge with cholecystokinin tetrapeptide differ between administration during REM and delta sleep. *Depress Anxiety* 2001; **14**: 141–4.

47. Geraci M, Anderson TS, Slate-Cothren S, Post R, McCann U. Pentagastrin-induced sleep panic attacks: Panic in the absence of elevated baseline arousal. *Biol Psychiatry* 2002; **52**: 1189–93.

48. McCann UD, Shiyoko O, Slate SO, Geraci M, Roscow-Terrill D, Uhde TW. A comparison of the effects of intravenous pentagastrin on patients with social phobia, panic disorder and healthy controls. *Neuropsychopharmacology* 1997; **16**: 229–37.

49. Uhde TW. Caffeine-induced anxiety: An ideal chemical model of panic disorder. In Asnis GM, van Praag HM (Eds), *Einstein Monograph Series in Psychiatry*. New York: Wiley-Liss, 1995; 181–205.

50. Balon R, Pohl R, Yeragani VK, Singareddy RK. Provocation of anxiety states in humans and its possible significance for the pathogenesis of these disorders. In Kasper S, den Boer JA, Sitsen JMA (Eds), *Handbook of Depression and Anxiety*, second edition. New York: Marcel Dekker, 2007; 703–32.

51. Nickell PV, Uhde TW. Anxiety disorders and epilepsy. In Devinsky O, Theodore WH (Eds), *Epilepsy and Behavior*. New York: Wiley-Liss, 1991; 67–84.

52. Mellman TA, Uhde TW. Patients with frequent sleep panic: Clinical findings and response to medication treatment. *J Clin Psychiatry* 1990; **51**: 513–6.

53. Mendez M, Radtke RA. Interactions between sleep and epilepsy. *J Clin Neurophysiology* 2001; **18**: 106–27.

54. Billiard M. Epilepsies and the sleep–wake cycle. In Sterman MB, Shouse MN, Passouant P (Eds), *Sleep and Epilepsy*. New York: Academic Press.

55. Janz D. Epilepsy and the sleeping–waking cycle. In Vincken PJ, Bruyn GW (Eds), *Handbook of Clinical Neurology. The Epilepsies*. Amsterdam: North-Holland Biomedical Press, 1974; 457–90.

56. Stein MB, Uhde TW. Infrequent occurrence of EEG abnormalities in panic disorder. *Am J Psychiatry* 1989; **146**: 517–20.

57. Edlund MJ, Swann AC, Clothier J. Patients with panic attacks and abnormal EEG results. *Am J Psychiatry* 1987; **144**: 508–09.

58. Sazgar M, Carlen PL, Wennberg R. Panic attack semiology in right temporal lobe epilepsy. *Epileptic Disord* 2003; **5**: 93–100.

59. Gambardella A, Messina D, Le Piane E, *et al*. Familial temporal lobe epilepsy autosomal dominant inheritance in a large pedigree from southern Italy. *Epilepsy Res* 2000; **38**: 127–32.

60. Wall M, Tuchman M, Mielke D. Panic attacks and temporal lobe seizures associated with a right temporal lobe arteriovenous malformation: Case report. *J Clin Psychiatry* 1985; **46**: 143–5.

61. Dantendorfer K, Frey R, Maierhofer D, Saletu B. Sudden arousals from slow wave sleep and panic disorder: Successful treatment with anticonvulsants – a case report. *Sleep* 1996; **19**: 744–6.

62. Gallinat J, Stotz-Ingenlath G, Lang UE, Hegerl U. Panic attacks, spike-wave activity, and limbic dysfunction. A case report. *Pharmacopsychiatry* 2003, **36**: 123–6.

63. Picardi A, Di Gennaro G, Meldolesi GN, Grammaldo LG, Esposito V, Quarato PP. Partial seizures due to sclerosis of the right amygdala presenting as panic disorder. *Psychopathology* 2007; **40**: 178–83.

64. Scalise A, Placidi F, Diomedi M, De Simone R, Gigli GL. Panic disorder or epilepsy? A case report. *J Neurol Sci* 2006; **246**: 173–5.

65. Uhde TW, Merritt-Davis O, Yaroslavsky Y, Glitz D, Singareddy RK, Cortese BM. *Sleep paralysis: Overlooked fearful arousal*. 159th Annual Meeting of the American Psychiatric Association, Toronto, Canada, May 20–25, 2006 in Syllabus & Proceedings Summary, 2006; Abstract #96D: 250–1.

66. Takeuchi T, Miyasita A, Sasaki Y, *et al.* Isolated sleep paralysis elicited by sleep interruption. *Sleep* 1992; **15**: 217–25.

67. Roland MMS, Baran AS, Richert AC. Sleep-related laryngospasm caused by gastroesophageal reflux. *Sleep Med* 2008; **9**: 451–3.

68. Broughton RJ. NREM arousal parasomnias. In Kryger M, Roth T, Dement W (Eds), *Principles and Practice of Sleep Medicine*, 3rd ed. Philadelphia: Saunders, 2000; 693–706.

69. Mold JW, Mathew MK, Belgore S, DeHaven M. Prevalence of night sweats in primary care patients: An OKPRN and TAFP-Net collaborative study. *J Fam Pract* 2002; **51**: 452–6.

70. Lopes FL, Nardi AE, Nascimento I, Valenca AM, Zin WA. Nocturnal panic attacks. *Arq Neuropsiquiatr* 2002; **60**: 717–20.

71. Craske MG, Lang AJ, Aikins D, Mystokowski JL. Cognitive behavioral therapy for nocturnal panic. *Behav Ther* 2005; **36**: 43–54.

72. Craske MG, Tsao JCI. Assessment and treatment of nocturnal panic attacks. *Sleep Med Rev* 2005; **9**: 173–84.

73. Krahn LE, Black JL, Silber MH. Narcolepsy: New understanding of irresistible sleep. *Mayo Clin Proc* 2001; **76**: 185–94.

74. Anic-Labat S, Guilleminault C, Kraemer HC, Meehan J, Arrigoni J, Mignot E. Validation of a cataplexy questionnaire in 983 sleep-disorders patients. *Sleep* 1999; **22**: 77–87.

75. Dauvilliers Y, Arnulf I, Mignot E. Narcolepsy with cataplexy. *Lancet* 2007; **369**: 499–511.

76. Hasler G, Buysse DJ, Gamma A, Ajdacic V, Eich D, Rössler W, Angst J. Excessive daytime sleepiness in young adults: A 20-year prospective community study. *J Clin Psychiatry* 2005; **66**: 521–9.

77. Theorell-Haglöw J, Lindberg E, Janson C. What are the important risk factors for daytime sleepiness and fatigue in women? *Sleep* 2006; **29**: 751–7.

78. Singareddy RK, Uhde TW. Nocturnal panic and depression: Relationship to sleep in panic disorder. 45th Annual Meeting of the American College of Neuropsychopharmacology, Hollywood, Florida, December 3–7, 2006 in *Neuropsychopharmacology* 2006; **31**: S228.

79. Flosnik DL, Cortese BM, Uhde TW. Cataplexy in anxious patients: Is sub-clinical narcolepsy under-recognized in anxiety disorders? *J Clin Psychiatry* 2009; in press.

80. Cortese BM, Uhde TW. Immobilization panic. *Am J Psychiatry* 2006; **163**: 1453–4.

Section 5 Chapter 30

Sleep-related movement disorders and other variants

Sleep-related epilepsy

Carl W. Bazil

Epilepsy is a common condition, affecting about 1% of the population [1]. Most patients with epilepsy have seizures while awake; however, some have seizures that predominantly or exclusively occur during sleep. This can lead to confusion with the diagnosis, and seizures may be mistaken for parasomnias. The reverse is also true: some parasomnias and even normal sleep phenomena can sometimes be confused with epilepsy. It is therefore important for all clinicians who treat sleep disorders to have some familiarity with epilepsy, particularly those types that occur predominantly during sleep.

History

An association between sleep and epilepsy has been noted at least since the time of Aristotle, who famously noted that "sleep is similar to epilepsy and in some way, sleep is epilepsy." Epilepsy itself is a diverse condition, but one that is very common and will therefore be encountered by any physician, but particularly by those treating sleep disorders. In ancient times, patients with epilepsy were thought to be possessed by demons or by Satan. One of the first descriptions of an epileptic seizure takes place in the New Testament, where Jesus cures a boy with epilepsy (Matthew 17:14–18, Mark 9:17–27, Luke 9:38–42). This was later immortalized in Raphael's masterpiece "The Transfiguration."

Epilepsy is among the most common of neurological disorders. Worldwide, it affects 1–3% of the population. Incidence is highest at the extremes of age; in the very young congenital and genetic abnormalities predominate, while over age 60 the most common causes are cerebrovascular diseases and degenerative diseases. In most cases, however, no definite cause is found and the brain appears structurally normal [1].

Epilepsy is actually a diverse condition, but all patients have in common the occurrence of sudden, unprovoked changes in behavior arising from abnormal electrical discharges in the brain. It is important to note that a provoked seizure (such as that caused by drug withdrawal or infection of the central nervous system) is *not* epilepsy, even when recurrent.

Epilepsy is divided into two main types: generalized and partial. In the former, patients have an overall hyperactivity of the brain, and electrical discharges seem to begin all over the brain at once. Many of these generalized epilepsy syndromes seem to have a genetic basis. Partial (or localization-related) epilepsy consists of a regional or localized hyperactivity, such that seizures begin in one area (or sometimes several areas) of the brain. The characteristics of these partial seizures are related to the area in which they begin. For example, a partial seizure beginning in the frontal lobe is likely to involve the motor system, manifest by uncontrolled movements of the opposite side of the body. Characterization of a patient as partial or generalized epilepsy is important in choosing the appropriate treatment.

Clinical findings, natural history, and management of various epilepsy syndromes

With epilepsy or conditions potentially confused with epilepsy, a careful history is by far the most important part of making a diagnosis. Both seizures and parasomnias can be paroxysmal, and in many cases have similar clinical semiology (see Tables 30.1 and 30.2). Those most commonly confused with epilepsy are cataplexy, sleep attacks (especially related to narcolepsy), night terrors, and REM behavior disorder.

The Parasomnias and Other Sleep-Related Movement Disorders, ed. M. J. Thorpy and G. Plazzi. Published by Cambridge University Press. © Cambridge University Press 2010.

Section 5: Sleep-related disorders and others

Table 30.1 Characteristics of specific NREM sleep disorders and seizures.

	Seizure	Sleep drunkenness	Sleep terrors	Somnambulism	Somniloquy	Sleep enuresis	PLMS RLS
Incontinence	+	–	–	–	–	+	–
Tongue biting	+	–	–	–	–	–	–
Confusion	+	+	+	+	+	–	–
Tonic–clonic movements	+	–	–	–	–	–	–
Drooling	+	–	–	–	–	–	–
Amnesia	+	+	–	+	+	–	–
Occur awake	+	–	–	–	–	–	–

PLMS, periodic limb movements of sleep; RLS, restless legs syndrome.

Table 30.2 Characteristics of specific REM sleep disorders and seizures.

	Seizure	Nightmare	Cataplexy	Sleep paralysis	Hypnic hallucinations	REM behavior disorder
Incontinence	+	–	–	–	–	–
Tongue biting	+	–	–	–	–	–
Confusion	+	–	–	–	–	–
Tonic–clonic movements	+	–	–	–	–	–
Drooling	+	–	–	–	–	–
Amnesia	+	–	–	–	–	–
Occur awake	+	–	+	+	+	–

Episodes that occur only during sleep should raise the suspicion of a sleep disorder, although cataplexy and sleep attacks occur with the patient awake. Additionally, many patients with sleep disorders have excessive daytime somnolence, and daytime attacks can occur during naps. Conversely, there are many epilepsy syndromes where attacks occur predominantly or exclusively during sleep (such as benign rolandic and nocturnal frontal lobe epilepsies). Excessive daytime somnolence is suggestive of an underlying sleep disorder, particularly narcolepsy but also restless legs syndrome, sleep apnea, and periodic limb movements. This can be helpful in diagnosis; however, frequent nocturnal seizures will also disrupt sleep and result in similar symptoms.

Generalized epilepsy syndromes

While most seizure types have the potential to occur during sleep, some have a particularly strong association. Awakening Grand Mal epilepsy and juvenile myoclonic epilepsy are often considered together with respect to sleep. Both potentially include multiple seizure types (absence, myoclonic, and generalized tonic–clonic). In both, seizures tend to occur in early morning hours shortly after awakening, although some patients have a second peak of occurrence in the early evening [2]. Myoclonic seizures can be subtle and overlooked for years as simple clumsiness, but they can be considerably debilitating. These patients may be exceedingly sensitive to sleep deprivation and alcohol consumption (from any cause, including co-existing sleep disorders). In a few cases strict adherence to sleep hygiene can virtually eliminate the occurrence of seizures. Most patients require medication but are easily controlled; however, the condition tends to persist throughout life and treatment must be continued even after many years of seizure freedom [2,3].

Figure 30.1 Repetitive centrotemporal spikes (arrows) in an 8-year-old boy with benign rolandic epilepsy.

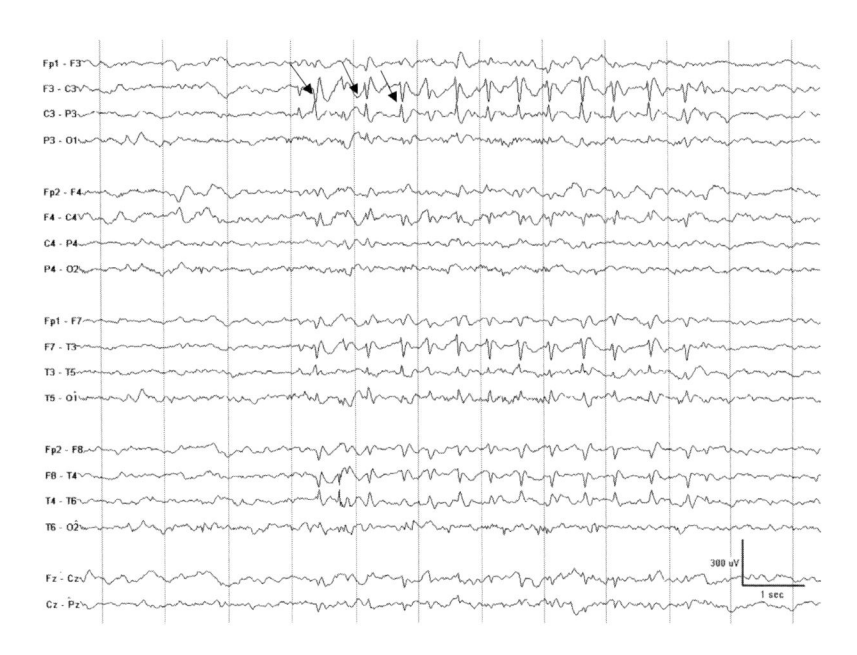

Benign rolandic epilepsy

Benign rolandic epilepsy, also known as benign epilepsy with centrotemporal spikes (BECTS), is a syndrome that typically begins in childhood and invariably remits in adolescence. It is characterized by seizures consisting of unilateral clonic jerking, often involving the face, and hypersalivation. Patients are often fully awake during the seizures. Seizures are predominantly nocturnal in all cases, and exclusively begin during sleep in about half [4,5]. The EEG shows characteristic spikes maximal in the central and temporal regions bilaterally and increasing dramatically during NREM sleep (Figure 30.1).

Landau–Kleffner syndrome and electrical status epilepticus during sleep

Landau–Kleffner syndrome (LKS) is a condition of acquired aphasia, frequently (but not always) with epileptic seizures and a markedly epileptiform EEG, particularly in sleep. Seizures are seen in approximately 70% of patients, but are typically easily controlled with medication [6]. O'Regan *et al.* [7] studied 25 children with an acquired disorder of communication and seizures, but not strictly meeting criteria for LKS. EEGs were uniformly epileptiform, usually (16/25) worsening with sleep. Most were considered to have a receptive aphasia. Language deficits have been hypothesized to result from the persistent epileptic discharges, as evidenced by hypometabolism on SPECT [7].

Electrical status epilepticus during sleep (ESES) is similar to LKS in age of onset and EEG findings. Both conditions demonstrate a normal EEG background during wakefulness, with generalized spike-wave discharges or sometimes focal epileptiform activity. However, in ESES discharges during sleep are generalized, while in LKS activity is more temporally located. In ESES, epileptiform activity becomes virtually continuous during NREM sleep such that it may be impossible to distinguish the sleep stage. REM sleep remains relatively preserved [8].

Localization-related epilepsy

In localization-related epilepsy, partial seizures tend to occur in both sleep and wakefulness, although the relative distribution varies according to site of onset. Clinically, an influence of sleep is widely accepted for frontal onset partial seizures. Three studies in patients with epilepsy support that frontal lobe seizures have been shown to occur more frequently during sleep compared to temporal lobe seizures [9–11]. In a review of 100 consecutive cases of nocturnal frontal lobe epilepsy (NFLE), 28% occurred in stage 3–4 sleep and only 3% during REM [12]. Clear epileptiform abnormalities on routine EEG occurred in less than half of patients. Only 42 patients showed a clear ictal discharge on polysomnography, adding to potential confusion with non-epileptic conditions including parasomnias.

Parasomnias frequently confused with epilepsy

As is the case with most parasomnias, a diagnosis of epilepsy is made mainly through history. Because patients may not recall some or all of a seizure event, this often depends upon the presence and reliability of an onlooker. When seizures occur mostly or exclusively at night, the history often becomes more incomplete and even misleading.

There are a large number of normal and abnormal sleep phenomena that can be confused with seizures. Sleep terrors can usually be distinguished from seizures by their exclusive occurrence in sleep combined with the characteristic dream imagery, predominant fear, and rapid recovery. Abnormal movements, prolonged confusion, drooling, and tongue biting are suspicious for seizure. Sleepwalking (somnambulism), somniloquy (sleep talking), and sleep enuresis (bedwetting) are also very common in childhood, and rare in adults. Nightmares consist of frightening dreams that often awaken the patient from sleep, and can be accompanied by agitation. A history usually identifies these as benign events; however, if specific dream imagery is not recalled, a history of sudden fear followed by confusion might be mistaken for nocturnal seizures.

REM behavior disorder is characterized by agitated, sometimes violent movements occurring during REM sleep [13,14]. Patients will typically report that a dream sequence occurs during the episode. The history of bizarre, semipurposeful behavior with confusion may be impossible to distinguish from seizures or post-ictal behavior. Unlike most partial seizures, REM behavior disorder will be restricted to sleep, and usually occurs in the early morning when REM is most prevalent. The memory of a dream sequence, if present, is helpful in distinguishing the two.

Effects of seizures on sleep

Intuitively, any seizure occurring during sleep has the potential to disrupt sleep structure. Most will cause at least a brief awakening, and normal sleep is unlikely during a post-ictal state. It may seem that such disruption could be relatively minor, but actually even brief seizures can result in prolonged alterations in sleep structure. Many studies have shown improvement in sleep with treatment of nocturnal seizures, including improved sleep efficiency, decreased arousals, and increased REM sleep [15,16]. The effects of individual temporal lobe seizures have been investigated on patients in an epilepsy monitoring unit, who were recorded with polysomnography under baseline conditions (seizure free), and following complex partial or secondarily generalized seizures [17]. With daytime seizures, there was a significant decrease in REM the following night (12% vs. 18% for baseline) without significant changes in other sleep stages or in sleep efficiency. When seizures occurred at night, this decrease in REM was more pronounced (7% vs. 16%) and there were increases in stage 1 and decreases in sleep efficiency. These effects were even more pronounced when seizures occurred early in the night. Therefore, seizures can have a profound effect on sleep lasting much longer than the apparent post-ictal period. This helps to explain a commonly seen clinical phenomenon: patients who have only nocturnal seizures, but report difficulty concentrating or even total inability to work on the days following a seizure.

Effect of sleep, sleep deprivation, and sleep disruption on the occurrence of seizures

The amount of baseline rhythmicity occurring in the brain differs considerably between the states of sleep and wakefulness. It is perhaps not surprising, then, that various seizure types begin preferentially in sleep as opposed to wakefulness or in specific stages of sleep. Crespel *et al.* [9] examined the occurrence of frontal and temporal lobe seizures in 30 patients, using 5 days of continuous video-EEG monitoring. Sixty-one per cent of frontal seizures began during sleep, compared with only 11% of temporal lobe seizures. In a larger study, Bazil and Walczak [10] retrospectively studied over a thousand seizures in 188 consecutive patients to look at patterns of onset in relationship to sleep. A

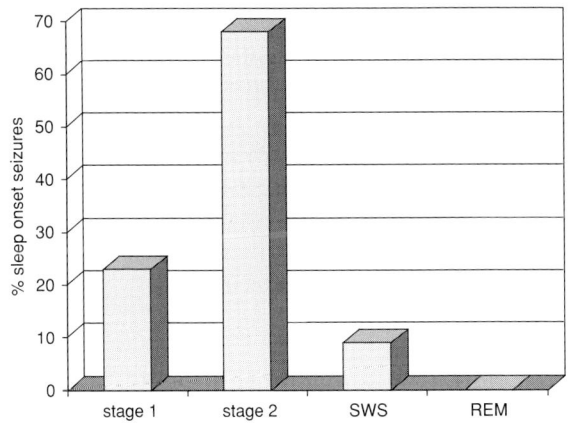

Figure 30.2 Percentage of sleep-onset partial seizures beginning in various sleep stages. SWS: slow-wave sleep. REM, REM sleep. Data from [11].

similar, prospective study was performed later in patients with partial seizures [11]. Both of these studies showed that, overall, 20% of seizures occurred during sleep. Frontal lobe seizures began during sleep more often than temporal lobe seizures, a finding which has been appreciated clinically. Both studies also showed that temporal lobe seizures were more likely to progress to secondarily generalized seizures when beginning during sleep, but frontal lobe seizures were not. This intriguing finding suggests differences in the pathways of spread in partial epilepsy, which could have implications for treatment if better understood. Seizures that occur only during sleep may represent an important, distinct class as these have a particularly good prognosis [18,19].

One of the most interesting and robust findings across many studies is the relative protection of REM against the occurrence of focal seizures. An analysis of 613 partial seizures in 133 patients showed that seizures begin commonly during the lighter stages of NREM sleep, but are rare during slow-wave sleep and none were recorded which began during REM (Figure 30.2) [11]. It is not known how the REM state inhibits the onset of seizures. Electrophysiologically, cerebral activity during REM most closely resembles wakefulness or light sleep; however the above studies show that seizures occur less frequently during REM than either of these states. It may be that relative hypersynchrony present during NREM sleep may facilitate onset and/or spread of certain partial seizures. This is an important area for future research, as understanding the mechanism whereby REM sleep inhibits seizure onset and propagation could lead to novel treatments for intractable epilepsy.

Sleep deprivation has long been thought to increase the risk of seizures, clinically readily apparent in a few syndromes such as juvenile myoclonic epilepsy. However, one controlled study of patients with refractory partial epilepsy failed to show such an effect [20]. This brings into question the common practice of sleep deprivation in epilepsy monitoring units in order to induce sciures. Sleep deprivation probably does increase the risk of seizures in most patients in the outpatient setting, particularly when chronic. This can be due to sleep disorders (as described above), from outside influences like poor sleep hygiene, or can be voluntary: patients simply restrict themselves to an inadequate sleep time, because of time constraints on other aspects of their lives. Any of these influences can result in increased seizures, further disrupting the already limited sleep time. A cycle of sleep disruption and intractable epilepsy can result, and seizures will not be controlled until the sleep disruption is also resolved.

Finally, certain circadian rhythms may influence seizures independently of sleep. Both rats with a model of limbic epilepsy and humans with medial temporal seizures have increased seizures during daylight, an effect not seen with human extratemporal seizures [21]. This is likely independent of sleep, of course, because rats are primarily nocturnal and humans diurnal. Humans with intractable temporal lobe epilepsy show abnormal secretion of melatonin, a sleep-related hormone with a characteristic circadian pattern [22]. Another study confirmed lower melatonin levels in epilepsy patients, and determined that this is true of both nocturnal and diurnal seizures [23]. Exogenous melatonin has been shown to help control seizures in a few small studies [24,25], raising the possibility that it may be useful in the treatment of some patients.

Effects of epilepsy drugs on sleep, and of sleep drugs on epilepsy

Early studies of anti-convulsant medications showed an increase in sleep stability with all agents. In retrospect, much of this effect was likely due to a reduction in seizure activity, rather than an independent effect of the drug. More recently, the effects of anti-convulsant drugs have been studied independently of seizures, showing different effects (both detrimental and beneficial) of various anti-convulsants on both sleep and specific sleep disorders.

Benzodiazepines and barbiturates are used less commonly for chronic treatment of seizure disorders, but have the most convincing evidence for detrimental effects on sleep structure. While both classes of medications reduce sleep latency, they also decrease the amount of REM sleep, and benzodiazepines also reduce slow-wave sleep [26,27]. Phenytoin increases light sleep and decreases sleep efficiency; most studies also show decreased REM sleep [26,28,29]. Findings for carbamazepine are more variable, but there also seems to be a reduction in REM sleep [28], particularly with acute treatment [30,31]. Valproate may increase stage 1 sleep [29] and (at least theoretically) could worsen obstructive sleep apnea through weight gain.

Studies of newer agents in general suggest fewer detrimental effects on sleep. Lamotrigine has been shown to have no effect on sleep in one study [30], but another showed decreases in slow-wave sleep [32]. Gabapentin, pregabalin, and tiagabine enhance slow-wave sleep and sleep continuity in patients with epilepsy [29,30] and in normal volunteers [27,33–37]. Furthermore, gabapentin is effective in the treatment of one common sleep disorder, restless legs syndrome [38], although carbamazepine and lamotrigine have also been used. A study of levetiracetam in epilepsy patients showed little effect [39]; studies in normal volunteers have either shown little effect [39], or an increase in sleep continuity and slow-wave sleep [40]. The effects of zonisamide, oxcarbazepine, and topiramate on sleep and sleep disorders are not known. Patients taking anti-convulsants known to disrupt sleep (phenobarbital, phenytoin, carbamazepine, or valproic acid) have increased drowsiness compared to epilepsy patients who are not taking anti-convulsants [41].

Effects of AEDs on sleep have been known, and sleep changes were known to affect memory and performance, but the most important aspect of this relationship is whether sleep changes due to AEDs actually affect performance. To date this has been shown only for tiagabine [37]. Thirty-eight healthy adults were restricted to 5 h of sleep for four consecutive nights, and randomized to tiagabine 8 mg at bedtime or placebo. In a measure of attention (psychomotor vigilance task), subjects on placebo deteriorated during sleep restriction but subjects receiving tiagabine did not. Subjects taking tiagabine also showed improved performance on the Wisconsin Card Sorting Task and reported more restorative sleep, but did not show improved wakefulness on the Multiple Sleep Latency Test and did not differ on several other measures of memory and alertness. However, it is intriguing that this drug, which enhanced slow-wave sleep, showed modest improvement in subjects who were sleep-deprived. It is not known whether these changes would correlate to improved performance in epilepsy patients, or if findings would generalize to other AEDs that improve slow-wave sleep.

Several drugs commonly used for sleep have a potential influence on seizures. Benzodiazepines and barbiturates, already mentioned, are used for both conditions. Nonbenzodiazepine hypnotics (zaleplon, zolpidem, eszopiclone) are not thought to carry risk of withdrawal seizures and therefore may be safer than these previous classes particularly in patients with a known history of seizures. There is also no indication that ramelteon, a melatonin agonist used for sleep, carries any risk in epilepsy.

Many patients with sleep disorders take anti-depressant drugs. While there are reports of increased seizures with tricyclic anti-depressants and selective serotonin reuptake inhibitors (SSRIs), any risk is probably minimal and these are not generally problematic. The same is true for trazadone, quetiapine, and doxepin. An exception may be bupropion, which carries a higher risk.

Anti-convulsant effects on various aspects of sleep and sleep disorders, and of sleep drugs on seizures, are summarized in Table 30.3.

Laboratory investigations

The primary tool for investigation of seizures is the electroencephalogram (EEG). This test records the change in electrical activity on the scalp over time. In routine polysomnography (PSG), only the central and occipital regions are recorded, and the parameters are set primarily for recognition of sleep structure. In a full EEG, all areas of the scalp are recorded.

For most patients with suspected epilepsy, a routine EEG is performed lasting about 30 min. While it is unlikely that an actual seizure will be recorded in that time, most patients will show inter-ictal abnormalities called "spikes" or "sharp waves." These markers

Table 30.3 Summary of AED effects on sleep and hypnotic effects on seizures.

	Effects on sleep		Effects on sleep disorders	
AED	Positive	Negative	Improves/treats	Worsens
Barbiturates	Decreased latency	Decreased REM	Sleep onset insomnia	OSA
Benzodiazepines	Decreased latency	Decreased REM, SWS	Sleep onset insomnia	OSA
Carbamazepine		Decreased REM?	RLS	RLS
Phenytoin	Decreased latency	Increased arousals and stage 1; decreased REM		NE
Valproic acid		Increased stage 1		OSA*
Felbamate	?	?	OSA*	Insomnia
Gabapentin	Increased SWS, decreased arousals	None	RLS	
Lamotrigine	None	Decreased SWS?		
Levetiracetam	Increased SWS	None		
Pregabalin	Increased SWS, decreased arousals	None	RLS?	OSA*
Tiagabine	Increased SWS	None		
Topiramate	?	?	OSA*	
Zonisamide	?	?		

	Effects on seizures	
Hypnotic	Positive	Negative
Benzodiazepines	Treats seizures, esp. acutely	Risk of withdrawal seizure
Non-benzodiazepine hypnotic (zolpidem, zaleplon, eszopiclone)	None	None
Anti-depressants (tricyclic, SSRI, atypical)	None	May be minimal risk of exacerbation
Buproprion	None	Mild risk of exacerbation

REM, REM sleep; RLS, restless legs syndrome; SWS, slow-wave sleep; ?: unknown; *indirectly, through weight change.

of epilepsy are present in up to 90% of patients with epilepsy [42], although repeated or prolonged studies may be needed to identify these [43]. Inter-ictal epileptiform discharges are rarely seen in individuals without epilepsy; these occur in about 2% of children and 0.5% of adults [44,45].

When the diagnosis remains in doubt, a definitive study is video-EEG monitoring. This is typically performed as an inpatient. EEG is recorded continuously, and the patient remains on a video camera until a typical episode takes place. In the case of rare episodes, patients may be weaned off medications, sleep-deprived, or stressed in other ways to encourage more frequent episodes. If episodes occur nearly every night, and particularly if other parasomnias are in the differential, video-EEG PSG may be performed as an outpatient. Most systems in current use for PSG have the potential to record a full EEG simultaneously with routine polysomnographic channels. The event(s) in question, once recorded, can then be examined using both techniques. Seizure activity may be difficult to confirm on a more limited PSG montage and setting but much clearer with a full EEG (Figure 30.3).

Section 5: Sleep-related disorders and others

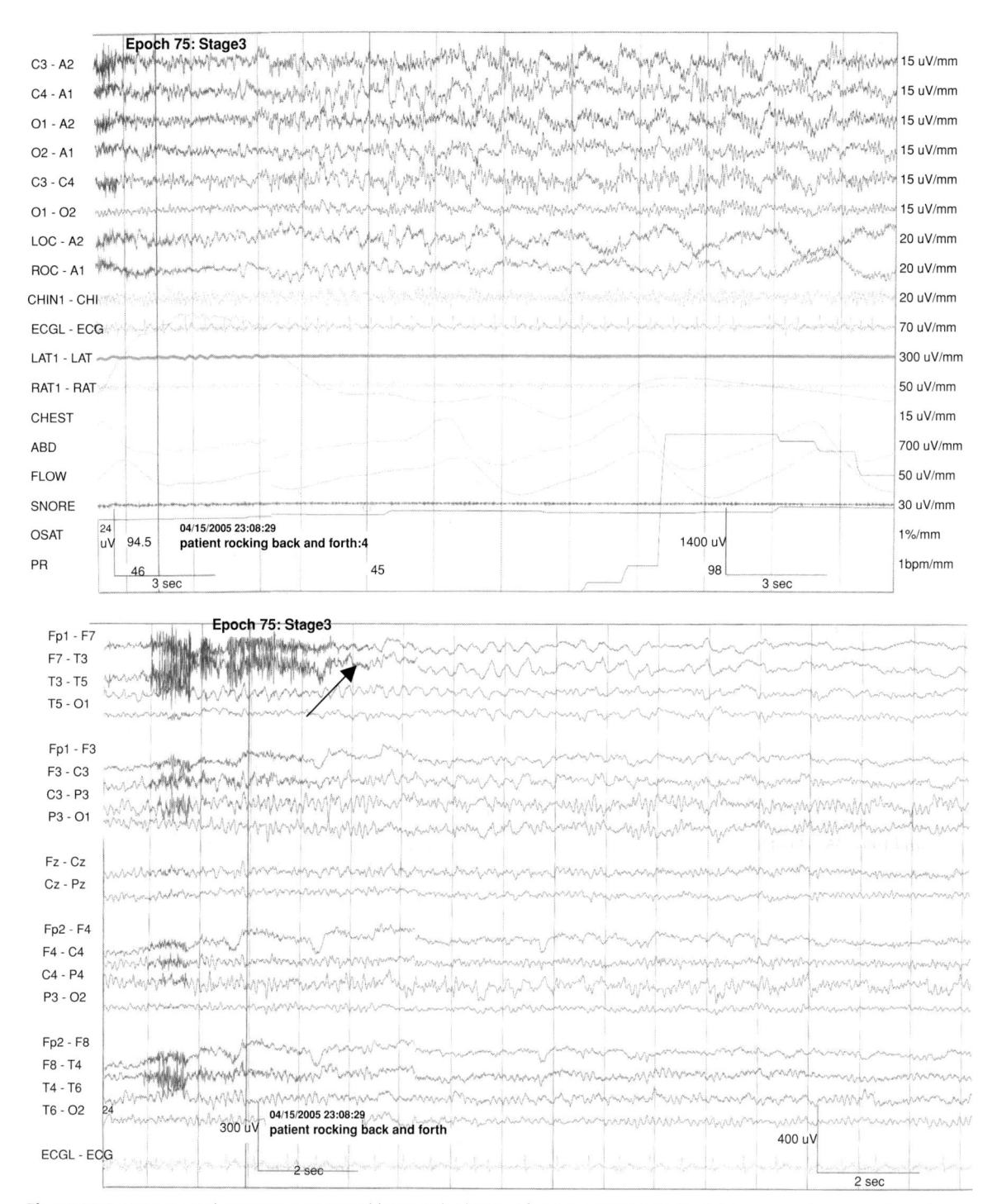

Figure 30.3 Unrecognized seizures in a 64-year-old man with a history of well-controlled epilepsy. Polysomnography was performed because of frequent episodes of nocturnal rocking. On polysomnography the nature of these is unclear (top); with EEG a rhythmic theta frequency discharge is seen maximal in the left temporal region and is diagnostic of a partial seizure (bottom; arrow).

Conclusions

Sleep-related epilepsy is common, and is important in the differential of paroxysmal behaviors seen during sleep. Seizures also have independent influences on sleep structure, and sleep deprivation (from sleep restriction, medication, or co-existing sleep disorders) can make seizures difficult to control or contribute to refractory epilepsy. It is therefore important for sleep clinicians to be aware of various nocturnal seizure types, and to consider full EEG montage during polysomnography when seizures may be present. If the diagnosis remains uncertain, prolonged video-EEG monitoring, perhaps with simultaneous polysomnographic recording, may be required. Finally, drugs used for sleep disorders may influence epilepsy, and drugs for epilepsy can impact sleep in both positive and negative ways; these are also considerations in many sleep patients.

References

1. Hauser WA, Annegers JF, Kurland LT. Prevalence of epilepsy in Rochester, Minnesota: 1940–1980. *Epilepsia* 1991; **32**: 429–45.
2. Wolf P, Schmitt JJ. Awakening epilepsies and juvenile myoclonic epilepsy. In Bazil CW, Sammaritano MR (Eds), *Sleep and Epilepsy: The Clinical Spectrum*. Amsterdam: Elsevier, 2002; 237–43.
3. Shinnar S, *et al*. Discontinuing antiepileptic drugs in children with epilepsy: A prospective study. *Ann Neurol* 1994; **35**: 534–45.
4. Blom S, Heijbel J. Benign epilepsy of children with centro-temporal EEG foci. Discharge rate during sleep. *Epilepsia* 1975; **16**: 133–40.
5. Blom S, Heijbel J, Bergfors PG. Benign epilepsy of children with centro-temporal EEG foci. Prevalence and follow-up study of 40 patients. *Epilepsia* 1972; **13**: 609–19.
6. Hirsch E, *et al*. Landau–Kleffner syndrome: A clinical and EEG study of five cases. *Epilepsia* 1990; **31**: 756–67.
7. O'Regan ME, *et al*. Epileptic aphasia: A consequence of regional hypometabolic encephalopathy? *Dev Med Child Neurol* 1998; **40**: 508–16.
8. Mendez M, Radtke RA. Interactions between sleep and epilepsy. *J Clin Neurophysiol* 2001; **18**: 106–27.
9. Crespel A, Baldy-Moulinier M, Coubes P. The relationship between sleep and epilepsy in frontal and temporal lobe epilepsies: Practical and physiopathologic considerations. *Epilepsia* 1998; **39**: 150–7.
10. Bazil CW, Walczak TS. Effects of sleep and sleep stage on epileptic and nonepileptic seizures. *Epilepsia* 1997; **38**: 56–62.
11. Herman ST, Walczak TS, Bazil CW. Distribution of partial seizures during the sleep–wake cycle: Differences by seizure onset site. *Neurology* 2001; **56**: 1453–9.
12. Provini F, *et al*. Nocturnal frontal lobe epilepsy. A clinical and polygraphic overview of 100 consecutive cases. *Brain* 1999; **122**: 1017–31.
13. Mahowald MW, Schenck CH. NREM sleep parasomnias. *Neurol Clin* 1996; **14**: 675–96.
14. Schenck CH, *et al*. Rapid eye movement sleep behavior disorder. A treatable parasomnia affecting older adults. *J Am Med Assoc* 1987; **257**: 1786–9.
15. Tachibana, N, *et al*. Supplementary motor area seizure resembling sleep disorder. *Sleep* 1996; **19**: 811–6.
16. Touchon J, *et al*. [Organization of sleep in recent temporal lobe epilepsy before and after treatment with carbamazepine]. *Rev Neurol (Paris)* 1987; **143**: 462–7.
17. Bazil CW, Castro LH, Walczak TS. Reduction of rapid eye movement sleep by diurnal and nocturnal seizures in temporal lobe epilepsy. *Arch Neurol* 2000; **57**: 363–8.
18. Yaqub BA, Waheed G, Kabiraj MM. Nocturnal epilepsies in adults. *Seizure* 1997; **6**: 145–9.
19. Park SA, *et al*. Clinical courses of pure sleep epilepsies. *Seizure* 1998; **7**: 369–77.
20. Malow BA, *et al*. Sleep deprivation does not affect seizure frequency during inpatient video-EEG monitoring. *Neurology* 2002; **59**: 1371–4.
21. Quigg M, *et al*. Temporal distribution of partial seizures: Comparison of an animal model with human partial epilepsy. *Ann Neurol* 1998; **43**: 748–55.
22. Bazil CW, *et al*. Patients with intractable epilepsy have low melatonin, which increases following seizures. *Neurology* 2000; **55**: 1746–8.
23. Yalyn O, *et al*. A comparison of the circadian rhythms and the levels of melatonin in patients with diurnal and nocturnal complex partial seizures. *Epilepsy Behav* 2006; **8**: 542–6.
24. Fauteck, J, *et al*. Melatonin in epilepsy: First results of replacement therapy and first clinical results. *Biol Signals Recept* 1999; **8**: 105–10.
25. Peled N, *et al*. Melatonin effect on seizures in children with severe neurologic deficit disorders. *Epilepsia* 2001; **42**: 1208–10.
26. Wolf P, Roder-Wanner UU, Brede M. Influence of therapeutic phenobarbital and phenytoin medication on the polygraphic sleep of patients with epilepsy. *Epilepsia* 1984; **25**: 467–75.

27. Hindmarch I, Dawson J, Stanley N. A double-blind study in healthy volunteers to assess the effects on sleep of pregabalin compared with alprazolam and placebo. *Sleep* 2005; **28**: 187–93.
28. Drake ME, Jr, *et al*. Outpatient sleep recording during antiepileptic drug monotherapy. *Clin Electroencephalogr* 1990; **21**: 170–3.
29. Legros B, Bazil CW. Effects of antiepileptic drugs on sleep architecture: A pilot study. *Sleep Med* 2003; **4**: 51–5.
30. Placidi F, *et al*. Effect of anticonvulsants on nocturnal sleep in epilepsy. *Neurology* 2000; **54**: S25–32.
31. Yang JD, *et al*. Effects of carbamazepine on sleep in healthy volunteers. *Biol Psychiatry* 1989; **26**: 324–8.
32. Foldvary N, *et al*. The effects of lamotrigine on sleep in patients with epilepsy. *Epilepsia* 2001; **42**: 1569–73.
33. Foldvary-Schaefer N, *et al*. Gabapentin increases slow-wave sleep in normal adults. *Epilepsia* 2002; **43**: 1493–7.
34. Bazil C, Battista J, Basner R. Gabapentin improves sleep in the presence of alcohol. *J Clin Sleep Med* 2005; **1**: 284–7.
35. Mathias S, *et al*. The GABA uptake inhibitor tiagabine promotes slow wave sleep in normal elderly subjects. *Neurobiol Aging* 2001; **22**: 247–53.
36. Walsh JK, *et al*. Dose–response effects of tiagabine on the sleep of older adults. *Sleep* 2005; **28**: 673–6.
37. Walsh JK, *et al*. Tiagabine is associated with sustained attention during sleep restriction: Evidence for the value of slow-wave sleep enhancement? *Sleep* 2006; **29**: 433–43.
38. Garcia-Borreguero D, *et al*. Treatment of restless legs syndrome with gabapentin: A double-blind, cross-over study. *Neurology* 2002; **59**: 1573–9.
39. Bell C, *et al*. The effects of levetiracetam on objective and subjective sleep parameters in healthy volunteers and patients with partial epilepsy. *J Sleep Res* 2002; **11**: 255–63.
40. Cicolin A, *et al*. Effects of levetiracetam on nocturnal sleep and daytime vigilance in healthy volunteers. *Epilepsia* 2006; **47**: 82–5.
41. Salinsky MC, Oken BS, Binder LM. Assessment of drowsiness in epilepsy patients receiving chronic antiepileptic drug therapy. *Epilepsia* 1996; **37**: 181–7.
42. Marsan CA, Zivin LS. Factors related to the occurrence of typical paroxysmal abnormalities in the EEG records of epileptic patients. *Epilepsia* 1970; **11**: 361–81.
43. Salinsky M, Kanter R, Dasheiff RM. Effectiveness of multiple EEGs in supporting the diagnosis of epilepsy: An operational curve. *Epilepsia* 1987; **28**: 331–4.
44. Gregory RP, Oates T, Merry RT. Electroencephalogram epileptiform abnormalities in candidates for aircrew training. *Electroencephalogr Clin Neurophysiol* 1993; **86**: 75–7.
45. Eeg-Olofsson O, Petersen I, Sellden U. The development of the electroencephalogram in normal children from the age of 1 through 15 years. Paroxysmal activity. *Neuropaediatrie* 1971; **2**: 375–404.

Section 6: Therapy of parasomnias

Section 6 Chapter 31

Therapy of parasomnias

Pharmacotherapy and parasomnias

Rafael Pelayo and Deepti Sinha

Introduction

This chapter will review pharmacological options in the treatment of parasomnias in both adults and children. A literature search using the terms *parasomnias* and *pharmacology* provides many references. Unfortunately, about two-thirds of these references will actually be for restless leg syndrome. Restless leg syndrome is not categorized as a parasomnia in the *International Classification of Sleep Disorders* and will not be covered in this chapter. The actual literature on the pharmacological treatment of parasomnias is relatively small considering the overall prevalence of these disorders. At the time of writing, there are no randomized placebo-controlled trials for adults with parasomnias. In children, only one such trial was found. A randomized study of the use of melatonin as an adjunct for children with epilepsy found a decrease in parasomnias on a questionnaire [1]. Clearly there is a paucity of randomized trials on the use of pharmacological agents in parasomnias. The use of any medication for parasomnias is largely predicated on clinical or anecdotal experience. The focus of the content in this chapter will be randomized trials. We will review separately the use of clonazepam, melatonin, tricyclic antidepressants and other medications for arousal parasomnias, REM behavior disorder and bruxism.

Off-label concerns

With regard to pharmacological treatment options the learning process for all clinicians, whether they predominately treat adults or children, is very similar. Ideally we first learn the normal physiology, then the pathophysiology for the condition. Pharmacological treatment options would then be understood within this framework. Without knowledge of sleep physiology and pathophysiology, rational pharmacological management and advancement is difficult. Despite their high prevalence, sleep disorders, and parasomnias in particular, are not emphasized during the typical medical school curriculum or residency training. This paucity of education may account for the relatively little information being available on the pharmacological management of parasomnias. The indications for pharmacotherapy in parasomnias are also limited, as behavioral approaches are used successfully most often, especially in children.

When medications are used to treat parasomnias, they are typically not FDA-approved for the specific sleep disorder. Since arousal parasomnias are particularly common among children, this is particularly troublesome among pediatric age range patients.

Pediatric considerations

Within a broader review of the pharmacology of parasomnias, a discussion of pertinent features in pediatric sleep pharmacology is important. Medications used in children can appear capricious. An example of this is clonidine. Clonidine is one of the most commonly prescribed medications for sleep in children despite the absence of any randomized control trials supporting its use. Pediatricians prescribe clonidine for children of all ages, infants through teens [2–4]. How can this drug be such a popular choice among pediatricians, particularly when it is rarely used to treat sleep disorders in adults? Is the pathophysiology of sleep disorders so different between adults and children that it is rational for an anti-hypertensive agent to be routinely used in children? Of note, despite the absence of evidence-based data, the use of medication for sleep disorders in children is increasing. Stojanovski and colleagues examined trends in physician prescribing of medications for children with sleep difficulties in outpatient settings

Section 6: Therapy of parasomnias

in the US [4]. The study used data from the National Ambulatory Medical Care Survey (NAMCS) collected from 1993 to 2004. The rate of medication prescriptions for children with sleep disorders appears to be increasing. The study found that approximately 18.6 million visits occurred for sleep-related difficulty in children. In this 12-year study period, 81% of patients with pediatric insomnia were prescribed a sleep medication: 33% received anti-histamines, and another 26% were prescribed alpha-2 agonists (presumably clonidine). The finding that 81% of children were prescribed a medication is particularly remarkable considering that only 48% of the adult patients suffering from insomnia were prescribed a medication [4].

The paucity of information on the pharmacological treatment of parasomnias in children may not be surprising given the inherent problems of the clinical situation. Most pharmacological guidelines were developed for sleep disorders in adults and must be empirically extrapolated to children. The physician is often forced to prescribe medications as an "off-label" indication. This may result in frustrating insurance reimbursement delays or denials for the family. These reimbursement problems may affect the availability of a specific medication, the family's compliance with the medication or force the physician to prescribe a less desirable alternative. The medication may not be available commercially in an easily administered form. Younger children may not be able to swallow pills, or ingest chewable tablets, requiring the local pharmacist to compound the medication into a suspension. In addition, due to the natural aversion among both parents and physicians to use medications for pediatric sleep disorders, medications are usually prescribed as a last resort or in the most refractory situations. At times, a decision to use medication in a child may be made not necessarily to assist the child as much as to help the parents or other family members sleep better. It is not unusual that parents may finally seek help for a child's long-standing sleep problem when they feel they can no longer put up with interruptions to their own sleep. The clinician needs to be aware of this situation, which may cause guilty feelings to arise in the family members.

Further complicating the pharmacological treatment of parasomnias in children is the general lack of specialized training in sleep disorders available to all health care providers, not just pediatricians, who are working with these children. Failure to consider or properly apply non-drug treatments as part of the comprehensive management of the child may also lead to unsatisfactory results for the patient and the family. These factors result in children that are not properly managed due to either underdosing or overdosing of medication, or incorrect medication selection.

A key principal in sleep pharmacology is not to equate sedation with normal, refreshing sleep. Perhaps the simplest and best-known example of this principal is alcohol. Consuming large amounts of alcohol can be very sedating, but we do not wake up feeling particularly refreshed after a night of excessive drinking. Indeed alcohol may increase the likelihood of parasomnias occurring. There may be an over-reliance on the effects of the medication by both the parents and health care provider without adequate understanding of the cause of the poor sleep or the appropriate application of behavioral techniques to help improve the child's sleep.

A common scenario in clinical practice is a parent's complaint of a child's paradoxical reaction to a hypnotic medication. "He did not sleep at all" or "he became hyper" may be the parent's complaint. From a physiological point of view, how can we explain that a child did not get sleepy when given a hypnotic agent? Is the child's brain missing the usual GABA receptors? Of course not, but the child's poor reaction to the medication is not typically questioned and the medication is simply removed from the limited list of pharmacological options available to the patient. A more physiological approach would be to understand why the medication failed to achieve the desired result. In the authors' experience the reason may not be due to the choice of medication per se, but due to the medication dose or time of administration.

When prescribing a medication for a child there is a natural inclination to give the lowest dose possible. However, children may have faster hepatic metabolism of the medication resulting in faster elimination. If the dose of the agent is too low, the medication may disinhibit a child but not make the child actually fall asleep. The parents would report unusual behavior. If a child typically fights their bedtime, for example due to fear of being alone in the dark, and the medication dose given to the child only makes that child drowsy but without falling asleep, frightening hypnagogic hallucinations may occur. This might be particularly disturbing in children with an underlying psychiatric or neurological condition, for whom the outside world may already be confusing. With the resulting confusion or disorientation caused by too low a dose of a sedating medication, it is not surprising that parents may report paradoxical reactions to the putative hypnotic.

Not only is the specific medication and dosage key, but the timing of administration is also very important, because of the circadian modulation of alertness. Humans typically experience an enhanced alertness in the evening, which is often referred to as a "second wind". During this circadian phase it is harder to fall asleep. If the hypnotic medication is given during this circadian time window, it may not work. If the medication is given too early while the child is not ready to sleep but rather has heightened alertness, dissociative phenomena such as frightening hypnagogic hallucinations may occur [5]. In the situation of children with neurological or psychiatric disorders they may not understand that the medication was meant to help them sleep. Typically hypnotics only shorten the usual falling asleep time (sleep latency) at most by only 20 or 30 min compared to placebo. Giving a medication 2 or 3 h prior to the usual falling asleep time could elicit this common scenario. This same medication and dose given at a more appropriate circadian time could be effective.

This lack of proper management of the sleep problem may be particularly common among children with neurological, psychiatric, behavioral or emotional disorders. The use of psychotropic medication in children has been increasing [6]. If the child cannot communicate what they feel is causing the sleep difficulty, incorrect assumptions may be made by the family and/or health care provider. In cases of insomnia, this can result in an escalating cycle of progressively more sedating agents with increasing likelihood of adverse effects. Concomitant daytime sedation may occur, which may interfere with the child's daytime therapeutic program and exacerbate the child's disabilities. In some situations, the fear of putative addiction may limit the physician or the family from using pharmacotherapy adequately to improve the child's sleep.

Benzodiazepines

There are no medications with an FDA indication for any of the 15 different parasomnias listed in the *International Classification of Sleep Disorders* [7]. Benzodiazepines, which have been used extensively in adults with insomnia, are the most commonly utilized agents for the off-label treatment of parasomnias. Benzodiazepines have been particularly useful for arousal parasomnias such as sleepwalking and REM sleep behavior disorder (RBD). The mechanism of action is based on activation of the gamma aminobutyric acid (GABA) receptor complex [8]. Benzodiazepines may have muscle relaxing properties and should be used with caution if comorbid sleep-disordered breathing is suspected. On a polysomnogram, benzodiazepines may alter the normal sleep stages referred to as sleep architecture. There can be drug-related artifacts such as atypical sleep spindles and suppression of slow-wave sleep.

Among the benzodiazepine class, clonazepam is the most common medication used in the treatment of parasomnias [9–11]. The popularity of the clinical use of clonazepam in parasomnias may be due to familiarity with the drug along with the putative clinical efficacy. The exact mechanism of action is unknown. The principal mechanism of clonazepam seems to be enhancement of the activity of GABA, acting as an allosteric modulator of the major inhibitory neurotransmitter GABA A complex, which is a chloride channel. GABA-independent mechanisms have been reported [12]. Clonazepam has also been reported to have anti-dopaminergic activity [13], and serotonergic properties [14,15]. Clonazepam specifically modulates the activity of thalamic reticular nucleus neurons which may explain some of its anti-convulsant properties [16]. Clonazepam is rapidly and completely absorbed after oral administration. Onset of action is 20–60 min. The time to peak level is 1–3 h. Duration of action is 6–8 h in children and up to 12 h in adults. The bioavailability is about 90%. Maximum plasma concentrations are reached within 1–4 h after oral administration. The half-life of clonazepam is typically 30–40 h. The half-life tends to be longer in adults compared to children. The metabolism is extensively hepatic and excreted in urine.

Benzodiazepines and arousal parasomnias

Clonazepam can be used to prevent parasomnias associated with partial arousals such as sleep terrors or sleepwalking. These parasomnias may decrease as the child gets older. When parasomnias are very frequent and disturbing to the patient and family, a low dose of clonazepam at 0.25–0.5 mg may be helpful. Clonazepam may increase the arousal threshold, allowing the child to sleep without interruption. Clonazepam is available in thin wafers that dissolve on the tongue, obviating the need for the child to swallow a pill.

Clonazepam is the drug of choice for parasomnias such as RBD and is also used for arousal parasomnias such as sleep terrors and sleepwalking. For arousal parasomnias in children, most are managed with reassurance or timed awakening and making the environment safe for the child. The frequency of episodes tends to lessen with age. Studies for the pharmacologic treatment of parasomnias in children have been done with the use of imipramine and diazepam, but not clonazepam. There are very limited studies in children, as most do not require pharmacological interventions. There has been a case report of a boy with Asperger's whose sleepwalking was successfully managed with melatonin [17]. For adults, treatment is recommended if the parasomnia is associated with injury or danger to the patient or others. Guilleminault et al. looked at 84 children with sleep terrors with and without sleepwalking, and found that 49 of these patients had sleep-disordered breathing and, with treatment, the parasomnias disappeared [18].

Clonazepam has been studied as pharmacotherapy for arousal parasomnias over the last two decades. It has predominantly been studied in adults and specifically in those who have had a sleep related injury. Schenck et al. studied 100 patients who presented to their sleep center with nocturnal injuries and diagnosed them with polysomnography [19]; 54 of these patients were diagnosed with either sleep terrors or sleepwalking (age of onset ranging from 3 to 58 years). Clonazepam was prescribed in 28 of these patients as well as 33 patients with RBD. Out of the 61 patients, 51 (83.6%) reportedly had significant improvement in sleep injury up to 6 years after starting treatment. In 1996, Schenck and Mahowald went on to study a further 170 adults with sleep-related injury between 1982 and 1994, of whom 69 had either sleepwalking or sleep terrors; other diagnoses included RBD, RLS and chronic insomnia [20]; 146 (86%) of these patients had complete or near-complete control of their symptoms. There have also been case reports of patients with behaviors such as driving and sleep violence who have been diagnosed with sleepwalking who have responded to clonazepam [20,21].

Benzodiazepines decrease sleep latency and episodes of wake after sleep onset. Clonazepam may therefore reduce arousability during slow-wave sleep in arousal parasomnias [22]. In terms of dose, most studies have used doses ranging from 0.25 to 2 mg. Schenck and Mahowald started at 0.25–0.5 mg taken 1–2 h before bedtime [20]. The dose was increased every few nights until symptoms were controlled or side effects occurred. Clonazepam is available in disintegrating wafers for children. Side effects reported with the use of clonazepam in this setting included daytime sleepiness (morning) and memory dysfunction, as well as alopecia. The side effects resolve with a reduction of dose in most cases.

Benzodiazepines and REM behavior disorder (RBD)

Clonazepam is the treatment of choice in adults with REM sleep behavior disorder [10,23]. Schenck and colleagues described a case series of 96 patients with chronic RBD in which clonazepam was "very effective" in controlling both the violent dream and behavioral sleep disturbances [24]. In this series, clonazepam showed complete benefit in 79% of patients, and partial benefit in an additional 11%. The initial dose was 0.5 mg at bedtime and was increased as high as 2 mg. The clinical response typically occurs within the first week.

Olson and colleagues reported a case series of 93 patients with RBD in which they found that treatment with clonazepam was completely or partially successful in 87% [25]. In this series clonazepam was prescribed in 57 out of 93 patients (61%) in doses of 0.25–1.5 mg before sleep. Of 38 patients on clonazepam therapy for whom information was available (mean follow-up 23.7 months), the medication was completely successful in 21 (55%), partially successful in 12 (32%) and unsuccessful in five (13%). Nine patients reported early morning sedation, which was usually dose-related. Two patients developed early morning motor incoordination, which reportedly resolved either spontaneously or with dose adjustment. One patient developed impotence, necessitating discontinuation of the drug. Clozapine was used by two patients with dementia in whom clonazepam had failed; RBD resolved completely in one patient and partially in the other. No medication was used in 34 patients (37%). The most common reason for not prescribing medication was that the symptoms were judged to be too mild to merit medication. In 6 out of 93 patients clonazepam was not prescribed due to concomitant obstructive sleep apnea syndrome or nocturnal stridor. Finally, only 4 of the 93 patients in the series refused medication after it was offered [25].

The overall clinical experience is that tolerance is infrequent and the beneficial effects of clonazepam usually persist for several years. Although the mechanism of action of clonazepam is unclear, it seems to work via suppression of clinical motor manifestations of REM sleep rather than reducing REM sleep muscle tone. Lapierre et al. reported that clonazepam reduced behavioral manifestations and decreased phasic EMG activity without restoring tonic REM sleep muscle activity [26]. The beneficial effects of clonazepam have been attributed in part to its serotonergic properties [15]. From the two large case series, clonazepam is ineffective in only approximately 10% of patients [24,25]. Although clonazepam is effective, many of these patients are elderly, and the possibility of worsening obstructive sleep apnea (OSA) and increasing the risk of confusion or falls must be taken into consideration in individual patients. There have been no reports describing the efficacy of other benzodiazepine medications in RBD. Alternative treatments for RBD are discussed below.

Benzodiazepines and sleep bruxism

Sleep bruxism treatment options include dental splints, behavioral techniques, and medications [27]. Several medications have been studied [28]. Sleep bruxism appears to be the only parasomnia in which placebo-controlled studies have been published. Given its ubiquitous nature in sleep medicine, it is not surprising that clonazepam is one of the studied drugs [29]. Salutu and colleagues reported a randomized trial on ten patients, six women and four men, with sleep bruxism. Of note, all the patients had a concomitant movement disorder. Six of them had restless legs syndrome and four had periodic leg movement disorder. After one adaptation night, patients received placebo or 1 mg clonazepam 30 min before lights out in a single-blind study design. Objective sleep quality was determined by polysomnography, subjective sleep and awakening quality by rating scales, and objective awakening quality by psychometric tests. As compared with placebo, 1 mg clonazepam significantly improved the mean bruxism index from 9.3 to 6.3/h of sleep. Furthermore, it significantly improved the total sleep period, total sleep time, sleep efficiency, sleep latency and time awake during the total sleep period. Periodic leg movements significantly decreased. The authors reported that while the apnea index and apnea–hypopnea index increased marginally it remained within normal limits. Subjective sleep quality improved as well, although no significant changes in the other scales were reported. The authors concluded that not only did acute clonazepam therapy significantly improve the bruxism index, but also the objective and subjective sleep quality [29].

Melatonin

Melatonin (N-acetyl-5-methoxytryptamine) is most well known for its use in circadian rhythm disorders such as delayed sleep phase syndrome, jetlag and in blind patients, to help synchronize the body clock with the surrounding environment and socially accepted norms. Its use for parasomnias has been studied in patients with RBD. A recent meta-analysis cast doubts on its efficacy in some sleep disorders [30].

Perhaps because it is readily available and generally perceived to be safe, melatonin is often tried by parents either with or without their pediatrician's advice to treat sleep disorders, particularly in children with disabilities [31]. Jan et al. published a case report describing a 12-year-old child with Asperger syndrome with sleep terrors and sleepwalking responding to melatonin [17]. The parasomnia episodes occurred 2–3 times almost every night. Oral administration of controlled release melatonin (5 mg), 30 min before the desired bed time, corrected the sleep phase onset within 2 days. The sleep terrors and the sleepwalking episodes abruptly disappeared and did not recur for over six months. The authors speculated that severe sleep deprivation triggered the parasomnias, and by improving the child's total sleep time with melatonin the parasomnia trigger was corrected [17].

Although the initial treatment of choice for RBD is typically clonazepam, concerns of side effects such as worsening of OSA, side effects and risk of falls in the elderly have prompted a search for alternatives. Melatonin is a possible alternative. Although to date there are no randomized, double-blind placebo-controlled trials on the use of melatonin in RBD, there are reports of its efficacy. Kunz and Bes published a case report in 1997 in a patient with RBD who had significant difficulties falling asleep in whom melatonin was given for its sedative properties [32]. In this case report, a 64-year-old man with RBD and hypertension was given 3 mg of melatonin 10–30 min before bedtime for 5 months. He had significant difficulties with falling asleep, night waking related to the RBD and daytime sleepiness. With treatment, he was noted to have preservation of REM atonia and a reduction in phasic muscle activity with improvement in symptoms, which slowly returned once melatonin was stopped.

The same authors reported an open-label trial in six RBD patients [33]. Results were promising with five patients responding and the sixth patient known to be non-compliant. In this study again the percentage of REM without atonia reduced with melatonin. Interest piqued in the use of melatonin in RBD because the effect of reduction of REM without atonia is not an effect seen by the use of clonazepam.

These results were replicated in a study in which 13 out of 15 patients responded with reduction in REM without atonia, with most patients (9 out of 13) having 25–50% improvement in symptoms and three having 75% improvement [34]. In this study, melatonin levels were monitored, and those with lower levels prior to melatonin administration tended to respond to exogenous melatonin. Further studies are required to determine if melatonin levels are able to predict those who will respond to therapy.

Boeve *et al.* studied 14 patients with RBD and associated neurological disorders such as dementia with Lewy bodies, Parkinsonism, narcolepsy and multisystem atrophy. In this study patients were taking melatonin alone or in conjunction with clonazepam [35]. Twelve out of 14 patients showed some improvement and, interestingly, of those who had marked improvement or complete resolution of symptoms, five used melatonin alone and five used clonazepam with melatonin. This study provides follow-up for an average of 14 months, and eight patients found melatonin to be effective treatment for at least 12 months, suggesting that melatonin may be useful for long-term administration.

Although these studies have all shown the potential benefit of use of melatonin in RBD, it is unclear as to the mechanism of action in these patients. Given that melatonin is known to help in synchronization of the circadian rhythm with the environment, it is hypothesized that in RBD, that synchrony is lost and that melatonin may restore the synchronization [33]. In terms of clinical effect, melatonin has been shown to restore atonia during REM sleep which alleviates the acting out of dreams. In one patient with RBD and Alzheimer's disease, sleep became more consolidated with melatonin [36].

Melatonin is currently not an FDA-approved drug and so is not regulated. Its availability is generally from health stores. The dose of melatonin which has been studied in RBD ranges from 3 to 12 mg before bed. Patients may be started at 3 mg and the dose increased incrementally as required to achieve relief of symptoms. As noted, some patients may combine melatonin with clonazepam for resolution of symptoms if either alone has not been successful.

Reported side effects from melatonin used in RBD range from excessive sedation in the morning to headache, muscle weakness and delusions or hallucinations [34,35]. The delusions/hallucinations occurred in one patient at a dose of 12 mg, with the headaches in two patients also occurring at this dose and both side effects resolved with a lower dose regime. Only one patient was noted to discontinue melatonin due to excessive sleepiness as a side effect.

With these reports, it appears that melatonin is relatively safe to use in RBD; however, larger, double-blind, placebo-controlled trials are required to evaluate its effectiveness.

Anti-depressants

Although much research has been done with benzodiazepines in parasomnias, other classes of medications have been trialed, mostly in small studies. Tricyclic anti-depressants such as imipramine have been studied for sleep terrors and sleepwalking. In 1979, a case report was published of imipramine helping a 62-year-old woman who was described as having sleep terrors with nocturnal behaviors including screaming and violence [37]. Although this case report gives the woman a diagnosis of sleep terrors, it is possible that the woman actually had RBD, given that no polysomnogram was done. Imipramine has also been tried successfully in seven children diagnosed with sleep terrors or sleepwalking [38]. All of the patients responded with cessation of their nocturnal events, with the longest follow-up being 6 months. The significant anti-cholinerigc side effects of tricyclic medications make them unlikely to be relied on as first-line treatment for arousal-type parasomnias; however, they can be an alternative when other medications such as clonazepam are contraindicated.

Amitriptyline inhibits the re-uptake of noradrenaline and serotonin. These two effects are considered to be the likely base of the anti-depressant effect of amitriptyline. The drug also has strong anti-cholinergic effects. The plasma half-life is 12–24 h. It has been considered a treatment option for sleep bruxism, but the results of randomized trials have been mixed and overall do not support its routine use for sleep bruxism.

In 1997, Mohamed and colleagues studied ten adults with sleep bruxism using a double-blind randomized experimental design [39]. Subjects were administered amitriptyline (25 mg/night) or placebo for one week each. No improvement in pain or change in nocturnal masseteric electromyographic activities was reported using the tricyclic anti-depressant. The authors concluded that small doses of amitriptyline "cannot be recommended for the control of sleep bruxism and associated discomforts" [39]. Since this was only a one-week study, it could be argued that a longer duration may have had different results. A longer trial is described below.

More recently, Raigrodski and colleagues published a 4-week long clinical pilot study to evaluate the effect of amitriptyline on the pain-intensity level and level of stress in bruxers [40]. Using a randomized, double-blind, cross-over experimental design, ten subjects received active treatment (amitriptyline 25 mg/night) and placebo. The administration of amitriptyline for 4 weeks did not significantly reduce pain intensity; however, it significantly reduced the level of stress perception. The authors concluded that their study did not support the administration of small doses of amitriptyline for the management of pain resulting from sleep bruxism; however, it did support the administration of small doses of amitriptyline for the management of the perception of stress levels associated with sleep bruxism [40]. The same group in another publication measured the effect of amitriptyline on nocturnal masseteric activity and duration of sleep in bruxers. Using a portable EMG integrator the nocturnal, unilateral, and cumulative myoelectrical activity of the masseter muscle was recorded during the fourth and eighth weeks of the study. The results showed that amitriptyline did not significantly decrease the mean EMG activity nor did it significantly increase the duration of sleep [41].

Paroxetine has also been studied for sleep terrors, nocturnal panic attacks and sleepwalking in a case report of a 46-year-old woman with a 30-year history of parasomnias [42]. She was described as having persistent sleep terrors despite using benzodiazepines. Her situation was further complicated by the ingestion of alcohol at bedtime. Paroxetine at 20 mg in the morning was added to her clonazepam. The dose was increased to 40 mg and she was weaned off the clonazepam. Paroxetine was chosen for its anxiolytic effect as well as the serotonergic effect on sleep promotion. Paroxetine has been found to provide symptomatic relief for post-traumatic stress disorder including nightmares and insomnia complaints in placebo-controlled studies [43].

Anti-hypertensives

Due to the potential role of a rise in sympathetic activity in the pathophysiology of sleep bruxism, sympatholytic medications have been investigated for their efficacy in treating sleep bruxism. A sleep research group from Montreal specifically studied propranolol, a non-selective adrenergic beta-blocker, and clonidine, a selective alpha2-agonist, medications to determine if they would decrease sleep bruxism and prevent the rise in sympathetic activity preceding the onset of sleep bruxism [44]. Using a randomized controlled crossover study design with placebo compared to propranolol 120 mg and clonidine 0.3 mg, they studied 25 subjects with sleep bruxism. Polysomnograms were done for four nights. The first night was used as a baseline habituation night. The sleep bruxism index was estimated using masseter muscle activity. Sympathetic activity was determined using heart rate variability measured with a spectral analysis of RR intervals. Sleep and sleep bruxism variables were not significantly influenced by propranolol. As expected, propranolol decreased the mean RR intervals; however, the bruxism index was not significantly improved. With clonidine there was a reduction in both sympathetic activity as well as the bruxism index. Clonidine was associated with increased duration of stage 2 sleep and a decrease in REM sleep. The sleep bruxism index was reduced by 61%. The authors concluded that clonidine decreased sympathetic tone in the minute preceding the onset of sleep bruxism, thus reducing sleep bruxism by preventing the sequence of autonomic to motor activation of sleep bruxism. They concluded that these results supported the role of sympathetic activity in the pathophysiology of sleep bruxism. They also warned of the possibility of clonidine-induced hypotension developing in this patient population [44].

For the suppression of nightmares the use of REM-suppressing medications such as tricyclic anti-depressants and SSRIs would appear to be a rational choice despite the paucity of randomized trials [45]. Of interest is a growing literature on the use of prazosin for suppression of nightmares, in particular among military victims of post-traumatic stress disorder (PTSD) [46–49]. While treating combat-related PTSD patients with prazosin for their complaints related to benign prostate hypertrophy, patients reported an unexpected reduction in combat-related nightmares [45]. Daly *et al.* published a clinical case series of soldiers recently returned from Operation Iraqi Freedom who self-reported distressing combat trauma-related nightmares. They were prescribed 1 mg of prazosin before bedtime. The dose was increased once a week by 1 mg based on treatment response. The highest effective dose was 5 mg. Of 23 soldiers, 20 were described as having experienced marked improvement including complete elimination of nightmares, two others experienced reduced nightmare frequency or intensity, and one experienced no change. The mechanism of action for the efficacy is hypothesized as prazosin alpha1-adrenergic antagonist action, since increased CNS norepinephrine outflow and alpha1-adrenergic receptor responsiveness appear to be involved in the pathophysiologic processes of trauma-related nightmares in PTSD [46].

L-Tryptophan

L-Tryptophan has been studied for both sleep bruxism and isolated sleep paralysis. Snyder and Hams reported that L-tryptophan was effective in controlling isolated sleep paralysis in three patients. The mechanism of action would be presumably via increasing serotonin levels [50].

Etzel and colleagues performed an experiment to study the effect of L-tryptophan on sleep bruxism [51]. Portable EMG recorders were used to monitor unilateral masseter muscle activity during sleep in eight patients identified as sleep bruxers. Following an initial baseline period, the patients were given, in a randomized double-blind study, either tryptophan (50 mg/kg of body weight) or a placebo for 8 days followed by an additional 8 days of reverse medication. Dietary patterns and food intake were monitored throughout the experimental period. No significant treatment differences in bruxing levels were found, suggesting that L-tryptophan supplementation in the absence of dietary manipulation is ineffective in the treatment of sleep bruxism [51].

Other medications

Bromocriptine, a dopamine D2 receptor agonist, has been studied for the treatment of sleep bruxism. Lavigne and colleagues performed a randomized, cross-over, double-blind, placebo-controlled study of bromocriptine in seven patients with what was described as "severe and frequent" sleep bruxism [52]. The study used a cross-over design that included 2 weeks of active treatment or placebo with a washout period of 1 week. The study included the use of single photon emission computed tomography (SPECT) under both placebo and bromocriptine regimens to further evaluate whether bromocriptine influences striatal D2 receptor binding. Bromocriptine did not reduce the frequency of episodes of bruxism during sleep or the amplitude of masseter muscle contractions. SPECT also failed to reveal that either treatment had any influence on striatal D2 binding. The authors concluded that "a nightly dose of bromocriptine did not exacerbate or reduce sleep bruxism motor activity" [52].

More recently, botulinum toxin has been studied in patients with sleep bruxism. Guarda-Nardini and colleagues reported a double-blind, placebo-controlled, randomized clinical trial with a six-month follow-up period of botulinum toxin type A to treat myofascial pain symptoms and to reduce muscle hyperactivity in a small group of patients with sleep bruxism [53]. Twenty patients with an age range of 25–45 years were enrolled along with ten control subjects given saline injections. Objective and subjective clinical parameters were assessed at baseline, one week, one month, and six-month follow-up appointments. An improved range of mandibular movements and decreased pain at rest and during chewing were found in the botulinum toxin treated group compared with placebo. Patients treated with botulinum toxin had a higher subjective improvement in their perception of treatment efficacy than did the placebo subjects. Despite the small sample size, the authors concluded that botulinum toxin was an effective treatment to reduce myofascial pain symptoms in bruxers and that larger trials were warranted [53].

The anti-convulsant topiramate has been reported to be effective for sleep-related eating disorder (SRED). This is a parasomnia characterized by partial or full awakenings from sleep with compulsive eating. Different medications have been tried with various successes, but topiramate seems to be the most promising currently [54,55]. Winkelman published a retrospective chart review of 25 consecutive patients treated in an open-label trial of topiramate for SRED in a sleep disorders clinic. The mean dose of topiramate was 135 mg (range 25–300 mg) over a mean period of approximately 1 year (range 1–42 months). Over two-thirds of the patients were considered topiramate responders. Twenty-eight per cent of the patients lost more than 10% of their body weight. Adverse events were reported by 84% of patients. The most common side effects were paresthesias, excessive daytime sleepiness and sexual dysfunction. Nearly half of the responders discontinued topiramate after a mean of 1 year. The author concluded that in this open-label retrospective trial, topiramate was very effective in reducing nocturnal eating in patients. However, tolerability of topiramate was "an issue in some patients" [54].

The selective dopamine agonist, pramipexole, has also been studied for SRED by Provini *et al.* [56]. They gave 11 consecutive patients with SRED pramipexole 0.18–0.36 mg or placebo for 2 weeks using a double-blind cross-over randomized protocol. Outcomes were based on actigraphic recording and subjective sleep diary evaluations. Pramipexole was described as being well tolerated without any patient withdrawing from the study. Pramipexole reduced night-time activity and increased the number of self reported nights of good sleep [56].

Schenck and Mahowald reported on the efficacy of a cocktail of bupropion–levodopa–trazodone therapy in two adults with sleep-related eating and sleep disruption with chemical dependency [57]. One of the patients was a physician and he gained control of the nocturnal eating using bupropion-SR, 150 mg three times a day; carbidopa/L-dopa, 50/200 mg qHS; and trazodone 200 mg qHS. The second patient was a woman with a childhood history of sleepwalking. She had entered a residential program for alcohol and cocaine abuse. Her nocturnal eating, excessive awakenings, and major depression were reportedly controlled for over 2 years on a regimen of bupropion 225 mg b.i.d.; carbidopa/L-dopa 75/300 mg qHS and carbidopa/L-dopa CR 50/200 mg qHS; and trazodone 150 mg qHS. The trazodone therapy was begun one month after the start of bupropion–levodopa therapy, in order to control excessive awakenings that had persisted despite control of nocturnal eating.

Conclusions

There is a need for greater information on the pharmacological management of parasomnias. With our current knowledge, benzodiazepines are useful in the treatment of arousal parasomnias, RBD and sleep bruxism. Melatonin may be an alternative for RBD, and anti-depressants have some role in the treatment of nightmares. Anti-hypertensives and botulinum toxin have potential for treatment of sleep bruxism. Various medications have been used for nocturnal eating syndrome, with topiramate, when tolerated, being a good choice. Pharmacological guidelines need to be developed not only for adults, but specifically for children. Ideally, these guidelines should be FDA-approved for the parasomnias. Development of easy to swallow, chewable or liquid forms of these medications may be needed. Training programs should play a leading role in enhancing the clinician's knowledge of the pharmacological treatment of parasomnias. Given the diversity of the different parasomnias, a surprisingly relatively narrow spectrum of medications has been reported to be effective. Is this wholly or in part due to an absence of pharmacological creativity or excessive caution on the part of clinicians, or is it perhaps that these seemingly disparate conditions have unidentified pathophysiologic mechanisms in common?

References

1. Gupta M, Aneja S, Kohli K. Add-on melatonin improves sleep behavior in children with epilepsy: Randomized, double-blind, placebo-controlled trial. *J Child Neurol* 2005; **20**: 112–5.

2. Schnoes CJ, Kuhn BR, Workman EF, Ellis CR. Pediatric prescribing practices for clonidine and other pharmacologic agents for children with sleep disturbance. *Clin Pediatr (Phila)* 2006; **45**: 229–38.

3. Owens JA, Rosen CL, Mindell JA. Medication use in the treatment of pediatric insomnia: Results of a survey of community-based pediatricians. *Pediatrics* 2003; **111**: e628–35.

4. Stojanovski SD, Rasu RS, Balkrishnan R, Nahata MC. Trends in medication prescribing for pediatric sleep difficulties in US outpatient settings. *Sleep* 2007; **30**: 1013–7.

5. Pelayo R, Chen W, Monzon S, Guilleminault C. Pediatric sleep pharmacology: You want to give my kid sleeping pills? *Pediatr Clin North Am* 2004; **51**: 117–34.

6. Zito JM, Safer DJ, dosReis S, Gardner JF, Boles M, Lynch F. Trends in the prescribing of psychotropic medications to preschoolers. *J Am Med Assoc* 2000; **283**: 1025–30.

7. AASM. *International Classification of Sleep Disorders.* 2nd ed. Westchester, Illinois: American Academy of Sleep Medicine, 2005.

8. Ashton H. Guidelines for the rational use of benzodiazepines. When and what to use. *Drugs* 1994; **48**: 25–40.

Section 6: Therapy of parasomnias

9. Wills L, Garcia J. Parasomnias: Epidemiology and management. *CNS Drugs* 2002; **16**: 803–10.
10. Mahowald MW, Schenck CH, Bornemann MA. Pathophysiologic mechanisms in REM sleep behavior disorder. *Curr Neurol Neurosci Rep* 2007; **7**: 167–72.
11. Schenck CH, Arnulf I, Mahowald MW. Sleep and sex: What can go wrong? A review of the literature on sleep related disorders and abnormal sexual behaviors and experiences. *Sleep* 2007; **30**: 683–702.
12. Paul V, Krishnamoorthy MS. The antimyoclonic action of clonazepam through a GABA-independent mechanism. *Indian J Physiol Pharmacol* 1989; **33**: 243–6.
13. Tenn CC, Niles LP. Mechanisms underlying the antidopaminergic effect of clonazepam and melatonin in striatum. *Neuropharmacology* 1997; **36**: 1659–63.
14. Jenner P, Pratt JA, Marsden CD. Mechanism of action of clonazepam in myoclonus in relation to effects on GABA and 5-HT. *Adv Neurol* 1986; **43**: 629–43.
15. Chadwick D, Hallett M, Harris R, Jenner P, Reynolds EH, Marsden CD. Clinical, biochemical, and physiological features distinguishing myoclonus responsive to 5-hydroxytryptophan, tryptophan with a monoamine oxidase inhibitor, and clonazepam. *Brain* 1977; **100**: 455–87.
16. Sohal VS, Keist R, Rudolph U, Huguenard JR. Dynamic GABA(A) receptor subtype-specific modulation of the synchrony and duration of thalamic oscillations. *J Neurosci* 2003; **23**: 3649–57.
17. Jan JE, Freeman RD, Wasdell MB, Bomben MM. A child with severe night terrors and sleep-walking responds to melatonin therapy. *Dev Med Child Neurol* 2004; **46**: 789.
18. Guilleminault C, Palombini L, Pelayo R, Chervin RD. Sleepwalking and sleep terrors in prepubertal children: What triggers them? *Pediatrics* 2003; **111**: e17–25.
19. Schenck CH, Milner DM, Hurwitz TD, Bundlie SR, Mahowald MW. A polysomnographic and clinical report on sleep-related injury in 100 adult patients. *Am J Psychiatry* 1989; **146**: 1166–73.
20. Schenck CH, Mahowald MW. Long-term, nightly benzodiazepine treatment of injurious parasomnias and other disorders of disrupted nocturnal sleep in 170 adults. *Am J Med* 1996; **100**: 333–7.
21. Schenck CH, Mahowald MW. Two cases of premenstrual sleep terrors and injurious sleep-walking. *J Psychosom Obstet Gynaecol* 1995; **16**: 79–84.
22. Remulla A, Guilleminault C. Somnambulism (sleepwalking). *Expert Opin Pharmacother* 2004; **5**: 2069–74.
23. Gagnon JF, Postuma RB, Montplaisir J. Update on the pharmacology of REM sleep behavior disorder. *Neurology* 2006; **67**: 742–7.
24. Schenck CH, Hurwitz TD, Mahowald MW. Symposium: Normal and abnormal REM sleep regulation. REM sleep behaviour disorder: An update on a series of 96 patients and a review of the world literature. *J Sleep Res* 1993; **2**: 224–31.
25. Olson EJ, Boeve BF, Silber MH. Rapid eye movement sleep behaviour disorder: Demographic, clinical and laboratory findings in 93 cases. *Brain* 2000; **123**: 331–9.
26. Lapierre O, Montplaisir J. Polysomnographic features of REM sleep behavior disorder: Development of a scoring method. *Neurology* 1992; **42**: 1371–4.
27. Lobbezoo F, Van Der Zaag J, van Selms MK, Hamburger HL, Naeije M. Principles for the management of bruxism. *J Oral Rehabil* 2008; **35**: 509–23.
28. Huynh NT, Rompre PH, Montplaisir JY, Manzini C, Okura K, Lavigne GJ. Comparison of various treatments for sleep bruxism using determinants of number needed to treat and effect size. *Int J Prosthodont* 2006; **19**: 435–41.
29. Saletu A, Parapatics S, Saletu B, *et al*. On the pharmacotherapy of sleep bruxism: Placebo-controlled polysomnographic and psychometric studies with clonazepam. *Neuropsychobiology* 2005; **51**: 214–25.
30. Buscemi N, Vandermeer B, Hooton N, *et al*. Efficacy and safety of exogenous melatonin for secondary sleep disorders and sleep disorders accompanying sleep restriction: Meta-analysis. *Br Med J* 2006; **332**: 385–93.
31. Sajith SG, Clarke D. Melatonin and sleep disorders associated with intellectual disability: A clinical review. *J Intellect Disabil Res* 2007; **51**: 2–13.
32. Kunz D, Bes F. Melatonin effects in a patient with severe REM sleep behavior disorder: Case report and theoretical considerations. *Neuropsychobiology* 1997; **36**: 211–4.
33. Kunz D, Bes F. Melatonin as a therapy in REM sleep behavior disorder patients: An open-labeled pilot study on the possible influence of melatonin on REM-sleep regulation. *Mov Disord* 1999; **14**: 507–11.
34. Takeuchi N, Uchimura N, Hashizume Y, *et al*. Melatonin therapy for REM sleep behavior disorder. *Psychiatry Clin Neurosci* 2001; **55**: 267–9.
35. Boeve BF, Silber MH, Ferman TJ. Melatonin for treatment of REM sleep behavior disorder in neurologic disorders: Results in 14 patients. *Sleep Med* 2003; **4**: 281–4.
36. Anderson KN, Jamieson S, Graham AJ, Shneerson JM. REM sleep behaviour disorder treated with melatonin

in a patient with Alzheimer's disease. *Clin Neurol Neurosurg* 2008; **110**: 492–5.

37. Beitman BD, Carlin AS. Night terrors treated with imipramine. *Am J Psychiatry* 1979; **136**: 1087–8.

38. Pesikoff RB, Davis PC. Treatment of pavor nocturnus and somnambulism in children. *Am J Psychiatry* 1971; **128**: 778–81.

39. Mohamed SE, Christensen LV, Penchas J. A randomized double-blind clinical trial of the effect of amitriptyline on nocturnal masseteric motor activity (sleep bruxism). *Cranio* 1997; **15**: 326–32.

40. Raigrodski AJ, Mohamed SE, Gardiner DM. The effect of amitriptyline on pain intensity and perception of stress in bruxers. *J Prosthodont* 2001; **10**: 73–7.

41. Raigrodski AJ, Christensen LV, Mohamed SE, Gardiner DM. The effect of four-week administration of amitriptyline on sleep bruxism. A double-blind cross-over clinical study. *Cranio* 2001; **19**: 21–5.

42. Lillywhite AR, Wilson SJ, Nutt DJ. Successful treatment of night terrors and somnambulism with paroxetine. *Br J Psychiatry* 1994; **164**: 551–4.

43. Stein DJ, Davidson J, Seedat S, Beebe K. Paroxetine in the treatment of post-traumatic stress disorder: Pooled analysis of placebo-controlled studies. *Expert Opin Pharmacother* 2003; **4**: 1829–38.

44. Huynh N, Lavigne GJ, Lanfranchi PA, Montplaisir JY, de Champlain J. The effect of two sympatholytic medications – propranolol and clonidine – on sleep bruxism: Experimental randomized controlled studies. *Sleep* 2006; **29**: 307–16.

45. van Liempt S, Vermetten E, Geuze E, Westenberg H. Pharmacotherapeutic treatment of nightmares and insomnia in posttraumatic stress disorder: An overview of the literature. *Ann NY Acad Sci* 2006; **1071**: 502–07.

46. Daly CM, Doyle ME, Radkind M, Raskind E, Daniels C. Clinical case series: The use of Prazosin for combat-related recurrent nightmares among Operation Iraqi Freedom combat veterans. *Mil Med* 2005; **170**: 513–5.

47. Peskind ER, Bonner LT, Hoff DJ, Raskind MA. Prazosin reduces trauma-related nightmares in older men with chronic posttraumatic stress disorder. *J Geriatr Psychiatry Neurol* 2003; **16**: 165–71.

48. Taylor F, Raskind MA. The alpha1-adrenergic antagonist prazosin improves sleep and nightmares in civilian trauma posttraumatic stress disorder. *J Clin Psychopharmacol* 2002; **22**: 82–5.

49. Raskind MA, Thompson C, Petrie EC, *et al*. Prazosin reduces nightmares in combat veterans with posttraumatic stress disorder. *J Clin Psychiatry* 2002; **63**: 565–8.

50. Snyder S, Hams G. Serotoninergic agents in the treatment of isolated sleep paralysis. *Am J Psychiatry* 1982; **139**: 1202–03.

51. Etzel KR, Stockstill JW, Rugh JD, Fisher JG. Tryptophan supplementation for nocturnal bruxism: Report of negative results. *J Craniomandib Disord* 1991; **5**: 115–20.

52. Lavigne GJ, Soucy JP, Lobbezoo F, Manzini C, Blanchet PJ, Montplaisir JY. Double-blind, cross-over, placebo-controlled trial of bromocriptine in patients with sleep bruxism. *Clin Neuropharmacol* 2001; **24**: 145–9.

53. Guarda-Nardini L, Manfredini D, Salamone M, Salmaso L, Tonello S, Ferronato G. Efficacy of botulinum toxin in treating myofascial pain in bruxers: A controlled placebo pilot study. *Cranio* 2008; **26**: 126–35.

54. Winkelman JW. Efficacy and tolerability of open-label topiramate in the treatment of sleep-related eating disorder: A retrospective case series. *J Clin Psychiatry* 2006; **67**: 1729–34.

55. Winkelman JW. Treatment of nocturnal eating syndrome and sleep-related eating disorder with topiramate. *Sleep Med* 2003; **4**: 243–6.

56. Provini F, Albani F, Vetrugno R, *et al*. A pilot double-blind placebo-controlled trial of low-dose pramipexole in sleep-related eating disorder. *Eur J Neurol* 2005; **12**: 432–6.

57. Schenck CH, Mahowald MW. Combined bupropion–levodopa–trazodone therapy of sleep-related eating and sleep disruption in two adults with chemical dependency. *Sleep* 2000; **23**: 587–8.

Section 6 Chapter 32

Therapy of parasomnias

Behavioral and psychiatric treatment of parasomnias

Shelby F. Harris and Michael J. Thorpy

Introduction

The successful management of parasomnias frequently requires a combination of pharmacologic, psychological and behavioral treatments. Oftentimes, these events are considered unimportant (or untreatable) events, but a knowledgeable clinician can use them as clues to uncover a significant sleep disorder and to generate a comprehensive treatment plan.

In the past, clinicians relied upon traditional pharmacologic agents (e.g. REM suppressants); however, a number of additional treatments are becoming available. With newer forms of psychotherapy, including various treatment approaches underneath the umbrella term "cognitive behavior therapy", as well as various other treatment options from hypnotherapy to scheduled awakenings, this chapter presents a review of the behavioral and pharmacological treatments commonly recommended for parasomnias (divided into NREM events, REM events, and events in transition between sleep and wakefulness, as treatment options are different depending upon the distinction). This chapter will also include a brief review of the literature, and the various treatment options will be discussed to give the clinician a better understanding of the current available treatment approaches.

Treatment of arousal disorders (sleepwalking, night terrors, confusional arousals, sleep-related eating, sleepsex)

Disorders of arousal generally encompass the following diagnoses: sleepwalking, night terrors, confusional arousals, sleepsex disorders and sleep-related eating disorders. The overall behavioral and pharmacological treatment for these disorders has significant overlap and will be discussed as a whole, with disorder-specific treatment recommendations mentioned throughout.

A high prevalence of arousal disorders exists in the general population, and these are mild, occur in childhood and resolve with time. Formal overnight polysomnography (PSG) should be limited to patients whose behaviors cause serious physical damage, are violent, or are extremely bothersome to other individuals. When determining the course of treatment for arousal disorders, the clinician should consider the overall frequency and severity of the episodes, as most arousal disorders are mild and pharmacological intervention is generally not indicated. Treatment may also be necessary for any other sleep disorders (e.g. sleep apnea) that occur concurrently and may trigger arousals.

Education

Education is paramount in addressing all disorders of arousal. All patients should be informed of the parasomnia diagnosis and educated about the pathophysiology and any associated features that might increase its chances of recurring. Patients and family should be advised that many disorders of arousal do not require intervention and that events will often reduce in frequency over time.

When working with children, it is especially important to educate parents about the diagnosis, as some parents may believe these events signal symptoms of underlying medical illness or psychological trauma. Note that while stress may be a factor in disorders of arousal, it should not be the clinician's first assumption – especially with children.

Chapter 32: Behavioral and psychiatric treatment

Table 32.1 Safety suggestions for patients with violent and dangerous behaviors during sleep.

Place mattress on floor
Remove obstructions from room
Remove and/or lock away dangerous objects
Remove coat hooks from door
Sleep in a separate bed from bed partner
Cover windows and glass doors with thick drapes
Lock doors with a double cylinder lock
Light outside hallways
Place gates at top of staircases and in doorways
Put bells on outside of doors
Install alarm systems to alert when someone has left the room or house

Refrain from engaging the patient mid-episode

Household members should be instructed to avoid confronting patients during events, and instead quietly guide the patient back to bed with the goal of not waking the patient. Engaging the patient can prolong the event and confrontation may worsen a patient's behavior, possibly resulting in violence.

Safety

Safety is most important when treating patients with disorders of arousal. Traditional problem-solving can prove beneficial when working with this patient population. No single solution works with every patient, and safety concerns must be addressed and tailored to each individual. Placing the mattress on the floor, sleeping in a separate bed from the bed partner, covering windows and glass doors with thick drapes and moving gates to the top of staircases and in doorways can help to reduce risk of injury. Refer to Table 32.1 for a list of safety suggestions that can be recommended to patients.

Practice good sleep hygiene and sleep scheduling

Good sleep hygiene can help to eliminate potential arousals. Regular sleep–wake times and obtaining sufficient sleep are important, as sleep deprivation has been linked to arousals. Sources of arousal, such as extraneous sound or light, should be minimized. Limiting extraneous sound through the use of ear plugs or a white noise machine is recommended. Blocking external light and noise by installing heavy light-blocking shades is also suggested. Exercise, drugs and alcohol in the evening should be avoided (see Chapter 6 for more information).

Scheduled awakenings

Several case studies have found scheduled awakenings helpful in reducing night-time events. Although the exact mechanism of its action remains unclear, scheduled awakenings may reduce the overall duration of slow-wave sleep [1,2]. One treatment that is most likely to be successful when the episodes occur nightly is to wake the patient (usually by the parent or a household member) 15 min before the time of the usual first arousal. A thorough sleep diary should be kept (by parents) on a nightly basis to document the time of each arousal episode. The patient must be awakened enough to be able to open the eyes and then say a few words. The parents/observers must continue to wake the patient in this fashion on a nightly basis before each arousal for one month, until the events subside. If the arousal events re-occur, the treatment is reinstated. One should proceed with caution when using this treatment, however, as this may worsen the arousals.

Psychotherapy

When underlying psychological issues are evident (such as anxiety, depression, trauma or heightened stress), psychotherapy has been reported to be useful in overall treatment of disorders of arousal [3]. Psychopathology is believed to be more frequent in adults presenting with arousal disorders and any adult should be assessed for specific psychiatric comorbidities. However, limited data exist on the overall efficacy of psychotherapy in the treatment of parasomnias, as its usefulness has primarily been demonstrated anecdotally through case studies. Kales and colleagues [3] present a series of three case studies of three adult male patients who were all married, had at least 12 years of education, and came to their sleep lab with long-standing disorders of arousal. Through treatment with an active and directive psychodynamic therapist, the night-terror patient develops an increased awareness of how he internalizes emotional states and acquires appropriate ways to express aggressive emotions. As the patient becomes better able to cope with stressful life events, he develops more self-esteem. As this occurs, he gradually becomes able to work through long-standing emotional conflicts, therefore reducing the internalized conflict and aggression that often present as night terrors.

Stress management

Stress management treatments are generally recommended as strain can precipitate events. The beneficial effects of muscle relaxation on disorders of arousal have been reported in both children and adults. Progressive muscle relaxation (PMR) [4], practiced just before bedtime, has been found to be helpful anecdotally and in case reports [5]. Limited larger-scale trials have demonstrated the efficacy of muscle relaxation on disorders of arousal.

Hypnosis

Hypnosis will be covered in more detail in Chapter 33. Several case studies and small case series have been reported in the literature documenting the usefulness of hypnosis in the treatment of disorders of arousal, particularly sleepwalking and night terrors [6–8]. Some have noted that the decrease in tonic levels due to the reduction induced through hypnosis may help to decrease events [9]. However, a recent publication by Hauri and colleagues [10] notes that hypnosis was found to be helpful at initial and five-year follow-up in most parasomnias, but was less beneficial for night terrors. Further study may delineate any role that hypnosis plays in the treatment of disorders of arousal.

Medications

Medications for parasomnias will be covered in more detail in Chapter 31. Pharmacological treatment becomes necessary when events become frequent, put the family and/or patient at risk of being harmed, or disturb family life. Benzodiazepines (e.g. clonazepam, diazepam and temazepam) have been successfully used to reduce both arousals and slow-wave sleep. They can be used continuously or during times when great risk for harm is suspected. Some patients have responded well to desipramine, paroxetine and imipramine, but few cases have been reported. Patients with sleep-related eating disorders have been reported to respond well to topiramate [11].

Treatment of REM-related parasomnias

Nightmares

Despite the widespread prevalence of nightmares and emerging availability of effective nightmare treatment options, many clinicians are still unaware of the psychiatric and medical toll that chronic nightmares can have on patients. Frequent nightmares can lead to disturbed sleep onset latency, awakenings, restless sleep, insomnia and a lower overall quality of life [12].

Psychotherapeutic approaches

Imagery rehearsal therapy

To date, cognitive behavioral treatments (CBT) for nightmares have received the most empirical support for nightmare treatment [13], with imagery rehearsal therapy (IRT) being the most researched of all interventions. As a result, IRT is often suggested as a first-line or adjunctive therapy for the treatment of nightmares [14,15].

Patients with chronic nightmares often feel as if they have lost control over their nightmares. IRT gives patients ways to be in command of the night-time. Originally developed to treat idiopathic nightmares, IRT is now often used to treat both idiopathic and post-traumatic nightmares. IRT consists of writing down a nightmare, changing it in any way the patient wishes, writing down the changed dream and rehearsing the new changed dream imaginally for between 5 and 20 min per day [16]. Ideally, participants are encouraged to begin with nightmares that are less distressing overall and (if applicable to the patient) not an exact replication of any trauma. As this can be modified into a generally simple technique, most research protocols have tested this treatment in a group format [16–19].

Krakow and colleagues [16] conducted a randomized wait-list-controlled trial that tested group-format IRT for chronic nightmares in 168 sexual assault survivors. Improvements were significant (compared to wait-list control) from baseline to 3-month follow-up in the IRT group in nightmares and PTSD severity with moderate improvements seen on sleep quality and post-treatment PTSD symptom severity.

This study was limited by its lack of a placebo control group, its large drop-out rates on follow-up, reliance on retrospective self-report measures and a sizeable number of participants being in psychotherapy or pharmacotherapy at the time of treatment, possibly adding a confounding variable.

Krakow and colleagues obtained similar results when they implemented IRT in a group of 62 crime victims with PTSD, nightmares and insomnia. IRT was combined with primary cognitive behavior therapy for insomnia (including sleep hygiene, stimulus control, sleep restriction and cognitive restructuring) [20]. Ten hours of group treatment were administered over a total of four sessions. At 3-month follow-up, significant reductions were noted in both nightmare frequency and insomnia with smaller reductions seen in PTSD symptoms.

In an expansion of IRT, Krakow et al. [21] more recently developed sleep dynamic therapy (SDT), a program consisting of CBT for insomnia, IRT, and emotional processing. Patients are also taught to compare their sleep to that of normal sleepers in order to help them recognize the markers of poor sleep quality, and also to identify any sleep movement disorders or sleep-disordered breathing. SDT was administered in one large group in six 2-h weekly group sessions to 66 fire evacuees, all of whom were experiencing PTSD, nightmares and insomnia. Results indicated moderate reductions in sleep quality, sleep efficiency and total sleep time, with only small effects at 12-week follow-up. These modest improvements at follow-up may be a result of the high number of sleep-disordered breathing in the population [21], as well as difficulties dealing with highly personal and emotional information in such a large group [22]. Since no control group was included, no definitive conclusions can be made regarding the SDT's overall effects.

Imagery rehearsal therapy is reported to be successful at reducing nightmares, with nightmare improvement in as many as 90% or more of individuals who use the technique [23]. Still, there are some limitations to the use of IRT. Some patients may find imagery to be too difficult or may be flooded by negative imagery. These patients may need initial structured guidance in positive imagery practice and specific cognitive behavioral interventions to help manage negative imagery that arises during subsequent IRT practice. In addition, most of the research on IRT has been conducted by the same research group [13]; further studies are warranted to compare IRT with other techniques such as exposure, pharmacological treatment (e.g. prazosin), and with larger samples for greater statistical power.

Psychodynamic psychotherapy

A variety of nightmare treatments have been reported in the literature. For many years, traditional models of psychotherapy viewed nightmares as a symptom of a larger primary psychiatric illness. The aim of this treatment was the primary psychiatric diagnosis through resolution of underlying internal conflict, with the understanding that the nightmares would ultimately resolve [24]. There is no empirical support demonstrating the use of traditional psychotherapeutic models in the treatment of nightmares [25], and a discussion of its effectiveness cannot be made presently.

Several studies have demonstrated that successful treatment of nightmares leads to improvements in both sleep quality and overall quality of life. This suggests that nightmares are not just a symptom of a primary psychiatric disorder, but may instead be a primary disorder [18,19]. This line of research has a number of implications for the traditional models of nightmare treatment, placing less emphasis on the nightmare as a symptom and more on nightmares as a sole diagnostic entity.

Prolonged exposure for PTSD

Nightmares are commonly seen in patients with PTSD [26]. While one might postulate that treating the underlying PTSD using well-established treatments for such a diagnosis might be warranted, the research does not presently maintain this viewpoint.

Prolonged exposure, a treatment developed by Foa and colleagues for PTSD [27], is a highly effective treatment for PTSD and has been studied in numerous well-controlled trials across a wide variety of trauma survivors. Prolonged exposure is often recommended as a first-line treatment for PTSD [28], although most studies have not investigated the impact of this intervention upon sleep disturbance (a common complaint reported in patients with PTSD).

Two studies have researched the effects of prolonged exposure on nightmares, and the results are inconclusive [29,30]. In both studies, CBT reduced recurrent and frequent nightmares, and in one of the studies, nearly half of the patients reported continuing difficulties with insomnia.

Continued research is warranted in this field, with a particular emphasis on sleep outcomes. This will ultimately help with modifications in overall treatment plans and aid in the understanding of what treatments best help patients with specific symptoms.

Relaxation strategies

Only a few studies exist which investigate relaxation strategies in the treatment of nightmare disorder [31,32]. Miller and DiPilato [31] compared PMR [4], systematic desensitization, and wait-list control in 32 patients with nightmares. Results from this study indicated that overall, both relaxation and systematic desensitization both showed reduction in nightmare intensity, with 80% reduction in nightmares in 63% of the clients. More favorable outcomes were noted for systematic desensitization at 25-week follow-up, with clients in this group reporting significantly reduced nightmare intensity.

Burgess and colleagues [32] researched PMR [4], self-exposure and wait-list control in 170 adults with primary nightmares. At both one- and six-month follow-up, the exposure group reported greater improvements in nightmare frequency than the other groups. The dropout rate was high in the self-exposure group, and in those that were single.

Exposure and systematic desensitization (SD)

Exposure therapy for nightmares generally consists of a patient writing down a nightmare and then "reliving" the nightmare in the imagination until the anxiety decreases. The patient is generally instructed to engage in daily practice of this nightmare imagining. Any anxiety produced from the nightmare practice comes to a peak and is recorded on a homework sheet. The patient continues the exercise until the anxiety has subsided by at least half of the peak. The goal is to expose the patient to the anxiety, sometimes working from least anxiety-arousing nightmares to the most feared ones so that the patient eventually habituates to the anxiety. The patient must avoid any distraction during the exercise, as any diversions will prevent the anxiety from properly habituating. While relaxation and other coping techniques may be taught before and after the exercise, their use during the exercise is discouraged to increase anxiety and heighten overall habituation.

Limited research exists to draw any specific conclusions regarding exposure therapy. As discussed in detail earlier, Burgess and colleagues [32] report the only straight exposure studies comparing exposure with self-relaxation. The exposure group reported improvement at both one- and six-month follow-up.

Systematic desensitization, developed by Wolpe [33], is another form of exposure therapy, but utilizes coping strategies such as relaxation techniques. To begin SD for nightmare treatment, the patient is first taught relaxation skills by a trained clinician with the understanding that these skills will help counter fear and anxiety responses. The therapist works with the patient to create a hierarchy of nightmares, from least to most feared (similar to traditional exposure). After the patient has learned relaxation techniques, the patient then learns to apply them while imagining nightmares (e.g. Cellucci and Lawrence [12] set a time limit on the practice for two imaginations for each nightmare, with the first practice of 10–15 s and the second for 25–30 s). The patient can also be taught additional coping strategies such as positive self-statements (e.g. "I can do this") or any cognitive therapy for overestimations or catastrophizing to use during the nightmare practice.

Traditional exposure (discussed earlier) is now generally favored over SD in most CBT treatment protocols for anxiety disorders in order to maximize habituation through denying coping strategies only during the exposure exercise. That being said, however, in nightmare treatment, there is a scarcity of research to draw any firm conclusions as SD has been shown to be effective. Future studies with ample power should compare traditional exposure to SD and IRT.

As noted earlier, Miller and DiPilato [31] compared relaxation training, SD and wait-list controls. Results indicate that although SD and PMR both faired well immediately post-treatment with nightmare reduction and intensity, SD had superior rates at 25-week follow-up as compared to relaxation.

Cellucci and Lawrence [12] contrasted SD to continuous nightmare self-recording and a placebo nightmare discussion group in a total sample of 29 patients over an 8-week period. Results indicated that short-term SD treatment was superior to both group discussion placebo and nightmare recording on measures of nightmare frequency and intensity.

One study compared IRT with SD and could not conclude that one treatment was more effective than the other [34]. Lancee [35] suggests that a trend may exist for IRT to reduce some affective difficulties and recommends further investigation with greater power comparing IRT to desensitization. Studies with larger sample sizes are also warranted.

Nightmare recording

Recording has inconsistently reduced nightmare frequency, and has not been shown to successfully reduce complaints commonly associated with chronic nightmares such as anxiety, depression and reduced quality of life [12,31,34].

Neidhart and colleagues compared IRT to nightmare recording in a group of 20 subjects with chronic nightmares. Both nightmare recording and IRT participants were instructed to write down their nightmares for a total of one month. Recording participants received no further treatment. IRT participants received one-session instructions of IRT with standard imagery rehearsal techniques. Results indicated a significant decrease in the nightmare frequency in both treatment groups. Neidhardt and colleagues are unsure of the reasons behind this given the inconsistency in previous research. Of note, self-rated distress decreased significantly in the IRT group.

Lucid dreaming treatment (LDT)

In LDT, nightmare sufferers learn to change the nightmare directly within the nightmare itself. Increased rates of lucid dreaming have been found in those with greater nightmare frequencies, and it has been suggested that nightmares may elicit lucid dreaming [36].

A few case studies have investigated the effects of LDT upon nightmares, and each has shown reductions in nightmare frequencies [37–39]. One study investigated LDT on a large scale [40]. Spoormaker and van den Bout randomly divided 23 nightmare sufferers into three groups: one group ($n = 8$) received one 2-h individual LDT session, a second group ($n = 8$) received one 2-h group LDT session, and the third group ($n = 7$) was placed on a wait-list. Significant, although modest, reductions in nightmare frequency were noted with LDT treatment as compared to wait-list controls. Those who were in individual LDT treatment appeared to have greater reductions in nightmare frequency than those who were in group LDT. The role of lucidity in dreaming is unclear as only 6 of the 16 patients were able to become lucid while having a nightmare and could then alter the dream. Five patients indicated a reduction in nightmares, but did so without any lucidity whatsoever. Although nightmare frequency was reduced in a number of patients, there was no reduction or change in PTSD symptom severity (although PTSD severity was quite low to begin with). The investigation of Spoormaker and van den Bout [40] was a pilot study and lacked statistical power. Longer-term follow-up data were not gathered. The effects of other therapeutic factors such as therapist attention, exposure, mastery and lucidity were not controlled for; therefore any conclusions regarding the chief therapeutic mode of action in LDT cannot be drawn. Given the lack of data on LDT overall, any conclusions regarding its efficacy should be made with caution.

Hypnosis

Hypnosis has been reported to be helpful in nightmare treatment [41]. Under hypnosis, the patient can gain mastery over the nightmare by changing a part of the dream or creating a less frightening ending [41]. Hauri and colleagues [10] report on a 5-year follow-up study of hypnosis with 36 patients (age range 6–16, mean age 32.7 years). Results indicate that hypnosis was an effective treatment in both short- and long-term follow-up with nightmares, with 67% of the patients being symptom-free or much improved at 5-year follow-up. Additional information on hypnosis in parasomnias is covered in Chapter 33.

Pharmacologic treatments for nightmares

Although some promising pharmacological treatments for nightmares are available, it should be noted that a number of common medications have been linked to causing or increasing nightmares. Such pharmacological agents include amphetamines, beta-blockers, sedative/hypnotics, and anti-depressants – especially those that react with norepinephrine, dopamine and serotonin [42].

Prazosin

Prazosin is a drug that blocks central alpha-1-adrenoceptors and is generally non-sedating. It has been safely used for many years in general medicine to treat hypertension. In their initial work with prazosin, Taylor and Raskind [43] suggest that CNS alpha-1 adrenergic receptor stimulation disrupts sleep physiology and leads to the heightened reactivity seen as the basis of PTSD. They hypothesize that a pharmacologic blockade of postsynaptic alpha-1 receptors could provide symptomatic relief from trauma nightmares, sleep disturbance and other PTSD symptoms [43].

An initial four patient, 6-week open-label trial of prazosin (1–4 mg/day) in patients with PTSD demonstrated reductions in sleep disruption and nightmares [43]. Follow-up research by Raskind and his team

[44] has evaluated prazosin (13.3 ± 3 mg/day) versus placebo in reducing nightmares, depressive symptoms, and insomnia in 40 combat veterans with PTSD. Results indicated that prazosin was superior to placebo in reducing trauma nightmares, insomnia and depressive symptomatology.

Early studies of prazosin have shown very clear and promising results for its use in nightmare treatment [43,44]. However, it appears that prazosin must be used continuously in order to maintain effects, otherwise nightmares will likely return upon drug withdrawal.

Anti-depressants

Older research investigating the use of anti-depressants on idiopathic nightmares has been poor, but their application to PTSD-related nightmares has been inconclusive at best and deserves more attention [45]. Certain SSRIs (e.g. sertraline) have been linked to insomnia, and further evaluation is needed to understand this side effect profile as well as their impact upon insomnia.

The Expert Consensus Guideline Series on the treatment of PTSD suggests that SSRIs should be the first-line treatment for patients with any variant of this disorder, placing emphasis upon paroxetine, fluoxetine and sertraline [28].

Some investigators have found fluvoxamine to be helpful in the treatment of nightmares. Neylan and colleagues [46] investigated fluvoxamine (150 mg/day; range 100–250 mg/day) in an open-label trial of 21 combat veterans with PTSD. The authors suggest that SSRIs may reduce nightmares by altering amygdala activation during REM sleep, as improvements were seen in PTSD symptomatology, depression, subjective sleep quality, trauma-related combat dreams and sleep maintenance.

Nefazodone, trazodone, and cyproheptadine – agents that potentiate serotonin while also acting as serotonin 5-HT2 receptor agonists – have also been demonstrated to improve sleep disturbances – especially in patients with PTSD [47].

Trazodone, approved by the FDA solely for the treatment of depression, is commonly used in psychiatry for its hypnotic side effects as a treatment for insomnia [28]. Research investigating trazodone in the use of nightmares is scarce, although two studies have successfully demonstrated its use as a treatment for patients with PTSD, insomnia and nightmares [48,49]. Conclusions regarding its future use as a treatment for nightmares should not be made until more research is conducted.

Mixed results have been found regarding TCAs and MAOIs for the treatment of nightmares; most studies have investigated their use in patients with PTSD, with phenelzine showing the best results [50]. Given poor patient compliance and adverse effect profiles, MAOIs and TCAs are not likely to be studied in greater detail. These medications are generally used as sedatives when all other treatments have failed. Clinicians should be aware of the limited data available regarding the effectiveness of MAOIs and TCAs.

REM sleep behavior disorder (RBD)

The current treatment of choice for RBD is clonazepam [51]. Melatonin [52], levodopa [53] and pramipexole [54] have also been reported to be useful treatments. Although RBD can be managed quite well with medication, behavioral measures can be useful for certain patients and should be put in place before medications take effect. Safety is paramount, and the same measures should be taken to keep the room safe as was suggested earlier in this chapter for disorders of arousal. The patient's bed partner should sleep in a separate bed until the episodes are well controlled. Education of the patient and family is important, as any violent episodes can cause strain in relationships due to misunderstanding and fear.

Treatment of events in transition between sleep and wakefulness

Nocturnal panic disorder

Cognitive behavioral therapy

CBT for nocturnal panic (NP) has recently been investigated by Craske and colleagues [55,56], and initial results support the efficacy of this approach. CBT is effective for the more general diagnosis of panic disorder, with 85–100% of individuals completing treatment being panic-free post-treatment [57]. However, NP has rarely been investigated as a specific outcome measure.

CBT for panic typically consists of 11 60-min sessions. Initial sessions focus upon education about panic attacks and provide patients with information regarding the physiological aspects of the fight/flight response in relation to both daytime and nocturnal panic attacks. Patients are taught the cycle of panic, leading from misattribution of internal sensations (e.g. increased heart rate) that might be catastrophized (e.g. heart attack). This increased anxiety may signal a panic attack, therefore further solidifying this belief. Patients begin to avoid specific situations that might lead to physiological arousal for fear that such situations will lead to a panic attack, which leads to certain situations becoming associated with panic attacks.

NP patients are taught that a heightened sensitivity to anxiety sensations leads them to notice subtle changes in physiology during sleep. Arousal then becomes increased because the patient fears the sensation, and one may be more susceptible to panic while asleep. The patient is educated on the wide range of reasons physiological changes occur during sleep.

Cognitive restructuring is taught to patients to help understand how their thoughts can lead to feelings such as fear. Patients are taught to evaluate the evidence behind their anxiety-based thoughts by using questions such as "what is the evidence for and against X?" Patients are encouraged to gather data, explore alternative explanations to their thoughts, and to examine realistic consequences and strategies to deal with the worst event that might occur (i.e. "What's the worst thing that would happen if I did awaken in a panic? How would I cope? Would I survive?").

Patients are also taught breathing exercises and are asked to breathe deeply through the diaphragm. These exercises, including a meditative component using the word "relax," are incorporated just before bedtime and upon awakening.

Interoceptive exposure consists of exercises that expose patients to the physical sensations of a panic attack and weaken the connection between internal bodily sensations and panic attacks. For patients with daytime panic, this might include spinning in a chair to induce dizziness or running in place to increase heart rate. For patients with nocturnal panic, Craske [55] suggests having patients practice deep relaxation or sleeping in hot, stuffy conditions – situations that are common triggers for NP sufferers.

Finally, exposure exercises that provoke anxious sensations (e.g. exercise, caffeine) are initiated in more natural settings, first within the therapy session and later at home. Patients create a hierarchy of feared situations and work their way up from least difficult to most (e.g. sleeping with the lights and TV on, sleeping with the TV on in the dark, sleeping in the dark only). Patients are to use cognitive restructuring exercises and relaxation before and after each exposure. For NP patients, a discussion of proper sleep hygiene is also necessary.

Pharmacotherapy

Although limited in data, case studies report successful treatment of NP with benzodiazepines (clonazepam, alprazolam) and anti-depressants (SSRIs, TCAs) [58]. Reports overall have been promising, but further double-blind placebo-controlled studies are needed to establish the overall efficacy of SSRIs and TCAs in NP.

Sleep-related dissociative disorders

Sleep-related dissociative disorders are commonly divided into three categories: dissociative identity disorder, dissociative fugue, and dissociative disorder not otherwise specified. During these states (which can vary greatly in length of time from minutes to hours), patients commonly have disturbances in consciousness, memory identity, and environmental awareness [59]. Nocturnal re-enactments can range greatly in severity, such as: acting out past physical and sexual abuse, sexualized behavior, driving an automobile, flying a plane, binging on high-caloric sweets, or eating uncooked foods [60]. The individual generally has no memory of the nocturnal event.

Patients often report having a history of sexual, physical and emotional abuse, and may have a history of mood disorders, borderline personality disorder, PTSD, numerous psychiatric hospitalizations and multiple suicide attempts [61].

Given these high rates of psychiatric comorbidity, patients with these events require a full psychological evaluation and no single treatment approach is accepted as the most effective in this population. For example, Briere [62] suggests that patients who use dissociation as a primary coping strategy as a result of traumatic childhood events would likely benefit from intensive psychotherapy that helps to develop stronger affective regulation. Schenck and colleagues [7] demonstrated promising effects with clonazepam (0.25–2 mg nightly) on 33 adult patients with dangerous nocturnal events.

Taken together, limited evidence exists regarding treatment of this population. A combined pharmacotherapy and psychotherapeutic approach is likely to be most effective. Treatment should be aimed at any underlying psychiatric disorders; pharmacotherapy should be directed towards any depression and/or anxiety and psychotherapy should be directed at tension management and reduction of stimuli that tend to provoke events.

Conclusion

Treatment of parasomnias continues to evolve as new treatments become available. No longer limited to older pharmacological agents, the treating clinician has a number of effective treatments available at hand from which to choose. The most effective behavioral treatments have been developed for arousal disorders, nightmares, PTSD, and panic disorder. Each treatment plan for a patient with parasomnias should be individualized to his or her specific treatment goals, and the provider must make sure the patient is educated about his or her disorder and the risks/benefits of the treatments being recommended. Overall, the ultimate goal in treating patients with parasomnias is to work together to tailor the treatment to the patient in order to reduce the risk of injury, increase safety for family members, and ultimately increase the patient's quality of life.

References

1. Lask, B. Novel and nontoxic treatment for night terrors. *Br Med J* 1988; **297**: 592.
2. Frank C, Spirito A. The use of scheduled awakenings to eliminate childhood sleepwalking. *J Ped Psychol* 1997; **22**: 345–53.
3. Kales JD, Cadieux RJ, Soldatos CR. Psychotherapy with night-terror patients. *Am J Psychother* 1982; **36**: 399–407.
4. Jacobsen E. *Progressive Relaxation*. Chicago: University of Chicago Press, 1929.
5. Kellerman J. Behavioral treatment of night terrors in a child with acute leukemia. *J Nerv Ment Dis* 1979; **167**: 182–5.
6. Guilleminault C, Moscovitch A, Leger D. Injury, violence and nocturnal awakenings. *Am J Forensic Psychiatry* 1995; **16**: 33–46.
7. Schenck CH, Milner D, Hurwitz TD, *et al*. A polysomnographic and clinical report of sleep related injury in 100 adult patients. *Am J Psychiatry* 1989; **146**: 1166–1173.
8. Zach GA. Hypnosis, Part II: Theories and structure. *Compendium* 1990; **11**: 360–4.
9. Kennedy GA. A review of hypnosis in the treatment of parasomnias: Nightmare, sleepwalking and sleep terror disorders. *Am J Clin Hypnosis* 2002; **2**: 99–155.
10. Hauri PJ, Silber MH, Boeve BF. The treatment of parasomnias with hypnosis: A 5-year follow-up study. *J Clin Sleep Med* 2007; **3**: 369–73.
11. Winkleman JW. Treatment of nocturnal eating syndrome and sleep-related eating disorder with topiramate. *Sleep Med* 2003; **4**: 243–6.
12. Celluci AJ, Lawrence P. The efficacy of systematic desensitization in reducing nightmares. *J Behav Therapy Exp Psychiatry* 1978; **9**: 109–14.
13. Wittman L, Schredl M, Kramer M. Dreaming in posttraumatic stress disorder: A critical review of phenomenology, psychophysiology and treatment. *Psychother Psychosom* 2007; **76**: 25–39.
14. Krakow B, Zadra A. Clinical management of chronic nightmares: Imagery rehearsal therapy. *Behav Sleep Med* 2006; **4**: 45–70.
15. Maher MJ, Rego SA, Asnis GM. Sleep disturbances in patients with post-traumatic stress disorder: Epidemiology, impact and approaches to management. *CNS Drugs* 2006; **20**: 567–90.
16. Krakow B, Hollifield M, Johnston L, *et al*. Imagery rehearsal therapy for chronic nightmares in sexual assault survivors with posttraumatic stress disorder: A randomized controlled trial. *J Am Med Assoc* 2001; **286**: 537–45.
17. Neidhardt EJ, Krakow B, Kellner R, Pathak D. The beneficial effects of one treatment session and recording of nightmares on chronic nightmare sufferers. *Sleep* 1992; **15**: 470–3.
18. Krakow B, Kellner R, Neidhardt EJ, *et al*. Imagery rehearsal treatment of chronic nightmares: With a thirty month follow-up. *J Behav Ther Exp Psychol* 1993; **24**: 325–30.
19. Krakow B, Kellner R, Pathak D, *et al*. Imagery rehearsal treatment for chronic nightmares. *Behav Res Ther* 1995; **33**: 837–43.
20. Krakow B, Johnston L, Melendrez D, *et al*. An open-label trial of evidence-based cognitive behavior therapy for nightmares and insomnia in crime victims with PTSD. *Am J Psychiatry* 2001; **158**: 2043–7.
21. Krakow B, Melendrez G, Johnston L, *et al*. Sleep dynamic therapy for Cerro Grande fire evacuees with posttraumatic stress symptoms: A preliminary report. *J Clin Psychiatry* 2002; **63**: 673–84.
22. Harvey AG, Jones C, Schmidt DA. Sleep and posttraumatic stress disorder: A review. *Clin Psych Rev* 2003; **23**: 377–407.
23. DeViva J, Zayfert C, Pigeon W, *et al*. Treatment of residual insomnia after CBT for PTSD: Case studies. *J Trauma Stress* 2005; **18**: 155–9.
24. Freud S. *The Interpretation of Dreams*. New York: Basic Books, 1955.

25. Coalson B. Nightmare help: Treatment of trauma survivors with PTSD. *Psychotherapy* 1995; **32**: 381–8.

26. Spoormaker VI, Montgomery P. Disturbed sleep in post-traumatic-stress disorder: Secondary symptom or core feature. *Sleep Med Rev* 2008; **12**: 169–84.

27. Foa EB, Davidson JRT, Frances A. *Effective Treatments for PTSD*. New York: Guilford Press, 2000.

28. Foa EB, Davidson JRT, Frances A. The expert consensus guideline series: Treatment of posttraumatic stress disorder. The Expert Consensus Panels for PTSD. *J Clin Psychiatry* 1999; **60**(Suppl 16): 3–76.

29. Zayfert C, DeViva JC. Residual insomnia following cognitive behavioral therapy for PTSD. *J Trauma Stress* 2004; **17**: 69–73.

30. Nishith P, Duntley SP, Domitrovich PP, et al. Effect of cognitive behavioral therapy on heart rate variability during REM sleep in female rape victims with PTSD. *J Trauma Stress* 2003; **16**: 247–50.

31. Miller WR, DiPilato M. Treatment of nightmares via relaxation and desensitization: A controlled evaluation. *J Consult Clin Psychol* 1983; **51**: 870–7.

32. Burgess M, Gill M, Marks I. Postal self exposure treatment of recurrent nightmares: A randomized controlled trial. *Br J Psychiatry* 1998; **172**: 257–62.

33. Wolpe J. *The Practice of Behavior Therapy*. New York: Pergamon Press, 1969.

34. Kellner R, Neidhardt J, Krakow B, Pathak D. Changes in chronic nightmares after one session of desensitization or rehearsal instructions. *Am J Psychiatry* 1991; **149**: 659–63.

35. Lancee J, Spoormaker VI, Krakow B, Van Den Bout J. A systematic review of cognitive-behavioral treatment for nightmares: Toward a well-established treatment. *J Clin Sleep Med* 2008; **4**: 475–80.

36. Schredl M, Erlacher D. Lucid dreaming frequency and personality. *Pers Ind Differ* 2004; **37**: 1463–73.

37. Halliday G. Direct psychological therapies for nightmares: a review. *Clin Psychol Rev* 1987; **7**: 501–23.

38. Zadra AL, Pihl RO. Lucid dreaming as a treatment for recurrent nightmares. *Psychother Psychosom* 1997; **66**: 50–5.

39. Spoormaker VI, Van Den Bout J, Meijer EJG. Lucid dreaming treatment for nightmares: A series of cases. *Dreaming* 2003; **13**: 181–6.

40. Spoormaker VI, Van Den Bout J. Lucid dreaming treatment for nightmares: A pilot study. *Psychother Psychosom* 2006; **75**: 389–94.

41. Kingsbury SJ. Brief hypnotic treatment of repetitive nightmares. *Am J Clin Hypnosis* 1993; **35**: 161–9.

42. Nielson TA. Dreaming disorders. In: *Principles and Practice of Sleep Medicine*. 4th edition. Philadelphia: Elsevier Saunders, 2005; 936–45.

43. Taylor F, Raskind MA. The alpha1-adrenergic antagonist prazosin improves sleep and nightmares in civilian trauma posttraumatic stress disorder. *J Clin Psychopharmacol* 2002; **22**: 82–5.

44. Raskind MA, Peskind ER, Hoff DJ, et al. A parallel group placebo controlled study of prazosin for trauma nightmares and sleep disturbance in combat veterans with posttraumatic stress disorder. *Biol Psychiatry* 2007; **8**: 928–34.

45. Van Liempt S, Vermetten E, Gueze E, Westenberg HGM. Pharmacotherapy for disordered sleep in post-traumatic stress disorder: A systematic review. *Int Clin Psychopharmacol* 2006; **21**: 193–202.

46. Neylan TC, Metzler TJ, Schoenfeld FB, et al. Fluvoxamine and sleep disturbances in posttraumatic stress disorder. *J Trauma Stress* 2001; **14**: 461–7.

47. Neylan TC, Lenoci M, Maglione ML, et al. The effect of nefazodone on subjective and objective sleep quality in posttraumatic stress disorder. *J Clin Psychiatry* 2003; **64**: 445–50.

48. Warner MD, Dorn MR, Peabody CA. Survey on the usefulness of trazodone in patients with PTSD with insomnia or nightmares. *Pharmacopsychiatry* 2001; **34**: 128–31.

49. Ashford J, Miller TW. Effects of trazodone on sleep in patients diagnosed with post-traumatic stress disorder (PTSD). *J Contemp Psychother* 1996; **26**: 221–33.

50. Lerer B, Bleich A, Kotler M, et al. Posttraumatic stress disorder in Israeli combat veterans: Effect of phenelzine treatment. *Arch Gen Psychiatry* 1987; **44**: 976–81.

51. Schenck CH, Mahowald MW. Polysomnographic, neurological, psychiatric, and clinical outcome report on 70 consecutive cases with REM sleep behavior disorder (RBD): Sustained clonazepam efficacy in 89.5% of 57 treated patients. *Cleve Clin J Med* 1990; **57**: S9–23.

52. Boeve BF, Silber MH, Ferman JT. Melatonin for treatment of REM sleep behavior disorder in neurologic disorders: Results in 14 patients. *Sleep Med* 2003; **4**: 281–4.

53. Tan A, Salgado M, Fahn S. Rapid eye movement sleep behavior disorder preceding Parkinson's disease with therapeutic response to levodopa. *Mov Disord* 1996; **11**: 214–6.

54. Fantini ML, Gagnon JF, Filipini D, Montplaisir J. The effects of pramipexole in REM sleep behavior disorder. *Neurology* 2003; **61**: 1418–20.

55. Craske MG, Tsao JCI. Assessment and treatment of nocturnal panic attacks. *Sleep Med Rev* 2005; **9**: 173–84.
56. Craske MG, Lang AAJ, Aikins D, Mystkowski JL. Cognitive behavioral therapy for nocturnal panic. *Behav Therapy* 2005; **36**: 45–54.
57. Barlow DH, Gorman JM, Shear MK, Woods SW. Cognitive-behavioral therapy, imipramine, or their combination for panic disorder: A randomized controlled trial. *J Am Med Assoc* 2000; **283**: 2529–36.
58. Mellman TA, Uhde TW. Patients with frequent sleep panic: Clinical findings and response to medication treatment. *J Clin Psychiatry* 1990; **51**: 513–6.
59. Rice E, Fisher C. Fugue states in sleep and wakefulness: A psychophysiological study. *J Nerv Mental Dis* 1976; **163**: 79–87.
60. Agarun M, Kara H, Ozer O, *et al*. Characteristics of patients with nocturnal dissociative disorders. *Sleep Hypnosis* 2001; **3**: 131–4.
61. Mellman TA, Kulick-Bell R, Ashlock LE, Nolan B. Sleep events among veterans with combat-related posttraumatic stress disorder. *Am J Psychiatry* 1995; **152**: 110–15.
62. Briere, J. Dissociative symptoms and trauma exposure: Specificity, affect dysregulation, and posttraumatic stress. *J Nerv Mental Dis* 2006; **194**: 78–82.

Section 6 Therapy of parasomnias

Chapter 33

Hypnotherapy and parasomnias

Gina Graci

Common parasomnia treatment approaches

The treatment of parasomnias involves several components: education, behavioral intervention (e.g. hypnosis, stress management, relaxation/imagery), and in certain circumstances, medication. The first treatment strategy begins with patient education. Patients need to learn how to recognize sleep problems, as well as how they and their provider team can help them. In the case of parasomnias, the potential for harm of self or bed partner necessitates treatment [1]. Educating patients on appropriate sleep hygiene behaviors is an essential step in treating the sleep disorder. Appropriate sleep hygiene behaviors can include maintaining a regular sleep routine (going to bed and waking up at the same time each day), keeping the home environment safe, and eliminating environmental disturbance (e.g. lights, noises, regulate room temperature, keeping pets out of the bedroom, etc.) [2]. Additional behaviors may include avoiding mentally and physically stimulating activities before bedtime and engaging in calming, sleep-enhancing behaviors one hour before bedtime, avoiding heavy meals and ingestion of caffeine and alcohol.

In addition to adapting appropriate sleep hygiene behaviors, engaging in behaviors that assist in the prevention of parasomnia is important. For instance, maintaining the same sleep schedule assists in avoiding sleep deprivation which can trigger some parasomnias. Figure 33.1 illustrates risk factors for parasomnias.

Patients are also likely to benefit from the understanding and use of a variety of relaxation techniques [1]. These range from relatively simple techniques that require 3–5 min of teaching to much more complex shifts in the patients' view of life which consume two months or more of teaching. Some of these techniques may include guided imagery, progressive muscle relaxation (PMR) and biofeedback. If the individual does not respond to education and behavioral management approaches, a more thorough pharmacological approach may be warranted, and the patient should consult with a physician. Treatment can be efficacious if the patient begins medication management.

To date, there is a paucity of empirical research pertaining to the use of hypnosis as a single treatment modality to treat sleep disturbance. However, there is a plethora of research suggesting that hypnosis in combination with cognitive behavioral therapy (CBT) is therapeutic for a variety of psychological, behavioral, and medical disorders. While relaxation therapies and self-hypnotic strategies have been investigated in the treatment of sleep disorders as single treatment modalities, hypnosis should be used as an adjunct to treatment. This gap in the literature is primarily due to the fact that clinicians trained in hypnotherapy generally do not have the appropriate training to treat sleep disorders, and vice versa. The goal of this chapter is to educate clinicians specializing in the treatment of hypnosis to become familiar with parasomnias and the use of therapeutic suggestions for the treatment of parasomnias.

Hypnosis and sleep

Many individuals erroneously believe that individuals are sleeping when in a hypnotic trance. Sleep and hypnosis are distinctly different from each other, even though they may appear similar [1]. A hypnotic trance can be viewed as a more highly suggestible state of relaxation, and a trance does not necessarily lead to sleep, whereas in sleep there is a perceptual disengagement and unresponsiveness to the environment

---

The Parasomnias and Other Sleep-Related Movement Disorders, ed. M. J. Thorpy and G. Plazzi. Published by Cambridge University Press. © Cambridge University Press 2010.

Section 6: Therapy of parasomnias

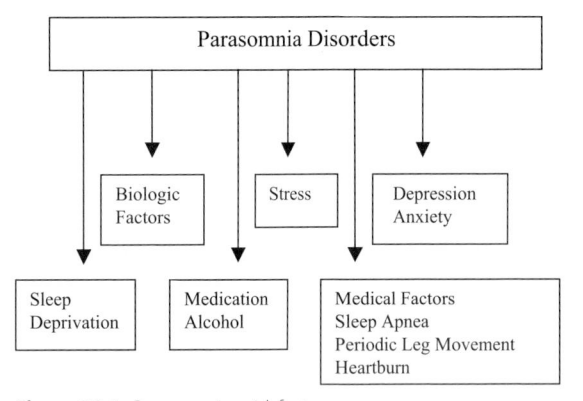

Figure 33.1 Parasomnia – risk factors.

[3]. Furthermore, hypnosis may be conceptualized as a state of increased concentration and awareness or an experience in changes in sensations, perceptions, thoughts, feelings, or behaviors [4]. Electrical recordings of brain waves called electroencephalographic (EEG) studies show that hypnosis is characterized by waking EEG patterns and not those of sleep [5]. Hypnosis promotes relaxation, which facilitates sleep in anxious or tense individuals.

It is important to note that hypnosis is a specialized technique/tool and not a therapy in itself [4]. Hypnosis should always be used as an adjunct to psychotherapy. Hypnosis is a highly efficacious tool, especially when integrated into a treatment plan. The utilization of hypnosis in hypnotherapy assists patients' in modifying their behavior and emotional processes [6].

Hypnosis in the treatment of parasomnias

The most common parasomnias that have been amenable to hypnosis/hypnotherapy include nightmare, sleep terror, sleepwalking, and night eating disorder [7]. Other parasomnias may be treated with hypnosis; however, treatment efficacy is lacking. Those sleep disorders with an organic or medical basis associated with them (e.g. REM sleep behavior disorder) may still be treated with hypnosis for the benefits of relaxation and stress management.

Clinical hypnosis is a safe and effective method of treating certain parasomnias because it allows the clinician to gain access to the underlying problem [8]. It may also be considered a tool that can be utilized to amplify the therapeutic effects of therapy [4]. Self-hypnosis is considered a voluntary relaxation technique [9] that is similar to meditation because it can ease the body and mind preparing the body for sleep [10]. Hypnosis and self-hypnosis offer rapid methods for managing anxiety and worry often associated with stressors, facilitating deep relaxation, and controlling mental overactivity and decreasing physiological arousal [1,11,12]. Hypnosis has been found to be effective in reducing stress and promoting relaxation which may or may not cause a reduction in sleep disturbance episodes. If it is determined that the parasomnias have a psychological contributor (e.g. nightmares, sleepwalking episodes related to a traumatic injury), they are very amenable to hypnotism.

There is only one case study series with a five-year follow-up investigating the effects of hypnotherapy on parasomnias. In 2007, Hauri *et al.* reported that one or two sessions of hypnosis is efficacious for the treatment of sleepwalking; nightmares, sleep terrors, nocturnal eating disorder, sleep-related grooming, and sleep talking [13]. Thirty-six patients diagnosed (by sleep specialists) with chronic parasomnias received either one or two hypnotherapy sessions and were followed by questionnaire for five years. Results indicated that at one month post-hypnotherapy, approximately 50% of the study respondents either denied experiencing parasomnia events or rated themselves as much improved. These improvement rates remained high after 5 years; that is, 41% of the respondents continued to deny experiencing a parasomnia episode. The authors speculated that the five-year statistic may not be due to hypnotherapy alone, because respondents may have sought additional treatments. However, the results are impressive and cannot be ignored, especially since one or two hypnotherapy treatments are a short, time-efficient treatment compared to the greater number of sessions required for other therapy modalities, such as CBT [1,13].

In 2002, Kennedy investigated the use of hypnosis in the treatment of nightmares, sleepwalking, and sleep terror disorders [14]. The results indicated that individuals experienced a reduction in parasomnias. The author suggested that for the treatment of nightmares, hypnosis was an efficacious tool, and the results may be attributable to the specific hypnotic suggestion used to alter the nightmare content. The effects of increased relaxation to maintain sleep throughout the night are also important. Furthermore, the author concluded that hypnosis was effective for treating sleepwalking and sleep terror disorders because of the reduction of tonic levels due to the anxiolytic effects associated with relaxation.

Treatment of nightmares

Children between the ages of 7 and 12 are susceptible to hypnotic suggestion, primarily at sleep onset or immediately upon awakening [4,15]. Parents can assist in the reduction of their child's nightmares by staying with their child as they put him/her to bed. At the signs and symptoms of sleep onset (e.g. heavy eyelids), the parent can begin to vocalize positive suggestions. For example, verbalizing the safety and security of their child [4]. Parents may also vocalize that their child will maintain a deep, calm, and peaceful sleep, minimizing the amount of movement during the night unless the child needs to use the bathroom, etc.

During hypnotherapy sessions, hypnotists may also suggest that the patient have a dream during hypnosis with a similar content to a daydream or nightdream. The therapist will use these dreams to learn about meaningful themes, problems or conflicts [4]. Hypnotic suggestions for nightmares or sleep terrors can include having happy dreams, tranquil dreams, pleasant dreams without waking up, and feeling very relaxed and calm when sleeping [16]. Additional suggestions can include that when the bad dream begins, the patient try to switch to a different (more positive) dream, or alter the dream content/ending [4,17].

Dr. Cartwright, the former director of the Rush Behavioral Sleep Disorders Center, during a didactic training session, discussed a case presentation of a child who experienced repeated nightmares of a frightening monster. During the session, the child was asked if he would be comfortable shaking hands with the monster and introducing himself. The child stated that he would be comfortable with talking to the monster because "when people introduce themselves, bad things don't happen". The suggestion was then given to the child that when the nightmare occurs again to approach the monster and introduce himself, ask for the monster's name and shake hands. When the child returned for his next session, he discussed having the dream and the monster was no longer frightening or problematic because once he shook hands with the monster, the monster was no longer frightening. The child denied experiencing nightmares again.

Dr. Cartwright also suggests using alternative endings. For instance, if a patient has a recurring dream that they are falling or they are driving an automobile and their brakes do not work, change the ending. In the case of falling, change the sequence of the dream as it occurs. For instance, an individual can suddenly have the ability to fly which would alter the ending – they can be rescued (e.g. by a large object), or when getting close to the ground, they can freeze in mid-air or dramatically slow the speed of their descent so they are able to safely land on their feet. In the case of the driving with faulty brakes, change the dream so that the individual does not get into the same car, or suddenly has the ability to slow the car down by inventing a magic button that they press and stop the car safely (similar to a James Bond car). In either scenario, the key element is that the suggestion(s) that are created for individuals will foster feelings of empowerment with enhanced feelings of self-control so that they can create an alternative ending.

Treatment of sleepwalking

In 1991, Hurwitz indicated that hypnosis was effective in the treatment of 27 adults with sleepwalking and sleep terror disorders [18]. Seventy-four per cent of these individuals reported improvement (much to very much improved) over a substantial time period (63 months). Post-hypnotic suggestions included those for anxiety reduction, increased feelings of security, restful sleep, and instructed patients to reiterate these post-hypnotic suggestions during self-hypnosis practice at home. These authors recommend one to six hypnosis treatments for reduction of parasomnia episodes.

For severe cases of sleepwalking where an individual is extremely agitated (e.g. running wildly and blindly into objects or walls), Weitzenhoffer suggests forgoing the sleep induction [19]. The rationale is that the sleep induction may trigger an agitated sleepwalking episode. This author recommends utilizing "active hypnosis" with patients.

Treatment of nocturnal enuresis

Hypnosis has been reported to successfully treat children and adolescents with primary nocturnal enuresis (bedwetting during nocturnal sleep) [4,15]. A typical session includes educating the patient (by drawings and verbal explanation) of how the bladder functions. Hypnotic induction follows, with the suggestion that a section of the brain will awaken the child when their bladder becomes full. Reduction or elimination of bedwetting during sleep occurs after a few sessions. This suggestion can also work with adults as long as there is not a medical condition associated with the nocturnal enuresis.

REM behavior disorder and sleep bruxism

In the treatment of REM sleep behavior disorder and sleep bruxism, research is scarce. If there is a biological basis for these disorders, hypnosis can still have a therapeutic effect by promoting relaxation, reducing physiological arousal, anxiety, and stressors. In the case of REM sleep behavior disorder, this sleep disorder can have significant psychosocial repercussions. Individuals diagnosed with Parkinson's disease experience many challenging (emotional, physical, functional, and social) issues and impairments that they encounter on a daily basis. In addition to having daytime issues, these individuals have to encounter significant sleep disturbance which can be an additional stressor. Restless sleep, with the potential to inflict self-injury or to injure their bed partner is of utmost concern. Relationship difficulties can ensue because the bed partner may become frightened to sleep with their significant other. Hypnosis will not alter the disease process; however, it can reduce sleep onset by promoting relaxation and decreasing physiological arousal. This effect of reduction in tonic levels may or may not decrease the sleep disturbance associated with REM sleep behavior disorder.

The key element in treating sleep disorders of this kind is essentially for symptom reduction and not cure. It is also important to consider whether the side effects of medications produce parasomnia symptoms, in which case hypnosis most likely will not have a therapeutic effect.

Suggestions and post-hypnotic suggestions

The use of post-hypnotic suggestion and the utilization of these suggestions by audiocassette tape (for self-hypnosis) reinforces the effectiveness of the direct suggestion [4]. Parasomnia treatment generally involves 1–2 sessions of hypnotherapy focusing on relaxation and self-hypnosis at bedtime. Treatment often accompanies medical intervention with prescription drugs in addition to hypnosis or relaxation/imagery [1,20]. Booster sessions may also be considered on an as needed basis.

Examples of post-hypnotic suggestions for parasomnias

You will experience feelings of safety and security during sleep and return safely to bed.

Your sleep will be restful sleep with minimal movement or awakenings.

When your feet touch the floor, you will awaken feeling calm and peaceful and return safely to bed.

When you touch your door knob or the lock on your door, you will awaken feeling calm and peaceful. You will calmly and safely return to bed.

When you touch your window, you will awaken feeling calm and peaceful and return safely to bed.

When you touch your refrigerator door, you will awaken feeling calm and peaceful and return safely to bed.

Therapeutic issues

Behavioral treatment approaches initially appear to be more time-consuming and more expensive than hypnotic medications; however, over the life span of total physician visits and prescriptions, it may be more cost-effective for patients to engage in behavioral treatments. Hypnotherapy has a role in the behavioral treatment of sleep disorders and it is beneficial for hypnotherapists to gain specialty training in the treatment of sleep disorders.

Despite the lack of research on the effects of hypnosis on the treatment of parasomnias, there is agreement that hypnosis is a non-invasive, inexpensive, side-effect-free, short-term treatment for the treatment of parasomnias [1,4,6,13,14,21]. Furthermore, hypnotherapy allows unconscious exploration of underlying functions/conflicts associated with the sleep disturbance [11].

The following cases represent an amalgamation of cases and groups that have been treated using the concepts, assessments and treatments for parasomnias.

Case one

Mrs. Jones was a 26-year-old Caucasian female referred for a sleep consult by her psychologist. Her presenting problem was frequent nocturnal arousals in which she would sit up in bed with her feet resting on the floor and begin to yell, scream, grab her throat, and experience shortness of breath with intense feelings of terror. She reported that when these events occur, she believes that she is dying with the inability to be consoled by any member of her family. Mrs. Jones denied remembering what caused the sleep arousal or the content of her dream. She brought two videos to the session which captured these "episodes".

Mrs. Jones had been married for 8 years and had 4 children, aged 1, 3, 5, and 6 years. Her sleep arousal problems were reported to occur for the last 3 years. However, the frequency and intensity of these sleep awakenings increased over time. A thorough sleep evaluation was conducted and the following information was collected. She reported no difficulty falling asleep; however, she frequently experienced early morning awakenings with inability to return to sleep during the week. She had a slender body habitus and her physical exam was negative for a diagnosis of sleep apnea.

Mrs. Jones had been a full-time homemaker and home schooled her children. She stated that she loved her husband and children. However, she always wanted to earn her college degree, but with the pregnancy and birth of each child, she stated that she realized this "dream" was never going to come to fruition. She portrayed herself as a daydreamer, often daydreaming about what it would be like to attend college, graduate with a psychology degree and possibly attend graduate school so that she could become a psychologist.

She described her husband as a dedicated husband and father who worked long hours as an engineer. Mrs. Jones repeatedly stated that she has shared her "dreams" of attending college with her husband before they were married and during their marriage, but he does not support her dreams/goals. He told her that being a wife and mother was the most "noble" profession and she should not want anything more. Mr. Jones was the main financial contributor to the family and he told her that they had everything that they could need or want because he "provides for his family". Overall, Mrs. Jones stated that she enjoyed her life, but rarely had energy or time for personal or social interests (e.g. private time, going out with friends). She also stated that at times she felt as if she was "suffocating" because she had so much work to do during the day and night.

Mrs. Jones' medical history was unremarkable. She was unable to provide an explanation for her arousals from sleep and voiced significant upset and frustration with these events. She stated that she was beginning to "fear" falling to sleep at night because when these "events" occurred they were so frightening that she would remain awake for several hours until she calmed down and relaxed. She denied symptoms of depression and the use of drugs, but endorsed experiencing anxiety because she had so much to accomplish on a daily basis and often did not get everything done that she needed to accomplish for the day. She denied drinking or smoking. She stated that she used to exercise but stopped exercising after the birth of her second child because of time constraints. She is of petite build and normal weight. Mrs. Jones reported nightly bedtimes between 10:30 and 11:00 p.m. Her reported wake up time was 6:00–6:30 a.m. daily. She endorsed experiencing sleepiness during the day but denied napping.

Mrs. Jones lived in a two-storey home, with her family and mother- and father-in-law. She stated that her in-laws were somewhat demanding but the relationship was "good". Her hobbies included reading, watching television, and taking walks. She indicated that she often did not have time for hobbies.

Mrs. Jones was unfamiliar with relaxation techniques; she indicated receptivity to learning hypnosis and to the logging of her sleep.

After a thorough sleep intake and assessment, Mrs. Jones was diagnosed with sleep terror disorder. Her treatment included two sessions of hypnosis and continued work with her psychologist.

In the first session, she indicated a willingness to "learn new things" and was attentive during the session. She complied with daily sleep log recordings. During hypnosis she was asked how she felt emotionally during the day and she replied, "I feel like I am being suffocated because I am so busy and there is no time for me." Mrs. Jones stated that she felt relaxed after the session, but home practice was not as relaxing. Hypnotic suggestions included falling into a deep sleep and maintaining this deep sleep throughout the night (unless she had to use the bathroom) and if awakened, she would feel safe and secure and the return to sleep would be easy. Suggestions also included that when she awakened and her feet touched the floor, she would awaken feeling calm and peaceful. Breathing would be slow and unlabored. She would take oxygen in and out of her lungs easily.

It was apparent that Mrs. Jones felt suffocated in her daytime life (performing motherly duties, homeschooling her children, cleaning and cooking, taking care of her in-laws and having to give up her dreams of attending college) and acted out these feelings in her sleep terror episodes. After two sessions, her sleep diary indicated that she was sleeping better and the frequency of these arousal episodes declined significantly. Mrs. Jones' psychologist continued to assist her in processing her conflicted feelings of being a mother and wanting to accomplish her dreams/goals. Within a year, Mrs. Jones denied having sleep terror episodes.

Case two

Ms. Tyler was a 38-year-old female presenting with sleepwalking episodes and nocturnal binge-eating episodes. These episodes occurred approximately three times per week and their initial onset began six years ago. Ms. Tyler was single and employed as a secretary. She had been involved in an on-again, off-again intimate relationship with her significant other for the last four years. She described herself as an "attention to detail" person and enjoyed her job. She had an active social life, attending social events with friends several times a week. Ms. Tyler was an avid cyclist and biked approximately 60 miles per week. She stated that "biking" was her primary stress release and she looked forward to biking on a daily basis. Furthermore, Ms. Tyler described herself as a restrictive eater, primarily eating low-fat, low-carbohydrate food. She stated that she enjoyed having dessert occasionally and will make sure that "she makes up for indulging" with her next biking session. She denied a significant medical history, but endorsed experiencing mild depression for the last 20 years and had been in psychotherapy for 6 years. She stated that she enjoyed the "supportive component" of therapy. Ms. Tyler was a tall, slender woman and denied experiencing symptoms of apnea, periodic leg movement disorder, restless leg syndrome or sleep paralysis.

The standard sleep interview indicated that during her sleepwalking episodes she has walked out of her home (she lives in a high-rise condominium), telephoned friends in the middle of the night, and has written emails. She repeatedly stated that she was embarrassed by these nightly behaviors, especially the nonsensical emails. Furthermore, she stated that during some of her sleepwalking events, she would go to her refrigerator and eat frozen leftovers. Ms. Tyler had also eaten entire frozen entrees with no recollection the following morning, except with the feeling of abdominal "fullness". She would find the empty food containers in the trash with no other visible evidence that she ate during the night. Ms. Tyler denied a childhood history of sleepwalking or sleep talking.

Prior to going to bed, Ms. Tyler would engage in mentally stimulating activities and often would have work issues on her mind. Typically, she would fall asleep within 30 min but within 2–3 h after sleep onset, she would engage in sleepwalking/sleep eating episodes. These episodes occurred 2–3 times per week.

Ms. Tyler was diagnosed with a sleepwalking disorder. Treatment was formulated from the information gathered during the intake and hypnotic suggestions were generated from this information.

Ms. Tyler was seen for two sessions. The first session included hypnotic suggestions for when her feet touched the floor, when she touched her laptop cover, when she touched the door knob to her door, and when she opened the refrigerator door, she would awaken feeling calm and safe and would return to bed. Suggestions for maintaining a deep and restorative sleep (with minimal movement) throughout the night were given to Ms. Tyler. This first session also included education on maintaining proper sleep hygiene behaviors. For instance, she was instructed not to exercise at least 4 h before bedtime, avoid sleep deprivation, avoid mentally stimulating activities at least 1 h prior to bedtime, etc. After the first session, she reported a significant decrease in sleepwalking/eating episodes with continued decline after the second session (she reported experiencing one sleepwalking/sleep eating episode for the month). Ms. Tyler continued to see her therapist and work on issues related to "the need to feel in control" and learn more effective methods for coping with stress(ors). Her therapist began to focus on the conscious/unconscious causes for her sleep disturbance.

References

1. Graci GM, Sexton-Radek K. Treating sleep disorders using cognitive behavioral therapy and hypnosis. In Chapman RA (Ed), *The Clinical Use of Hypnosis in Cognitive Behavior Therapy: A Practitioner's Casebook*. New York: Springer, 2005; 348.
2. Sexton-Radek K, Graci GM. *Combatting Your Sleep Problems*. Westport, CT: Praeger, 2007; 152.
3. Kryger MH, Roth T, Dement WC. Principles and practice of sleep medicine. *Depress Anxiety* 2001; **13**: 157.

4. Beng-Yeong N, Tih-Shih L. Hypnotherapy for sleep disorders. *Ann Acad Med Singapore* 2008; **37**: 683–8.

5. Evans FJ. Hypnosis and sleep: The control of altered states of awareness. *Sleep Hypnosis* 1999; **1**: 232–7.

6. Insight. Hypnotherapy shows promise of sleep for sleep disorders. 2007 October 27, 2007 [cited 2008 December 12].

7. Sharma S. Parasomnias. 2007 April 4, 2007 [cited 2008 December 12].

8. Modlin T. Sleep disorders and hypnosis: To cope or cure? *Sleep Hypnosis* 2002; **4**: 39–46.

9. Dement W, Vaughan C. *The Promise of Sleep*. New York, NY: Random House, 2000; 524.

10. Kryger M. *A Woman's Guide to Sleep Disorders*. New York, NY: McGraw-Hill, 2004.

11. Hammond D. Sleep disorders. In Hammond D (Ed), *Handbook of Hypnotic Suggestions and Metaphors*. New York, NY: W.W. Norton & Company, 1990; 220–1.

12. Bauer KE, McCanne TR. An hypnotic technique for treating insomnia. *Int J Clin Exp Hypnosis* 1980; **28**: 1–5.

13. Hauri P, Silber M, Boeve B. The treatment of parasomnias with hypnosis: A 5-year follow-up study. *J Clin Sleep Med* 2007; **15**: 369–73.

14. Kennedy GA. A review of hypnosis in the treatment of parasomnias: Nightmare, sleepwalking, and sleep terror disorders. *Austral J Clin Exp Hypnosis* 2002; **30**: 99–155.

15. Olness K, Kohen DP. *Hypnosis and Hypnotherapy with Children*. 3rd ed. New York: The Guilford Press, 1996; 457.

16. De Rios M, Friedman J. Suggestions when there are sleep problems. In Hammond D (Ed), *Handbook of Hypnotic Suggestions and Metaphors*. New York, NY: W.W. Norton & Company, 1990; 337.

17. Cartwright R. *Children and Dreams* (ed. G. Graci). Chicago: Rush University Medical Center, 2001.

18. Hurwitz T, Mahowald MW, Schenck CH, Schluter JL, Bundlie SR. A retrospective outcome study and review of hypnosis as treatment of adults with sleepwalking and sleep terror. *J Nerv Mental Dis* 1991; **179**: 228–33.

19. Weitzenhoffer A. The induction of hypnosis. In *The Practice of Hypnotism*. New York: John Wiley & Sons, 2000.

20. Cohen J. Parasomnia – Causes, symptoms, information with treatment. 2007 October 18, 2007 [cited 2008 December 12].

21. Quan S. Podcast of the *Journal of Clinical Sleep Medicine. J Clin Sleep Med* 2006; **1**: 1–3.

Index

abuse and parasomnias 25
acephalgic migraines 197
acute focal pontine inflammatory lesions 54–5
ADHD, association with RMD 272, 275
Adolescent Dissociative Experiences Scale 170–1
agrypnia excitata 54
alcohol
 and parasomnias 49–50
 and seizures 91–2
 and sleep-related violence 91
 and the law 92
alcoholic blackout 92
alternating leg muscle activation (ALMA) 233
Alzheimer's disease
 and RBD 5, 55
 neuroimaging 17
American Academy of Sleep Medicine atlas of sleep scoring 131, 132–3
amitriptyline 46, 306–7
amyotrophic lateral sclerosis (ALS) 55, 57
anti-depressants 306–7
 and parasomnias 46
 nightmare disorder treatments 319
anti-hypertensives 307–8
anxiety disorders 29
APOE e4 variant 17
arousal disorders see disorders of arousal
arterial blood gas tests 30
asthma 26–7, 282
autism spectrum disorders 55, 272, 274
automatism, and violent behavior 83–4, 85–7
autoscopy 145, 147

autosomal dominantly inherited spinocerebellar ataxia type 2 and 3 (SCA2, SCA3) 55, 57

bed partner, information from 19, 20
bed-wetting see sleep enuresis
Belicki scale of nightmare distress 154
benign rolandic epilepsy 291
benign sleep myoclonus of infancy 233
benzodiazepines 4, 303–5
 and arousal parasomnias 303–4
 and RBD 304–5
 and sleep bruxism 305
 and sleepwalking 46–7
 and SRED 47–8
 clonazepam 303–5, 306
 effects on SWS 47
Big Five Factor model of personality 155
binge-eating disorder (BED) 208
bipolar disorder 43, 44, 45
blackouts, alcohol-related 92
"blip" syndrome 231
blood pressure (BP) monitoring 40
blood tests 30
body rocking RMD 271
body rolling RMD 270
Bonkalo, Alexander 81, 99, 105
Bonnet, Charles 194 see also Charles Bonnet syndrome
botulinum toxin 308
brain, iron depletion and RLS 14
brain volumetric changes, neuroimaging 14–15
brainstem lesions and RBD 5
bromocriptine 308
bruxism see sleep bruxism
brycose see sleep bruxism

bulimia nervosa 29
bupropion–levodopa–trazodone therapy 309

caffeine and parasomnias 50
capnograph 39
cardiovascular system examination 26
caregivers, information from 19–20
cataplexy 142
catathrenia (sleep-related groaning) 184–92
 clinical findings 184–9
 differential diagnosis 189–91
 distinction from snoring 190–1
 epidemiology 9–10
 future directions for research 192
 genetic factors 191
 history 184
 ICSD-2 classification 184
 laboratory investigations 189–91
 management 192
 natural history 189
 pathology 191–2
 terminology 184
central apnea 190
cerebral metabolic rate for glucose (CMRgl) 17
Charles Bonnet syndrome 194, 195–6
 hallucinations 23, 28
Child Dissociative Checklist 171
children
 confusional arousals 100–2
 pharmacological treatment of parasomnias 301–3, 305
 sleep terrors 8–9
 sleepwalking 3–4, 8, 112, 115, 116
children with disabilities, pharmacotherapy and parasomnias 305
chloral hydrate 43
chlorpromazine 46

Index

chlorprothixene 46
chronic obstructive pulmonary disease (COPD) 26, 27
circadian rhythms 207, 293, 306
classifications of parasomnias and parasomnia-like events 7, 19, 20
clinical evaluation 19–31
    arterial blood gas tests 30
    blood tests 30
    characterizing the sleep disturbance 19–21
    chief complaint 19
    classification of parasomnias and parasomnia-like events 7, 19, 20
    differential diagnosis 19, 21, 23, 27
    electroencephalogram (EEG) 29
    evoked potential studies 30
    family history 23–4
    heart monitoring 30
    laboratory investigations 29
    legal implications 24–5
    need for extensive evaluation 29
    neuroimaging 29
    normal behaviors 21
    patient education about diagnosis 30
    patient history 19–21
    patient's functional status and mood 23
    physical examination 25–7
    polysomnogram 29
    precipitating factors 21–3, 25
    psychiatric assessment 23
    pulmonary function tests 30
    serum ferritin level 30
    sleep log or diary 25
    sleep questionnaires 25
    systematic approach 19
    testing for drug abuse 30
    thyroid function tests 30
    timing of abnormal events 21
    treatment 30
    urine screening 30
    violent parasomnias 24–5
Clinical Global Impression of Improvement measure 208
clonazepam 47, 303–5, 306, 319
clonidine 307
    prescription in children 301
clozapine 304
cognitive behavioral therapy (CBT)
    nightmare disorder 314–16
    nocturnal panic disorder 318–19

complex nocturnal visual hallucinations (CNVH) 194, 195–6
complex partial seizures 28 see also epilepsy; sleep-related epilepsy
compression neuropathies 28–9
confusional arousals 99–107
    continuum of arousal disorders 100
    definition 99
    distinction from sleep panic arousals 282
    Elpenor syndrome 99, 105
    epidemiology 7–8
    history 99
    terminology 99–100
    violent behavior 8
    see also disorders of arousal
confusional arousals in adults 102–6
    associations with other conditions 103–4
    associations with other sleep disorders 103, 104
    clinical manifestations 103
    complications 105–6
    diagnosis 104–5
    differential diagnosis 104–5
    forensic implications 105–6
    hypersomnia 104
    predisposing and precipitating factors 103
    prevalence 103
    prognosis 106
    sleep-related sexual behavior 103, 105–6
    sleep-related violence 103, 105–6
    treatment 106
confusional arousals in children 100–2
    clinical features 102
    features of arousal disorders in childhood 100–2
    genetic predisposition 101
    management of 101–2
    precipitating factors 101
conversion disorders 29
Crown–Crisp experiential index 121
culpability for sleep-related violence 83–4
culture-bound syndromes, recurrent isolated sleep paralysis (RISP) 150
cyclic alternating pattern (CAP) scoring system 4

de novo parasomnias 42–3, 51
delirium tremens 54
delta sleep 43 see also slow-wave sleep (SWS)
dementia with Lewy bodies (DLB) and RBD 5, 56
    link with dream-enactment behavior (DEB) 17
    hallucinations 196, 198
desipramine hydrochloride 43
developmental disabilities and RMD 271, 272, 274
diazepam 304
differential diagnosis 19, 21, 23, 27 see also clinical evaluation
disorders of arousal (ICSD-2) 7–9
    continuum 100
    differential diagnosis 27
    in childhood 100–2
    see also confusional arousals; sleep terrors; sleepwalking
disorders of arousal, treatments 312–14
    avoid engaging the patient mid-episode 313
    benzodiazepines 303–5
    education of patient and family 312
    good sleep hygiene 313
    hypnosis 314
    medications 314
    progressive muscle relaxation (PMR) 314
    psychotherapy 313–14
    safety 313
    scheduled awakenings 313
    sleep scheduling 313
    stress management 314
dissociation, medico-legal context 92–3
dissociative disorders 29 see also sleep-related dissociative disorders
Dissociative Experiences Scale 171
Dissociative Processes Scale 171
dopamine system
    role in RBD 16
    role in RLS/PLMD 13–14
dream-enactment behavior 5
    link with dementia with Lewy bodies 17
    neuroimaging 17
    see also REM sleep behavior disorder (RBD)

331

Index

drugs
  and RBD 5
  interactions 42, 44–5
  iatrogenic RBD 5
  testing for drug abuse 30
  violence related to 91, 92
  see also parasomnias due to medications or substances

DSM IV-TR
  classification of parasomnias and parasomnia-like events 20
  criteria for nightmares 153–4
  dissociative disorders 29, 163, 164

Eating Attitudes Test (EAT) 206

eating disorders 28–9 see also sleep-related eating disorder (SRED)

education of patient and family 312

electrical status epilepticus during sleep (ESES) 291

electrocardiogram (ECG) 39–40

electroencephalogram (EEG) 29, 38
  CAP analysis 4
  quantified 4
  use of sleep EEG in parasomnias 4

electromyogram (EMG) 29, 38–9

electrooculogram (EOG) 38

Elpenor syndrome 99, 105 see also confusional arousals

end-stage renal disease, and RLS 215

endoesophageal pressure measurement 39

enuresis, nocturnal, early studies 3, 4
  see also sleep enuresis

epidemiology of parasomnias 7–10
  catathrenia 9–10
  classification of parasomnias 7
  confusional arousals 7–8
  disorders of arousal (ICSD-2) 7–9
  exploding head syndrome 9
  nightmare disorder 9
  other parasomnias (ICSD-2) 9–10
  parasomnia due to drug or substance 9
  parasomnia due to medical condition 9
  parasomnias associated with REM sleep (ICSD-2) 9
  recurrent isolated sleep paralysis 9
  REM sleep behavior disorder (RBD) 9
  sleep enuresis 9, 10
  sleep-related dissociative disorders 9
  sleep-related hallucinations 9, 10
  sleep terrors 8–9
  sleepwalking 8
  unspecified parasomnia 9

epilepsy
  complex partial seizures 28
  epileptic hallucinations 196–7
  nocturnal 3
  sleep-related violence 90–1
  see also seizure disorders; sleep-related epilepsy

episodic nocturnal phenomena, early studies 3

Epworth Sleepiness Scale 25

essential startle disease 234

eszopiclone (Lunesta) 42, 49

ethnicity and parasomnias 10

evoked potential studies 30

excessive daytime sleepiness 142

excessive fragmentary hypnic myoclonus (EFHM) 233, 237

excessive fragmentary myoclonus (EFM)
  characteristics 237
  clinical findings 237–8
  FM index (FMI) 239
  future directions for research 241–2
  genetics 241
  ICSD-2 classification 241
  laboratory investigations 241
  management 241
  natural history 241
  pathology 241

excessive sleep inertia see confusional arousals

expert opinion in legal cases 87–9

exploding head syndrome 29, 194, 199, 229
  clinical findings 199
  epidemiology 9
  genetics 198
  history 195
  ICSD-2 classification 194
  laboratory investigations 197
  management 198
  natural history 199
  pathophysiology 199

exposure therapy, nightmare disorder 316

familial patterns in parasomnias 3–4
  see also genetic factors in parasomnias

familial periodic paralyses 29

families
  education about the condition 312
  information from 20
  learning how to react to behaviors 30

family history 23–4

fatal familial insomnia 54, 55

fatigue severity scale 25

Feinberg, Joel 83

fictive motor movements 145

finger plethysmograph (FP) 40

flip-flop model of RISP 144–5

flunitrazepam 47

fluoxetine 50–1

flurazepam 46, 47

forensic opinions 87–9

fragmentary myoclonus 237–42
  clinical findings 237–41
  FM index (FMI) 239
  future directions for EFM research 241–2
  genetics 241
  history 237
  laboratory investigations 241
  management of EFM 241
  natural history of EFM 241
  pathology 241
  physiologic hypnic myoclonias (PHM) 237–42
  terminology 237

fragmentary NREM myoclonus 237

Freud, theory about night terrors 119

Gastaut, Henri 3

genetic factors in parasomnias 10, 23–4
  catathrenia (sleep-related groaning) 191
  confusional arousals in children 101
  excessive fragmentary myoclonus (EFM) 241
  exploding head syndrome 198
  mouse models of SRED 207
  nightmares 9
  predisposition to parasomnias 43
  propriospinal myoclonus 267

Index

recurrent isolated sleep paralysis (RISP) 150
REM sleep behavior disorder (RBD) 138
RLS 7, 217–8
sleep bruxism (SB) 254
sleep enuresis 10, 176–7
sleep-related dissociative disorders 171
sleep-related hallucinations 198
sleep terrors 124
sleepwalking 115
vulnerability to abnormal arousals 51

groaning in sleep *see* catathrenia

group A xeroderma pigmentosus 55

Guillain–Barré syndrome 55

hallucinations
  legal implications 25
  RISP hallucinoid experiences 145
  sleep-related 10
  see also hypnagogic hallucinations; hypnopompic hallucinations; sleep-related hallucinations

Hardy, Thomas 106

head banging (jactatio capitis nocturna) RMD 270

head rolling RMD 270

headache syndromes 29

heart monitoring 30

hereditary hyperekplexia syndrome 234

history, patient *see* patient history

history of parasomnia studies 3–5

homicide, during sleepwalking/sleep terrors 8

hypersomnia 104

hypnagogic foot tremor 233

hypnagogic hallucinations 10, 54, 58, 142, 194, 195 *see also* hallucinations; sleep-related hallucinations

hypnagogic jerks *see* sleep starts

hypnic jerks 21 *see also* sleep starts

hypnic myoclonus *see* fragmentary myoclonus

hypnic starts *see* sleep starts

hypnopompic hallucinations 10, 54, 58, 194, 195 *see also* hallucinations; sleep-related hallucinations

hypnosis and sleep 323–4

hypnotherapy and parasomnias 323–8
  arousal disorders 314
  case studies 326–7
  nightmares 317, 325
  nocturnal enuresis 325–6
  post-hypnotic suggestions 326
  REM sleep behavior disorder (RBD) 326
  sleep bruxism 326
  sleepwalking 325
  suggestions 326
  therapeutic issues 326

iatrogenic RBD 5

ICD-9-CM classification of parasomnias and parasomnia-like events 20

ICSD-2 classification
  catathrenia (sleep-related groaning) 184
  confusional arousals 99, 103
  excessive fragmentary myoclonus (EFM) 241
  nightmares 153–4
  parasomnias 19
  parasomnias due to medications or substances 42–3
  REM sleep behavior disorder (RBD) 131, 132
  sexsomnias 70
  sleep bruxism (SB) 252
  sleep-related dissociative disorder 29
  sleep-related eating disorder (SRED) 203
  sleep-related movement disorders 19
  sleep-related rhythmic movement disorder (RMD) 271

ICSD-R, parasomnias due to medications or substances 42

idiopathic hypersomnia 104

idiopathic RBD 5, 132, 133, 135–6

idiopathic RLS (iRLS) 14

imagery rehearsal therapy (IRT) 156, 314–15, 316

imipramine 50, 304, 306

incontinence 175 *see also* sleep enuresis

incubus hallucinations 119, 120, 145–6, 148, 149

infants, breathing patterns 191

infective diseases and parasomnias 59

injuries *see specific conditions*

insanity defense for sleep-related violence 84–5

insomnia
  and PTSD 64–5
  and trauma 64–5

International Children's Continence Society (ICCS) 175

International Classification of Sleep Disorders 2nd edition (ICSD-2) 7

International Restless Legs Syndrome Study Group (IRLSSG) diagnostic criteria 213–14

intruder hallucinations 145–6, 148, 149

iron depletion in RLS 14

iron status and secondary RLS 219–20, 221

iron-deficiency anemia, and RLS 215

isolated sleep paralysis (ISP), definition 142 *see also* recurrent isolated sleep paralysis (RISP)

jactatio capitis nocturna (head banging RMD) 270

Karolinska Sleepiness Scale 25

Kleine–Levin syndrome 28, 44

Klüver–Bucy syndrome 28

l'ivresse du sommeil *see* confusional arousals

L-tryptophan 308

laboratory investigations 29

Landau–Kleffner syndrome 291

leg cramps *see* sleep-related leg cramps

legal implications of parasomnias 24–5 *see also* medico-legal consequences of parasomnias

legal responsibility, alcohol and parasomnias 49

levodopa 309, 318

Lewy bodies and RBD 5

Lewy body dementia *see* dementia with Lewy bodies

333

Index

limbic encephalitis and RBD 55, 57
lithium carbonate 44, 45–6
lucid dreaming treatment (LDT), nightmare disorder 317

McNaghten Rules 84
malingering 29
  and sexsomnias 75–6
  distinction from RBD 135
  medico-legal context 93
mater puerorum 119, 120
medical conditions *see* parasomnias due to medical and neurological disorders
medications
  and sleep terrors 8–9
  and sleepwalking 8–9
  see also parasomnias due to medications or substances; pharmacotherapy and parasomnias
medico-legal consequences of parasomnias 81–93
  alcohol and substance-related violence 91–2
  assessment of sleep-related violence 89–93
  automatism 83–4, 85–7
  conditions associated with sleep-related violence 82, 89–93
  culpability 83–4
  dissociation 92–3
  expert opinion 87–9
  insanity defense 84–5
  McNaghten Rules 84
  malingering 93
  role of the sleep expert 87–9
  sleep-related violence 81–2
  the law and forensic parasomnias 85–7
  UK and common law 82–3, 84, 85–7, 88–9
  US law 83–4, 85, 87–8
melatonin 304, 305–6, 318
mental illness
  and nocturnal eating syndrome (NES) 58
  and sleep-related eating disorder (SRED) 58
methaqualone 46
migraine 29, 58–9, 116
migraine equivalents 197

migraine-related hallucinations 197
Minnesota Multiphasic Personality Inventory (MMPI) 23, 121
mirtazapine 50
mood stabilizers and parasomnias 44–5
Morvan's fibrillary chorea 54, 55
motor activity sensors 38–9
multiphase sleep–wake schedule (MPS) 143
multiple medications 42, 44–5
multiple sclerosis 54, 57
multiple system atrophy (MSA) and RBD 5, 55, 56
  neuroimaging 16
Munchausen by proxy 29
myoclonic seizures, distinction from sleep starts 233
myoclonus, history of the term 261

narcolepsy 9, 54
  comorbidity with RBD 134
  loss of orexin neurons 144
  narcoleptic tetrad 142
  treatment 149
narcoleptic tetrad 142
National Ambulatory Medical Care Survey (NAMCS) 302
neurodegenerative diseases
  and parasomnias 55–8
  association with RBD 134, 135–6, 138
neuroimaging of healthy human sleep 13
neuroimaging of parasomnias 13–7
  dream-enactment behavior 17
  periodic limb movement disorders (PLMD) 13–14
  REM sleep behavior disorder (RBD) 15–17
  restless legs syndrome (RLS) 13–15
  sleepwalking 15
  use in clinical evaluation 29
neurological examination 27
neurological syndromes
  and RBD 5
  see also parasomnias due to medical and neurological disorders
night eating syndrome (NES) *see* nocturnal eating syndrome (NES)

night shift paralysis 143–4
night sweats, distinction from sleep panic arousals 283
night terrors *see* sleep terrors
night-time eating *see* sleep-related eating disorder (SRED)
nightmare disorder *see* nightmares/nightmare disorder
nightmare recording 317
nightmares/nightmare disorder 9, 153–8
  and PTSD 65
  and sleep physiology 154–5
  and sleep quality 154
  and trauma 65
  Belicki scale of distress 154
  case report (adult) 156–7
  case report (child) 157–8
  clinical findings 153
  diagnostic criteria for nightmare disorder 153–4
  differential diagnosis 28, 153
  distinction from sleep panic arousals 282
  etiology 155–6
  frequency vs. distress 154
  history 153
  history of the concept 3
  nature of 153
  prevalence 155
nightmares/nightmare disorder management 156, 329–33
  anti-depressants 318
  cognitive behavioral therapy (CBT) 314–16
  exposure therapy 316
  hypnotherapy 317, 325
  imagery rehearsal therapy (IRT) 156, 314–15, 316
  lucid dreaming treatment (LDT) 317
  nightmare recording 317
  pharmacologic treatments 317–18
  prazosin 317–18
  progressive muscle relaxation (PMR) 316
  prolonged exposure for PTSD 315–16
  psychodynamic psychotherapy 315
  psychotherapeutic approaches 314–17
  relaxation strategies 316
  sleep dynamic therapy (SDT) 315
  systematic desensitization (SD) 316
  therapeutic principles 156
nocturnal angina 281
nocturnal asthma 282

Index

nocturnal bruxism *see* sleep bruxism

nocturnal eating syndrome (NES) 202–3
   demographics 205
   differential diagnosis 204–5
   in obesity and mental illness 58
   neuroendocrine studies 207
   pharmacologic treatments 207–8
   treatment 207–8

nocturnal eating/drinking syndrome (NEDS) 203

nocturnal frontal lobe epilepsy (NFLE) 90–1
   distinction from RBD 134–5
   distinction from RMD 274
   see also sleep-related epilepsy

nocturnal gastroesophageal reflux, distinction from sleep panic arousals 282

nocturnal panic attacks 29, 153

nocturnal panic disorder 318–19
   cognitive behavioral therapy (CBT) 318–19
   pharmacotherapy 319

nocturnal psychogenic dissociative disorders, distinction from RBD 135

nocturnal seizures
   differential diagnosis 28
   distinction from sleep panic arousals 280–1
   distinction from sleep starts 233
   see also sleep-related epilepsy

non-familial hyperekplexia 234

normal sleep phenomena 21

NREM parasomnias
   and medications 43–9, 50
   and substances 49–50
   differential diagnosis 27–8
   distinction from RBD 134
   Push/Pull model 49
   spectrum of disorders 27–8

NREM partial arousals, distinction from sleep panic arousals 282

NREM sleep
   early studies 3
   instability 4

obesity
   and nocturnal eating syndrome (NES) 58
   and sleep-related eating disorder (SRED) 58

obstructive sleep apnea (OSA) syndrome
   physical examination 25, 26, 27
   and parasomnias 4
   and violent behavior 7–8

obstructive sleep apnea with agitated arousals, distinction from RBD 135

olanzapine 46

"old hag" attacks *see* recurrent isolated sleep paralysis (RISP)

oneirism 131 *see also* REM sleep behavior disorder (RBD)

oronasal air flow sensors 39

other parasomnias (ICSD-2) 9–10

out-of-body experiences 145, 146, 147

overlap disorders 28, 42, 51, 133

panic arousals *see* sleep panic arousals (SPA)

paradoxical sleep without atonia *see* REM sleep behavior disorder (RBD)

paraphilias 75

parasomnia overlap disorders 28, 42, 51, 133

parasomnias
   common approaches to treatment 323
   consequences for patients 19
   derivation of the term 3
   early studies 3–5
   history of the concept 3

parasomnias associated with REM sleep (ICSD-2) 9

parasomnias due to medical and neurological disorders 9, 27, 54–9
   agrypnia excitata 54
   disorders associated with RBD 54–7
   hypnagogic and hypnopompic hallucinations 54, 58
   infective diseases 59
   migraine 58–9
   neurodegenerative diseases 54–7
   nocturnal eating syndrome (NES) in obesity and mental illness 58
   pharmacologically induced RBD 58–9
   REM sleep without atonia (RSWA) 55, 56, 57
   secondary sleep parasomnias 54
   sleep disordered breathing 58
   sleep-related eating disorder (SRED) in obesity and mental illness 58
   sleepwalking 59
   symptomatic RBD 54–7
   synucleinopathies 55–6
   tauopathies 55, 56–7

parasomnias due to medications or substances 9, 27, 42–51
   alcohol 49–50
   amitriptyline 46
   anti-depressants 46
   benzodiazepines 46–8
   caffeine 50
   chloral hydrate 43
   chlorpromazine 46
   chlorprothixine 46
   de novo parasomnias 42–3, 51
   desipramine hydrochloride 43
   diagnostic criteria 42–3
   disorders of arousal (DOA) 42
   drug interactions 42, 44–5
   effects of psychiatric medications 43–6
   effects of stopping smoking 42
   effects on a specific sleep stage or marker 43
   eszopiclone (Lunesta) 42, 49
   flunitrazepam 47
   fluoxetine 50–1
   flurazepam 46, 47
   genetic predisposition to parasomnias 43
   genetic vulnerability to abnormal arousals 51
   ICSD-R and ICSD-2 criteria 42–3
   imipramine 50
   imprecise nature of early studies 43
   lithium carbonate 43, 44–5
   methaqualone 46
   mirtazapine 50
   mood stabilizers 44–5
   NREM parasomnias and medications 43–9, 50
   NREM parasomnias and substances 49–50
   olanzapine 46
   overlap disorder 42, 51
   paroxetine 46
   patients taking multiple medications 42, 44–5
   perphenazine 43, 45–6
   prolixin 43
   RBD and associated medications 42, 50–1
   sexsomnia 48
   sleep disorder patients 46–9
   sleep-related eating disorder (SRED) 42, 43, 47, 48–9, 206–7

Index

parasomnias (cont.)
  sleepwalking 43, 46–51
  sleepwalking in psychiatric patients 44–6
  thioridazine hydrochloride 43, 45
  timing of the onset of parasomnia 42
  triazolam 45
  venlafaxine 50
  zolpidem (Ambien) 42, 48–53, 206–9

Parkinson's disease (PD)
  and RBD 5, 55, 132–40
  and parasomnias 54, 59
  assessment for signs of 27
  hallucinations 194, 196
  neuroimaging 13

parkinsonism
  and RBD 50
  assessment for signs of 41

paroxetine 60, 321

paroxysmal nocturnal dyspnea, distinction from sleep panic arousals 295

patient
  education about diagnosis 44, 326
  functional status and mood 23–4

patient history 19–21
  characterizing the sleep disturbance 19–21
  chief complaint 19
  information from bed partner 19, 20
  information from family or caregivers 19, 20
  timing of abnormal events 21

pavor nocturnus 119, 120

peduncular hallucinosis 28, 196

periodic leg/limb movement disorder (PLMD) 13–14, 213

periodic leg/limb movements during sleep (PLMS) 14, 213, 214, 234

periodic leg movements (PLM) 213

periodic leg movements during wake (PLMW) 213, 214

perphenazine 43, 44–5, 46

personality and parasomnias 23

pharmacologically induced RBD 52–8

pharmacotherapy and parasomnias 4, 32, 301–9
  amitriptyline 306–7
  anti-depressants 306–7
  anti-hypertensives 307–8

benzodiazepines 303–5
botulinum toxin 308
bromocriptine 308
bupropion–levodopa–trazodone therapy 309
children with disabilities 305
clonazepam 303–5, 306
clonidine 301–7
clonidine prescription in children 301
clozapine 304
diazepam 304
imipramine 304, 306
L-tryptophan 308
melatonin 304, 305–6
off-label concerns 301, 302
paroxetine 307
pediatric considerations 301–3
pramipexole 309
prazosin 307–8
propranolol 307
topiramate 308–9
see also specific conditions

physical examination 25–7

physiologic fragmentary or partial hypnic myoclonus (PFHM) 232

physiologic hypnic myoclonias (PHM) 237–41 see also fragmentary myoclonus

Pittsburgh Sleep Quality Index 25

polysomnographic recording 36–8
  digital resolution 37
  sampling rate 37–8
  telemetry recording 37

polysomnography
  nocturnal 5
  sleepwalking 112–14
  use in clinical evaluation 29
  see also video-polysomnography

post-sigh apnea 190

post-traumatic re-enactments, distinction from nightmares 153

post-traumatic stress disorder (PTSD) 23, 64–7
  and RBD 57, 134
  and REM sleep 65–6
  body/limb movement during sleep 66
  clinical course 64
  combat-related 318–19
  comorbidities 57, 64, 134
  diagnostic criteria (DSM-IV) 64
  insomnia 64–5
  nightmares 64, 158
  parasomnias 66–7
  prevalence 64

prolonged exposure therapy 315–16
  sleep disturbances 64–7
  symptoms 64

pramipexole 33, 309

prazosin 317–18, 307–8

precipitating factors for parasomnias 21–3, 24, 30

pregnancy
  and parasomnias 54
  and RLS 215

progressive muscle relaxation (PMR) 314, 316

progressive supranuclear palsy and RBD 56

prolixin 43

prolonged exposure for PTSD 315–16

propranolol 307

propriospinal myoclonus 261–7
  clinical findings 262–5
  differential diagnosis 266–7
  future directions for research 267
  genetics 267
  history 261–2
  ICSD-2 classification 262
  laboratory investigations 265–6
  management 267
  natural history 265
  pathology 267
  terminology 261–2

propriospinal myoclonus at sleep onset (PSM) 232

pseudo-RBD 135

psychiatric disorders
  and parasomnias 23
  differential diagnosis 29

psychiatric medications and parasomnias 43–6

psychodynamic psychotherapy 315

psychotherapy
  arousal disorders 313–14
  nightmare disorder 314–17

PTSD see post-traumatic stress disorder

pulmonary function tests 30

pulse oximeter 39

Push/Pull model of NREM parasomnias 49

RBD see REM sleep behavior disorder (RBD)

recurrent isolated sleep paralysis
 (RISP) 142–51
  age of onset 147–8
  cognitive arousal and sleep pressure
   143–4
  culture-bound syndrome 150
  definition 142
  definition of isolated sleep paralysis
   (ISP) 142
  definition of sleep paralysis 142
  education of the public and health
   professionals 151
  effects of sleeping position 147
  epidemiology 9
  fear associated with 148–9
  flip-flop model of RISP 144–5
  frequency and severity 142–3
  frequency of episodes 148, 150
  genetic factors 150
  hallucinations 142, 145–7, 148, 149
  incubus hallucinations 145–6, 148,
   149
  intruder hallucinations 145–6, 148,
   149
  management 149
  neurophysiology 144–5
  night shift paralysis 143–4
  prevalence 142–3
  PTSD patients 149
  relation to affective disorders
   148–9
  relation to nightmares 149
  research questions 150–1
  severity and distress 150
  severity and frequency 142–3
  sex differences 148
  sleep onset REM periods
   (SOREMPS) and timing 143
  terminology 142
  threat-activated vigilance system
   (TAVS) 146, 149
  timing of episodes 143
  vestibular–motor hallucinations
   145, 146–7, 148
relaxation strategies 314, 316
REM parasomnias, differential
 diagnosis 28
REM sleep, and PTSD 65–6
REM sleep behavior disorder (RBD) 5,
 131–9
  AASM scoring criteria 131, 132–3
  acute form 131
  age of onset 131, 135
  alternative names for 131
  and alcohol 49–50
  and Alzheimer's disease 56
  and Lewy body dementia 54, 55
  and limbic encephalitis 55, 57

and multiple system atrophy (MSA)
 55, 56
and neurodegenerative diseases
 55–6, 134, 135, 136, 139
and Parkinson's disease 55
and parkinsonism 55
and post-traumatic stress disorder
 (PTSD) 57, 134
and progressive supranuclear palsy
 56
and synucleinopathies 5, 55–6, 131,
 134, 135, 136–8
and tauopathies 55, 56–7
and violent behavior 9
benzodiazepines 314–15
chronic form 131
clinical findings 131–3
clinical–pathophysiological
 subtypes 133
co-existing pathologies 133–4
diagnostic criteria 132–3
differential diagnosis 27, 134–5
disorders associated with 54–7
distinction from epileptic nocturnal
 seizures 134–5
distinction from malingering 135
distinction from nocturnal frontal
 lobe epilepsy (NFLE) 134–5
distinction from nocturnal
 psychogenic dissociative
 disorders 135
distinction from NREM
 parasomnias 134
distinction from OSA with agitated
 arousals 135
distinction from pseudo-RBD 135
distinction from rhythmic
 movement disorder (RMD) 134
distinction from sleep panic
 arousals 283
due to medications or substances 42
epidemiology 9
future directions in research 139
genetic factors 138
history 131
hypnotherapy 326
iatrogenic 5
ICSD-2 criteria 131, 132
idiopathic 5, 131, 132, 135–6
injuries caused by 131
laboratory investigations 136–8
management 139
narcolepsy comorbidity 133
natural history 135–6
neuroimaging 15–17, 136–8
neuropathological studies 138
neurotransmission abnormalities
 138
parasomnia overlap disorder 133

pathology 138–9
pharmacological therapy 139
pharmacologically induced 50–1,
 57–8
physiopathogenesis 138–9
polysomnography 136, 137
possible role of mirror neurons 139
preclinical RBD 133, 136
prevalence 131
prodromes 135
role of the dopamine system 14
sexual or sexualised behaviors 77–8
sleep-related violence 90
status dissociatus 133, 135
structural and functional
 abnormalities 138
subclinical RBD 133, 136
symptomatic 54–7, 131, 135, 136
see also REM sleep without atonia
REM sleep motor parasomnia see REM
 sleep behavior disorder (RBD)
REM sleep without atonia (RSWA) 55,
 56, 57 see also REM sleep
 behavior disorder (RBD)
respiratory activity sensors 39
restless legs syndrome (RLS) 213–26
  A11 system 219
  age of onset 215–16
  and brain volumetric changes 14–15
  anti-convulsants (alpha-2 delta
   medications) 224–5
  associations with iron depletion 14
  augmentation on medication 224
  autopsy evaluations 219
  blood tests 217
  brain imaging 219
  clinical presentation 215
  CSF studies 219
  diagnosis 213–14
  differential diagnosis 214–15
  discomfort correlated with brain
   function 15
  distinction from sleep starts 234–5
  dopamine agonist treatments 222–4
  dopamine pathology 218–19, 220
  endogenous opioid release 15
  epidemiology 216–17
  evaluation and treatment 221–5
  frequency, time and intensity of
   symptoms 221
  future directions for research 225–6
  genetic factors 217, 218–19
  history 213
  hormones and RLS 218
  idiopathic RLS (iRLS) 14
  iron status and secondary RLS
   219–20

restless legs syndrome (RLS) (cont.)
  iron treatments 221
  laboratory investigations 217
  laboratory tests 221
  management 221–5
  medical and medication history 221
  morbidity 217
  natural history 215–17
  neuroimaging 13–15
  opioid treatments 225
  pathology 218–20
  pharmacological response 218
  pharmacological treatments 222
  polysomnograms 217
  risk factors 216–17
  role of the dopamine system 13–14
  secondary causes 215
  secondary RLS and iron 219–20
  secondary RLS evaluation and treatment 221
  secondary vs. primary RLS 215
rhythmic masticatory muscle activity (RMMA) 252
rhythmic movement disorder (RMD)
  distinction from RBD 134
  distinction from sleep starts 214
  see also sleep-related rhythmic movement disorder (RMD)
rhythmic movements of sleep (RMS) 271
RLS see restless legs syndrome (RLS)
Roger, Henri 3

safety
  arousal disorders 213
  sleep environment 30
scheduled awakenings 313
schizoaffective disorder 44, 45
Schlaftrunkenheit see confusional arousals
secondary sleep parasomnias 54
seizure disorders
  differential diagnosis 27
  link with episodic nocturnal events 3
  sleep-related 4–5
  see also epilepsy; sleep-related epilepsy
seizures, and alcohol 91–2
serum ferritin level test 30
sexsomnias 70–8
  clinical course 74–5

clinical features of NREM parasomnias 71–2
clinical features of sexsomnias 72–3
conditions with sexual behavior during sleep 75–8
confusional arousals in adults 103, 105–6
diagnosis 73–4
differential diagnosis 75–8
due to medications or substances 48
forensic implications 74–5
historical overview 70–1
ICSD-2 classification 70
paraphilias 75
pharmacological interventions 74
RBD 77–8
safe sleeping arrangements 74
sexual behavior in sleep (SBS) 70
sleep-related penile erections (SRE) 72
suspected malingering 75–8
terminology 70–1
treatment objectives 74–5
see also disorders of arousal

sexual behavior in sleep (SBS) 70 see also sexsomnias

sexualized behavior during sleep, sleep-related dissociative disorders 168–9

sleep apnea, distinction from sleep panic arousals 282

sleep bruxism (SB) 4, 252–7
  ambulatory recordings 254
  arousal-related SB episodes 255
  benzodiazepines 305
  clinical features 252–3
  clinical findings 252–3
  differential diagnosis 253
  etiology 255–6
  genetics 254
  history 252
  hypnotherapy 326
  ICSD-2 classification 252
  laboratory investigations 254
  lifestyle and sleep hygiene 256
  management 256–7
  natural history 253–4
  neurochemical link 255
  normal RMMA 255
  pathophysiology 255–6
  pharmacologic treatment 257
  physiologic sequence 255
  prevention of damage 256–7
  rhythmic masticatory muscle activity (RMMA) 252, 253, 254, 255
  risk factors 253
  sleep hygiene 256

sleep-disordered breathing 256
swallowing 255–6
sleep disorder patients, parasomnias due to medications 46–9
sleep disordered breathing (SDB) and parasomnias 4, 58
sleep disorders, and PTSD 64–7
sleep disturbance, characterization 19–21
sleep drunkenness 21 see also confusional arousals
sleep dynamic therapy (SDT) 315
sleep enuresis (SE) 175–81
  behavioral therapy 179
  bladder control training 179
  clinical findings 175–6
  conditioning therapy 179
  definition 175
  diagnosis and treatment 177–81
  differential diagnosis 27
  enuresis monitoring 40
  epidemiology 9, 10
  genetic factors 176–7
  hereditary component 10
  hypnotherapy 325–6
  incontinence alarms 30
  laboratory investigations 176
  management 177–81
  motivational therapy 177
  natural history 176
  pathophysiology 177
  pharmacological therapy 179–81
  primary and secondary conditions 175–6
  relationship to sleep disorders 181
  sleep diary 176
sleep environment, safety issues 30
sleep expert, role in legal cases 87–9
sleep history see patient history
sleep hygiene 30, 313
sleep inertia 21 see also confusional arousals
sleep log or diary 25
sleep panic arousals (SPA) 278–85
  clinical features 278–9
  cognitive behavioral therapy (CBT) 284–5
  comorbidity 279
  definition 278
  differential diagnosis 280–3
  epidemiology 278
  future directions for research 285
  management 283–5

Index

pathophysiological considerations 280
patient education and reassurance 284
pharmacological treatment 284
phenomenology 278
polysomnography 279
sleep hygiene 285

sleep paralysis 9
  definition 142
  distinction from sleep panic arousals 282
  see also isolated sleep paralysis (ISP); recurrent isolated sleep paralysis (RISP)

sleep paralysis without narcolepsy see isolated sleep paralysis (ISP)

sleep questionnaires 25

sleep-related dissociative disorders 31, 163–72
  and sexualized behavior during sleep 168
  and sleepwalking/sleep terrors 165
  and violent sexual behavior during sleep 169
  case presentations 165–8, 169
  clinical findings 164
  clinical presentations 165–9
  differential diagnosis 169–70
  dissociative disorder NOS 163, 164
  dissociative fugue 163, 164
  dissociative identity disorder 163, 164
  DSM-IV-TR classification 163, 164
  epidemiology 10
  evaluation questionnaires 165–6
  familial clustering of dissociative disorders 171
  genetic factors 171
  history 163–4
  indicators of psychiatric distress 172
  investigations 170–1
  management 172
  natural history 164–9
  nature of dissociation 163–4
  pathology 171
  trauma-related distress 163
  treatments 319–20

sleep-related eating disorder (SRED) 202–8
  association with eating disorders 206
  association with mood disorders 206
  association with sleep disorders 206
  comorbid sleep disorders 206
  consequences 205

definition and characteristics 203–4
demographics 205
differential diagnosis of SRED and NES 204–5
due to medications or substances 45, 46, 50, 51–2, 216–17
genetic studies (mouse models) 207
historical perspective 202–3
ICSD-2 definition 203
in obesity and mental illness 58
mouse models 207
neuroendocrine studies in NES 207
night-eating syndrome (NES) 202–3, 204–5
pharmacologic treatments 207–8
physiology of SRED 206–7
role of circadian rhythms 202
treatment 207–8
weight gain 205
see also disorders of arousal

sleep-related epilepsy 289–97
  benign rolandic epilepsy 291
  differential diagnosis 289–90, 292
  distinction from RBD 134–5
  distinction from RMD 274
  effects of epilepsy drugs on sleep 293–4
  effects of seizures on sleep 292
  effects of sleep deprivation on seizures 292, 293
  effects of sleep disruption on seizures 292, 293
  effects of sleep drugs on epilepsy 294
  effects of sleep on seizures 292–3
  electrical status epilepticus during sleep (ESES) 291
  generalized epilepsy syndromes 290
  history 289
  sleep-related violence 90
  influence of circadian rhythms 293
  laboratory investigations 294–6
  Landau–Kleffner syndrome 291
  localization-related epilepsy 289, 291, 292
  parasomnias frequently confused with epilepsy 292
  partial seizures 289, 291, 292

sleep-related groaning see catathrenia

sleep-related hallucinations 194–9
  Charles Bonnet syndrome 194, 195–6
  clinical findings 195, 196, 197
  complex nocturnal visual hallucinations (CNVH) 194, 195, 196
  definitions 194, 195
  dementia with Lewy bodies 195, 196

epidemiology 10
epileptic hallucinations 196, 197
exploding head syndrome 194, 199
genetics 198
historical perspective 194
hypnagogic and hypnopompic hallucinations 194, 195
laboratory investigations 197
management 198
migraine-related hallucinations 197
natural history 195, 197
Parkinson's disease 194, 196
pathophysiology 198
peduncular hallucinosis 196
see also hallucinations; hypnagogic hallucinations; hypnopompic hallucinations

sleep-related laryngospasm, distinction from sleep panic arousals 282

sleep-related leg cramps 244–50
  anti-epileptic medications 250
  calcium channel blocker therapy 249
  definition 244
  diagnosis 245–6
  epidemiology 244
  gabapentin therapy 250
  magnesium sulfate therapy 248–9
  naftidrofuryl oxalate therapy 250
  non-pharmacologic treatments 246–7
  orphenadrine citrate therapy 250
  pathophysiology 244–5
  phenytoin therapy 250
  quinine sulfate therapy 247–8
  risk factors 245
  stretching exercises 246–7
  treatments 246–50
  vitamin B complex therapy 250
  vitamin E therapy 249
  work-up 246

sleep-related movement disorders 21, 213

sleep-related penile erections (SRE) 72

sleep-related rhythmic movement disorder (RMD) 270–5
  association with ADHD 272, 275
  body rocking 271
  body rolling 270
  characteristics 270
  clinical manifestations of RMD 270–1
  comorbidity of RMD 272
  complications of RMD 272
  conditions which mimic RMD 274–5
  diagnostic criteria 271

339

Index

sleep-related rhythmic (*cont.*)
  differential diagnosis 274–5
  epidemiology of RMD 271–2
  head banging (jactatio capitis nocturna) 270
  head rolling 270
  ICSD-2 diagnostic criteria 271
  natural history of RMD 271–2
  polysomnography in RMD 272–3
  postulated causes of RMD 273–4
  treatment of RMD 275

sleep-related twitching 237

sleep-related violence 81–2
  alcohol-related 91–2
  alcoholic blackout 92
  conditions associated with 82, 89–93
  confusional arousals in adults 102–3
  dissociation 92–3
  drug-related 91, 92
  epilepsy 90–1
  forensic assessment 89–91
  malingering 93
  nocturnal frontal lobe epilepsy (NFLE) 90–1
  parasomnias 89–90
  RBD 90
  sleep terrors 123
  sleepwalking 8, 89, 90
  substance-related 91, 92
  see also violent behavior; violent parasomnias

sleep scheduling 313

sleep starts 229–35
  acoustic sleep starts 232
  "blip" syndrome 231
  clinical subtypes and descriptions 229–32
  conditions mimicking sleep starts 232–4
  differential diagnosis 232–4
  exploding head syndrome 231
  history 229
  intensified hypnic jerks 230–1
  motor sleep starts ("hypnic jerks") 229–30
  pathophysiology 234–5
  polysomnographic findings 234–5
  pure sensory sleep starts 230
  repetitive spells in neurologically impaired children 231–2
  sensory-motor types 230
  treatment 235

sleep terrors 119–26
  age of onset 122–3

and sleep-related dissociative disorders 165–8
  clinical evaluation 123–4
  clinical findings 120–2
  diagnostic criteria 122
  differential diagnosis 121
  distinction from nightmares 153
  distinction from sleep panic arousals 182
  early studies 3, 4
  epidemiology 7–8
  Freudian theory 119
  genetic predisposition 124
  history 119–20
  laboratory investigations 123–4
  management 124–6
  natural history 122–3
  precipitating factors 122–3
  treatment 124–6
  triggers 8–9
  violent behavior and injury 8, 123

sleepsex *see* disorders of arousal; sexsomnias

sleepwalking (somnambulism) 109–16
  and sleep-related dissociative disorders 165–8
  and thyrotoxicosis 59
  associated conditions 115–16
  children 112, 115, 116
  clinical presentation 109–10
  comorbid sleep disorders 111
  diagnostic considerations 110–12
  due to medications or substances 42, 43–4, 45, 46, 47, 48
  early studies 3–4
  epidemiology 8
  familial patterns 3–4, 8
  genetic predisposition 115
  hypnotherapy 325
  injury to self and others 8, 109–10
  management 116
  natural history 112
  neuroimaging 15
  NREM sleep parasomnia classification 109
  pathophysiology 115–16
  polysomnography 112–14
  precipitating factors 111, 112
  psychiatric patients 44–7
  sleep laboratory investigations 110–14
  triggers 9–10
  violent behavior 8, 109–10
  see also disorders of arousal

sleepwalking polysomnography 112–14

hypersynchronous delta waves 113
NREM sleep instability 112–13
post-arousal EEG activity 113–14
slow-wave activity 113

slow-wave sleep (SWS) 43, 46–7, 51

smoking, effects of stopping 42

snoring 190–1

somnambulism *see* sleepwalking

somniloquy (sleep talking) 21

somnolescent starts *see* sleep starts

spasmus nutans 274

sporadic Creutzfeldt–Jacob disease 54

stage 1 REM 137 *see also* REM sleep behavior disorder (RBD)

Stanford Sleepiness Scale 25

status dissociatus 28, 133, 135

stereotypic movement disorder 274

stress management, arousal disorders 314

stridor 190

substances *see* parasomnias due to medications or substances

substantia nigra iron depletion, role in RLS 14

sudden unexplained nocturnal death syndrome (SUNDS) 123

sympathetic skin response (SSR) monitoring 40

symptomatic RBD 54–7, 131, 135, 136

synucleinopathies and RBD 55–6, 131, 134, 136, 138

systematic desensitization (SD), nightmare disorder 316

tauopathies and RBD 55, 56–7

teeth grinding *see* bruxism

thioridazine hydrochloride 45, 46

threat-activated vigilance system (TAVS) 146, 149

thyroid function tests 30

thyrotoxicosis and sleepwalking 59

timing of abnormal events 21

tonic immobility 147

tooth grinding/clenching *see* sleep bruxism

topiramate 308–9

Index

Tourette's syndrome 55, 116
tracheal microphone 35
trauma 64–5
   and nightmares 65
   and parasomnias 23
   see also post-traumatic stress disorder (PTSD)
trazodone 318
treatment for parasomnias 30 *see also specific conditions*
triazolam 47
tricyclic antidepressants and RBD 5
triggers for parasomnias 23–4, 25, 30
twin studies 4–5
two-oscillator model of breathing 192

UK and common law, consequences of parasomnias 82–3, 84, 85–7, 88–9
unspecified parasomnia (ICSD-2) 9
upper airway resistance syndrome (UARS) 190
urine screening 30
US law, consequences of parasomnias 82–3, 84, 85–88

venlafaxine 50
vestibular–motor hallucinations 145, 146–7, 148
video-polysomnography 34–40
   blood pressure (BP) 40
   capnograph 39
   diagnostic use 34
   electrocardiogram (ECG) 39–40
   electroencephalogram (EEG) 38
   electromyogram (EMG) 38–9
   electrooculogram (EOG) 38
   endoesophageal pressure measurement 39
   enuresis monitoring 40
   environmental microphone 35
   features of the video camera(s) 35
   file size and quality of the video recording 36
   finger plethysmograph (FP) 40
   fundamental elements 34
   infrared lights 35
   motor activity sensors 38–9
   oronasal air flow sensors 39
   polysomnographic recording 36–8
   pulse oximeter 39
   recorded parameters 38–9, 40
   recording room 34
   research use 34
   respiratory activity sensors 39
   role of the technician 34, 40
   sleep stages recording 38
   sympathetic skin response (SSR) 40
   telemetry recording 43
   tracheal microphone 39
   video recording 34–6
violent behavior
   confusional arousals 7–8
   obstructive sleep apnea 7–8
   RBD 9
   sleep terrors 8
   sleepwalking 8
   substance-related 91, 92
   see also sleep-related violence
violent parasomnias
   distinction from mindful criminal acts 25
   legal implications 24–5
   see also sleep-related violence
violent sexual behavior during sleep, sleep-related dissociative disorders 169
vitiligo and parasomnias 59

zolpidem (Ambien) 42, 48–9, 50, 51, 206–7